Current Research in Behavioral Neurology

Current Research in Behavioral Neurology

Editor: Catelyn Wilkerson

FOSTER
ACADEMICS

www.fosteracademics.com

www.fosteracademics.com

FOSTER
ACADEMICS

Cataloging-in-Publication Data

Current research in behavioral neurology / edited by Catelyn Wilkerson.
p. cm.
Includes bibliographical references and index.
ISBN 978-1-63242-717-5
1. Clinical neuropsychology. 2. Neuropsychiatry. 3. Neuropsychology.
I. Wilkerson, Catelyn.
RC341 .C87 2019
612.8--dc23

Foster Academics,
118-35 Queens Blvd., Suite 400,
Forest Hills, NY 11375, USA

ISBN 978-1-63242-717-5 (Hardback)

Printed and bound in China.

Contents

Preface IX

Chapter 1 **Effects of Early-Life Stress on Social and Anxiety-Like Behaviors in Adult Mice: Sex-Specific Effects** 1
Natalya P. Bondar, Arina A. Lepeshko and Vasiliy V. Reshetnikov

Chapter 2 **Delusions in Patients with Dementia with Lewy Bodies and the Associated Factors** 14
Ray-Chang Tzeng, Ching-Fang Tsai, Ching-Tsu Wang, Tzu-Yuan Wang and Pai-Yi Chiu

Chapter 3 **Morphological Biomarker Differentiating MCI Converters from Nonconverters: Longitudinal Evidence based on Hemispheric Asymmetry** 22
Xiaojing Long, Chunxiang Jiang and Lijuan Zhang

Chapter 4 **Evaluating the Utility of a Structured Clinical Protocol for Reducing the Impact of Behavioural and Psychological Symptoms of Dementia in Progressive Neurological Diseases** 31
Nicholas P. Ryan, Laura Scott, Maryanne McPhee, Susan Mathers, Marie-Claire Davis, Roxanne Maule and Fiona Fisher

Chapter 5 **The Effects of Transcranial Direct Current Stimulation on the Cognitive Functions in Older Adults with Mild Cognitive Impairment** 40
Pablo Cruz Gonzalez, Kenneth N. K. Fong and Ted Brown

Chapter 6 **Biochanin A Reduces Inflammatory Injury and Neuronal Apoptosis following Subarachnoid Hemorrhage via Suppression of the TLRs/TIRAP/MyD88/NF-κB Pathway** 54
Ling-yun Wu, Zhen-nan Ye, Zong Zhuang, Yongyue Gao, Chao Tang, Chen-hui Zhou, Chun-xi Wang, Xiang-sheng Zhang, Guang-bin Xie, Jing-peng Liu, Meng-liang Zhou, Chun-hua Hang and Ji-xin Shi

Chapter 7 **Scoping Review of the Driving Behaviour of and Driver Training Programs for People on the Autism Spectrum** 64
Nathan J. Wilson, Hoe C. Lee, Sharmila Vaz, Priscilla Vindin and Reinie Cordier

Chapter 8 **Neurohealth Properties of *Hericium erinaceus* Mycelia Enriched with Erinacines** 81
I-Chen Li, Li-Ya Lee, Tsai-Teng Tzeng, Wan-Ping Chen, Yen-Po Chen, Young-Ju Shiao and Chin-Chu Chen

Chapter 9 **Risk Factors for the Progression of Mild Cognitive Impairment in Different Types of Neurodegenerative Disorders** 91
Pei-Hao Chen, Shih-Jung Cheng, Hui-Chi Lin, Chuo-Yu Lee and Chih-Ho Chou

Chapter 10 **Mining EEG with SVM for Understanding Cognitive Underpinnings of Math Problem Solving Strategies** 98
Paul Bosch, Mauricio Herrera, Julio López and Sebastián Maldonado

Chapter 11 **Social Cognition Dysfunctions in Neurodegenerative Diseases: Neuroanatomical Correlates and Clinical Implications** 113
Foteini Christidi, Raffaella Migliaccio, Hernando Santamaría-García, Gabriella Santangelo and Francesca Trojsi

Chapter 12 **Determination of Care Burden of Caregivers of Patients with Multiple Sclerosis in Turkey** 131
Serpil Özmen and Afife Yurttaş

Chapter 13 **Neural Basis of Depression Related to a Dominant Right Hemisphere: A Resting-State fMRI Study** 138
Mi Li, Hongpei Xu and Shengfu Lu

Chapter 14 **A Comparative Study of Conventional Physiotherapy versus Robot-Assisted Gait Training Associated to Physiotherapy in Individuals with Ataxia after Stroke** 147
Marcia Belas dos Santos, Clarissa Barros de Oliveira, Arly dos Santos, Cristhiane Garabello Pires, Viviana Dylewski and Ricardo Mario Arida

Chapter 15 **Effect of Voluntary Wheel Running on Striatal Dopamine Level and Neurocognitive Behaviors after Molar Loss in Rats** 153
Linlin Zhang, Yi Feng, Wenliang Ji, Jianzhang Liu and Kun Liu

Chapter 16 **The Effect of Gentle Handling on Depressive-Like Behavior in Adult Male Mice: Considerations for Human and Rodent Interactions in the Laboratory** 159
Caroline Neely, Christina Lane, Julio Torres and Jane Flinn

Chapter 17 **Mechanism of Restoration of Forelimb Motor Function after Cervical Spinal Cord Hemisection in Rats: Electrophysiological Verification** 165
Takumi Takeuchi, Masahito Takahashi, Kazuhiko Satomi, Hideaki Ohne, Atsushi Hasegawa, Shunsuke Sato and Shoichi Ichimura

Chapter 18 **Allergic Rhinitis in Rats is Associated with an Inflammatory Response of the Hippocampus** 176
Shasha Yang, Jing Wu, Qinxiu Zhang, Xinrong Li, Daien Liu, Bin Zeng, Zhiqing Liu, Haoran Kang and Zhendong Zhong

Chapter 19 **Metabolic Risk Factors of Alzheimer's Disease, Dementia with Lewy Bodies, and Normal Elderly** 183
Chih-Kuang Cheng, Yu-Chien Tsao, Yuan-Chih Su, Fung-Chang Sung, Hsu-Chih Tai and Woon-Man Kung

Chapter 20 **Glucose Metabolic Brain Network Differences between Chinese Patients with Lewy Body Dementia and Healthy Control** 191
Danyan Chen, Jiaying Lu, Hucheng Zhou, Jiehui Jiang, Ping Wu, Qihao Guo, Jingjie Ge, Huiwei Zhang, Kuangyu Shi and Chuantao Zuo

Chapter 21 **Cerebral Responses to Acupuncture at GV24 and Bilateral GB13 in Rat Models of Alzheimer's Disease** 203
Shaoyang Cui, Mingzhu Xu, Jianting Huang, Qing Mei Wang, Xinsheng Lai, Binbin Nie, Baoci Shan, Xun Luo, John Wong and Chunzhi Tang

Chapter 22 **Screening for Emotional Expression in Frontotemporal Dementia** 213
Andrew R. Carr, Mark M. Ashla, Elvira E. Jimenez and Mario F. Mendez

Chapter 23 **Mediational Model of Multiple Sclerosis Impairments, Family Needs and Caregiver Mental Health in Guadalajara, Mexico** 219
Melody N. Mickens, Paul B. Perrin, Adriana Aguayo, Brenda Rabago, Miguel A. Macías-Islas and Juan Carlos Arango-Lasprilla

Chapter 24 **Age- and Gender-based Differences in Nest-Building Behavior and Learning and Memory Performance Measured using a Radial Six-Armed Water Maze in C57BL/6 Mice** 230
Xiang-Dong Xiong, Wei-Dong Xiong, Shang-Shen Xiong and Gui-Hai Chen

Chapter 25 **Functional Connectivity Changes in Behavioral, Semantic and Nonfluent Variants of Frontotemporal Dementia** 237
P. Reyes, M. P. Ortega-Merchan, A. Rueda, F. Uriza, Hernando Santamaria-García, N. Rojas-Serrano, J. Rodriguez-Santos, M. C. Velasco-Leon, J. D. Rodriguez-Parra, D. E. Mora-Diaz and D. Matallana

Chapter 26 **Dynamic Evaluation of Notch Signaling-Mediated Angiogenesis in Ischemic Rats using Magnetic Resonance Imaging** 247
Jia-qi Tian, Jia-jun Zheng, Xiao-zhu Hao, Le-kang Yin, Xiao-xue Zhang, Chan-chan Li, Xiao-yuan Feng, Min Jiang, Hua-ping Sun, Kang Zheng and Yan-mei Yang

Chapter 27 **Sleep Quality and Emotion Regulation Interact to Predict Anxiety in Veterans with PTSD** 255
Janna Mantua, Steven M. Helms, Kris B. Weymann, Vincent F. Capaldi II and Miranda M. Lim

Permissions

List of Contributors

Index

Preface

Every book is initially just a concept; it takes months of research and hard work to give it the final shape in which the readers receive it. In its early stages, this book also went through rigorous reviewing. The notable contributions made by experts from across the globe were first molded into patterned chapters and then arranged in a sensibly sequential manner to bring out the best results.

Behavioral neurology is a specialization of neurology, which is concerned with the study of the impact of neurological diseases and damage on cognitive function, behavior and memory. It also deals with the treatment of all such damages and conditions. Some of the diseases and disorders under study in behavioral neurology are amnesia, aprosodia, autism, dementia, apraxia, psychosis, traumatic brain injury, attention deficit/hyperactivity disorder, etc. In vivo neuroimaging techniques are widely used for the understanding of structural and functional correlations of brain lesions with behavioral dysfunction in individuals. This book is a valuable compilation of topics, ranging from the basic to the most complex advancements in the field of behavioral neurology. It presents this complex subject in the most comprehensible language. With state-of-the-art inputs by acclaimed experts of this field, this book targets students and professionals.

It has been my immense pleasure to be a part of this project and to contribute my years of learning in such a meaningful form. I would like to take this opportunity to thank all the people who have been associated with the completion of this book at any step.

Editor

1

Effects of Early-Life Stress on Social and Anxiety-Like Behaviors in Adult Mice: Sex-Specific Effects

Natalya P. Bondar, [1,2] **Arina A. Lepeshko**, [1,2] **and Vasiliy V. Reshetnikov** [1]

[1] *Laboratory of Gene Expression Regulation, Institute of Cytology and Genetics, Siberian Branch of the Russian Academy of Sciences, 10 Prospect Lavrentyeva, Novosibirsk 630090, Russia*
[2] *Novosibirsk National Research State University, 2 Pirogova Street, Novosibirsk 630090, Russia*

Correspondence should be addressed to Natalya P. Bondar; nbondar@bionet.nsc.ru

Academic Editor: Giuseppe Biagini

Stressful events in an early postnatal period have critical implications for the individual's life and can increase later risk for psychiatric disorders. The aim of this study was to investigate the influence of early-life stress on the social behavior of adult male and female mice. C57Bl/6 mice were exposed to maternal separation (MS, 3 h once a day) or handling (HD, 15 min once a day) on postnatal day 2 through 14. Adult male and female mice were tested for social behavior in the social interaction test and for individual behavior in the plus-maze and open-field tests. Female mice exposed to maternal separation had increased social behavior and increased anxiety. MS male mice had no changes in social behavior but had significantly disrupted individual behavior, including locomotor and exploratory activity. Handling had positive effects on social behavior in males and females and decreased anxiety in males. Our results support the hypothesis that brief separation of pups from their mothers (handling), which can be considered as moderate stress, may result in future positive changes in behavior. Maternal separation has deleterious effects on individual behavior and significant sex-specific effects on social behavior.

1. Introduction

There is a wealth of data demonstrating that exposure to stressful events early in life can increase the risk for psychiatric disorders, including mood and anxiety disorders [1–4]. The neural basis of the consequences of early-life stress is poorly understood, and stressful events are supposed to cause structural and functional disturbances in brain regions responsible for emotional behavior in humans [5–7]. Adults with a history of mistreatment in childhood have reductions of medial prefrontal cortex volume [8], decreased hippocampal volume [9, 10], hyperactivity of the hypothalamic-pituitary-adrenal axis [11], and an associated deterioration of sensory and cognitive functions [12]. Animal models of early-life stress also demonstrate disturbances in neuronal activities and brain plasticity [13–17].

Maternal separation (MS) is the most commonly used rodent model of early-life stress [18, 19]. Separation of pups from their dams and nest for 3 or more hours once a day during the first two postnatal weeks produces increased anxiety-like behavior and exaggerated hypothalamic-pituitary-adrenal (HPA)-axis responses to stress in adulthood as well as behavioral and cognitive disturbances [20–24]. These effects have well been studied in rats, while behavioral changes in MS mice remain inconsistent [18, 25].

Nevertheless, consequences of early-life stress in mice are significantly sex-biased. Maternal separation of pups from their dams generally increases anxiety in adult male mice [26–28], while females tend to have a stable anxiety level [25, 27, 29, 30]. Few studies have found increased anxiety in adult female mice after early-life stress [28, 31]. Neither male nor female mice have changes in the level of depression in the forced swim test [25, 26, 32–34]. In mice, MS in combination with restraint stress for mothers during pup separation enhanced the expression of depressive symptoms in the form of decreased sucrose solution preference in both male and female offspring [29]. If maternal separation was combined with early weaning, the authors observed persistent behavioral disturbances in male mice, including enhanced anxiety-like behavior and depressive behavior [35–37]. Apparently, mice require more stress to attain changes in emotion-related behavior and stress reactivity similar to those in rats [25].

In humans, psychiatric disorders such as depression and anxiety are highly comorbid with social dysfunction, and disturbances in social behavior generally appear before these disorders. Therefore, studying dysfunctional social interactions is important for understanding the development of the stress response [38]. However, the influence of maternal separation on social behavior is poorly studied. Studies on males usually find no changes in social behavior in mice [39–41] and rats [42, 43]. A small proportion of the studies reports either slightly intensified social interaction in male mice [29] or, the other way round, decreased social behavior [44] under the influence of early-life stress. Female studies are few, and they provide inconsistent observations: some state that maternal separation results in decreased time investigating other mice [31], while others suggest that it has no effect on social behavior [29]. Thus, effects of early-life stress on adult social behavior remain evasive, especially in their sex-specific aspect.

Interestingly, brief separation of rat pups from their dams (10–15 min per day) often has an opposite effect on later behavioral and stress-related responses compared to prolonged separation [21, 22, 45]. Some mouse studies show decreased anxiety and increased exploratory activity in males [46, 47] and none of these effects in females [25, 30]. The influence of brief separation in early life on mouse social behavior has not yet been investigated.

Here, we attempt to characterize the effects of early-life stress on the social behavior of adult male and female mice and to see if there are correlations between changes and disturbances of individual behavior. A brief (15 min/day) and a prolonged separation (3 h/day) paradigm were used to identify possible positive and negative consequences of early-life adversity.

2. Materials and Methods

2.1. Animals. C57BL/6J mice were housed in the Center for Genetic Resources of Laboratory Animals (RFMEFI61914X0005 and RFMEFI62114X0010), Institute of Cytology and Genetics, the Siberian Branch of the Russian Academy of Sciences, Novosibirsk, Russia. The animals were housed under standard conditions (12 : 12 h light/dark cycle, lights on at 8.00 a.m.; feed pellets and water were available ad libitum). All procedures were approved by the Ethics Committee of the Institute of Cytology and Genetics SB RAS (Protocol number 25, December 2014) in conformity with EU Directive 2010/63/EU for animal experiments.

2.2. Maternal Separation. Virgin males and females were used for mating. Pregnant females were individually housed with paper nesting material during their third week of gestation. Only litters containing 4–6 pups were used for experiments. All stress procedures were carried out from 1 to 4 pm, in the light phase of day. Offspring were separated from dams on PND 2 through PND 14 (the day of birth was PND 0). At first, each dam was removed from her home cage and placed into a clean cage. Pups were then removed from its home cage and placed together into a small box filled with bedding (one litter for one box). After that, the dam was placed back into the home cage. In the brief separation condition [handling (HD)] the pups were separated from their dams for 15 min once a day, while at the prolonged separation [maternal separation (MS)], the pups were separated for 180 min once a day. The temperature in the MS cages was kept at 31 ± 2°C using infrared heat lamps to prevent thermoregulatory distress. No heat lamps were used on HD pups. The control pups were not separated from their dams. All cages were cleaned on a weekly basis. After weaning on PND 30, the offspring were housed in sibling groups of 2 to 4 animals of the same sex under standard housing conditions. Experimental groups consisted of 27 males (11 control, 10 HD, and 6 MS) and 25 females (11 control, 6 HD, and 8 MS), each group included mice from at least three litters. The behavioral tests were conducted on PND 85–PND 110 in the following order: plus-maze, open-field, and the social interaction test (one test per day). 24 h after the last behavioral test, the animals were euthanized and the adrenal glands and thymus were removed and weighted. Schema of the experiment was presented on Figure 1(a).

2.3. Behavioral Tests

2.3.1. Plus-Maze Test. The elevated plus-maze test was performed according to the established procedure [48, 49]. The maze consisted of two opposite open arms (25 cm × 5 cm) and two opposite enclosed arms (25 cm × 5 cm × 15 cm) and had an open roof. The maze was set at 50 cm above the floor. All measurements were made in a dimly lit experimental room. The test apparatus was thoroughly cleaned between tests with different animals. During a 5 min test period, the following parameters of anxiety-like behavior were recorded: the percentage of entries into the open arms, closed arms, and central platform and the percentage of time spent in the open arms, closed arms, and central platform. These parameters were reported as the percentage of total entries and the percentage of testing time, respectively. The additional parameters were the latency of the first exit from the central platform, the number of head-dips, and the number of passages from one closed arm to another.

2.3.2. Open-Field Test. The open field (OF) consisted of a square arena (80 cm × 80 cm) with a white floor and 25 cm high walls. The arena was brightly illuminated and had a central zone (40 cm × 40 cm) and a peripheral zone (anywhere between the central zone and the walls). Each mouse was placed individually in the central zone, and the following behavioral parameters were recorded during a 5 min test period: the total distance traveled; the latency of the first exit from the central zone; the number of visits to the central zone; the time spent in the central and the peripheral zone; the number of rearing and self-grooming episodes; and total activity state (activity level of mouse was determined by the software as a function of pixel changes, EthoVision XT

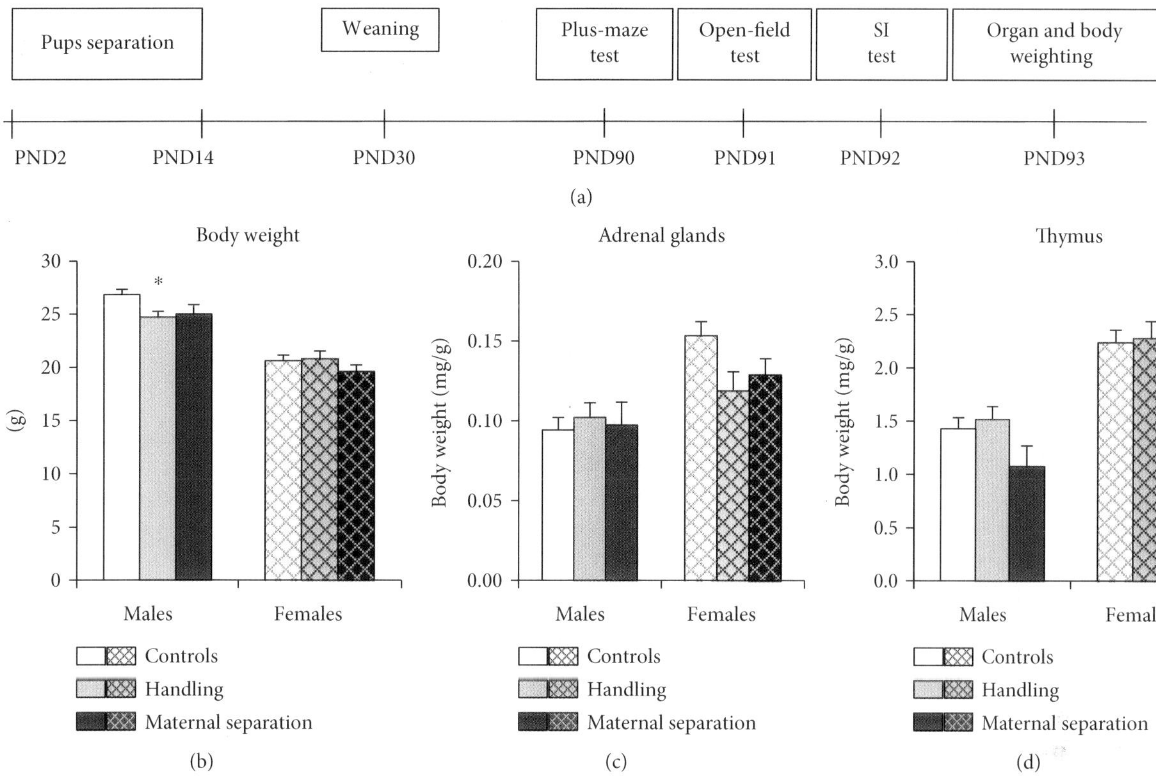

FIGURE 1: Timeline of the experiment (a), weights of the body (b), relative weights of adrenal glands (c), and thymus (d) in adult male and female mice. Handling decreased the weight of the body in males but not females. Females have the only tendency to reduce relative adrenal weight under early postnatal stress. Relative weights of adrenal glands and thymus are shown as organ weight in mg per gram of body weight. Data present as mean ± standard error of the mean (SEM). White box: controls (males $n = 11$, females $n = 11$); grey box: HD (males $n = 10$, females $n = 6$), black box: MS (males $n = 6$, females $n = 8$); open columns: males; cross-hatched columns: females. $^{*}p < 0.05$ compared to controls.

threshold for activity—0.2%). The OF arena was thoroughly cleaned between tests with different animals.

2.3.3. Social Interaction Test. A square plastic arena (40 cm × 40 cm × 25 cm) was used for the social interaction test. A small perforated plastic target box (10 cm × 10 cm) was placed near the center of one of the walls. The test consisted of two trials (5 min each). At the beginning of each trial, an experimental mouse was placed in the zone opposite to the target box, face to the wall. In the adaptation trial, the target box was empty and the animal was habituated to the novel environment for 5 min. In the interaction trial, an unfamiliar partner of the same sex was placed into the target box and the reaction of the experimental mouse to the social target was investigated. Between the trials, the mouse was placed to a neutral cage. The following parameters were recorded during each trial: the total distance traveled, the number of visits to the interaction zone (a 5 cm zone around the target box), the time spent in the interaction zone, and the latency of the first contact with the target box. The interaction ratio was calculated as 100*(time in the interaction zone, partner present)/(time in the interaction zone, partner absent).

2.4. Characterization of Estrous Phase. Vaginal smears from each female were taken every day after behavioral tests to determine the phase of the estrous cycle. Based on vaginal cytology, females were divided into two groups: diestrous (those in diestrus and metaestrus) and estrous (those in estrus and proestrus).

2.5. Statistical Analysis. All tests were videotaped and manually scored by the free open-source software BORIS (Behavioral Observation Research Interactive Software, http://www.boris.unito.it) [50]. The distance traveled in the OF test was scored using EthoVision XT v.10.0 (Noldus Information Technology, Netherlands).

Normal distribution and homogeneity of variances were tested using Shapiro–Wilk's and Levene's tests, respectively. As most behavioral data were not normally distributed, nonparametric tests were used. The statistical analysis of behavioral data was performed using Kruskal–Wallis one-way ANOVA, with the type of stress as a factor separately for males and females. Pairwise comparisons were performed by the Mann–Whitney U test. The statistical significance threshold was set at $p < 0.05$.

3. Results

3.1. Body, Adrenal Glands, and Thymus Weight. Males had more body weight and less relative weights of adrenals and thymus than females (effect of sex: for body weight H $(1, 52) = 18.8$, $p < 0.001$; for adrenals H $(1, 52) = 29.1$,

$p < 0.001$; for thymus H (1, 52) = 35.9, $p < 0.001$) (Figure 1). Early postnatal stress has an effect on body weight in males (H (2, 27) = 6.8, $p = 0.03$); in HD males, the body weight is reduced in comparison with the control ($p = 0.017$), and MS males also have a tendency to reduce the body weight ($p = 0.0841$). Females have the only tendency to reduce relative adrenal weight under early postnatal stress (H (1, 19) = 3.3, $p = 0.069$).

3.2. Plus-Maze Behavior. Generally, males were less anxious than females (more time spent in open arms (H (1, 52) = 6.6, $p = 0.01$) and center (H (1, 52) = 19.9, $p < 0.001$)) and have higher locomotor activity than females (more total number of entries (H (1, $N = 52$) = 15.9, $p = 0.0001$); more passages (H (1, $N = 52$) = 6.2, $p = 0.0126$)).

Early-life stress had no effect on plus-maze behavior in male mice (Figure 2). However, stress in early life led to significant anxiogenic effect in MS females. MS females had increased latency to exit the central platform compared with controls (effect of stress: H (2, 24) = 9.9, $p = 0.007$; Mann–Whitney U test: $U = 8$, $p = 0.006$) and spent less time in the open arms than controls (effect of stress: H (2, 24) = 8.6, $p = 0.013$; Mann–Whitney U test: $U = 16$, $p = 0.041$) and HD mice ($U = 3$, $p = 0.01$). Stress has a weak effect on the number of entries into the closed (a trend, H (2, 24) = 5.1, $p = 0.077$) and open (a trend, H (2, 24) = 5.1, $p = 0.077$) arms. Nevertheless, the percentage of entries into the open arms was decreased ($U = 17$, $p = 0.05$) and the percentage of entries into the closed arms was increased ($U = 17$, $p = 0.05$) in MS females compared to controls. Anxious effect was not caused by a decrease in locomotor activity of females (total entries, $p > 0.05$), and MS females even had a higher number of passages between the closed arms compared to controls ($U = 12.5$, $p = 0.018$). HD females had only increased latency to exit the central platform compared with controls ($U = 11.5$, $p = 0.031$).

Females were grouped by the phase of the estrous cycle to assess its effect on plus-maze behavior. However, an insufficient number of mice in each phase does not allow a correct statistical analysis. MS females tended to have increased anxiety both in estrus and diestrus (Figure 3).

3.3. Open-Field Behavior. Males have higher locomotor activity than females (longer distance travelled: H (1, 52) = 17.8, $p < 0.001$, higher total activity: H (1, 52) = 24.7, $p < 0.001$) and more often go to the central zone (H (1, 52) = 9.3, $p = 0.002$), indicating that males are less anxious than females in OF.

3.3.1. Males. In the OF test, maternal separation had the greatest effect on the locomotor and exploratory activities of animals (Figure 4). Stress had an influence on total activity (H (2, 27) = 6.5; $p = 0.038$); parameters reflecting any movements of mice and the total activity of MS males were lower than in the control ($U = 7.0$; $p = 0.031$) and HD group ($U = 3.0$; $p = 0.016$). Decrease in activity is accompanied by decreasing distance travelled (stress effect: H (2, 27) = 5.0; $p = 0.083$; $U = 9.0$; $p = 0.05$ compared to control; $U = 6.0$; $p = 0.048$ compared to the HD group). The MS group has less the duration of rearing (H (2, 27) = 8.6; $p = 0.013$; $U = 8.0$; $p = 0.04$) than the controls that reflects a decrease exploratory activity under prolonged postnatal stress.

Brief postnatal stress (handling) has an effect, mainly, on anxiety-like behavior. The number of visits (effect of stress: H (2, 27) = 5.6; $p = 0.062$; $U = 28.5$; $p = 0.022$) and time spent in the central zone (effect of stress: H (2, 27) = 5.2; $p = 0.075$; $U = 25.0$; $p = 0.013$) in the HD group were increased to compare with controls, reflecting a slight decrease in anxiety. Moreover, the duration of rearing were decreased in the HD groups compared to controls ($U = 23.0$; $p = 0.009$), as in the MS group. Parameters of locomotor activity were unchanged in the HD group.

3.3.2. Females. The analysis did not reveal any significant differences between groups (Figure 4). Estrous phase did not influence behavior in the OF test. However, diestrous HD females were slightly more anxious than MS females (Figure 5).

3.4. Social Interaction Test. Social interaction test assesses the level of sociability, which is measured by comparing the time a mouse spends in an interaction zone with a social target to the time in that zone in the absence of a social target. Males spend more time than females in the interaction zone both with an empty box and with a social target (effect of sex: H (1, 52) = 6.2, $p = 0.012$; H (1, 52) = 4.6, $p = 0.033$, resp.).

3.4.1. Males. Behaviors in an adaptation trial of the SI test, when a mouse can investigate a new place, confirm the decline locomotor and exploratory activities in the MS group. MS males covered significantly less distance than controls (effect of stress: H (2, 27) = 5.5, $p = 0.064$; $U = 8.0$; $p = 0.042$) and HD males ($U = 4.0$; $p = 0.024$) (Figure 6). The number of rearing was lower in MS males than in controls (effect of stress: H (2, 27) = 8.1, $p = 0.017$; $U = 4.0$; $p = 0.012$) and HD males ($U = 0.5$; $p = 0.006$).

In the interaction trial, when an unknown mouse was introduced into the small box, all groups had increased time spent in the interaction zone (interaction score > 100%, Figure 6). A significant effect of stress was revealed on the time spent in the interaction zone (H (2, 27) = 8.1, $p = 0.018$); HD males spent more time responding to the social target than controls ($U = 30.0$; $p = 0.03$). The MS group did not differ from controls and the HD group.

3.4.2. Females. Early-life stress has no significant effect on behavioral parameters in the adaptation trial. In the interaction trial, all groups had increased time spent in the interaction zone when a partner was presented (interaction score > 100%, Figure 7). Surprisingly, the interaction scores in HD and MS females were higher than in controls (effect of stress: H (2, 25) = 10.3, $p = 0.006$; $U = 8.0$; $p = 0.012$ and $U = 11.0$; $p = 0.006$, resp.), indicating that both stressed females groups increased sociability. MS females have enhanced not only score but also time spent near the social target compared to controls (effect of stress: H (2, 25) = 4.7, $p = 0.096$; $U = 17.0$; $p = 0.026$). And, apparently, this increased sociability led to an increase in the distance traveled in MS females compared to controls (effect of stress: H (2, 25) =6.0, $p = 0.049$; $U = 17.0$; $p = 0.026$).

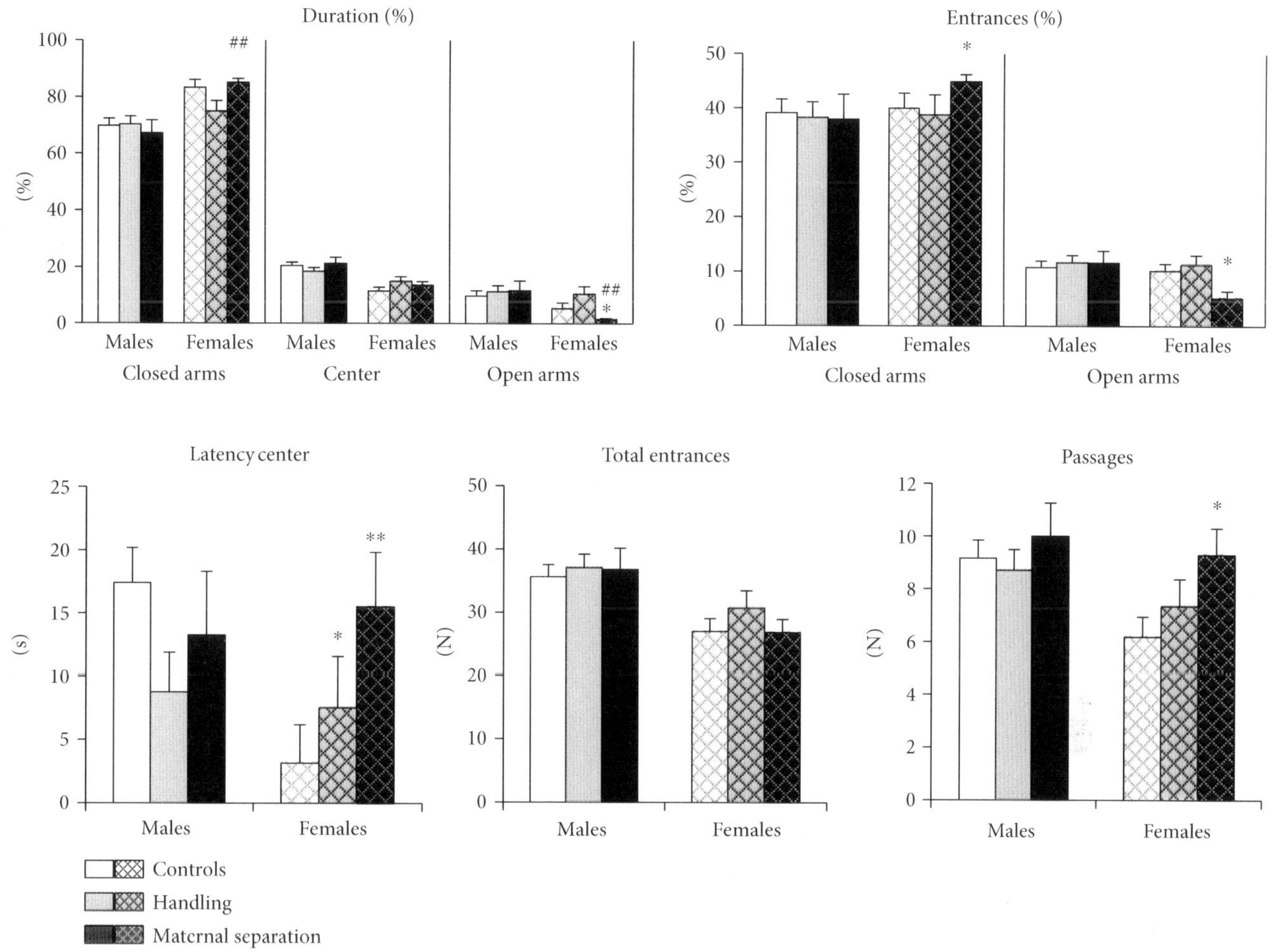

FIGURE 2: Effects of early-life stress on the behavior of adult mice in the plus-maze test. Early-life stress had no effect on plus-maze behavior in male mice but led to significant anxiogenic effect in MS females. Data present as mean ± standard error of the mean (SEM). White box: controls (males $n = 11$, females $n = 11$); grey box: HD (males $n = 10$, females $n = 6$), black box: MS (males $n = 6$, females $n = 8$); open columns: males; cross-hatched columns: females. $^{*}p < 0.05$, $^{**}p < 0.01$ compared to controls; $^{\#\#}p < 0.01$ compared to HD.

Figure 8 shows behavioral parameters depend on estrus and diestrus. There was only one estrous HD female in the test, which complicated the statistical analysis of the estrous cycle.

4. Discussion

Our study focused on the effects of maternal separation on the social behavior of adult mice and compared changes with changes in individual behavior. We showed that early postnatal stress had different effects on males and females.

The study of individual female behavior in the MS group revealed significantly increased anxiety in the elevated plus maze. Females avoided the open arms of the maze, but their locomotor activity was the same as that of controls. The OF test also did not reveal changes in the locomotor activity of MS females. In contrast to females, MS male anxiety in our experiments remained unchanged. The lack of MS effect on male emotional behavior was accompanied by changes in locomotor and exploratory activity. The OF test showed a significantly less distance traveled and reduced total and exploratory activity. Moreover, less distance was covered in the SI test during the adaptation trial, when the mice explore a new field without any additional social stimulus. So we have found gender-specific influence of prolonged maternal separation on anxiety and locomotion. There are few works in which both males and females of the C57BL6 mice were simultaneously studied. Some of them found the same effects of MS on anxiety in males and females [28, 30], whereas one study revealed sex-specific influence on anxiety [27], but different from our results. Various results can be explained by the differences in methodology of maternal separation. So, for example, in the study of Romeo and colleagues [27], separated pups were kept at the ambient temperature of the vivarium during 3 hours without additional heating that can lead to a pup's hypothermia. Some of the works used sexually experienced females (having two or three litters before) [25, 30]. Procedures for checking health and gender of pups as well as culling the pups at first postnatal day are stress factors for dams and pups and can affect results of the experiment [28]. So, minor differences in methodological aspects lead to a significant disagreement in the results.

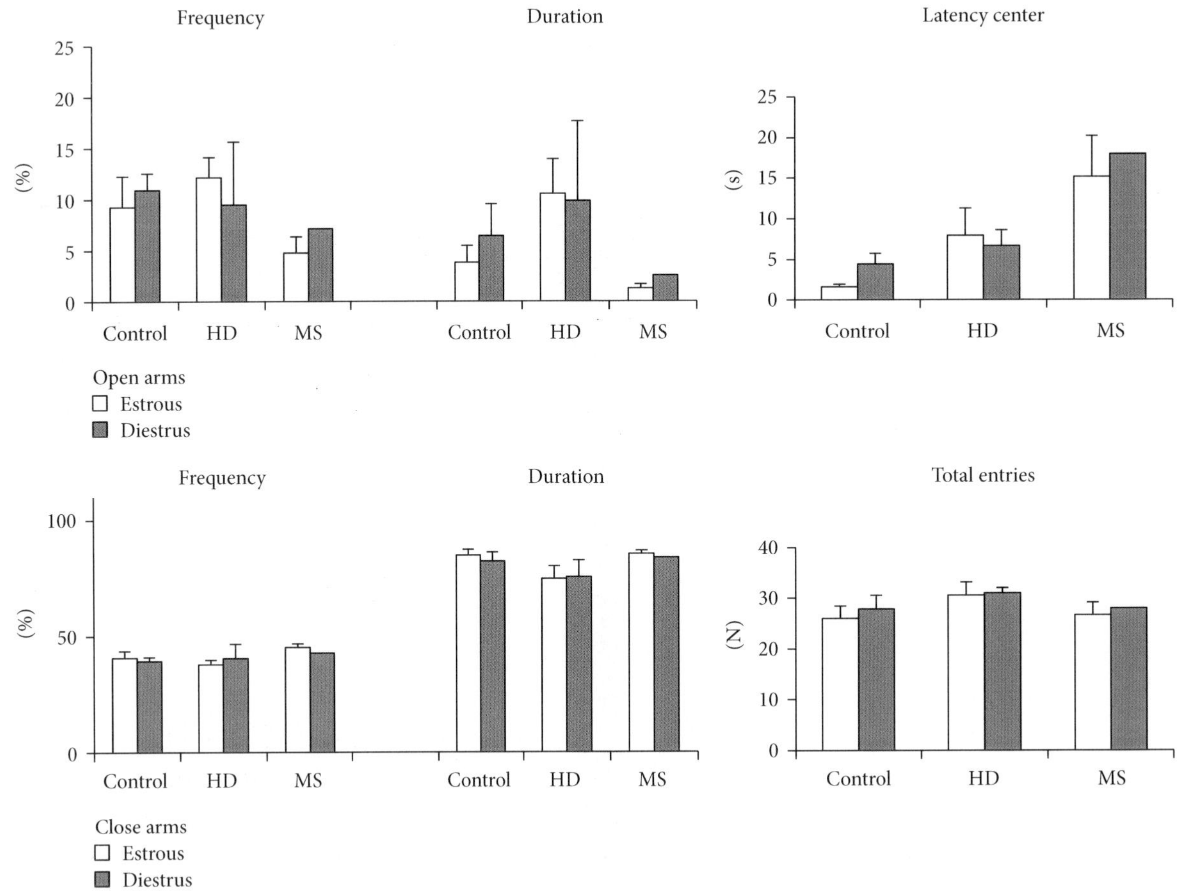

Figure 3: The influence of early-life stress on the behavior of adult female mice in plus-maze test in different phases of estrous cycle. Data present as mean ± standard error of the mean (SEM). White box: estrous (5 female controls, 4 HD group, and 6 MS group), gray box: diestrus (6 female controls, 2 HD group, and 1 MS group). Insufficient number of mice in each phase did not allow a correct statistical analysis.

These disagreements and other inconsistent results [31, 32, 51–55] suggest that effects on anxiety in mice are highly variable and depend even on small variations in environmental conditions during the postnatal period. Similarly, Millstein and Holmes [25] have concluded that repeated postnatal MS did not produce clear changes in anxiety- or depression-related behaviors in any of the five mouse strains studied. However, even in the lack of MS effects on behavior, it may alter the feedback regulation of response to a subsequent stress event, for example, resulting in a more pronounced and prolonged elevation of corticosterone levels [56–58] or a greater decrease in GR expression in the frontal cortex and hippocampus [59, 60].

The study of social behavior revealed somewhat unexpected results in females with prolonged maternal separation. The social interaction test showed increased sociability in MS females: the females responded to a novel conspecific more actively than the controls. However, this is not consistent with a high level of anxiety observed in females given the plus-maze test. High anxiety normally inhibits exploratory or social activity in animals. Here, we can hypothesize that the adaptation trial, during which the animals are familiarizing themselves with the experimental field, reduces anxiety. As is known, animals in familiar situations are less anxious and tend to have longer social contacts [61]. Additionally, longer testing decreases the fear of new space and stimulates exploratory behavior [62, 63]. As is known, anxiety in new, unfamiliar situations ("state" anxiety) does not necessarily correlate with anxiety shown in familiar situations ("trait" anxiety) [64, 65]. Some kinds of stress, for example, repeated aggression experience, induce enhanced anxiety [66] as observed in the plus-maze together with enhanced exploratory activity towards a new neutral stimulus [67]. It is possible that early-life stress in MS females increases "state," but not "trait" anxiety, and that these females, when in a familiar situation, can display a high level of social behavior. However, this hypothesis requires scrutiny.

Interestingly, in contrast to females, the social behavior of adult males was absolutely unaffected by prolonged maternal separation, and the level of reaction to the presentation of another mouse remained the same as in controls, which is consistent with some other social behavioral studies in males [39, 40].

Thus, in our experiment, separating the pups from their dams for 3 hours in an early postnatal period has a pronounced sex-specific effect on both social and individual mice behavior. Females are more sensitive to

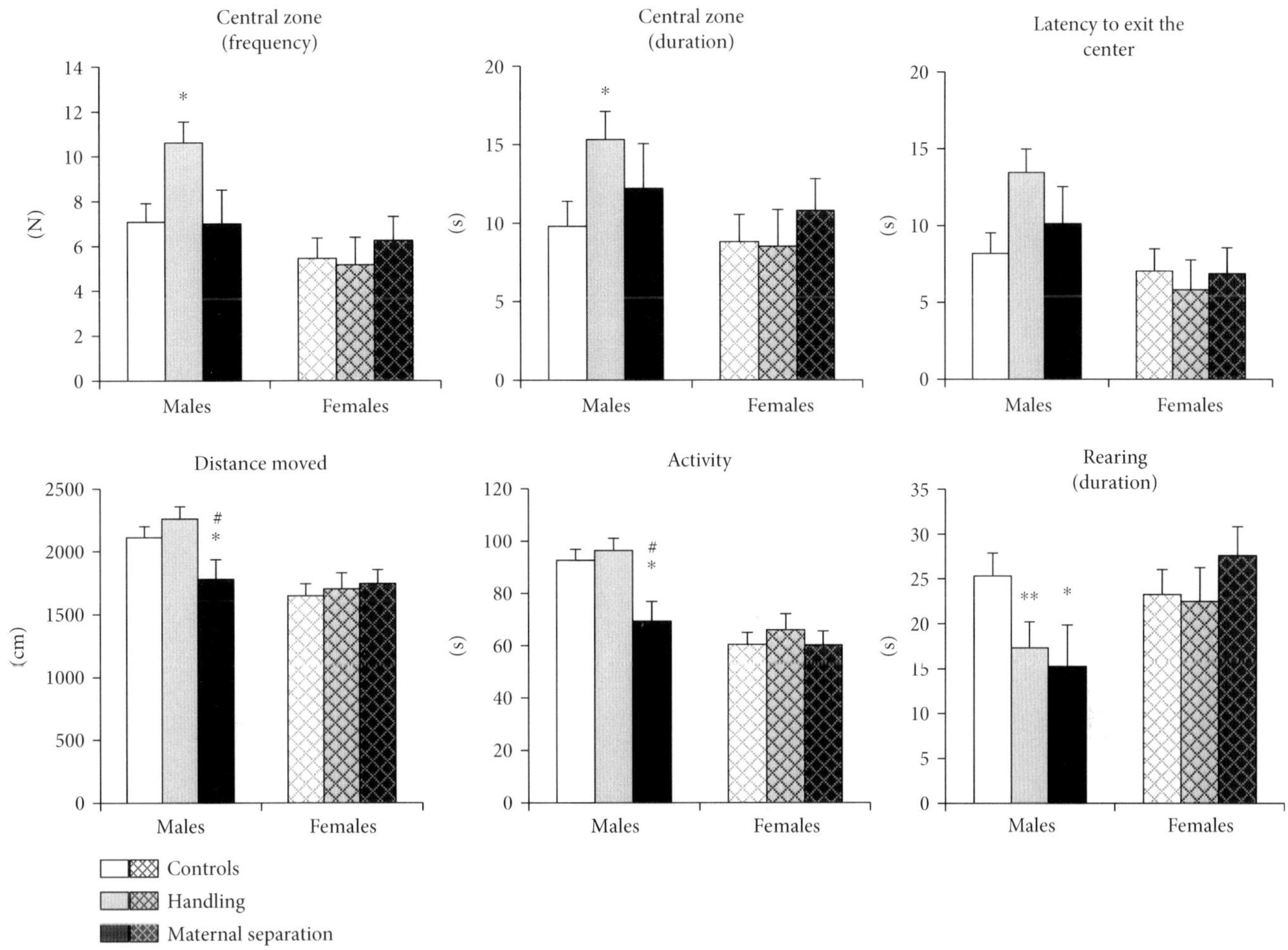

Figure 4: Effects of early-life stress on the behavior of adult mice in the open-field test. Male mice showed decreased locomotor and exploratory activities of MS males and decreased anxiety-like behavior in HD males. Females did not show the behavioral changes in the test. Data present as mean ± standard error of the mean (SEM). White box: controls (males $n = 11$, females $n = 11$); grey box: HD (males $n = 10$, females $n = 6$), black box: MS (males $n = 6$, females $n = 8$); open columns: males; cross-hatched columns: females. $^{*}p < 0.05$, $^{**}p < 0.01$ compared to controls; $^{\#}p < 0.05$ compared to HD.

stress than males, and maternal separation has contrasting effects (increased anxiety versus increased sociability) on the former.

Results of rat experiments demonstrated that brief maternal separation, or handling, which can be considered moderately stressful for pups, can result in positive behavioral changes and even tolerance to more intensive stress [21, 22, 45, 56, 68]. In our experiment, we also have found a positive effect of handling—HD males demonstrated a decreased anxiety in the OF test and increased sociability in the SI test. Males were not afraid of visiting the central part of the open field and spent more time there than the controls or the MS group, and HD males also spent more time in the interaction zone when the unknown partner was presented. Brief separation of females had no effect on anxiety or individual and exploratory behavior but also an increased level of sociability—HD females had the highest interaction score, which reflects the difference between a reaction to a partner and a reaction to an empty box. There are few works on the impact of handling on subsequent behavior of adult mice. Unlike rat studies, the vast majority of studies of HD stress have not found significant changes in anxiety or individual behavior in male and female C57BL6 mice [25, 30, 69]. Only one study has found decreased anxiety in male mice induced by brief separation [46], which is similar to our results. Our study has shown for the first time, to our knowledge, that brief maternal separation may positively affect social behavior in mice. Both males and females showed increased sociability in the form of a more active reaction to the same-sex partner in the social interaction test.

Our study has shown that female mice have more pronounced positive and negative consequences of both maternal separation and neonatal handling compared to their male conspecifics. Compared to male rodents, female rodents are known to have greater corticosterone release under basal conditions [70] and in response to stress [71–74]. Female mice were shown to be more sensitive to unpredictable chronic mild stress [75], subchronic variable stress [76], and even acute stress [77]. Also, females have longer consequences of social defeat stress than males [78, 79]. These findings explain the higher sensitivity of females to early-life stress consequences.

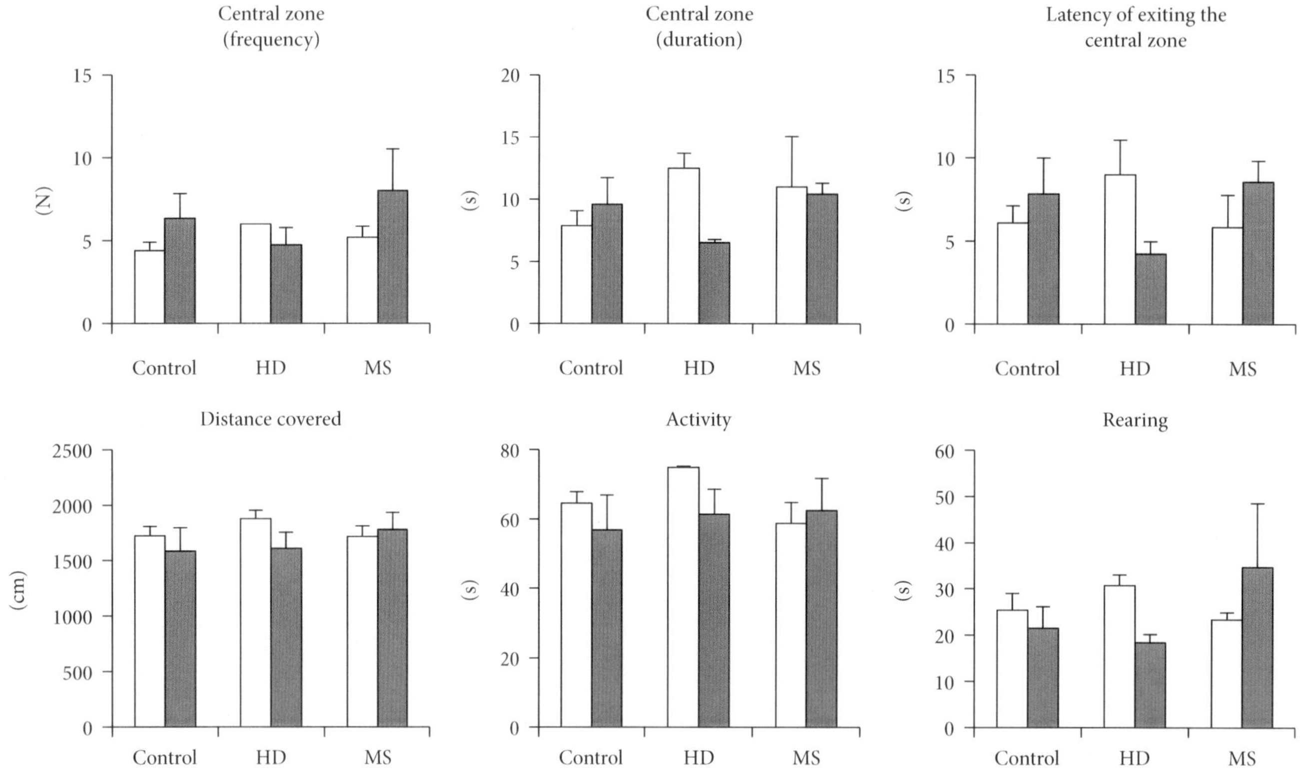

FIGURE 5: The influence of early-life stress on the behavior of adult female mice in open-field test in different phases of estrous cycle. Data present as mean ± standard error of the mean (SEM). White box: estrus (5 female controls, 2 HD group, and 5 MS group), gray box: diestrus (6 female controls, 4 HD group, and 3 MS group). Insufficient number of mice in each phase did not allow a correct statistical analysis.

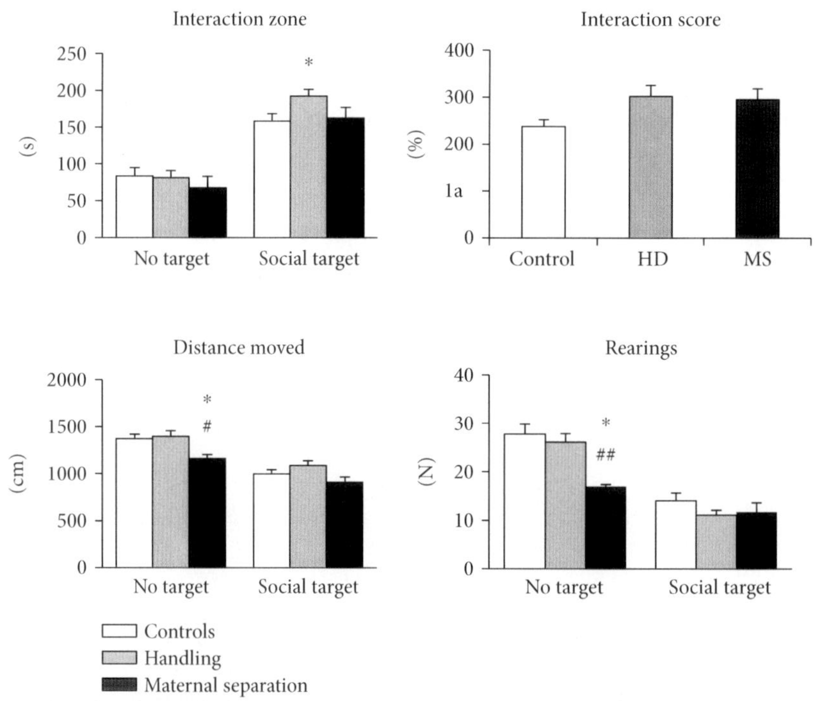

FIGURE 6: Effects of early-life stress on the social behavior of adult male mice. Handling have increased sociability of males, whereas maternal separation had no effects on social behavior. Data present as mean ± standard error of the mean (SEM). White box: controls (males, $n = 11$); grey box: HD (males, $n = 10$), black box: MS (males, $n = 6$); no target: the adaptation trial with an empty target box; social target: the interaction trial with an unfamiliar partner in the target box. $^{*}p < 0.05$ compared to controls; $^{\#}p < 0.05$; $^{\#\#}p < 0.01$ compared to HD.

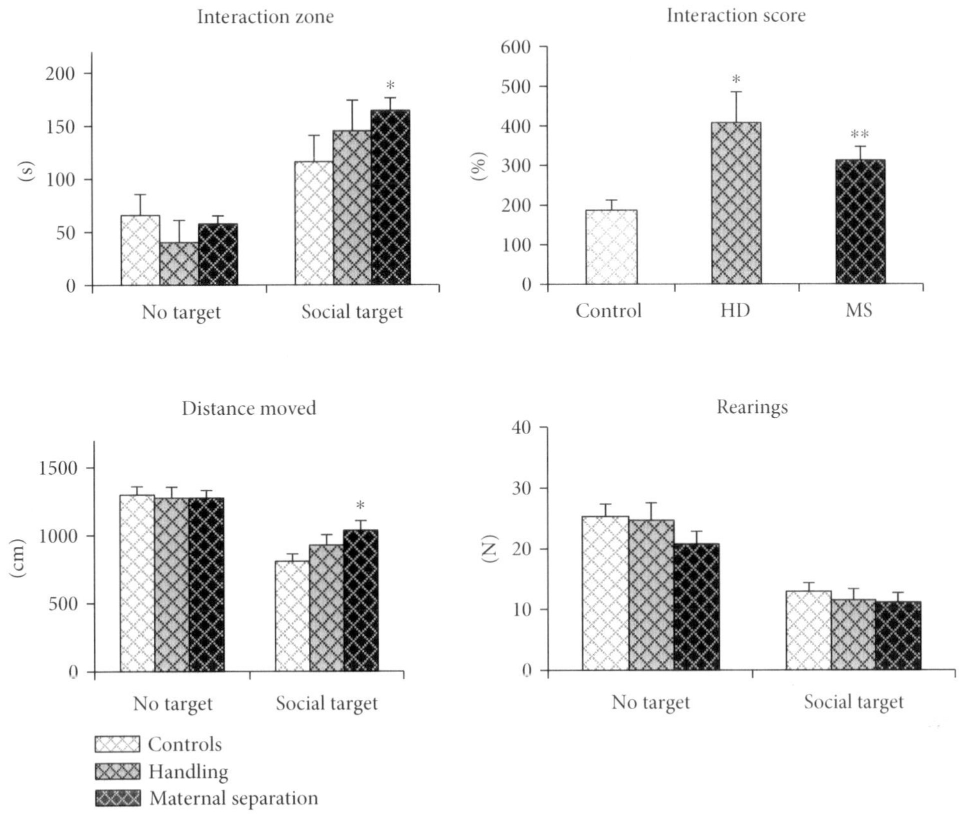

FIGURE 7: Effects of early-life stress on the social behavior of adult female mice. Both stressed females groups increased sociability in the test. Data present as mean ± standard error of the mean (SEM). White box: controls (females $n = 11$); grey box: HD (females $n = 6$), black box: MS (females $n = 8$); no target: the adaptation trial with an empty target box; social target: the interaction trial with an unfamiliar partner in the target box. $^{*}p < 0.05$, $^{**}p < 0.01$ compared to controls.

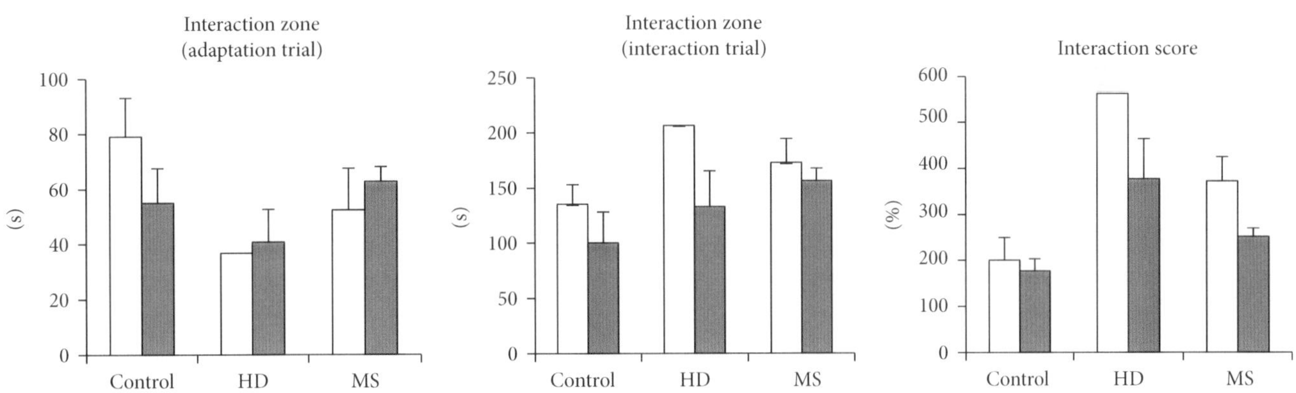

FIGURE 8: The influence of early-life stress on the behavior of adult female mice in social interaction test in different phases of estrous cycle. Data present as mean ± standard error of the mean (SEM). White box: estrus (5 control females, 1 HD group, and 4 MS group), gray box: diestrus (6 control females, 5 HD group, and 4 MS group). Insufficient number of mice in each phase did not allow a correct statistical analysis.

According to a systematic review [18], female studies nearly always show positive or deleterious effects of early stress on anxiety, depressiveness, or cognitive functions, while male studies do not reveal significant effects of stress on these psychoemotional traits in about 30% of cases. The analysis of maternal separation consequences [18] suggests that, in most (but not all) cases, stress results in higher anxiety and cognitive deterioration in both males and females. However, a sex-specific difference is sometimes observed in the studies. The study by Romeo and colleagues [27] showed opposite changes in the locomotor activity of males and females, and another study [28] identified contrasting changes in aggressive behavior. Increased social behavior after maternal separation that we have discovered is typical of females only, while males have the same reaction to the partner as controls. Notably, brief separation has the same effect on social behavior both in males and females. Thus, the influence of early-life stress on behavior in adulthood is gender-dependent.

Multiple studies in sex hormone effects on emotional behavior and stress response [80, 81] suggest that estrous cycle should be taken into account in female experiments. Although emotional behavior and especially the level of anxiety in females are sensitive to the level of sex hormones [82, 83], only few studies on female behavior after early-life stress [27, 84] take into account the phase of the estrous cycle. Most researchers believe that daily vaginal smears are too stressful for animals or that the selections of females used in the studies are insufficiently representative to analyze [25, 28–30]. However, studies often find no correlation between behavior and cycle phase [85, 86]. The reason may be that hormonal influence is not very strong, and the stress of testing hides possible behavior dependence on hormones. We have not detected an influence of cycle phase on the behavioral traits studied. Proper statistical analysis was impeded by a low number of animals in the groups. However, the direction of change was the same in the estrous and diestrous phases, that is, hormonal level had an insignificant effect on emotional behavior, locomotor, and exploratory activity.

5. Conclusion

Thus, the present study shows that the social and individual behavior of adult mice can be modified by early-life events in a sex-specific manner. We have found no changes in the anxiety or social behavior of MS males. Disrupted individual behavior has been the only consequence of early stress. The intensity of stress may have been insufficient to produce later effects in males. Females have been more sensitive to stress. Maternal separation has led to increased female anxiety and social behavior. Brief separation of pups from their mothers resulted in positive behavioral changes in males and females. Both sexes had increased social behavior, and males had decreased anxiety, which confirms the hypothesis that mild early-life stress has a positive effect on later emotional behavior.

Acknowledgments

This work was supported by the Russian Science Foundation [Grant no. 16-15-10131]. The authors thank Pavlov K.S. (Laboratory of Experimental Models of Neurodegenerative Processes, Institute of Physiology and Basic Medicine, Novosibirsk, Russia) for his technical assistance with EthoVision XT, v.10.0.

References

[1] J. G. Johnson, P. Cohen, M. S. Gould, S. Kasen, J. Brown, and J. S. Brook, "Childhood adversities, interpersonal difficulties, and risk for suicide attempts during late adolescence and early adulthood," *Archives of General Psychiatry*, vol. 59, no. 8, pp. 741–749, 2002.

[2] A. M. Vaiserman, "Epigenetic programming by early-life stress: evidence from human populations," *Developmental Dynamics*, vol. 244, no. 3, pp. 254–265, 2015.

[3] F. Varese, F. Smeets, M. Drukker et al., "Childhood adversities increase the risk of psychosis: a meta-analysis of patient-control, prospective- and cross-sectional cohort studies," *Schizophrenia Bulletin*, vol. 38, no. 4, pp. 661–671, 2012.

[4] C. Heim, P. M. Plotsky, and C. B. Nemeroff, "Importance of studying the contributions of early adverse experience to neurobiological findings in depression," *Neuropsychopharmacology*, vol. 29, no. 4, pp. 641–648, 2004.

[5] H. J. Krugers and M. Joels, "Long-lasting consequences of early life stress on brain structure, emotion and cognition," *Current Topics in Behavioral Neurosciences*, vol. 18, pp. 81–92, 2014.

[6] M. H. Teicher, A. Tomoda, and S. L. Andersen, "Neurobiological consequences of early stress and childhood maltreatment: are results from human and animal studies comparable?," *Annals of the New York Academy of Sciences*, vol. 1071, no. 1, pp. 313–323, 2006.

[7] M. Vythilingam, C. Heim, J. Newport et al., "Childhood trauma associated with smaller hippocampal volume in women with major depression," *The American Journal of Psychiatry*, vol. 159, no. 12, pp. 2072–2080, 2002.

[8] A. L. van Harmelen, P. J. de Jong, K. A. Glashouwer, P. Spinhoven, B. W. Penninx, and B. M. Elzinga, "Child abuse and negative explicit and automatic self-associations: the cognitive scars of emotional maltreatment," *Behaviour Research and Therapy*, vol. 48, no. 6, pp. 486–494, 2010.

[9] U. Rao, L. A. Chen, A. S. Bidesi, M. U. Shad, M. A. Thomas, and C. L. Hammen, "Hippocampal changes associated with early-life adversity and vulnerability to depression," *Biological Psychiatry*, vol. 67, no. 4, pp. 357–364, 2010.

[10] M. H. Teicher, C. M. Anderson, and A. Polcari, "Childhood maltreatment is associated with reduced volume in the hippocampal subfields CA3, dentate gyrus, and subiculum," *Proceedings of the National Academy of Sciences of the United States of America*, vol. 109, no. 9, pp. E563–E572, 2012.

[11] A. Danese and B. S. McEwen, "Adverse childhood experiences, allostasis, allostatic load, and age-related disease," *Physiology & Behavior*, vol. 106, no. 1, pp. 29–39, 2012.

[12] P. Dawes, K. J. Cruickshanks, D. R. Moore et al., "The effect of prenatal and childhood development on hearing, vision and cognition in adulthood," *PLoS One*, vol. 10, no. 8, article e0136590, 2015.

[13] A. Chocyk, B. Bobula, D. Dudys et al., "Early-life stress affects the structural and functional plasticity of the medial prefrontal cortex in adolescent rats," *The European Journal of Neuroscience*, vol. 38, no. 1, pp. 2089–2107, 2013.

[14] M. Rincel, A. L. Lepinay, Y. Janthakhin et al., "Maternal high-fat diet and early life stress differentially modulate spine density and dendritic morphology in the medial prefrontal cortex of juvenile and adult rats," *Brain Structure and Function*, 2017.

[15] Y. Janthakhin, M. Rincel, A. M. Costa, M. Darnaudery, and G. Ferreira, "Maternal high-fat diet leads to hippocampal and

amygdala dendritic remodeling in adult male offspring," *Psychoneuroendocrinology*, vol. 83, pp. 49–57, 2017.

[16] N. P. Bondar and T. I. Merkulova, "Brain-derived neurotrophic factor and early-life stress: multifaceted interplay," *Journal of Biosciences*, vol. 41, no. 4, pp. 751–758, 2016.

[17] I. Herpfer, H. Hezel, W. Reichardt et al., "Early life stress differentially modulates distinct forms of brain plasticity in young and adult mice," *PLoS One*, vol. 7, no. 10, article e46004, 2012.

[18] S. G. Tractenberg, M. L. Levandowski, L. A. de Azeredo et al., "An overview of maternal separation effects on behavioural outcomes in mice: evidence from a four-stage methodological systematic review," *Neuroscience & Biobehavioral Reviews*, vol. 68, pp. 489–503, 2016.

[19] A. Kaffman and M. J. Meaney, "Neurodevelopmental sequelae of postnatal maternal care in rodents: clinical and research implications of molecular insights," *Journal of Child Psychology and Psychiatry*, vol. 48, no. 3-4, pp. 224–244, 2007.

[20] E. R. de Kloet, R. M. Sibug, F. M. Helmerhorst, and M. V. Schmidt, "Stress, genes and the mechanism of programming the brain for later life," *Neuroscience & Biobehavioral Reviews*, vol. 29, no. 2, pp. 271–281, 2005.

[21] S. Levine, "Influence of psychological variables on the activity of the hypothalamic-pituitary-adrenal axis," *European Journal of Pharmacology*, vol. 405, no. 1–3, pp. 149–160, 2000.

[22] C. R. Pryce and J. Feldon, "Long-term neurobehavioural impact of the postnatal environment in rats: manipulations, effects and mediating mechanisms," *Neuroscience & Biobehavioral Reviews*, vol. 27, no. 1-2, pp. 57–71, 2003.

[23] M. V. Schmidt, "Molecular mechanisms of early life stress—lessons from mouse models," *Neuroscience & Biobehavioral Reviews*, vol. 34, no. 6, pp. 845–852, 2010.

[24] G. Biagini and E. M. Pich, "Corticosterone administration to rat pups, but not maternal separation, affects sexual maturation and glucocorticoid receptor immunoreactivity in the testis," *Pharmacology, Biochemistry, and Behavior*, vol. 73, no. 1, pp. 95–103, 2002.

[25] R. A. Millstein and A. Holmes, "Effects of repeated maternal separation on anxiety- and depression-related phenotypes in different mouse strains," *Neuroscience & Biobehavioral Reviews*, vol. 31, no. 1, pp. 3–17, 2007.

[26] M. Mehta and C. Schmauss, "Strain-specific cognitive deficits in adult mice exposed to early life stress," *Behavioral Neuroscience*, vol. 125, no. 1, pp. 29–36, 2011.

[27] R. D. Romeo, A. Mueller, H. M. Sisti, S. Ogawa, B. S. McEwen, and W. G. Brake, "Anxiety and fear behaviors in adult male and female C57BL/6 mice are modulated by maternal separation," *Hormones and Behavior*, vol. 43, no. 5, pp. 561–567, 2003.

[28] A. H. Veenema, R. Bredewold, and I. D. Neumann, "Opposite effects of maternal separation on intermale and maternal aggression in C57BL/6 mice: link to hypothalamic vasopressin and oxytocin immunoreactivity," *Psychoneuroendocrinology*, vol. 32, no. 5, pp. 437–450, 2007.

[29] M. Kundakovic, S. Lim, K. Gudsnuk, and F. A. Champagne, "Sex-specific and strain-dependent effects of early life adversity on behavioral and epigenetic outcomes," *Frontiers in Psychiatry*, vol. 4, p. 78, 2013.

[30] J. D. Bailoo, R. L. Jordan, X. J. Garza, and A. N. Tyler, "Brief and long periods of maternal separation affect maternal behavior and offspring behavioral development in C57BL/6 mice," *Developmental Psychobiology*, vol. 56, no. 4, pp. 674–685, 2014.

[31] M. C. Tsuda and S. Ogawa, "Long-lasting consequences of neonatal maternal separation on social behaviors in ovariectomized female mice," *PLoS One*, vol. 7, no. 3, article e33028, 2012.

[32] H. M. Savignac, T. G. Dinan, and J. F. Cryan, "Resistance to early-life stress in mice: effects of genetic background and stress duration," *Frontiers in Behavioral Neuroscience*, vol. 5, p. 13, 2011.

[33] E. Binder, K. Malki, J. L. Paya-Cano et al., "Antidepressants and the resilience to early-life stress in inbred mouse strains," *Pharmacogenetics and Genomics*, vol. 21, no. 12, pp. 779–789, 2011.

[34] J. J. Dimatelis, I. M. Vermeulen, K. Bugarith, D. J. Stein, and V. A. Russell, "Female rats are resistant to developing the depressive phenotype induced by maternal separation stress," *Metabolic Brain Disease*, vol. 31, no. 1, pp. 109–119, 2016.

[35] E. D. George, K. A. Bordner, H. M. Elwafi, and A. A. Simen, "Maternal separation with early weaning: a novel mouse model of early life neglect," *BMC Neuroscience*, vol. 11, no. 1, p. 123, 2010.

[36] B. C. Carlyle, A. Duque, R. R. Kitchen et al., "Maternal separation with early weaning: a rodent model providing novel insights into neglect associated developmental deficits," *Development and Psychopathology*, vol. 24, no. 04, pp. 1401–1416, 2012.

[37] I. Gracia-Rubio, M. Moscoso-Castro, O. J. Pozo, J. Marcos, R. Nadal, and O. Valverde, "Maternal separation induces neuroinflammation and long-lasting emotional alterations in mice," *Progress in Neuro-Psychopharmacology and Biological Psychiatry*, vol. 65, pp. 104–117, 2016.

[38] A. Lin, S. J. Wood, and A. R. Yung, "Measuring psychosocial outcome is good," *Current Opinion in Psychiatry*, vol. 26, no. 2, pp. 138–143, 2013.

[39] E. Ognibene, W. Adriani, A. Caprioli et al., "The effect of early maternal separation on brain derived neurotrophic factor and monoamine levels in adult heterozygous reeler mice," *Progress in Neuro-Psychopharmacology and Biological Psychiatry*, vol. 32, no. 5, pp. 1269–1276, 2008.

[40] M. C. Tsuda, N. Yamaguchi, and S. Ogawa, "Early life stress disrupts peripubertal development of aggression in male mice," *Neuroreport*, vol. 22, no. 6, pp. 259–263, 2011.

[41] T. B. Franklin, N. Linder, H. Russig, B. Thony, and I. M. Mansuy, "Influence of early stress on social abilities and serotonergic functions across generations in mice," *PLoS One*, vol. 6, no. 7, article e21842, 2011.

[42] M. R. Farrell, F. H. Holland, R. M. Shansky, and H. C. Brenhouse, "Sex-specific effects of early life stress on social interaction and prefrontal cortex dendritic morphology in young rats," *Behavioural Brain Research*, vol. 310, pp. 119–125, 2016.

[43] H. J. Hulshof, A. Novati, A. Sgoifo, P. G. Luiten, J. A. den Boer, and P. Meerlo, "Maternal separation decreases adult hippocampal cell proliferation and impairs cognitive performance but has little effect on stress sensitivity and anxiety in adult Wistar rats," *Behavioural Brain Research*, vol. 216, no. 2, pp. 552–560, 2011.

[44] M. Niwa, Y. Matsumoto, A. Mouri, N. Ozaki, and T. Nabeshima, "Vulnerability in early life to changes in the

rearing environment plays a crucial role in the aetiopathology of psychiatric disorders," *The International Journal of Neuropsychopharmacology*, vol. 14, no. 04, pp. 459–477, 2011.

[45] M. J. Meaney, "Maternal care, gene expression, and the transmission of individual differences in stress reactivity across generations," *Annual Review of Neuroscience*, vol. 24, no. 1, pp. 1161–1192, 2001.

[46] D. B. Parfitt, J. R. Walton, E. A. Corriveau, and D. L. Helmreich, "Early life stress effects on adult stress-induced corticosterone secretion and anxiety-like behavior in the C57BL/6 mouse are not as robust as initially thought," *Hormones and Behavior*, vol. 52, no. 4, pp. 417–426, 2007.

[47] A. Luchetti, D. Oddi, V. Lampis et al., "Early handling and repeated cross-fostering have opposite effect on mouse emotionality," *Frontiers in Behavioral Neuroscience*, vol. 9, p. 93, 2015.

[48] R. G. Lister, "The use of a plus-maze to measure anxiety in the mouse," *Psychopharmacology*, vol. 92, no. 2, pp. 180–185, 1987.

[49] R. J. Rodgers and J. C. Cole, "Influence of social isolation, gender, strain, and prior novelty on plus-maze behaviour in mice," *Physiology & Behavior*, vol. 54, no. 4, pp. 729–736, 1993.

[50] O. Friard and M. Gamba, "BORIS: a free, versatile open-source event-logging software for video/audio coding and live observations," *Methods in Ecology and Evolution*, vol. 7, no. 11, pp. 1325–1330, 2016.

[51] S. Macri and G. Laviola, "Single episode of maternal deprivation and adult depressive profile in mice: interaction with cannabinoid exposure during adolescence," *Behavioural Brain Research*, vol. 154, no. 1, pp. 231–238, 2004.

[52] D. B. Parfitt, J. K. Levin, K. P. Saltstein, A. S. Klayman, L. M. Greer, and D. L. Helmreich, "Differential early rearing environments can accentuate or attenuate the responses to stress in male C57BL/6 mice," *Brain Research*, vol. 1016, no. 1, pp. 111–118, 2004.

[53] H. Toda, S. Boku, S. Nakagawa et al., "Maternal separation enhances conditioned fear and decreases the mRNA levels of the neurotensin receptor 1 gene with hypermethylation of this gene in the rat amygdala," *PLoS One*, vol. 9, no. 5, article e97421, 2014.

[54] I. C. Weaver, M. J. Meaney, and M. Szyf, "Maternal care effects on the hippocampal transcriptome and anxiety-mediated behaviors in the offspring that are reversible in adulthood," *Proceedings of the National Academy of Sciences of the United States of America*, vol. 103, no. 9, pp. 3480–3485, 2006.

[55] J. Lehmann and J. Feldon, "Long-term biobehavioral effects of maternal separation in the rat: consistent or confusing?," *Reviews in the Neurosciences*, vol. 11, no. 4, pp. 383–408, 2000.

[56] G. Biagini, E. M. Pich, C. Carani, P. Marrama, and L. F. Agnati, "Postnatal maternal separation during the stress hyporesponsive period enhances the adrenocortical response to novelty in adult rats by affecting feedback regulation in the CA1 hippocampal field," *International Journal of Developmental Neuroscience*, vol. 16, no. 3–4, pp. 187–197, 1998.

[57] P. M. Plotsky and M. J. Meaney, "Early, postnatal experience alters hypothalamic corticotropin-releasing factor (CRF) mRNA, median eminence CRF content and stress-induced release in adult rats," *Molecular Brain Research*, vol. 18, no. 3, pp. 195–200, 1993.

[58] M. Lippmann, A. Bress, C. B. Nemeroff, P. M. Plotsky, and L. M. Monteggia, "Long-term behavioural and molecular alterations associated with maternal separation in rats," *The European Journal of Neuroscience*, vol. 25, no. 10, pp. 3091–3098, 2007.

[59] C. O. Ladd, R. L. Huot, K. V. Thrivikraman, C. B. Nemeroff, and P. M. Plotsky, "Long-term adaptations in glucocorticoid receptor and mineralocorticoid receptor mRNA and negative feedback on the hypothalamo-pituitary-adrenal axis following neonatal maternal separation," *Biological Psychiatry*, vol. 55, no. 4, pp. 367–375, 2004.

[60] S. Navailles, R. Zimnisky, and C. Schmauss, "Expression of glucocorticoid receptor and early growth response gene 1 during postnatal development of two inbred strains of mice exposed to early life stress," *Developmental Neuroscience*, vol. 32, no. 2, pp. 139–148, 2010.

[61] S. E. File and J. R. Hyde, "Can social interaction be used to measure anxiety?," *British Journal of Pharmacology*, vol. 62, no. 1, pp. 19–24, 1978.

[62] D. Drai, N. Kafkafi, Y. Benjamini, G. Elmer, and I. Golani, "Rats and mice share common ethologically relevant parameters of exploratory behavior," *Behavioural Brain Research*, vol. 125, no. 1–2, pp. 133–140, 2001.

[63] E. Fonio, Y. Benjamini, and I. Golani, "Short and long term measures of anxiety exhibit opposite results," *PLoS One*, vol. 7, no. 10, article e48414, 2012.

[64] D. F. Avgustinovich, T. V. Lipina, N. P. Bondar, O. V. Alekseyenko, and N. N. Kudryavtseva, "Features of the genetically defined anxiety in mice," *Behavior Genetics*, vol. 30, no. 2, pp. 101–109, 2000.

[65] G. Griebel, C. Belzung, R. Misslin, and E. Vogel, "The free-exploratory paradigm: an effective method for measuring neophobic behaviour in mice and testing potential neophobia-reducing drugs," *Behavioural Pharmacology*, vol. 4, no. 6, pp. 637–644, 1993.

[66] N. N. Kudryavtseva, N. P. Bondar, and D. F. Avgustinovich, "Association between experience of aggression and anxiety in male mice," *Behavioural Brain Research*, vol. 133, no. 1, pp. 83–93, 2002.

[67] T. V. Lipina and N. N. Kudriavtseva, "The study of exploratory behavior in CBA/Lac male mice under influence of positive and negative social interactions," *Zhurnal Vyssheĭ Nervnoĭ Deiatelnosti Imeni I P Pavlova*, vol. 58, no. 2, pp. 194–201, 2008.

[68] D. M. Lyons, K. J. Parker, and A. F. Schatzberg, "Animal models of early life stress: implications for understanding resilience," *Developmental Psychobiology*, vol. 52, no. 5, pp. 402–410, 2010.

[69] Y. Bian, L. Yang, Z. Wang, Q. Wang, L. Zeng, and G. Xu, "Repeated three-hour maternal separation induces depression-like behavior and affects the expression of hippocampal plasticity-related proteins in C57BL/6N mice," *Neural Plasticity*, vol. 2015, Article ID 627837, 7 pages, 2015.

[70] H. C. Atkinson and B. J. Waddell, "Circadian variation in basal plasma corticosterone and adrenocorticotropin in the rat: sexual dimorphism and changes across the estrous cycle," *Endocrinology*, vol. 138, no. 9, pp. 3842–3848, 1997.

[71] A. Iwasaki-Sekino, A. Mano-Otagiri, H. Ohata, N. Yamauchi, and T. Shibasaki, "Gender differences in corticotropin and corticosterone secretion and corticotropin-releasing factor mRNA expression in the paraventricular nucleus of the hypothalamus and the central nucleus of the amygdala in response

to footshock stress or psychological stress in rats," *Psychoneuroendocrinology*, vol. 34, no. 2, pp. 226–237, 2009.

[72] G. L. Hermes, L. Rosenthal, A. Montag, and M. K. McClintock, "Social isolation and the inflammatory response: sex differences in the enduring effects of a prior stressor," *American Journal of Physiology. Regulatory, Integrative and Comparative Physiology*, vol. 290, no. 2, pp. R273–R282, 2006.

[73] I. Kloehn, S. B. Pillai, L. Officer, C. Klement, P. J. Gasser, and J. A. Evans, "Sexual differentiation of circadian clock function in the adrenal gland," *Endocrinology*, vol. 157, no. 5, pp. 1895–1904, 2016.

[74] R. Verma, Y. P. Balhara, and C. S. Gupta, "Gender differences in stress response: role of developmental and biological determinants," *Industrial Psychiatry Journal*, vol. 20, no. 1, pp. 4–10, 2011.

[75] R. Shepard, C. E. Page, and L. Coutellier, "Sensitivity of the prefrontal GABAergic system to chronic stress in male and female mice: relevance for sex differences in stress-related disorders," *Neuroscience*, vol. 332, pp. 1–12, 2016.

[76] G. E. Hodes, M. L. Pfau, I. Purushothaman et al., "Sex differences in nucleus accumbens transcriptome profiles associated with susceptibility versus resilience to subchronic variable stress," *The Journal of Neuroscience*, vol. 35, no. 50, pp. 16362–16376, 2015.

[77] D. F. Avgustinovich, I. L. Kovalenko, and L. A. Koryakina, "Effects of single episodes of severe stress on the behavior of male and female CBA/Lac and C57BL/6J mice," *Neuroscience and Behavioral Physiology*, vol. 37, no. 7, pp. 731–737, 2007.

[78] M. Q. Steinman, N. Duque-Wilckens, G. D. Greenberg et al., "Sex-specific effects of stress on oxytocin neurons correspond with responses to intranasal oxytocin," *Biological Psychiatry*, vol. 80, no. 5, pp. 406–414, 2016.

[79] B. C. Trainor, M. C. Pride, R. Villalon Landeros et al., "Sex differences in social interaction behavior following social defeat stress in the monogamous California mouse (*Peromyscus californicus*)," *PLoS One*, vol. 6, no. 2, article e17405, 2011.

[80] J. P. ter Horst, E. R. de Kloet, H. Schachinger, and M. S. Oitzl, "Relevance of stress and female sex hormones for emotion and cognition," *Cellular and Molecular Neurobiology*, vol. 32, no. 5, pp. 725–735, 2012.

[81] P. Palanza, L. Gioiosa, and S. Parmigiani, "Social stress in mice: gender differences and effects of estrous cycle and social dominance," *Physiology & Behavior*, vol. 73, no. 3, pp. 411–420, 2001.

[82] A. A. Walf and C. A. Frye, "Estradiol decreases anxiety behavior and enhances inhibitory avoidance and gestational stress produces opposite effects," *Stress*, vol. 10, no. 3, pp. 251–260, 2007.

[83] F. K. Marcondes, K. J. Miguel, L. L. Melo, and R. C. Spadari-Bratfisch, "Estrous cycle influences the response of female rats in the elevated plus-maze test," *Physiology & Behavior*, vol. 74, no. 4–5, pp. 435–440, 2001.

[84] R. W. Rhees, E. D. Lephart, and D. Eliason, "Effects of maternal separation during early postnatal development on male sexual behavior and female reproductive function," *Behavioural Brain Research*, vol. 123, no. 1, pp. 1–10, 2001.

[85] H. Meziane, A. M. Ouagazzal, L. Aubert, M. Wietrzych, and W. Krezel, "Estrous cycle effects on behavior of C57BL/6J and BALB/cByJ female mice: implications for phenotyping strategies," *Genes, Brain, and Behavior*, vol. 6, no. 2, pp. 192–200, 2007.

[86] J. P. Ter Horst, J. Kentrop, M. Arp, C. J. Hubens, E. R. de Kloet, and M. S. Oitzl, "Spatial learning of female mice: a role of the mineralocorticoid receptor during stress and the estrous cycle," *Frontiers in Behavioral Neuroscience*, vol. 7, p. 56, 2013.

2

Delusions in Patients with Dementia with Lewy Bodies and the Associated Factors

Ray-Chang Tzeng,[1] Ching-Fang Tsai,[1] Ching-Tsu Wang,[1] Tzu-Yuan Wang,[2] and Pai-Yi Chiu[3]

[1]*Department of Neurology, Tainan Municipal Hospital (Managed by Show Chwan Medical Care Corporation), Tainan, Taiwan*
[2]*Division of Endocrinology and Metabolism, Department of Internal Medicine, China Medical University Hospital, Taichung, Taiwan*
[3]*Department of Neurology, Show Chwan Memorial Hospital, Changhua, Taiwan*

Correspondence should be addressed to Pai-Yi Chiu; paiyibox@gmail.com

Academic Editor: Hiroshi Yoshizawa

Objective. Delusions are common neuropsychiatric symptoms in patients with dementia with Lewy bodies (DLB). The aim of this study was to investigate the associated factors of delusions in patients with DLB. *Method.* A retrospective study of outpatients with DLB registered in a regional hospital's database was performed. The associated factors including cognitive performance, clinical features, vascular risk factors, and neuropsychiatric symptoms between delusional and nondelusional patients with DLB were compared. *Results.* Among 207 patients with DLB, 106 (51.2%) were delusional and 101 (48.8%) were not. Delusion of other persons are stealing was the most common symptom (35.3%). The delusional group had a significantly higher diagnostic rate of probable than possible DLB, higher disease severity, poorer cognitive performance, more severe neuropsychiatric symptoms, and higher caregiver burden (all $p < 0.05$). In addition, the delusional group had a significantly lower frequency of diabetes compared to the nondelusional group (odds ratio = 0.28, $p < 0.001$). *Conclusion.* Delusion of other persons are stealing was the most common delusional symptom. The patients with DLB who presented with delusions had poorer cognitive function and more severe neuropsychiatric symptoms. A novel finding is that the DLB patients with diabetes had a lower frequency of delusions.

1. Introduction

Dementia with Lewy bodies (DLB) is the second most common degenerative dementia. According to the first consensus criteria for the diagnosis of DLB in 1996, it accounts for about 20% of all clinical and autopsy cases of degenerative dementia [1]. In a more recent systemic review of studies on the incidence and prevalence of DLB in 2005, it was reported to account for 0 to 30.5% of all dementia cases [2]. Delusions are among the most common neuropsychiatric features in patients with dementia, especially in those with DLB. Therefore, delusions become one of the supportive features for the clinical diagnosis of DLB [1, 3]. Studies on delusions in dementia have shown that delusions are seldom observed in the predementia stage; however, delusions increase in frequency from the early through the later stages of dementia [4–8].

Clinical studies of delusions in dementia have reported different frequencies and characteristics of delusions among different types of dementia [9]. Psychotic symptoms including delusions and hallucinations have been reported to be significantly more frequent in patients with DLB than in patients with Alzheimer's disease (AD) or other dementia [9–14]. Delusional misidentification is significantly more characteristic of DLB than AD, while paranoid delusions are not specifically associated with DLB [12]. Patients with DLB have more psychotic and mood symptoms; therefore, the carers of patients with DLB experience more stress than those caring for patients with AD and vascular dementia [9].

Pathophysiological studies of delusions in dementia have revealed specific neural substrates that may be associated with delusions in patients with DLB [12, 15–17]. In a study on correlations between cholinergic dysfunction and neuropsychiatric symptoms of dementia, the authors found that defective cholinergic activity in patients with DLB was correlated with hallucinations and delusions [15]. An autopsy study revealed that delusions in DLB are associated with elevated M_1 binding in Brodmann area 36 [16]. Unlike AD, DLB has been reported to be significantly inversely associated with tangle burden and psychosis [12]. A genetic study reported that the 5-HTTLPR polymorphism is associated with delusions in Lewy body dementias including DLB and Parkinson's disease dementia (PDD) [17].

There is robust evidence of the contribution of vascular risk factors (VRFs) to the incidence and prevalence of AD and vascular dementia (VaD) [18–21]. Diabetes is among the most important VRFs, and a recent meta-analysis reviewed 28 studies and revealed that diabetes has a relative risk (RR) of 1.76 for developing all types of dementia [18]. A case-control study of the risk factors for AD, PD, and DLB by Boot et al. found no association of diabetes with DLB [22]. Some studies demonstrated that most of the risk factors appeared in midlife and that they may increase the risk of dementia later in life [21, 23]. However, associations of VRF with the clinical presentation of dementia have seldom been discussed, and studies on the relationship between VRF and the clinical presentation of DLB even less so [22].

The aim of this study was to investigate factors including clinical features, cognitive performance, neuropsychiatric symptoms, and vascular risk factors between delusional and nondelusional patients with DLB.

2. Methods

2.1. Database. This is a retrospective study of outpatients with DLB registered in a health system's dementia database. The following information from this database was used for this study:

(1) Diagnosis of dementia according to the criteria for primary degenerative dementia in the fourth edition of the Diagnostic and Statistic Manual of Mental Disorders (DSM-IV). Diagnosis of DLB according to the revised consensus criteria for probable or possible DLB developed by the third report of the DLB consortium [3]

(2) Age, gender, education, dementia severity, and medications at the time of entry

(3) Clinical DLB features including fluctuation, parkinsonism, visual hallucinations, REM sleep behavior disorder (RBD), and severe neuroleptic sensitivity

(4) Cognitive performance on the Cognitive Abilities Screening Instrument, Chinese version (CASI C-2.0) with the following domains: long-term memory, short-term memory, attention, mental manipulation, orientation, abstract thinking, language, drawing, and verbal fluency [24]

(5) Neuropsychiatric symptoms in the 12-item version of the Neuropsychiatric Inventory (NPI) including delusions, hallucinations, agitation, depression, anxiety, euphoria, apathy, disinhibition, irritation, aberrant motor behavior, night behavior, and eat/appetite behavior on the basis of observations within the past month [25]

(6) Clinically relevant vascular risk comorbidities including hypertension, arrhythmia, coronary artery disease, diabetes, hyperlipidemia, and cerebrovascular disease (history of stroke/transient ischemic attack or the diagnosis of vascular encephalopathy in brain imaging)

2.2. Assessment of Clinical Features and Diagnosis of DLB. In the dementia clinic, all of the patients and their main caregivers were interviewed by a behavioral neurologist for the assessment of core and suggestive features. Fluctuation was diagnosed when a clinical history of fluctuation in cognition and a Mayo Fluctuation Composite Score (MFCS) > 2 [26] were both present. Visual hallucinations (VHs) were diagnosed when a clinical history of recurrent complex VHs were present. Parkinsonism was diagnosed when at least two of the following were present: bradykinesia, tremor, rigidity, and postural instability. RBD was diagnosed when the minimal criteria for REM sleep behavior disorder according to the International Classification of Sleep Disorders (ICSD) [27] was met. Severe neuroleptic sensitivity was diagnosed when a clinical history was established for both the usage of neuroleptic drugs and an obvious association of adverse events with the neuroleptic drugs. Because dopamine transporter uptake imaging was not available in our hospital until 2010, the suggestive feature "low dopamine transporter uptake in basal ganglia" in the revised consensus criteria could not be evaluated and was thus not included in this study. This may have resulted in a lower diagnostic rate for probable DLB and a higher diagnostic rate for possible DLB.

2.3. Assessment of Delusions and Other Neuropsychiatric Symptoms. All of the patients and their main caregivers were interviewed by a trained neuropsychologist for assessment of the NPI domain of delusions, including ratings on eight individual forms of delusions for the past one month. The NPI is a validated, standardized, and widely used instrument that was developed specifically to evaluate the neuropsychiatric symptoms of dementia. All of the 12 NPI domains were rated for symptom frequency from 1 (occasionally) to 4 (very frequently), symptom severity from 1 (mild) to 3 (severe), and caregiver burden from 0 (none) to 5 (extremely) [25].

2.4. Assessment of Disease Severity and Cognitive Function. The global severity of dementia was assessed according to the Clinical Dementia Rating (CDR) scale and sum of boxes of the CDR (CDR-SB) [28]. Cognitive functions were assessed with the CASI and the Mini-Mental State Examination (MMSE) modified from the CASI [24]. Motor functions were assessed with motor score of the Unified Parkinson's Disease Rating Scale (UPDRS-m) [29], and all patients were rated under medication. Cognitive tests of all patients were performed by a trained neuropsychologist. Dementia and subtypes of dementia were diagnosed by a consensus meeting composed of three neurologists, one geriatric psychiatrist, and one neuropsychologist. All patients received at least cerebral computed tomography or cerebral magnetic resonance imaging and also a set of blood screening tests for dementia.

2.5. Data Analysis. The Chinese version of SPSS 19.0 for Windows (IBM, SPSS Inc., Chicago) was used for statistical analyses. Comparisons between delusional and nondelusional DLB groups in demographic data, CASI, MMSE, motor score of the UPDRS, and composite scores (frequency × severity) of the NPI were analyzed using the independent t-test. Gender, CDR, clinical features, clinical history of VRFs, current use of antipsychotics, and current use of antiparkinsonian drugs were analyzed using the chi-square test. To compare the associations of clinical features, cognitive performance, neuropsychiatric symptoms, and VRFs between the delusional and nondelusional groups, we used both model 1 analysis (odds ratios (OR) adjusted for age and gender) and model 2 analysis (OR adjusted for age, gender, disease severity according to the CDR, antipsychotics, and antiparkinsonian drugs).

2.6. Ethical Considerations. The Committee for Medical Research Ethics of Show Chwan Memorial Hospital reviewed the project, and the Data Inspectorate approved it.

3. Results

From October 1, 2015, to June 21, 2017, a total of 207 patients who fulfilled the criteria for DLB and had complete data were analyzed. Among them, 106 (51.2%) were delusional and 101 (48.8%) were nondelusional (Figure 1). The delusion of other persons are stealing was the most common (35.3%), followed by delusions of self is in danger (21.3%), house is not his/her home (10.8%), spouse is having an affair (7.2%), family plans to abandon him/her (4.8%), an unwelcome guest is living in the house (2.9%), media persons are in the house (2.9%), and others are not who they claim (1.0%). The frequency of delusions increased as disease severity increased (28.6% in CDR 0.5, 47.5% in CDR 1, and 63.0% in CDR 2–3; $\chi^2 = 12.776, p = 0.002$). The severity of delusions among the delusional patients according to the composite score of delusion in the NPI was not different among the CDR groups (4.8 ± 3.7 in CDR 0.5, 4.6 ± 2.1 in CDR 1, and 4.9 ± 2.9 in CDR 2–3; $f = 0.481, p = 0.620$).

Comparisons of the demographic data are summarized in Table 1. The delusional group had a significantly higher diagnostic rate of probable DLB (74.5% in the delusional groups versus 60.4% in the nondelusional group, $p = 0.030$), higher disease severity according to CDR stage ($\chi^2 = 12.776, p = 0.002$) and CDR-SB ($t = 3.779, p = 0.002$), poorer cognitive performance according to the MMSE ($t = -2.623$, $p = 0.009$) and CASI ($t = -2.629$, $p = 0.009$), worse neuropsychiatric symptoms according to the NPI composite score ($t = 7.144$, $p < 0.001$), and higher caregiver burden scale in the NPI ($t = 10.113, p < 0.001$).

Comparisons of cognitive performance of each domain in the CASI are summarized in Table 2. The delusional group had poorer performance in the domains of mental manipulation (OR = 0.86, $p = 0.002$) and orientation (OR = 0.93, $p = 0.008$) in model 1 analysis, whereas no cognitive domain was associated with the delusional group in model 2 analysis.

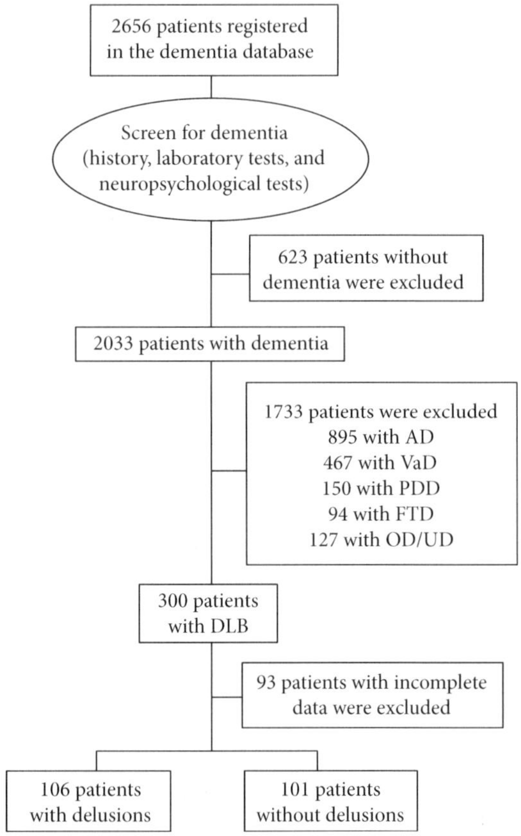

FIGURE 1

Comparisons of core and suggestive features are summarized in Table 3. The delusional group had a higher frequency of fluctuations (OR = 1.83, $p = 0.032$) and VH (OR = 2.99, $p < 0.001$) in model 1 analysis; however, only VH (OR = 2.31, $p = 0.019$) was significantly higher in the delusional group in model 2 analysis.

A comparison of a history of vascular risk factors demonstrated that the delusional group were significantly less associated with diabetes in both model 1 (OR = 0.36, $p = 0.002$) and model 2 (OR = 0.28, $p < 0.001$) analyses (Table 3). We further analyzed the delusional symptoms that were associated with diabetes after adjusting for age, gender, and disease severity according to the CDR and found that delusions of other persons are stealing (OR = 0.32, $p = 0.018$) and self is in danger (OR = 0.42, $p = 0.021$) were significantly lower in the patients with diabetes.

Comparisons of neuropsychiatric symptoms of each domain in the NPI are summarized in Table 4. The delusional group had higher frequencies of hallucinations (OR = 3.27, $p < 0.001$), agitation (OR = 2.40, $p = 0.003$), anxiety (OR = 2.49, $p = 0.002$), disinhibition (OR = 5.28, $p < 0.001$), irritation (OR = 4.85, $p < 0.001$), and aberrant motor behavior (OR = 2.93, $p = 0.001$) in model 1 analysis. In model 2 analysis, the delusional group had higher frequencies of hallucinations (OR = 2.59, $p = 0.003$), agitation

Table 1: Demographic and background characteristics between the delusional and nondelusional patients with DLB.

	Delusional	Nondelusional	t/χ^2	p
N	106	101		
Gender, male/female	53/53	62/39	2.716	NS
Age, years (SD, range)	78.9 (6.8, 62–91)	77.6 (6.8, 51–90)	−1.301	NS
Education, years (SD, range)	5.8 (5.2, 0–18)	6.6 (5.0, 0–19)	−1.047	NS
Duration, years (SD, range)				
Dementia	3.0 (3.0, 0–20)	2.8 (2.8, 0–15)	0.358	NS
Parkinsonism	3.0 (3.0, 0–20)	2.6 (2.3, 0–10)	1.019	NS
Psychiatric disorder	4.0 (5.1, 0–40)	3.2 (3.6, 0–25)	1.251	NS
RBD	5.0 (9.5, 0–50)	5.5 (11.0, 0–50)	−0.225	NS
DLB probable/possible	79/27	61/40	4.719	0.030
CDR 0.5/1/2–3	10/38/58	25/42/32	12.776	0.002
CDR-SB (SD, range)	9.3 (3.3, 1.5–17.0)	7.5 (3.8, 1.5–16.0)	3.779	<0.001
MMSE (SD, range)	14.0 (7.0, 0–29)	16.9 (8.0, 0–29)	−2.623	0.009
CASI (SD, range)	44.7 (23.1, 0–95)	53.7 (25.9, 0–94)	−2.629	0.009
NPI (SD, range)	34.3 (14.6, 3–77)	19.4 (15.4, 0–79)	7.144	<0.001
NPI burden (SD, range)	17.9 (6.7, 0–32)	9.1 (5.8, 0–25)	10.113	<0.001
UPDRS-m (SD, range)	17.7 (11.3, 0–63)	18.1 (11.4, 0–48)	−0.279	NS
Antipsychotics, n (%)	22 (20.8%)	12 (11.9%)	2.967	NS
Antiparkinsonian, n (%)	41 (38.7%)	42 (41.6%)	0.182	NS
LED (SD, range)	146 (237, 0–1050)	181 (276, 0–1158)	0.977	NS

NS: not significant; DLB: dementia with Lewy bodies; RBD: REM sleep behavior disorder; psychiatric disorder: psychosis or mood disorders; DLB probable/possible: diagnosis of probable DLB/possible DLB; CDR: Clinical Dementia Rating scale; CDR-SB: sum of boxes of CDR; MMSE: Mini-Mental State Examination; CASI: Cognitive Abilities Screening Instrument; NPI: total score of the 12-domain Neuropsychiatric Inventory; NPI burden: total caregiver burden scale in the NPI; UPDRS-m: motor score of the Unified Parkinson's Disease Rating Scale; antipsychotics: current using antipsychotics; antiparkinsonian: current use of antiparkinsonian agents; LED: levodopa equivalent dose, mg/day.

Table 2: Two models of risk estimates (odds ratios) for cognitive domains in CASI between the delusional and nondelusional patients with DLB.

Features	Mean (SD, range)		Model 1		Model 2	
	Delusional	Nondelusional	OR (95% CI)	p	OR (95% CI)	p
N	106	101				
Remote memory	6.6 (3.3, 0–10)	7.3 (3.2, 0–10)	0.95 (0.87–1.04)	NS	1.05 (0.94–1.17)	NS
Recent memory	4.2 (3.4, 0–12)	5.4 (3.7, 0–12)	0.92 (0.85–1.00)	NS	1.00 (0.90–1.10)	NS
Attention	5.2 (2.2, 0–8)	5.4 (2.2, 0–8)	0.98 (0.86–1.12)	NS	1.09 (0.94–1.27)	NS
Mental manipulation	2.5 (2.9, 0–10)	4.0 (3.5, 0–10)	**0.86 (0.77–0.95)**	**0.002**	0.91 (0.81–1.03)	NS
Orientation	6.7 (4.8, 0–18)	9.0 (6.0, 0–18)	**0.93 (0.88–0.98)**	**0.008**	0.99 (0.92–1.06)	NS
Abstract thinking	4.1 (2.8, 0–11)	4.8 (3.0, 0–12)	0.95 (0.85–1.05)	NS	1.04 (0.91–1.08)	NS
Language	6.8 (3.1, 0–10)	7.1 (3.0, 0–10)	0.98 (0.89–1.07)	NS	1.08 (0.96–1.20)	NS
Draw	4.8 (3.8, 0–10)	5.9 (3.9, 0–10)	0.94 (0.87–1.01)	NS	1.01 (0.92–1.10)	NS
Animal naming (verbal fluency)	4.0 (3.0, 0–10)	4.8 (3.3, 0–10)	0.94 (0.86–1.03)	NS	1.02 (0.92–1.14)	NS

DLB: dementia with Lewy bodies; CASI: Cognitive Abilities Screening Instrument; NS: not significant. The odds ratio (OR) and 95% confidence interval (CI) were calculated with the nondelusional group as reference. Model 1 ORs were adjusted for age, gender, and education; model 2 ORs were adjusted for age, gender, education, disease severity, antipsychotics, and antiparkinsonian agents.

(OR = 1.87, $p = 0.048$), anxiety (OR = 2.64, $p = 0.002$), disinhibition (OR = 4.81, $p = 0.003$), irritation (OR = 4.50, $p < 0.001$), and aberrant motor behavior (OR = 2.36, $p = 0.010$).

4. Discussion

In this study, about half (51.2%) of all patients had a delusion, and the delusion of other persons are stealing (35.3%) was the most common, followed by delusion of self is in danger (21.3%). These findings are consistent with the results from most of the previous studies on DLB [10–13] and also clinical study on AD [8]. The finding of higher frequency of delusions in more severe dementia is probably because delusions are highly associated with the ability of source memory monitoring, and this ability is gradually deteriorated as disease progresses [30]. In this study, although only a cognitive

Table 3: Two models of risk estimates (odds ratios) for core and suggestive features between the delusional and nondelusional patients with DLB.

Features	*N* (%) Delusional	Nondelusional	Model 1 OR (95% CI)	*p*	Model 2 OR (95% CI)	*p*
N	106	101				
Clinical features						
Fluctuation	62 (58.5%)	44 (43.6%)	**1.83 (1.05–3.17)**	**0.032**	1.52 (0.84–2.73)	NS
Visual hallucinations	65 (61.3%)	35 (34.7%)	**2.99 (1.70–5.27)**	**<0.001**	**2.26 (1.21–4.21)**	**0.010**
Parkinsonism	96 (90.6%)	87 (86.1%)	1.54 (0.65–3.66)	NS	1.26 (0.49–3.25)	NS
RBD	44 (41.5%)	45 (44.6%)	0.88 (0.51–1.53)	NS	1.18 (0.66–2.12)	NS
Neuroleptic sensitivity*	12 (11.3%; 54.5%)	7 (6.9%; 58.3%)	1.71 (0.65–4.55)	NS	1.72 (0.61–4.83)	NS
Vascular risk factors						
Hypertension	52 (49.1%)	45 (44.6%)	1.10 (0.63–1.92)	NS	1.17 (0.65–2.09)	NS
Diabetes	21 (19.8%)	40 (39.6%)	**0.36 (0.19–0.68)**	**0.002**	**0.28 (0.14–0.56)**	**<0.001**
Coronary artery disease	7 (6.6%)	7 (6.9%)	0.93 (0.31–2.81)	NS	0.82 (0.26–2.60)	NS
Hyperlipidemia	4 (3.8%)	5 (5.0%)	0.84 (0.22–3.26)	NS	0.80 (0.20–3.21)	NS
Arrhythmia	9 (8.5%)	13 (12.9%)	0.67 (0.27–1.67)	NS	0.55 (0.21–1.46)	NS
Cerebrovascular disease	16 (15.1%)	19 (18.8%)	0.58 (0.33–1.02)	NS	0.63 (0.29–1.38)	NS

DLB: dementia with Lewy bodies; RBD: REM sleep behavior disorder; NS: not significant. The odds ratio (OR) and 95% confidence interval (CI) were calculated with the nondelusional group as reference. *Severe neuroleptic sensitivity (among all patients; among those who had ever used antipsychotics). Model 1 ORs were adjusted for age and gender. Model 2 ORs were adjusted for age, gender, disease severity, antipsychotics, and antiparkinsonian agents.

Table 4: Two models of risk estimates (odds ratios) for neuropsychiatric symptoms in the NPI between the delusional and nondelusional DLB groups.

Neuropsychiatric symptoms	Mean (SD, range) Delusional	Nondelusional	Model 1 OR (95% CI)	*p*	Model 2 OR (95% CI)	*p*
N	106	101				
Hallucinations	71 (67.0%)	37 (36.6%)	**3.27 (1.83–5.85)**	**<0.001**	**2.59 (1.39–4.80)**	**0.003**
Agitation	52 (49.1%)	30 (29.7%)	**2.40 (1.34–4.30)**	**0.003**	**1.87 (1.01–3.48)**	**0.048**
Depression	76 (71.7%)	65 (64.4%)	1.31 (0.72–2.38)	NS	1.19 (0.64–2.22)	NS
Anxiety	72 (67.9%)	45 (44.6%)	**2.49 (1.40–4.43)**	**0.002**	**2.64 (1.45–4.81)**	**0.002**
Euphoria	2 (1.9%)	2 (2.0%)	1.22 (0.14–9.02)	NS	0.62 (0.77–4.96)	NS
Apathy	72 (67.9%)	59 (58.4%)	1.58 (0.88–2.82)	NS	1.26 (0.68–2.32)	NS
Disinhibition	24 (22.6%)	5 (5.0%)	**5.28 (1.91–14.44)**	**<0.001**	**4.81 (1.71–13.53)**	**0.003**
Irritation	62 (58.5%)	24 (23.8%)	**4.85 (2.62–8.99)**	**<0.001**	**4.50 (2.39–8.46)**	**<0.001**
Aberrant motor behavior	50 (47.2%)	23 (22.8%)	**2.93 (1.59–5.38)**	**0.001**	**2.36 (1.23–4.51)**	**0.01**
Sleep	91 (85.8%)	78 (77.2%)	1.72 (0.83–3.55)	NS	1.56 (0.74–3.30)	NS
Eat/appetite	47 (44.3%)	30 (29.7%)	1.54 (0.87–2.74)	NS	1.36 (0.75–2.46)	NS

DLB: dementia with Lewy bodies; NPI: Neuropsychiatric Inventory; NS: not significant. The odds ratio (OR) and 95% confidence interval (CI) were calculated with the nondelusional group as reference. Model 1 ORs were adjusted for age and gender; model 2 ORs were adjusted for age, gender, disease severity, antipsychotics, and antiparkinsonian agents.

screening tool was used to study the association of cognitive functions with delusions [24], our patients with DLB and delusions had poorer cognitive function, especially in the domain of mental manipulation, which is also regarded to be an executive function [31]. Studies on the mechanism and interaction of delusions with cognition had demonstrated that delusions are highly associated with cognitive impairment and especially with impairments in source monitoring [30] and are regarded to involve source memory and executive functions [30, 32]. A recent study on the interaction of cognitive functions and delusions in patients with AD also reported that psychosis is influenced by executive function [33]. In addition, relationships between behavioral syndromes and cognitive domains in patients with AD showed that psychosis was significantly associated with impaired working memory [33]. In previous studies of DLB and according to the consensus criteria, cognitive impairments in the domains of executive function, visuospatial function, and attention in patients with DLB have been noted in the early stage of disease [1, 3]. Therefore, it is reasonable to find a high frequency of delusions in patients with DLB.

Previous studies have shown that neuropsychiatric symptoms in patients with DLB are more severe and more frequent than in other types of dementia [9–14]. These symptoms are salient in the early stage of DLB, and they are manifested as delusions, visual hallucinations, REM sleep behavior disorder, and depression [1, 3]. Our patients with mild DLB had a high frequency of delusions (22.7% with CDR 0.5 and 39.5% with CDR 1), which is consistent with our previous study on delusions in different stages of AD [8]. The current study also demonstrated that the delusional patients generally had more severe neuropsychiatric symptoms and were associated with a higher frequency of hallucinations, agitation/aggression, anxiety, irritation, and aberrant motor behavior.

Previous studies on the association between vascular risk factors and degenerative and/or vascular disorders have focused on controlling risk factors in midlife to prevent morbidity and mortality in late life. In general, these factors are regarded to be important risk factors for both small and large vessel diseases, and most of the vascular risk factors, including diabetes, in midlife have been associated with increased neurodegenerative dementia and vascular dementia in late life [21, 23]. However, the association between the incidence of dementia or cognitive decline and diabetes in late life is still controversial. The contribution of vascular risk factors has seldom been studied in patients with DLB. A previous study on the risk factors for DLB compared to the risk factors for AD showed no differences in stroke or diabetes between the two groups [22]. A novel finding of the current study is that the patients with DLB comorbid with diabetes had a lower frequency of delusions. A possible explanation for this finding is that, similar to findings from a study of animals with diabetes, levels of muscarinic acetylcholine receptors (mAChRs) subtype M1 are decreased in the cerebral cortex of patients with diabetes [34]. The M1 subtype of mAChRs is the most abundant type in the human cerebral cortex and hippocampus [35]. In general, M1 immunoreactivity is markedly reduced in the brains of patients with AD and DLB [34]. However, in a study of autopsy cases, Ballard et al. reported that delusions in patients with DLB are associated with elevated M1 binding in Brodmann area 36 [12]. Another study found decreased levels of total muscarinic and muscarinic M1 receptors in animals with diabetes [34]. Based on these findings, we proposed that patients with DLB comorbid with diabetes may have decreased levels of M1 receptors in the brain, which may lead to a lower frequency of delusions. Further studies are warranted to clarify the pathophysiology and causal relationship among diabetes, antidiabetes drugs, and delusions in patients with DLB.

In conclusion, delusions and other neuropsychiatric symptoms were evaluated in a relatively large sample of patients with DLB in this study. We found that the frequency of delusions increased as the severity of dementia increased in patients with DLB. We use multidimensional analysis of the associated factors of delusions and found that the patients with DLB and delusions had a poorer cognitive function and more severe neuropsychiatric symptoms. The novel finding of this study is that the patients with DLB comorbid with diabetes had a lower frequency of delusions.

Additional Points

Significant Outcomes. (1) Neuropsychiatric symptoms were evaluated in a relatively large sample of patients with dementia with Lewy bodies (DLB). (2) We use multidimensional analysis of the associated factors of delusions in patients with DLB. (3) A novel finding is that patients with DLB comorbid with diabetes had fewer delusions. *Limitations.* (1) This study was conducted in 3 hospitals in Taiwan. Therefore, the findings may not be generalizable to all patients with DLB. (2) The comparison of associated factors between the delusional and nondelusional patients with DLB in this study was cross-sectional. Therefore, causal relationships of the factors and dementia could not be ascertained. (3) Because of a lack of measurable data including the glucose level, glycated hemoglobin level, blood pressures, and medications on vascular risk factors and the associated medications of the patients, further studies are needed to evaluate the contribution of these factors on the presentation of delusions in patients with DLB. (4) Because less than 20% of our participants had received dopamine transporter uptake imaging, this may have resulted in a lower diagnostic rate for probable DLB in this study.

Authors' Contributions

Ray-Chang Tzeng undertook the literature search and data analysis and edited the author contributions and was mainly responsible for revisions and drafts of the manuscript. Pai-Yi Chiu participated in the data analysis and contributed to revisions and the final draft of the manuscript. Tzu-Yuan Wang participated in data analysis and contributed to revisions of the manuscript. Ching-Fang Tsai contributed to revisions of the manuscript. Ching-Tsu Wang undertook the literature search and contributed to revisions.

Acknowledgments

The authors would like to thank Professor Shu-Hui Sue at the National Taichung University of Science and Technology and Professor Tsung-Lin Cheng at the National Changhua University of Education for their feedback and suggestions during the experimental design and statistical analysis.

References

[1] I. G. McKeith, D. Galasko, K. Kosaka et al., "Consensus guidelines for the clinical and pathologic diagnosis of dementia with Lewy bodies (DLB): report of the consortium on DLB international workshop," *Neurology*, vol. 47, no. 5, pp. 1113–1124, 1996.

[2] J. Zaccai, C. Mccracken, and C. Brayne, "A systematic review of prevalence and incidence studies of dementia with Lewy bodies," *Age and Ageing*, vol. 34, no. 6, pp. 561–566, 2005.

[3] I. G. McKeith, D. W. Dickson, J. Lowe et al., "Diagnosis and management of dementia with Lewy bodies: third report of the DLB Consortium," *Neurology*, vol. 65, no. 12, pp. 1863–1872, 2005.

[4] S. Van der Mussele, N. Le Bastard, Y. Vermeiren et al., "Behavioral symptoms in mild cognitive impairment as compared with Alzheimer's disease and healthy older adults," *International Journal of Geriatric Psychiatry*, vol. 28, no. 3, pp. 265–275, 2013.

[5] Y. E. Geda, R. O. Roberts, M. M. Mielke et al., "Baseline neuropsychiatric symptoms and the risk of incident mild cognitive impairment: a population-based study," *The American Journal of Psychiatry*, vol. 171, no. 5, pp. 572–581, 2014.

[6] C. G. Lyketsos, O. Lopez, B. Jones, A. L. Fitzpatrick, J. Breitner, and S. DeKosky, "Prevalence of neuropsychiatric symptoms in dementia and mild cognitive impairment: result from the Cardiovascular Health Study," *JAMA*, vol. 288, no. 12, pp. 1475–1483, 2002.

[7] L. G. Apostolova, L. J. Di, E. L. Duffy et al., "Risk factors for behavioral abnormalities in mild cognitive impairment and mild Alzheimer's disease," *Dementia and Geriatric Cognitive Disorders*, vol. 37, no. 5-6, pp. 315–326, 2014.

[8] P. Y. Chiu and C. L. Chung, "Delusions in patients with very mild, mild and moderate Alzheimer's disease," *Acta Neurologica Taiwanica*, vol. 15, no. 1, pp. 21–25, 2006.

[9] M. Caputo, R. Monastero, E. Mariani et al., "Neuropsychiatric symptoms in 921 elderly subjects with dementia: a comparison between vascular and neurodegenerative types," *Acta Psychiatrica Scandinavica*, vol. 117, no. 6, pp. 455–464, 2008.

[10] C. Ballard, C. Holmes, I. McKeith et al., "Psychiatric morbidity in dementia with Lewy bodies: a prospective clinical and neuropathological comparative study with Alzheimer's disease," *The American Journal of Psychiatry*, vol. 156, no. 7, pp. 1039–1045, 1999.

[11] D. Aarsland, C. Ballard, J. P. Larsen, and I. Mckeith, "A comparative study of psychiatric symptoms in dementia with Lewy bodies and Parkinson's disease with and without dementia," *International Journal of Geriatric Psychiatry*, vol. 16, no. 5, pp. 528–536, 2001.

[12] C. G. Ballard, R. Jacoby, T. del Ser et al., "Neuropathological substrates of psychiatric symptoms in prospectively studied patients with autopsy-confirmed dementia with Lewy bodies," *The American Journal of Psychiatry*, vol. 161, no. 5, pp. 843–849, 2004.

[13] A. Suárez-González, A. Serrano-Pozo, E. M. Arroyo-Anlló et al., "Utility of neuropsychiatric tools in the differential diagnosis of dementia with Lewy bodies and Alzheimer's disease: quantitative and qualitative findings," *International Psychogeriatrics*, vol. 26, no. 3, pp. 453–461, 2014.

[14] D. R. Lee, I. McKeith, U. Mosimann, A. Ghosh-Nodyal, and A. J. Thomas, "Examining carer stress in dementia: the role of subtype diagnosis and neuropsychiatric symptoms," *International Journal of Geriatric Psychiatry*, vol. 28, no. 2, pp. 135–141, 2013.

[15] C. Marra, D. Quaranta, P. Profice et al., "Central cholinergic dysfunction measured "in vivo" correlates with different behavioral disorders in Alzheimer's disease and dementia with Lewy body," *Brain Stimulation*, vol. 5, no. 4, pp. 533–538, 2012.

[16] C. Ballard, M. Piggott, M. Johnson et al., "Delusions associated with elevated muscarinic binding in dementia with Lewy bodies," *Annals of Neurology*, vol. 48, no. 6, pp. 868–876, 2000.

[17] B. Creese, C. Ballard, D. Aarsland, E. Londos, S. Sharp, and E. Jones, "Determining the association of the 5HTTLPR polymorphism with delusions and hallucinations in Lewy body dementias," *The American Journal of Geriatric Psychiatry*, vol. 22, no. 6, pp. 580–586, 2014.

[18] K. Gudala, D. Bansal, F. Schifano, and A. Bhansali, "Diabetes mellitus and risk of dementia: a meta-analysis of prospective observational studies," *Journal of Diabetes Investigation*, vol. 4, no. 6, pp. 640–650, 2013.

[19] J. A. Luchsinger, C. Reitz, L. S. Honig, M. X. Tang, S. Shea, and R. Mayeux, "Aggregation of vascular risk factors and risk of incident Alzheimer disease," *Neurology*, vol. 65, no. 4, pp. 545–551, 2005.

[20] P. B. Gorelick, "Risk factors for vascular dementia and Alzheimer disease," *Stroke*, vol. 35, no. 11, Supplement 1, pp. 2620–2622, 2004.

[21] M. Kivipelto, T. Ngandu, L. Fratiglioni et al., "Obesity and vascular risk factors at midlife and the risk of dementia and Alzheimer disease," *Archives of Neurology*, vol. 62, no. 10, pp. 1556–1560, 2005.

[22] B. P. Boot, C. F. Orr, J. E. Ahlskog et al., "Risk factors for dementia with Lewy bodies: a case-control study," *Neurology*, vol. 81, no. 9, pp. 833–840, 2013.

[23] N. S. Shah, J. S. Vidal, K. Masaki et al., "Midlife blood pressure, plasma β-amyloid, and the risk for Alzheimer disease: the Honolulu Asia Aging Study," *Hypertension*, vol. 59, no. 4, pp. 780–786, 2012.

[24] E. L. Teng, K. Hasegawa, A. Homma et al., "The Cognitive Abilities Screening Instrument (CASI): a practical test for cross-cultural epidemiological studies of dementia," *International Psychogeriatrics*, vol. 6, no. 1, pp. 45–58, 1994.

[25] J. L. Cummings, M. Mega, K. Gray, S. Rosenberg-Thompson, D. A. Carusi, and J. Gornbein, "The Neuropsychiatric Inventory: comprehensive assessment of psychopathology in dementia," *Neurology*, vol. 44, no. 12, pp. 2308–2314, 1994.

[26] T. J. Ferman, G. E. Smith, B. F. Boeve et al., "DLB fluctuations specific features that reliably differentiate DLB from AD and normal aging," *Neurology*, vol. 62, no. 2, pp. 181–187, 2004.

[27] American Academy of Sleep Medicine, *International Classification of Sleep Disorders, Revised: Diagnostic and Coding Manual*, p. 179, American Sleep Disorders Association, Rochester, MN, USA, 2001.

[28] J. C. Morris, "Clinical dementia rating: a reliable and valid diagnostic and staging measure for dementia of the Alzheimer type," *International Psychogeriatrics*, vol. 9, Supplement 1, pp. 173–176, 1999.

[29] Movement Disorder Society Task Force on Rating Scales for Parkinson's Disease, "The Unified Parkinson's Disease Rating Scale (UPDRS): status and recommendations," *Movement Disorders*, vol. 18, no. 7, pp. 738–750, 2003.

[30] S. Moritz, T. S. Woodward, J. C. Whitman, and C. Cuttler, "Confidence in errors as a possible basis for delusions in schizophrenia," *The Journal of Nervous and Mental Disease*, vol. 193, no. 1, pp. 9–16, 2005.

[31] R. Q. Freeman, T. Giovannetti, M. Lamar et al., "Visuoconstructional problems in dementia: contribution of executive systems functions," *Neuropsychology*, vol. 14, no. 3, pp. 415–426, 2000.

[32] G. D. Barba, Z. Nedjam, and B. Dubois, "Confabulation, executive functions, and source memory in Alzheimer's disease," *Cognitive Neuropsychology*, vol. 16, no. 3-5, pp. 385–398, 1999.

[33] J. Koppel, T. E. Goldberg, M. L. Gordon et al., "Relationships between behavioral syndromes and cognitive domains in Alzheimer disease: the impact of mood and psychosis," *The American Journal of Geriatric Psychiatry*, vol. 20, no. 11, pp. 994–1000, 2012.

[34] G. Gireesh, S. K. Reas, M. Jobin, and C. S. Paulose, "Decreased muscarinic M1 receptor gene expression in the cerebral cortex of streptozotocin-induced diabetic rats and *Aegle marmelose* leaf extract's therapeutic function," *Journal of Ethnopharmacology*, vol. 116, no. 2, pp. 296–304, 2008.

[35] K. Shiozaki, E. Iseki, H. Hino, and K. Kosaka, "Distribution of m1 muscarinic acetylcholine receptors in the hippocampus of patients with Alzheimer's disease and dementia with Lewy bodies-an immunohistochemical study," *Journal of the Neurological Sciences*, vol. 193, no. 1, pp. 23–28, 2001.

Morphological Biomarker Differentiating MCI Converters from Nonconverters: Longitudinal Evidence based on Hemispheric Asymmetry

Xiaojing Long, Chunxiang Jiang, and Lijuan Zhang

Paul C. Lauterbur Research Center for Biomedical Imaging, Shenzhen Institutes of Advanced Technology, Chinese Academy of Sciences, 1068 Xueyuan Avenue, Shenzhen 518055, China

Correspondence should be addressed to Lijuan Zhang; lj.zhang@siat.ac.cn

Academic Editor: Hwee L. Lee

Identifying subjects with mild cognitive impairment (MCI) who may probably progress to Alzheimer's disease (AD) is important for better understanding the disease mechanisms and facilitating early treatments. In addition to the direct volumetric and thickness measurement based on high-resolution magnetic resonance imaging (MRI), hemispheric asymmetry could be a potential index to detect morphological variations in MCI patients with a high risk of conversion to AD. The present study collected a set of longitudinal MRI data from 53 MCI converters and nonconverters and investigated the asymmetry differences between groups. Asymmetry variation was observed in the medial temporal lobe, especially in the entorhinal cortex, between converters and nonconverters 3 years before the former developed AD. The proposed asymmetry analysis was observed to be sensitive to detect morphological changes between groups as compared to the methods of voxel-based morphometry (VBM) and thickness measurement. Hemispheric asymmetry in specific brain regions as a neuroimaging biomarker can provide helpful information for prediction of MCI conversion.

1. Introduction

Alzheimer's disease (AD) is the most common form of dementia with a rapidly rising prevalence worldwide as a result of global aging. There are currently no treatments available that can provide a cure for AD. However, major scientific advances in genetical, biochemical, cell biological, and neuroscience studies over the last decades offer hope that effective therapeutic intervention is likely to be developed and to largely change the life quality of AD patients if the disease is detected prior to the onset of overt symptoms and signs [1].

Mild cognitive impairment (MCI) manifests as an intermediate stage between the expected cognitive decline in normal aging and the more serious decline in age-associated dementia [2]. It causes a slight but measurable decline in cognitive abilities; nevertheless, it does not significantly impact patients' daily functioning. People with MCI may be three to five times more likely to develop AD or other types of dementia relative to those without MCI [3]. However, not all people with MCI get worse and some even get better. Identifying the subjects with MCI who will end up with AD (referred to as "MCI converters") is of great importance in terms of better understanding the disease mechanisms and initiating early treatments for the patients.

Combined with the clinical tests of cognition or behaviors, biomarkers from structural and functional magnetic resonance imaging (MRI) have been employed for the disease characterization. Volumetric analysis for the whole brain, hippocampus, and ventricles has demonstrated different atrophy or enlargement rate in annual change between MCI converters and subjects with stable MCI with a larger tissue loss in MCI converters [4–8]. Voxel-based morphometry (VBM) and tensor-based morphometry (TBM), which allow 3D mapping of focal differences in brain anatomy, have detected significantly faster tissue reduction in the medial temporal lobe, posterior cingulate gyrus, and hippocampus [9–12]. Surface-based analysis which provides insight into the cortical morphological variations has identified shape differences between MCI converters and nonconverters in the inferior parietal cortex and both lateral and medial temporal cortices, especially in the entorhinal cortex [11, 13, 14].

Previous studies have also demonstrated asymmetrical cerebral atrophy in AD and MCI. Barnes et al. [15] and Shi et al. [16] have, respectively, reported asymmetric atrophy in the hippocampus. Derflinger et al. have found that lobar asymmetry of the temporal, parietal, and occipital lobes is different from healthy controls to AD patients [17]. In our earlier study, significant asymmetry alterations in limbic structures were identified among healthy elderly, MCI converters, and AD patients [18], suggesting that structural asymmetry difference may embed biomarkers that distinguish MCI converters from nonconverters.

In this study, a multivariate model that collectively takes into account the effects of multiple morphological variables, including the cortical thickness, surface area, and curvature index, was used to investigate the hemispheric asymmetry on a longitudinal database to distinguish MCI converters from nonconverters. Images from 5 visits (1 baseline and 4 follow-ups) were examined to determine the earliest time point at which converters can be differentiated from nonconverters. The results were compared to those of the VBM and vertex-based thickness analyses for a sensitivity evaluation among different methods in discriminating patients of a high risk.

2. Materials and Methods

2.1. Subjects and MR Scanning. Data of 26 MCI converters (15 males, aged 73.35 ± 6.71 years) and 27 nonconverters (21 males, aged 73.01 ± 7.47 years) was retrieved from the Alzheimer's Disease Neuroimaging Initiative (ADNI) database (http://adni.loni.usc.edu/), phases 1, Go, and 2. ADNI is the result of efforts of many investigators from a broad range of academic institutions and private corporations, and subjects have been recruited from over 50 sites across the US and Canada. The ADNI study was approved by the IRB of all participating sites. All subjects and, if applicable, their legal representatives gave written informed consent prior to the collection of clinical, genetic, and imaging data. The dataset follows the rigor establishment with careful quality control, detailed documentation, and full anonymization prior to data analysis. Approval for public sharing of the anonymized data was obtained.

The subjects are right handed and had taken at least five follow-up visits with MR scanning at an interval of roughly one year. The MCI nonconverters were not diagnosed with probable AD in any of the visits. The MCI converters remained in the MCI category for at least 3 consecutive visits before conversion to AD and maintained mild AD status for at least 2 consecutive visits after conversion.

High-resolution T1-weighted images (T1WI) were obtained using the MP-RAGE sequence with typical parameters of TR = 6.5~9.5 ms (GE)/2300~3000 ms (SIEMENS), TE = 3.0~4.0 ms, FA = 8°, FOV = 256 × 256, and in-plane resolution = 1 mm × 1 mm × 1.2 mm. The ADNI MRI core has established strict guidelines and procedures to ensure similar image qualities across sites and platforms over time. A customized MP-RAGE pulse sequence was developed for the GE platform to minimize vendor-to-vendor differences [19].

2.2. Hemispheric Asymmetry Analysis. Data were processed with the "recon-all" pipeline of FreeSurfer software (Version 5.0.0, http://surfer.nmr.mgh.harvard.edu/). Images were first intensity normalized, skull stripped, aligned to a standard space, and segmented into gray matter (GM), white matter (WM), and cerebrospinal fluid (CSF). The cortical surface and WM surface were constructed, inflated, topologically corrected, and projected to the standard spherical coordinate system defined by the FreeSurfer brain atlas. Then, the cerebral cortex was automatically divided into 34 gyral-based regions of interest (ROI) [20–22]. The surface area, mean curvature index, and cortical thickness were calculated on each ROI of each hemisphere. ROI-wise multivariate analysis of covariance (MANCOVA) was performed to test the compositive morphological differences between the left and right hemispheres for each group. For each ROI, the surface area, curvature index, and cortical thickness were introduced as collective response variables with gender and age as covariates. Regions with significant asymmetry were identified as $P < 0.05$. Correction was performed in multiple comparison procedures to control the false discovery rate (FDR) at 0.05. P values were mapped onto the cortical surface of the left hemisphere of FreeSurfer *fsaverage* template for visualization.

The asymmetry index (AI) of each ROI for each subject was defined as

$$\mathrm{AI}^j = \sum_i \frac{L_i^j - R_i^j}{L_i^j + R_i^j}, \tag{1}$$

and the group asymmetry index of each ROI was defined as

$$\mathrm{AI} = \mathrm{avg}_j \left(\sum_i \frac{L_i^j - R_i^j}{L_i^j + R_i^j} \right), \tag{2}$$

where L_i^j denotes the ith variable of the left hemisphere for the jth subject and R_i^j denotes the ith variable of the right hemisphere for the jth subject, $\mathrm{avg}_j(x)$ denotes an average of x across the group. $\mathrm{AI} > 0$ indicates leftward lateralization, and $\mathrm{AI} < 0$ indicates rightward lateralization. Between-group difference for a specific region was computed using the two-sample t-test on the asymmetry index AI^j with gender and age effects being regressed out. The significance level was set at 0.05.

2.3. Voxel-Based Morphometry (VBM). Cross-sectional VBM analysis was performed for each time point. SPM8 was used for voxel-based morphometry (http://www.fil.ion.ucl.ac.uk/spm/). Images from all groups were first roughly aligned via a rigid body transformation and segmented into gray matter, white matter, and CSF [23]. The template image used for spatial normalization was created by averaging across the study cohort. The segmented gray matter tissue map was

Table 1: Baseline demographic information of MCI converters and nonconverters.

Groups	Number of subjects (m/f)	Age	APOE A1	APOE A2	MMSE score
Converters	26 (15/11)	73.35 ± 6.71	3.19 ± 0.49	3.73 ± 0.45	27.19 ± 2.05
Nonconverters	27 (21/6)	73.01 ± 7.47	2.93 ± 0.47	3.41 ± 0.5	28.07 ± 1.33

aligned from the individual space to the template space, scaled by the Jacobian field, and smoothed with the full width at the half maximum (FWHM) of 10 mm, followed by a modulation step to correct for volume change [24]. A design matrix was constructed, and the general linear model (GLM) was fitted to the data with gender and age as covariates. Voxel-wise parametric statistical tests were performed to compare the GM differences between MCI converters and nonconverters. Corrections for multiple comparisons were conducted using the theory of Gaussian random fields (GRF) as the preprocessed images were spatially smoothed and voxels were correlated with their neighbors. Significant voxels with corrected $P < 0.05$ were displayed on the MNI brain template for visualization.

2.4. Vertex-Based Thickness Analysis. Cross-sectional thickness analysis was performed for each time point. FreeSurfer software (Version 5.0.0, http://surfer.nmr.mgh.harvard.edu/) was used for image processing and group analysis. Processing steps were conducted as introduced in hemispheric asymmetry analysis. Surface-based normalization was computed to map thickness data of each subject onto a common group space that allows the thickness to be compared across subjects at homologous points on the cortex. The thickness is then smoothed with FWHM = 10 mm, and the GLM was fitted to the data with gender and age as covariates (*FreeSurfer_Qdec*). Vertex-wise statistical test was performed to compare the thickness differences between converters and nonconverters for each hemisphere. Corrections for multiple comparisons were conducted to control the FDR at 0.05. The corrected significance map with $P < 0.05$ was finally overlapped onto the *fsaverage* brain template surface for visualization.

3. Results

No significant difference was found in age and MMSE scores at the baseline visit between converters and nonconverters (Table 1).

3.1. Hemispheric Asymmetry Analysis. Both MCI converters and nonconverters featured leftward lateralization in the transverse temporal gyrus, as well as rightward lateralization in the lateral orbitofrontal gyrus and inferior parietal lobule (Figure 1). Different asymmetry patterns were identified in the medial side of the brain, specifically located in the limbic system including the anterior cingulate cortex and the entorhinal cortex. Leftward lateralization was observed in the entorhinal cortex in MCI nonconverters from baseline to the last visit, as well as in the rostral anterior cingulate gyrus in converters during all visits. Rightward lateralization in the caudal anterior cingulate gyrus was detected at the baseline and the 2nd and 4th follow-up visits in MCI nonconverters.

Calculation of the group asymmetry index of each ROI at all visits showed that a certain of the 34 cortical regions that underwent asymmetry decreases with the mean asymmetry index trending towards zero over time (Figure 2). Those regions included the language-related areas such as the banks of the superior temporal sulcus, caudal middle frontal gyrus, inferior parietal lobule, and pars triangularis, as well as the memory-related areas such as the entorhinal cortex and parahippocampal gyrus (Figure 3). MCI converters exhibited a more notable decreasing trend than nonconverters, especially in areas of the banks of the superior temporal sulcus, the entorhinal cortex, and the pars triangularis. In some other regions, including the posterior cingulate, superior parietal lobule, fusiform, precentral gyrus, and precuneus, group asymmetry indices varied slightly over 5 visits and the values approximately equal zero (Figure 2). Two-sample t-test analysis demonstrated that significant between-group differences were found in the entorhinal cortex, frontal pole, and rostral anterior cingulate. No significant between-group difference was observed in other ROIs.

3.2. Voxel-Based Morphometry. The MCI converters were observed with greater tissue shrinkage from the baseline scanning to follow-ups in the bilateral hippocampus, amygdala, parahippocampal gyrus, and entorhinal cortex, compared with nonconverters (Figure 4). Significant volume reduction in converters was also observed in the precentral gyrus, superior frontal gyrus, middle temporal gyrus, and nucleus accumbens at the first two visits.

3.3. Vertex-Based Thickness Analysis. No significant thickness difference was found between the MCI converters and nonconverters in the first two visits. From 1 year before the converters progressed to AD, we observed thinner cortices mainly located in the bilateral occipital and temporal lobes, specifically in the lateral occipital gyrus, entorhinal cortex, temporal pole, and cingulate gyrus (Figure 5).

4. Discussion

In this study, cross-sectional hemispheric asymmetry analysis as well as VBM and vertex-based thickness analyses was performed for different time points to identify regions that could discriminate MCI converters from nonconverters and how early they could work for differentiation. The results demonstrated that asymmetry and VBM analyses were sensitive to morphological differences between the two cohorts, which can be used to dissociate MCI converters 3 years prior to conversion.

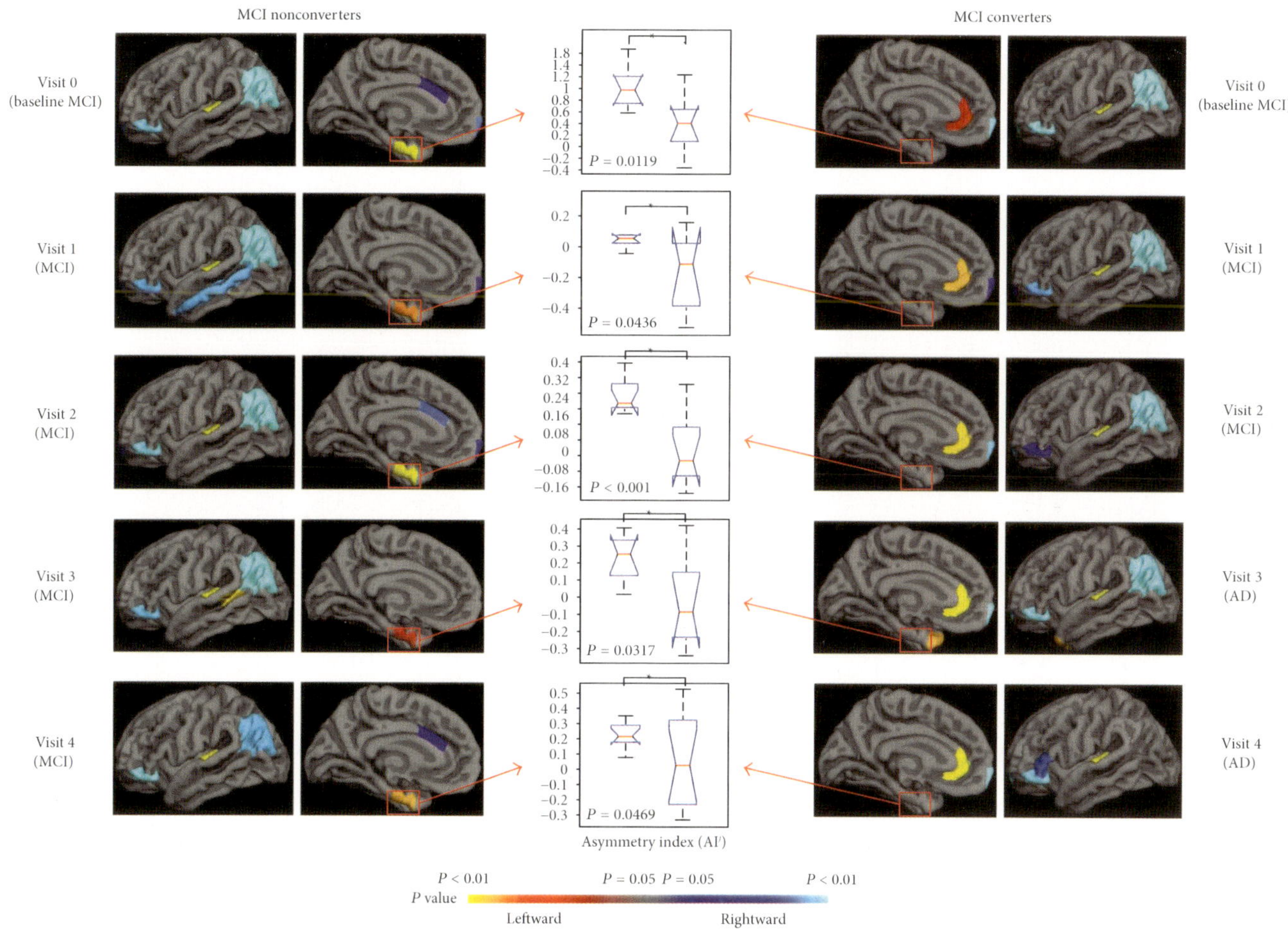

FIGURE 1: Hemispheric asymmetry analysis demonstrated different patterns in the medial side of the brain between the MCI nonconverters and converters at all time points. The MCI nonconverters showed leftward lateralization in the entorhinal cortex, while the converters showed rightward lateralization in the rostral cingulate gyrus. Significant between-group difference of the asymmetry index AI^j was observed in these two regions with t-test analysis (middle column).

VBM and vertex-based thickness analyses have been commonly used to capture the dynamics of gray matter atrophy and cortical thickness reduction in AD and MCI patients [12, 25, 26]. Chételat et al. have found significantly greater gray matter loss in MCI converters relative to nonconverters 18 months prior to their conversion in a longitudinal VBM study [12]. Risacher et al. have reported that MCI converters demonstrated higher atrophy progression with more severe reduction in gray matter density from baseline to 1 year [25]. They have also shown that annual thickness changes in MCI converters were significantly greater than those in nonconverters. In this work, we applied both VBM and thickness analyses along with the proposed asymmetry method on the same set of longitudinal data to detect the morphological differences between MCI converters and nonconverters. The VBM study identified remarkable volume reduction in MCI converters 3 years before they progressed to AD, whereas vertex-based thickness analysis only detected significant cortical thinning in converters 1 year before conversion. Hutton et al. showed that thickness analysis provided a more sensitive measure of age-associated decline in gray matter compared with VBM [27]. However, the present study demonstrated that VBM works better in differentiating slight variation between age-matched brains, which may be attributable to the difference in methodology that thickness analysis selectively investigates cortical thickness while VBM provides a mixed measure of gray matter including cortical surface area or cortical folding, as well as cortical thickness [27]. The proposed asymmetry method has also shown great power of sensitively detecting group differences. In our previous study, we have found that multivariate analysis that combined multiple morphological measures including the surface area, curvature index, and cortical thickness was more sensitive in picking up subtle alterations of hemispheric asymmetries than each individual measure [18]. None of the individual measures have acted as the pivotal contributor [28], but the compositive effect of all measures enhanced the performance. Studies have illustrated that gray matter atrophy is asymmetric in AD and MCI [17, 18]. The present work showed a consistent result but further demonstrated that the asymmetric tissue shrinkage occurred at least 3 years earlier to the conversion of AD. The asymmetry alteration could be a novel and sensitive imaging marker that can distinguish MCI

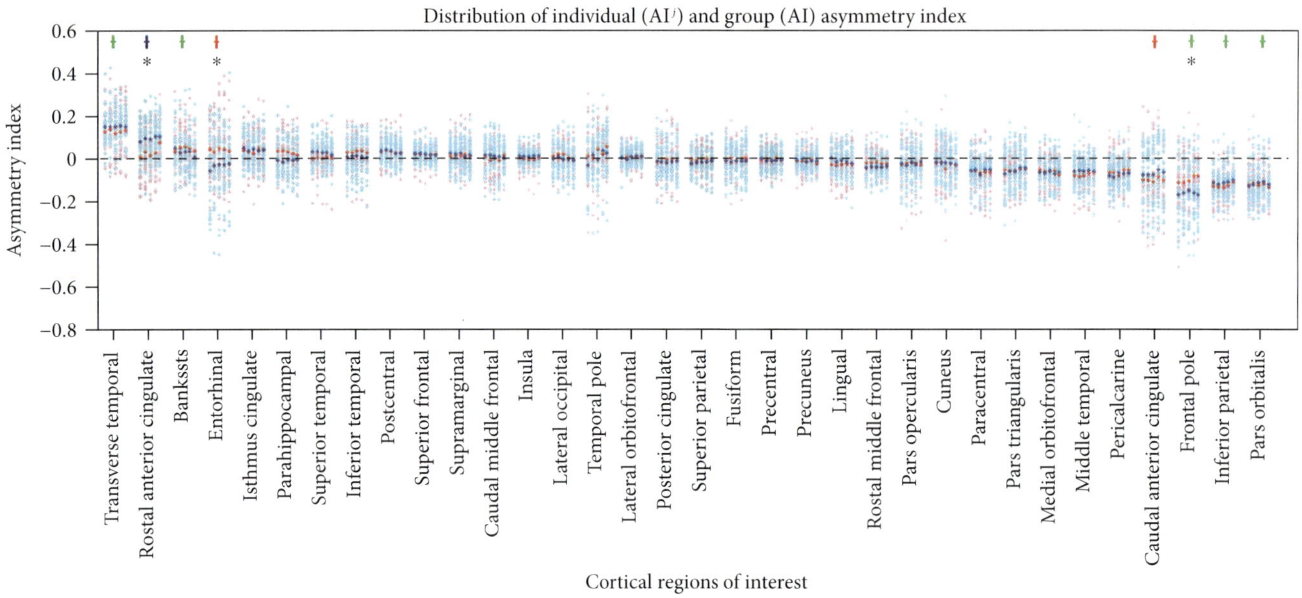

FIGURE 2: Distribution of individual and group asymmetry indices for 34 cortical regions. For each region, a column represented indices of one visit. Pink and red dots, respectively, represented individual and intragroup mean asymmetry indices of MCI nonconverters. Cyan and blue dots, respectively, represented individual and intragroup mean asymmetry indices of converters. Colored crosses denoted that significant asymmetry was observed in the corresponding region in either or both groups, where red crosses denoted significant asymmetry in nonconverters, blue denoted asymmetry in converters, and green denoted asymmetry in both groups. Black asterisks denoted that significant between-group difference was observed in the corresponding region. Bankssts: banks of the superior temporal sulcus.

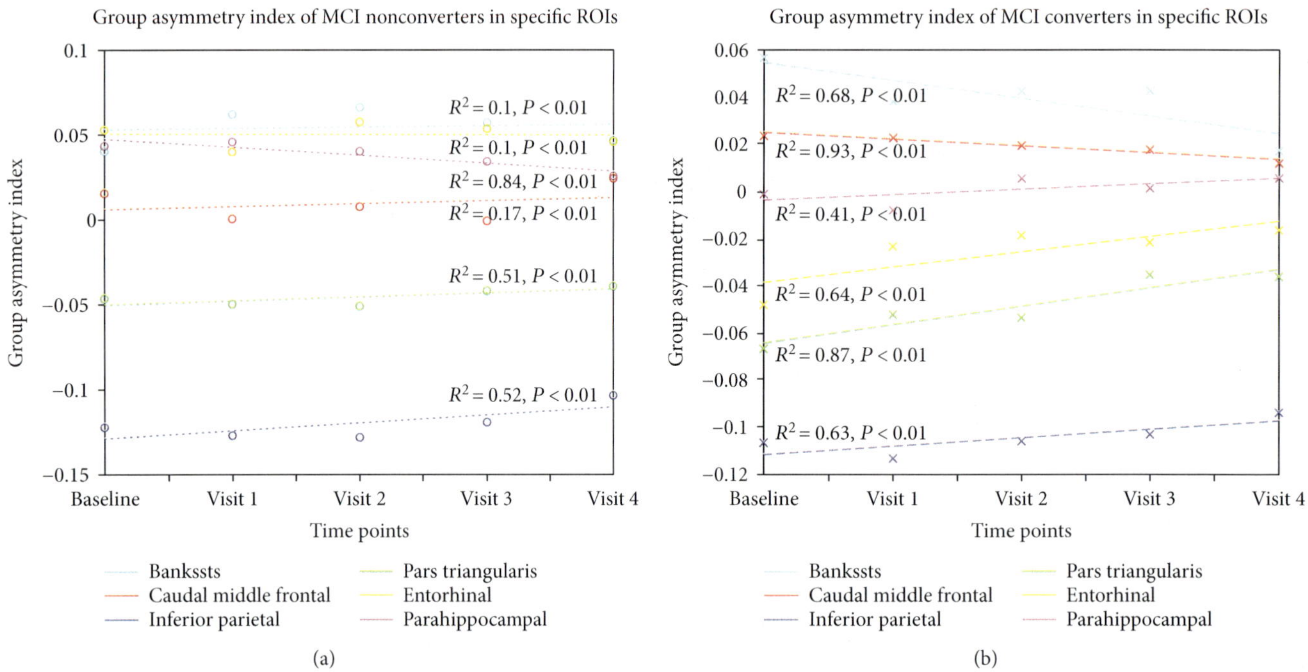

FIGURE 3: Regression of group asymmetry indices for MCI nonconverters and converters in five selected ROIs, including the banks of the superior temporal sulcus (cyan), caudal middle frontal gyrus (red), inferior parietal lobule (blue), pars triangularis (green), entorhinal cortex (yellow), and parahippocampal gyrus (pink). Group asymmetry indices decreased more notably to 0 in MCI converters from baseline to follow-up visits compared to nonconverters. Bankssts: banks of the superior temporal sulcus.

patients with a high risk of conversion to AD at an early time point.

Brain asymmetry is believed to be evolutionally adaptive, enabling more specialized and efficient functioning of the brain [29]. Gómez-Robles et al. have suggested that morphological asymmetry of the human brain enhances cognition compared to that of nonhuman primates [30]. Plessen et al. have assessed the correlation of cognitive

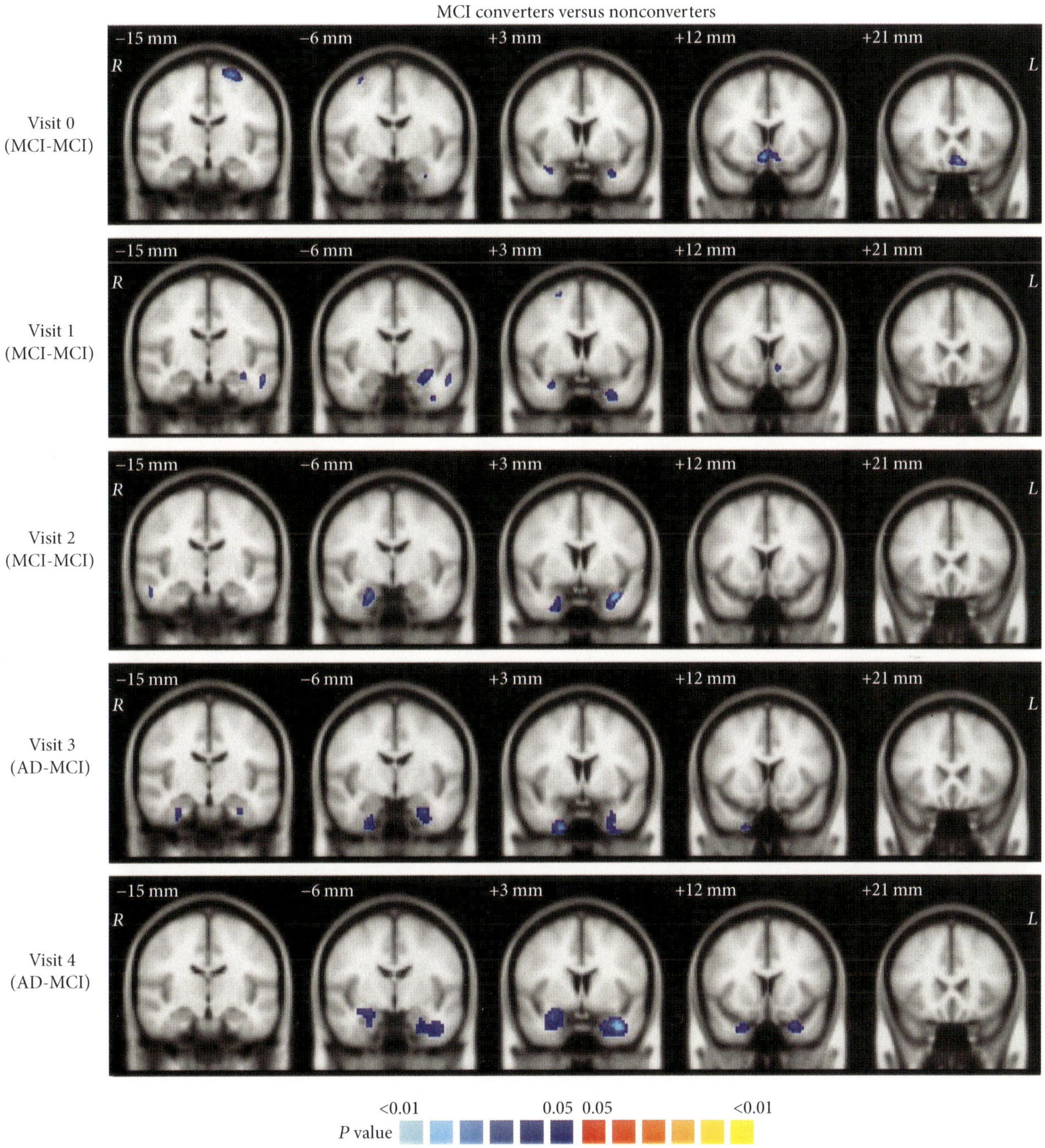

Figure 4: Voxel-based morphometry demonstrated notable and consistent volume reduction located in the hippocampus, amygdala, entorhinal cortex, and parahippocampal gyrus in the MCI converters from the baseline to the last visit.

performance with measures of cortical thickness asymmetry in children and adults and reported that asymmetry in cortical thickness is correlated with human cognitive function [31]. In this study, regression analysis of group asymmetry indices demonstrated a more pronounced decreasing trend from baseline to follow-up visits in MCI converters, compared with nonconverters, in the language-related and memory-related cortical regions, including the banks of the superior temporal sulcus, caudal middle frontal gyrus, inferior parietal lobule, pars triangularis, entorhinal cortex, and parahippocampal gyrus. The observation is consistent with the common understanding that AD is characterized by progressively worsening deficits in language [32] and memory [33]. Among the aforementioned cortical regions, the asymmetry indices of the entorhinal cortex, banks of the superior temporal sulcus, and pars triangularis demonstrated the sharpest decline in converters yet gentle variations in nonconverters, which agreed with our previous finding that hemispheric asymmetry was better preserved in these regions in healthy elderly and in the early stage of MCI converters but lost in AD patients [18]. Killiany et al. have reported that MRI measures of the entorhinal cortex and the banks of the superior temporal sulcus were most useful in predicting the follow-up status of MCI subjects [34]. These evidences

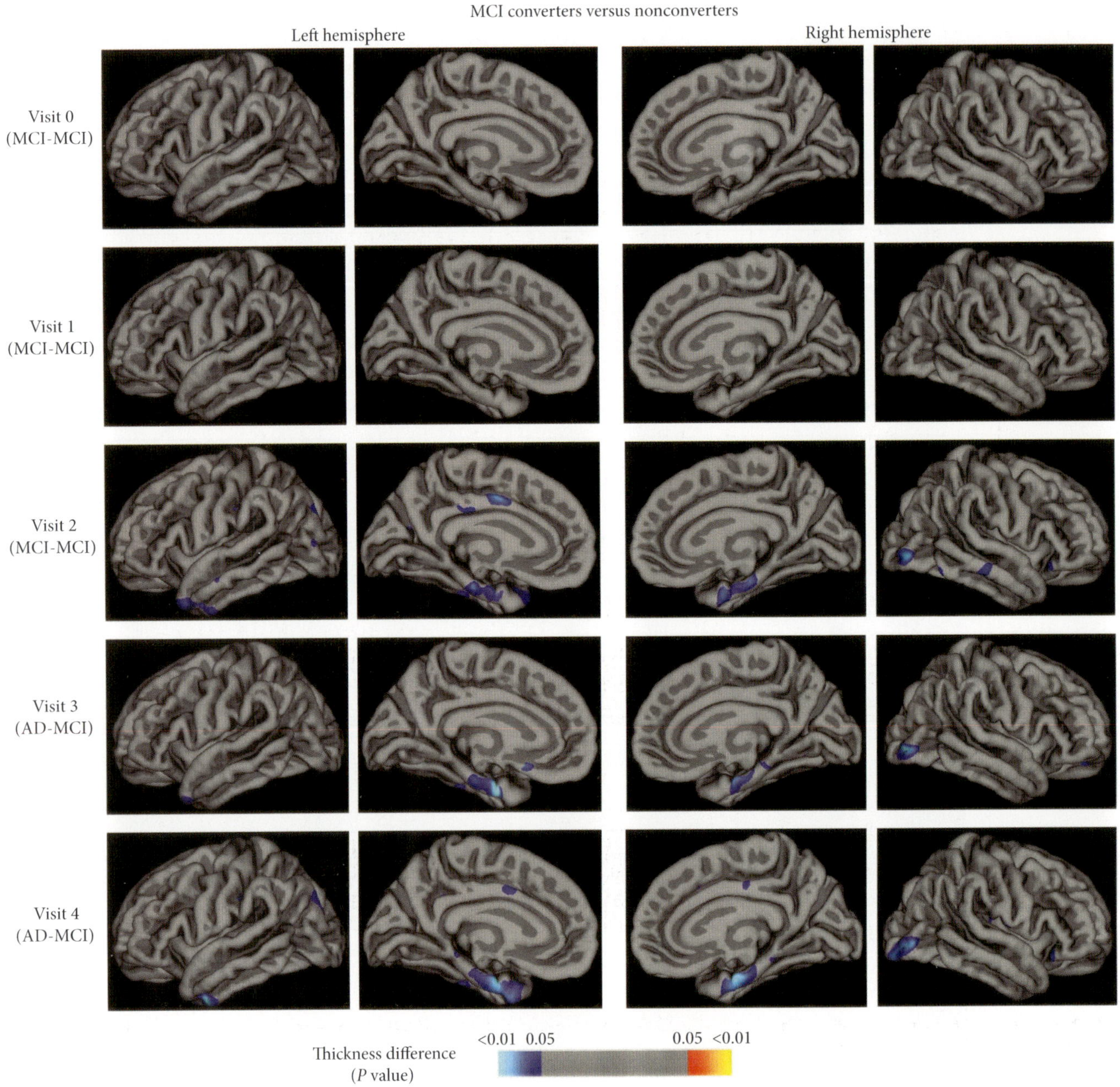

Figure 5: Vertex-based thickness analysis demonstrated bilateral thinner cortices in the lateral occipital gyrus, entorhinal cortex, temporal pole, and cingulate cortex in MCI converters from 1 year before they progressed to AD, where the entorhinal cortex presented the most severe shrinkage.

suggested that the discriminative characteristics of the featured regions may consist not only in the volume reduction of corresponding structures but also in the imbalance of tissue atrophy. Although converters and nonconverters were both diagnosed with MCI with a degree of cognitive decline at the baseline visit, the brain morphological patterns of the two groups have differed at an earlier time point.

Asymmetry indices in the posterior cingulate gyrus, superior parietal lobule, fusiform, precentral gyrus, and precuneus smoothly ranged around zero in both MCI converters and nonconverters, indicating very mild asymmetry from baseline to follow-ups. Nevertheless, the results may arise from different situations. Regions such as the fusiform, precentral gyrus, and precuneus presented no significant asymmetry in young adults and healthy elderly [18, 35], suggesting that the absence of asymmetry may intrinsically exist and may not be affected by aging or cognition decline. However, pronounced asymmetry was observed in regions such as the posterior cingulate and superior parietal lobule in young adult brain [18, 35] while it disappeared in healthy elderly and MCI subjects, which may imply that asymmetry in these regions varies over time but is not distinctive to differentiate between healthy elderly, MCI converters, and nonconverters.

Converging evidence has demonstrated that gray matter shrinkage in prodromal AD mainly occurred in the medial temporal lobe (MTL), specifically in the hippocampus, parahippocampal gyrus, and entorhinal cortex. By measuring the hippocampal and entorhinal volume, deToledo-Morrell et al. have shown that the volumes of these two regions can well differentiate MCI converters from nonconverters, especially the right hemisphere entorhinal cortex that best predicted conversion with an accuracy of 93.5% [36]. Risacher et al. have reported that the degree of degeneration of MTL tissue was the best antecedent MRI marker of conversion, where hippocampal volume decreases were the most robust [11]. Another study has found that cortical thickness was significantly reduced in MCI within the MTL network [37]. The results showed in the present study that the MTL structures, especially the entorhinal cortex, are the best predictor to identify MCI patients with a high risk for AD which was consistent with previous findings [38]. As a system specifically important for declarative memory [39], the MTL is the first brain area to succumb to neurofibrillary tau pathology in AD [40]. Significant morphological changes in MTL, which were detected in MCI converters 3 years before they progressed to AD, could be an effective biomarker for early diagnosis or prediction of AD.

In conclusion, hemispheric asymmetry analysis identified the entorhinal cortex as a significant morphological biomarker to differentiate MCI converters from nonconverters. Asymmetry variation demonstrated the ability to identify morphological changes in MCI converters 3 years prior to conversion. Focal hemispheric asymmetry decreases progressively from an early time point of prodromal AD, which provides helpful information that facilitates the prediction of MCI conversion and the patient management in the clinical practice.

Acknowledgments

Data used in this study were obtained from the Alzheimer's Disease Neuroimaging Initiative (ADNI) database (http://adni.loni.usc.edu/). The ADNI was launched in 2003 by the National Institute on Aging (NIA), the National Institute of Biomedical Imaging and Bioengineering (NIBIB), the Food and Drug Administration (FDA), private pharmaceutical companies, and nonprofit organizations, as a $60 million, 5-year public-private partnership. The primary goal of ADNI has been to test whether serial magnetic resonance imaging (MRI), positron emission tomography (PET), other biological markers, and clinical and neuropsychological assessment can be combined to measure the progression of mild cognitive impairment (MCI) and early Alzheimer's disease (AD). For up-to-date information, see http://www.adni-info.org. The study was partly supported by National Natural Science Foundation of China (Grant nos. 81301285 and 81371359), the Scientific Research Program of the Shenzhen Science and Technology Innovation Committee (JCYJ20150401163247205 and JCYJ20150521094519463), the Natural Science Foundation of Guangdong Province (2014A030312006), and the Key Laboratory for Magnetic Resonance and Multimodality Imaging of Guangdong Province (2014B030301013).

References

[1] D. M. Holtzman, J. C. Morris, and A. M. Goate, "Alzheimer's disease: the challenge of the second century," *Science Translational Medicine*, vol. 3, no. 77, article 77sr1, 2011.

[2] F. Jessen, S. Wolfsgruber, B. Wiese et al., "AD dementia risk in late MCI, in early MCI, and in subjective memory impairment," *Alzheimer's & Dementia*, vol. 10, no. 1, pp. 76–83, 2014.

[3] A. M. Weinstein, C. Barton, L. Ross, J. H. Kramer, and K. Yaffe, "Treatment practices of mild cognitive impairment in California Alzheimer's Disease Centers," *Journal of the American Geriatrics Society*, vol. 57, no. 4, pp. 686–690, 2009.

[4] M. C. Evans, J. Barnes, C. Nielsen et al., "Volume changes in Alzheimer's disease and mild cognitive impairment: cognitive associations," *European Radiology*, vol. 20, no. 3, pp. 674–682, 2010.

[5] L. K. McEvoy, C. Fennema-Notestine, J. C. Roddey et al., "Alzheimer disease: quantitative structural neuroimaging for detection and prediction of clinical and structural changes in mild cognitive impairment," *Radiology*, vol. 251, no. 1, pp. 195–205, 2009.

[6] C. Misra, Y. Fan, and C. Davatzikos, "Baseline and longitudinal patterns of brain atrophy in MCI patients, and their use in prediction of short-term conversion to AD: results from ADNI," *NeuroImage*, vol. 44, no. 4, pp. 1415–1422, 2009.

[7] S. M. Nestor, R. Rupsingh, M. Borrie et al., "Ventricular enlargement as a possible measure of Alzheimer's disease progression validated using the Alzheimer's Disease Neuroimaging Initiative database," *Brain*, vol. 131, no. 9, pp. 2443–2454, 2008.

[8] P. N. Wang, H. C. Liu, J. F. Lirng, K. N. Lin, and Z. A. Wu, "Accelerated hippocampal atrophy rates in stable and progressive amnestic mild cognitive impairment," *Psychiatry Research Neuroimaging*, vol. 171, no. 3, pp. 221–231, 2009.

[9] A. D. Leow, I. Yanovsky, N. Parikshak et al., "Alzheimer's Disease Neuroimaging Initiative: a one-year follow up study using tensor-based morphometry correlating degenerative rates, biomarkers and cognition," *NeuroImage*, vol. 45, no. 3, pp. 645–655, 2009.

[10] M. A. Trivedi, A. K. Wichmann, B. M. Torgerson et al., "Structural MRI discriminates individuals with mild cognitive impairment from age-matched controls: a combined neuropsychological and voxel based morphometry study," *Alzheimer's & Dementia*, vol. 2, no. 4, pp. 296–302, 2006.

[11] S. L. Risacher, A. J. Saykin, J. D. West et al., "Baseline MRI predictors of conversion from MCI to probable AD in the ADNI cohort," *Current Alzheimer Research*, vol. 6, no. 4, pp. 347–361, 2009.

[12] G. Chételat, B. Landeau, F. Eustache et al., "Using voxel-based morphometry to map the structural changes associated with rapid conversion in MCI: a longitudinal MRI study," *NeuroImage*, vol. 27, no. 4, pp. 934–946, 2005.

[13] Y. Cui, B. Liu, S. Luo et al., "Identification of conversion from mild cognitive impairment to Alzheimer's disease using multivariate predictors," *PLoS One*, vol. 6, no. 7, article e21896, 2011.

[14] E. Lebed, A. Trouvé, and M. F. Beg, "Cortical thickness analysis in Alzheimer's onset," *Alzheimer's & Dementia*, vol. 8, no. 4, pp. P157–P158, 2012.

[15] J. Barnes, R. I. Scahill, J. M. Schott, C. Frost, M. N. Rossor, and N. C. Fox, "Does Alzheimer's disease affect hippocampal asymmetry? Evidence from a cross-sectional and longitudinal volumetric MRI study," *Dementia and Geriatric Cognitive Disorders*, vol. 19, no. 5-6, pp. 338–344, 2005.

[16] F. Shi, B. Liu, Y. Zhou, C. Yu, and T. Jiang, "Hippocampal volume and asymmetry in mild cognitive impairment and Alzheimer's disease: meta-analyses of MRI studies," *Hippocampus*, vol. 19, no. 11, pp. 1055–1064, 2009.

[17] S. Derflinger, C. Sorg, C. Gaser et al., "Grey-matter atrophy in Alzheimer's disease is asymmetric but not lateralized," *Journal of Alzheimer's Disease*, vol. 25, no. 2, pp. 347–357, 2011.

[18] X. Long, L. Zhang, W. Liao, C. Jiang, B. Qiu, and The Alzheimer's Disease Neuroimaging Initiative, "Distinct laterality alterations distinguish mild cognitive impairment and Alzheimer's disease from healthy aging: statistical parametric mapping with high resolution MRI," *Human Brain Mapping*, vol. 34, no. 12, pp. 3400–3410, 2013.

[19] C. R. Jack Jr., M. A. Bernstein, N. C. Fox et al., "The Alzheimer's Disease Neuroimaging Initiative (ADNI): MRI methods," *Journal of Magnetic Resonance Imaging*, vol. 27, no. 4, pp. 685–691, 2008.

[20] A. Dale, B. Fischl, and M. Sereno, "Cortical surface-based analysis: I. Segmentation and surface reconstruction," *NeuroImage*, vol. 9, no. 2, pp. 179–194, 1999.

[21] A. Dale and M. Sereno, "Improved localizadon of cortical activity by combining EEG and MEG with MRI cortical surface reconstruction: a linear approach," *Journal of Cognitive Neuroscience*, vol. 5, no. 2, pp. 162–176, 1993.

[22] B. Fischl, M. Sereno, and A. Dale, "Cortical surface-based analysis: II: inflation, flatting, and a surface-based coordinate system," *NeuroImage*, vol. 9, no. 2, pp. 195–207, 1999.

[23] J. Ashburner and K. J. Friston, "Voxel-based morphometry—the methods," *NeuroImage*, vol. 11, no. 6, pp. 805–821, 2000.

[24] C. D. Good, I. S. Johnsrude, J. Ashburner, R. N. A. Henson, K. J. Friston, and R. S. J. Frackowiak, "A voxel-based morphometric study of ageing in 465 normal adult human brains," *NeuroImage*, vol. 14, no. 1, pp. 21–36, 2001.

[25] S. L. Risacher, L. Shen, J. D. West et al., "Longitudinal MRI atrophy biomarkers: relationship to conversion in the ADNI cohort," *Neurobiology of Aging*, vol. 31, no. 8, pp. 1401–1418, 2010.

[26] M. Bozzali, M. Filippi, G. Magnani et al., "The contribution of voxel-based morphometry in staging patients with mild cognitive impairment," *Neurology*, vol. 67, no. 3, pp. 453–460, 2006.

[27] C. Hutton, B. Draganski, J. Ashburner, and N. Weiskopf, "A comparison between voxel-based cortical thickness and voxel-based morphometry in normal aging," *NeuroImage*, vol. 48, no. 2, pp. 371–380, 2009.

[28] W. Liao, X. Long, C. Jiang et al., "Discerning mild cognitive impairment and Alzheimer disease from normal aging. Morphologic characterization based on univariate and multivariate models," *Academic Radiology*, vol. 21, no. 5, pp. 597–604, 2014.

[29] A. W. Toga and P. M. Thompson, "Mapping brain asymmetry," *Nature Reviews Neuroscience*, vol. 4, no. 1, pp. 37–48, 2003.

[30] A. Gómez-Robles, W. D. Hopkins, and C. C. Sherwood, "Increased morphological asymmetry, evolvability and plasticity in human brain evolution," *Proceedings of the Royal Society B: Biological Science*, vol. 280, no. 1761, article 20130575, 2013.

[31] K. J. Plessen, K. Hugdahl, R. Bansal, X. Hao, and B. S. Peterson, "Sex, age, and cognitive correlates of asymmetries in thickness of the cortical mantle across the life span," *The Journal of Neuroscience*, vol. 34, no. 18, pp. 6294–6302, 2014.

[32] S. H. Ferris and M. Farlow, "Language impairment in Alzheimer's disease and benefits of acetylcholinesterase inhibitors," *Clinical Interventions in Aging*, vol. 8, pp. 1007–1014, 2013.

[33] C. A. Gold and A. E. Budson, "Memory loss in Alzheimer's disease: implications for development of therapeutics," *Expert Review of Neurotherapeutics*, vol. 8, no. 12, pp. 1879–1891, 2008.

[34] R. J. Killiany, T. Gomez-Isla, M. Moss et al., "Use of structural magnetic resonance imaging to predict who will get Alzheimer's disease," *Annals of Neurology*, vol. 47, no. 4, pp. 430–439, 2000.

[35] E. Goldberg, D. Roediger, N. E. Kucukboyaci et al., "Hemispheric asymmetries of cortical volume in the human brain," *Cortex*, vol. 49, no. 1, pp. 200–210, 2013.

[36] L. deToledo-Morrell, T. R. Stoub, M. Bulgakova et al., "MRI-derived entorhinal volume is a good predictor of conversion from MCI to AD," *Neurobiology of Aging*, vol. 25, no. 9, pp. 1197–1203, 2004.

[37] S. Das, J. Pluta, L. Mancuso, D. Kliot, P. Yushkevich, and D. A. Wolk, "Involvement of anterior and posterior medial temporal lobe networks in early Alzheimer's disease," *Alzheimer's & Dementia*, vol. 10, no. 4, article P822, 2014.

[38] P. J. Visser, F. R. Verhey, P. A. Hofman, P. Scheltens, and J. Jolles, "Medial temporal lobe atrophy predicts Alzheimer's disease in patients with minor cognitive impairment," *Journal of Neurology, Neurosurgery, & Psychiatry*, vol. 72, no. 4, pp. 491–497, 2002.

[39] L. R. Squire, C. E. Stark, and R. E. Clark, "The medial temporal lobe," *Annual Review of Neuroscience*, vol. 27, no. 1, pp. 279–306, 2004.

[40] G. A. Kerchner, J. D. Bernstein, M. C. Fenesy et al., "Shared vulnerability of two synaptically-connected medial temporal lobe areas to age and cognitive decline: a seven tesla magnetic resonance imaging study," *The Journal of Neuroscience*, vol. 33, no. 42, pp. 16666–16672, 2013.

4

Evaluating the Utility of a Structured Clinical Protocol for Reducing the Impact of Behavioural and Psychological Symptoms of Dementia in Progressive Neurological Diseases

Nicholas P. Ryan,[1,2] Laura Scott,[1] Maryanne McPhee,[1] Susan Mathers,[1] Marie-Claire Davis,[1] Roxanne Maule,[1] and Fiona Fisher[1]

[1] *Calvary Health Care Bethlehem, South Caulfield, VIC, Australia*
[2] *Melbourne School of Psychological Sciences, The University of Melbourne, Parkville, VIC, Australia*

Correspondence should be addressed to Nicholas P. Ryan; nicholas.ryan@calvarycare.org.au and Fiona Fisher; Fiona.Fisher@calvarycare.org.au

Academic Editor: Leungwing Chu

Objectives. Behavioural and psychological symptoms of dementia (BPSD) cause significant distress to both aged care residents and staff. Despite the high prevalence of BPSD in progressive neurological diseases (PNDs) such as multiple sclerosis, Huntington's disease, and Parkinson's disease, the utility of a structured clinical protocol for reducing BPSD has not been systematically evaluated in PND populations. *Method.* Staff ($n = 51$) and individuals with a diagnosis of PND ($n = 13$) were recruited into the study, which aimed to evaluate the efficacy of a PND-specific structured clinical protocol for reducing the impact of BPSD in residential aged care (RAC) and specialist disability accommodation (SDA) facilities. Staff were trained in the clinical protocol through face-to-face workshops, which were followed by 9 weeks of intensive clinical supervision to a subset of staff ("behaviour champions"). Staff and resident outcome measures were administered preintervention and immediately following the intervention. The primary outcome was frequency and severity of BPSD, measured using the Neuropsychiatric Inventory-Nursing Home Version (NPI-NH). The secondary outcome was staff coping assessed using the Strain in Dementia Care Scale (SDCS). *Results.* In SDA, significant reductions in staff ratings of job-related stress were observed alongside a statistically significant decrease in BPSD from T1 to T2. In RAC, there was no significant time effect for BPSD or staff coping; however, a medium effect size was observed for staff job stress. *Conclusions.* Staff training and clinical support in the use of a structured clinical protocol for managing BPSD were linked to reductions in staff job stress, which may in turn increase staff capacity to identify indicators of resident distress and respond accordingly. Site variation in outcomes may relate to organisational and workforce-level barriers that may be unique to the RAC context and should be systematically addressed in future RCT studies of larger PND samples.

1. Introduction

Behavioural and psychological symptoms of dementia (BPSD) represent a significant challenge in the clinical care and management of individuals living with progressive neurological diseases (PNDs). About 300 per 100,000 people are affected by the two most common conditions in this group: multiple sclerosis (MS) and idiopathic Parkinson's disease (PD). A further significant proportion of people are affected by Huntington's disease (6–14 per 100,000) and motor neurone disease (4–8 per 100,000) [1]. These conditions generally affect individuals from early to late midlife and are associated with complex patterns of physical, cognitive, and behavioural impairment [2].

Though the nature and correlates of BPSD in PNDs are not well characterised, challenging behaviours such as aggression, irritability, shouting, repetitive questions, and sexual disinhibition are common and may underlie high rates of carer distress and burnout in these populations [3]. Not surprisingly, BPSD represent one of several factors that prompt a decision to move individuals with PNDs into residential facilities, where prevalence of BPSD is also high [4, 5].

In the Australian context, BPSD are linked to stress and burnout among nursing care staff [6], many of whom are poorly paid and lack specialist skills required to effectively manage these behaviours [7]. Specifically, research shows that inadequate staff training is associated with staff stress and burnout, which in turn increases risk for resident BPSD [8, 9].

Additionally, BPSD are costly and resource intensive. For instance, these symptoms typically prompt referrals to external support agencies and represent a leading cause of emergency calls to mental health services [10]. Owing to the substantial psychosocial and financial impact of BPSD, evidence-based protocols to reduce the impact of BPSD are required, particularly among PND populations where the evidence base for nonpharmacological interventions is scarce [11, 12].

BPSD in individuals with PNDs represent a complex multidimensional construct, likely reflecting an interplay of aetiological factors that precipitate and maintain symptoms. The complexity of BPSD is reflected in recent international guidelines (e.g., International Psychogeriatric Association Complete Guide to BPSD [13]), which delineate multiple aetiologies for BPSD, including genetic, psychosocial, neurobiological, medical, and physical factors which interact dynamically to give rise to challenging behaviours. This dynamic interplay of variables is particularly salient for individuals living with progressive neurological diseases, for whom the onset of symptoms occurs relatively early in life.

Although BPSDs may present in a superficially similar way across patients, the complex mix of causal factors underlying BPSDs in PND populations means that there is substantial variability in the specific factors that trigger and perpetuate BPSDs within the individual patient [14]. In keeping with this model, it follows that addressing case-specific causal factors (i.e., using a personalized individual approach) would be a critical component of an evidence-based treatment model for BPSD. That is, while genetic and neurobiological variables may not be currently treatable, psychosocial and acute/subacute physical and medical factors are potentially malleable to nonpharmacological interventions. For instance, factors such as pain or depression [15], loneliness [16], cognitive impairment [17], sensory impairment [18], overstimulation [19], and even the way personal care is carried out [20] are all potential contributing factors to BPSD in PNDs. All these variables represent modifiable targets for individualized, person-centred interventions that aim at addressing treatable causes of resident suffering. In keeping with this biopsychosocial perspective, Brechin et al. [21] argue for a stepped-care model of assessment and intervention, which centres on a case-specific approach to determine the factors related to BPSD, and implement appropriate interventions, primarily from a psychosocial perspective.

In the Australian context, person-centred, nonpharmacological treatments for BPSD have received preliminary support from a recent randomized controlled trial (RCT), which examined the efficacy of a structured clinical protocol for managing challenging behaviours in patients with older-onset dementia [22]. This study found that compared to an active control condition involving staff training *alone*, staff training and concurrent clinical support were associated with sustained improvements in both staff coping and resident behaviour. These promising results suggest that compared to standalone staff training programs which are typically associated with mixed results [14], there appear to be measurable added benefits of providing concurrent clinical support in using a structured clinical protocol. Despite these promising findings, research is yet to evaluate the utility of this biopsychosocial model for treating BPSD in individuals with PNDs in whom BSPDs are often underrecognised and untreated over a typically protracted disease course.

In addressing this substantial gap in knowledge, we developed a PND-specific structured clinical protocol that emphasised a person-centred, biopsychosocial approach targeting case-specific causal factors in BPSD in PNDs. In keeping with recent evidence that the benefits of staff training in BPSD clinical protocols are not maintained in the absence of clinical support [22], the three-tier training program involved (i) intensive staff training workshops delivered to all consenting facility staff; (ii) 9 weeks of intensive clinical support for a subgroup of facility staff ("behaviour champions"); and (iii) development and implementation of tailored procedures and resources intended to incorporate these principles into the organisational policy framework. "Behaviour champions" received intensive clinical supervision to implement the structured clinical protocol for residents living with PNDs. This intensive staff training program was grounded in the model for treatment of BPSD outlined by Brechin et al. [21], designed to empower staff with the skills and knowledge to more effectively manage the impact of BSPDs, and thus reduce reliance on external mental health services. A summary of the clinical protocol is provided in Figure 1, and further details are available from the corresponding author on request.

Due to the progressive and severely debilitating nature of PNDs, individuals with these conditions often require access to residential accommodation facilities that can provide high levels of specialist care and support. However, in the Australian context, facilities can differ markedly in terms of organisational culture and model of care, level of staff training and skills, and staff to resident ratios. Some individuals with PNDs may have access to specialist disability accommodation facilities tailored to high care needs of individuals under the age of 65. These specialist facilities typically benefit from smaller numbers of beds, higher staff to resident ratios, and an organisational ethos that promotes community participation and "living well." Given the limited availability of specialist disability accommodation facilities, many people with PNDs reside in large residential aged care facilities (RAC), which predominantly cater for older adults (over

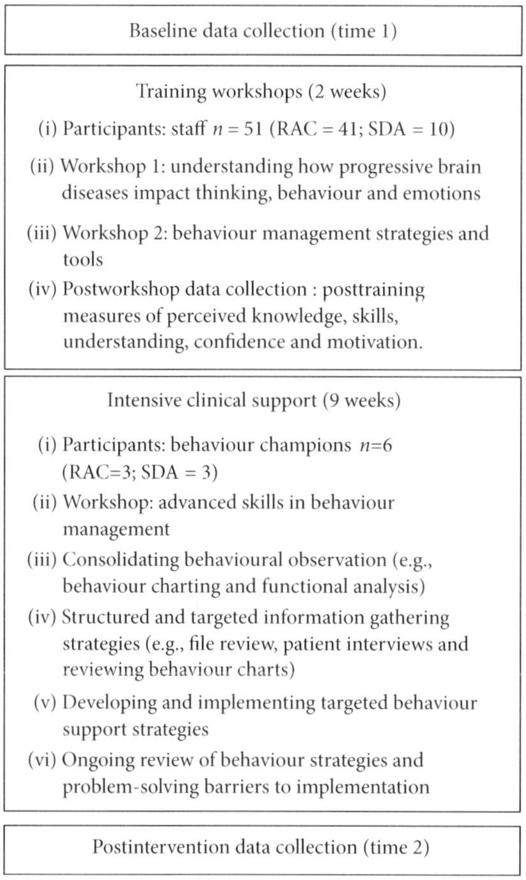

Figure 1: Timeline and protocol.

the age of 65) with high dependency needs. These facilities generally have fewer residents with young-onset PNDs, and individuals with PNDs typically enter these facilities during the later stages of illness when their need for physical, social, and emotional support is greatest [23].

Since different residential accommodation settings present distinct challenges and opportunities, this study aimed to evaluate the utility of the structured clinical protocol in both RAC and SDA. Since intensive training and clinical support would offer the substantial input required to change the clinical culture of the RAC, we hypothesised that the intervention would be associated with significant reductions in resident BPSD and improvements in staff coping, in both the RAC and SDA. The primary outcome measure was changes in resident BPSD, and the secondary outcome measure was changes in staff coping.

2. Method

2.1. Participants

2.1.1. Residents. Residents were recruited from a residential aged care (RAC) facility and a specialist disability accommodation (SDA) facility located in metropolitan Melbourne, Australia. The RAC comprised 45 beds (including 15 PND-specific beds) and 62 direct care staff. The SDA comprised a 6-bed, PND-specific facility employing 10 direct care staff.

At both facilities, all residents with a diagnosis of PND were approached to participate in the study. Residents provided informed consent after receiving information packs detailing the study. Accounting for resident deaths or removal from facilities during the study, the final sample comprised 13 individuals, 7 residing in the RAC (M age = 58.29 years, SD = 13.74) and 6 in the SDA (M age = 49.83 years, SD = 5.49).

2.1.2. Staff. Staff at each facility were recruited through project scoping sessions conducted by a registered clinical neuropsychologist. At project scoping sessions, staff were provided a verbal summary of the project goals and processes, as well as a comprehensive participant information and consent form. At these meetings, informed written consent was obtained from 51 staff members (RAC: $n = 41$; SDA: $n = 10$).

2.2. Materials

2.2.1. Resident Demographic Data. Demographic data, including age, gender, time residing at the facility, PND diagnosis, and other relevant diagnoses, were obtained from the residents' medical files at preintervention baseline.

2.2.2. Resident BPSD. The *Neuropsychiatric Inventory-Nursing Home Version (NPI-NH)* was used to assess the frequency of BPSD as rated by the behaviour champions. The NPI-NH is a modified version of the original Neuropsychiatric Inventory [24] designed to measure BPSD symptoms in geriatric patients. A structured interview format is used in both instruments to assess 12 areas of BPSD symptomatology commonly found in dementing illnesses (i.e., delusions, hallucinations, agitation/aggression, depression, anxiety, euphoria/elation, apathy/indifference, disinhibition, irritability/lability, aberrant motor behaviour, night-time behaviour, and appetite/eating changes).

Staff provide ratings of symptom frequency and severity, and rate the degree of organisational disruption (i.e., extra staff stress and workload) caused by the presenting symptoms. Frequency scores range from 0 to 4, and severity scores range from 0 to 3. A symptom subscale score is calculated from the product of the severity and the frequency scores for each domain, with scores ranging from 0 to 12. The sum of the subscale scores is calculated to form the total score, ranging from 0 to 144. High scores on each scale represent a higher level of behavioural symptoms. A major study on the validity of the NPI-NH has been published [25]. These researchers demonstrated that licensed vocational nurses provided more accurate ratings than certified nurses' aides, supporting the use of the patients' primary nurse (i.e., behaviour champion) in the present study.

2.2.3. Staff Demographic and Outcome Measures. Demographic data, including age, gender, and years worked at the facility, were obtained at baseline from each participating staff member. Self-reported confidence, knowledge, motivation, absenteeism, and use of employee support programs were measured using an in-house questionnaire.

Job strain, not related to specific residents, was measured using the 27-item *Strain in Dementia Care Scale (SDCS)* [7]. This measure was developed specifically for use in dementia care settings. The SDCS contains items relating to frustrated empathy, difficulty in understanding residents, balancing competing needs, balancing emotional involvement with residents, and perceived lack of appreciation from others. Staff rated how frequently a situation or feeling related to care of residents was experienced, from 1 (never/rarely) to 4 (very often), and how much stress the situation or feeling caused when it did occur, from 1 (none/hardly any) to 4 (high stress). A total score was calculated for frequency of strains and stress associated with items above. Internal reliability was high in this study, at $a = 0.88$ for the total frequency score and $a = 0.93$ for the total stress score.

All staff outcome measures were completed at preintervention baseline (T1) and immediately following the 11-week intervention program (T2).

2.3. Procedure. Ethics approval for the study was obtained from Calvary Health Care Bethlehem (CHCB) Human Research Ethics Committee and Melbourne Health Human Research Ethics Committee.

We conducted a pilot study to evaluate the utility of a structured clinical protocol for reducing the impact of BPSDs in residents living with PND. Data was collected at preintervention baseline, pre- and postworkshop training, and immediately following the roll-out of the entire 11-week intervention package which involved facility-wide staff workshop training (2 weeks) and an advanced training program involving a workshop and clinical supervision/support to a smaller subset of "behaviour champions" (9 weeks). The intervention protocol is described in the sections that follow and summarised in Figure 1.

2.3.1. Recruitment. Residents were recruited through consultation with senior staff at both facilities. The inclusion criteria required a positive diagnosis of progressive neurological.

2.3.2. Staff Training Workshops. All enrolled staff ($n = 51$) attended two ninety-minute training workshop sessions, which covered core components of the structured clinical protocol. Pre- and posttraining self-report questionnaires were administered to all staff that attended training sessions. Using a four-point Likert scale (1 = none to 4 = excellent), staff rated their perceived knowledge, understanding, skills, confidence, and motivation to engage in person centred, context-sensitive behaviour management approaches.

2.3.3. Intensive Clinical Support. A clinical neuropsychologist experienced in working with BPSD provided an additional 9-week advanced training package for behaviour champions enrolled at each site. The program involved a 90-minute advanced training workshop (week 1), followed by clinical support provided over eight weeks, with supervision provided weekly for the first month and fortnightly for the second month. Clinical supervision sessions focused on assisting staff in implementing the structured clinical protocol to manage resident BPSD (see Figure 1).

2.4. Data Analysis. All data were analysed using IBM SPSS 22.0 and screened for violations of normality.

Normality plots indicated that primary and secondary outcome measures (NPI-NH and SDCS, resp.) were normally distributed, and preliminary analysis indicated no violation of assumptions across analyses unless otherwise stated.

Site comparisons (RAC versus SDA) were conducted using independent samples t-tests for the following descriptive variables: resident age, baseline BPSD, staff age, and prior training. Chi-square analysis was conducted to determine whether there was sex differences in residents and staff between sites. Percentages and frequencies are reported for the following characteristics: prior training (yes/no). For primary and secondary outcome analyses, repeated measures t-tests were conducted for each outcome measure (baseline T1 scores–postintervention T2 scores) at both sites.

3. Results

3.1. Resident Characteristics. Descriptive statistics for the resident sample are provided in Table 1. Univariate analyses revealed that the RAC and SDA did not significantly differ on baseline total NPI-NH scores ($t(1, 11) = 1.07$, $p = 0.307$), such that residents at each facility had comparable levels of BPSD at baseline. No significant differences were identified for age or gender.

3.2. Staff Characteristics

3.2.1. Demographics by Site. Descriptive statistics for the staff sample are provided in Table 2. Groups differed in number of years worked in the facility, such that RAC staff reported longer tenure at the facility than those at the SDA. However, this difference did not reach statistical significance ($p = 0.078$).

3.2.2. Staff Perceptions of Self and Organisational Efficacy by Site. Table 2 presents baseline measures of staff self- and organisational efficacy, as assessed by staff ratings of their own knowledge, skills, confidence, and motivation to manage BPSD, in addition to perceptions of organisational efficacy in addressing BPSD. Staff at the RAC endorsed lower levels of motivation to manage BPSD ($M = 3.46$; $SD = 1.31$) than SDA staff ($M = 4.20$; $SD = 0.79$); however, the difference did not reach statistical significance ($p = 0.095$). Both groups were comparable on other measures of self-efficacy including baseline perceptions of knowledge/skills, understanding of policies/procedure, confidence, and support.

Analysis of staff perceptions of organisational efficacy revealed significant group differences, such that RAC staff endorsed lower levels of support from family carers of residents ($p = 0.023$). RAC staff also endorsed lower levels of organisational success in reducing distress in residents with BPSD; however, this difference did not reach statistical significance ($p = 0.054$).

3.3. Workshop Training Outcomes by Site

3.3.1. Workshop 1: Understanding How Progressive Brain Diseases Impact Thinking, Behaviour, and Emotions. For RAC, paired t-tests revealed significant posttraining increases

TABLE 1: Demographic and behavioural data for PND resident sample.

	Intervention setting		
	RAC	SDA	p value
Number of residents enrolled	7	6	—
Age (SD)	58.29 (13.74)	49.83 (5.49)	0.187
Females, n (%)	5 (71)	6 (100)	0.462
PND diagnosis, n (%)			
Multiple sclerosis	5 (72)	6 (100)	—
Huntington's disease	1 (14)	—	—
Parkinson's disease	1 (14)	—	—
Baseline total NPI	19.57 (9.18)	25.67 (11.34)	0.307
Baseline NPI disruption	7.86 (4.26)	8.67 (5.09)	0.760

on measures of staff perceived knowledge ($p < 0.001$), skills ($p = 0.038$), understanding ($p = 0.001$), confidence ($p = 0.008$), and motivation ($p = 0.040$) to identify and manage cognitive, behavioural, and emotional symptoms in people with progressive neurological diseases. Similarly, staff at the SDA reported significant posttraining increases in knowledge ($p = 0.015$), skills ($p = 0.040$), and motivation ($p = 0.041$) in this area of competence. There were no significant changes observed in staff ratings of confidence at the SDA.

3.3.2. Workshop 2: Behaviour Management Strategies and Tools. For RAC, paired t-tests revealed significant posttraining increases on measures of staff perceived knowledge ($p = 0.002$), skills ($p = 0.002$), understanding ($p < 0.001$), and motivation ($p = 0.001$) in completing behaviour charts and implementing behaviour support plans. Similarly, staff at the SDA reported significant posttraining increases in knowledge ($p = 0.035$); however, increases in perceived skills did not reach statistical significance ($p = 0.074$).

3.4. Outcomes by Site: BPSD Ratings

3.4.1. RAC. As shown in Table 3, for NPI-NH ratings, there was no significant time effect for BSPSDs from T1 to T2 ($t(1,6) = 1.18$, $p = 0.283$, $d = 0.33$). Similarly, there was no significant reduction in perceived level of organisational disruption associated with the behaviours ($t(1,6) = 0.536$, $p = 0.611$, $d = 0.13$).

3.4.2. SDA. Analyses of NPI-NH ratings revealed a significant reduction in BPSD from T1 to T2 ($t(1,5) = 2.58$, $p = 0.049$, $d = 0.84$). Reductions were also observed in perceived levels of organisational disruption associated with the behaviours; however, this change did not reach statistical significance ($t(1,5) = 1.97$, $p = 0.108$, $d = 1.13$).

3.5. Outcomes by Site: Staff Coping

3.5.1. RAC. Longitudinal analyses of the Strain in Dementia Care Scale (SDCS) ratings included follow-up data collected from 25 of the 41 staff (61%) initially enrolled at T1. Analyses of demographic and psychological characteristics of participating versus nonparticipating staff at T2 revealed no significant group differences in age, gender, or ratings of motivation, skills, or knowledge as assessed at T1.

As shown in Table 4, no significant time effect was found on the total frequency (of perceived job strains) scale ($t(1,24) = 1.56, p = 0.131, d = 0.32$). Though reductions in total stress (associated with perceived job strains) did not reach statistical significance ($t(1,24) = 1.77$, $p = 0.090$), a medium effect size was observed ($d = 0.50$).

3.5.2. SDA. Longitudinal analyses of the Strain in Dementia Care Scale (SDCS) ratings included follow-up data collected from 7 of the 10 staff (70%) initially enrolled at T1. Paired t-tests revealed no significant time effect on the total frequency (of perceived job strains) scale ($t(1,6) = -0.17$, $p = 0.872$, $d = 0.12$). In contrast, there was a statistically significant reduction in total stress (associated with job strains) from T1 to T2 ($t(1,6) = 2.66$, $p = 0.045$, $d = 0.85$).

3.6. Additional Analyses by Diagnostic Group. To account for potential variation in the behavioural profile and disease progression of MS and non-MS residents, data were reanalysed after excluding the non-MS residents. We found that exclusion of these residents did not significantly alter the results on the primary NPI-NH outcome measure.

4. Discussion

To our knowledge, this is the first study of its kind to evaluate the efficacy of training and clinical support in implementing a structured clinical protocol to reduce the impact of behavioural and psychological symptoms of dementia (BPSD) in progressive neurological diseases (PNDs). Due to the progressive and severely debilitating nature of PNDs, individuals with these conditions frequently require access to residential accommodation facilities that can provide high levels of care and support. In the Australian context, specialist disability accommodation facilities are limited, and when access is not available, these patients are typically placed into general residential aged care facilities, which often differ markedly in terms of staff expertise, ethos, and model of care. To account for these differences and ensure the generalisability of findings, we aimed to evaluate the feasibility and efficacy of the structured clinical protocol in both residential aged care (RAC) and specialist disability accommodation (SDA).

Grounded in Brechin et al.'s [21] model of treatment for BPSD, which emphasises a proactive, person-centred approach to identifying and targeting contextual environmental causes and risks for BPSD, we expected that the combination of training plus intensive clinical support would offer the substantial input required to change clinical culture in both types of facilities. We therefore hypothesised that the intervention would be associated with significant reductions in BPSD and improvement in staff coping, in both the RAC and SDA.

Results partially support our expectations. While findings provide preliminary support for the feasibility and efficacy of

TABLE 2: Demographic and psychological characteristics of participating staff.

	RAC	SDA	p value
Demographics			
N	41	10	—
Age, M (SD)	46.24 (12.55)	43.70 (9.43)	0.552
Tenure (years), M (SD)	8.58 (8.30)	3.77 (2.52)	0.078
Days absent	0.73 (2.54)	0.80 (1.32)	0.935
Baseline perceptions			
BPSD self-efficacy total ∗	19.07 (4.08)	19.70 (1.77)	0.639
Training provided	2.95 (0.92)	2.80 (0.63)	0.626
Skills/knowledge	3.10 (0.77)	2.80 (0.63)	0.263
Policy/procedures	3.07 (1.19)	3.20 (0.63)	0.747
Confidence	3.17 (0.70)	3.30 (0.82)	0.616
Motivation	3.46 (1.31)	4.20 (0.79)	0.095
Support	3.32 (0.82)	3.40 (1.17)	0.794
BPSD organisational efficacy total ∗	11.20 (2.74)	13.00 (2.83)	0.069
Reducing frequency	3.00 (0.89)	3.20 (0.63)	0.509
Research driven	2.63 (0.92)	3.00 (1.33)	0.307
Reducing distress	2.93 (0.79)	3.50 (0.97)	0.054
Supported by family/carers	2.63 (0.83)	3.30 (0.68)	0.023

∗ denotes the total score (composite measure) derived from subscales assessing perceived self and organisational efficacy in managing BPSDs.

TABLE 3: Means, standard deviations, and effect sizes on the NPI-NH.

	T1 baseline M (SD)	T2 follow-up M (SD)	Effect size d	Sig T1-T2
RAC ($n = 7$)				
NPI total	19.57 (9.18)	16.71 (7.87)	0.33	0.283
NPI disrupt	7.86 (4.26)	7.29 (4.35)	0.13	0.611
SDA ($n = 6$)				
NPI total	25.67 (11.34)	16.33 (10.78)	0.84	0.049
NPI disrupt	8.67 (5.09)	4.50 (1.05)	1.13	0.108

TABLE 4: Means, standard deviations, and effect sizes on the SDCS.

Facility	T1 baseline, M (SD)	T2 follow-up, M (SD)	Effect size d	Sig T1-T2
RAC				
Frequency of strains	58.80 (7.50)	56.56 (6.27)	0.32	0.131
Total stress	54.04 (12.48)	47.96 (11.64)	0.50	0.090
SDA				
Frequency of strains	48.00 (6.03)	48.67 (5.54)	0.12	0.872
Total stress	46.00 (10.00)	38.33 (7.99)	0.85	0.045

a PND-specific structured clinical protocol, we found that outcomes markedly differed between intervention settings. Encouragingly, and in keeping with expectations, we found that in the SDA setting, the 11-week program was associated with statistically significant reductions in BPSD. Findings also revealed significant improvements in staff coping in the SDA setting, as indicated by significant reductions in total job-related stress from T1 to T2. Contrary to expectations, training and intensive clinical support were not associated with a reduction in BPSD and staff stress at the RAC. Interestingly, while there was no effect of time on BPSD, reductions in job-related stress approached statistical significance.

While the significant effect of staff training and intensive clinical support was found only in the SDA setting, these results from a small sample of individuals with PNDs have important clinical and theoretical significance. Firstly, these findings add to an emerging body of research supporting the efficacy of nonpharmacological approaches to management of BPSD [21, 22]. Since existing research in this area has been limited only to a single RCT of a structured clinical protocol for BPSD in individuals with older-onset dementia of the Alzheimer's type [22], our findings extend on this earlier work to suggest that this intervention model may be an acceptable and efficacious approach to management of BPSD associated with young-onset PNDs, at least in the SDA setting.

From a theoretical standpoint, these findings suggest that BPSD are amenable to change via context-sensitive, behaviourally focused approaches that aim to respond to the individual's unmet psychological, social, and emotional needs [11, 21]. As such, based on this data, it seems reasonable to infer that when delivered in isolation, pharmacological approaches are likely insufficient to address the multiple aetiologies for BPSD in PNDs, including genetic, psychosocial, neurobiological, medical, and physical factors, which interact dynamically to give rise to a complex constellation of symptoms that are unique to the individual [3, 21, 22]. Current findings are also in keeping with recent international guidelines (e.g., International Psychogeriatric Association Complete Guide to BPSD, 2012), which suggest that non-pharmacological treatments may be useful to integrate into usual care for people with PNDs.

In keeping with expectations, significant decreases in staff job stress at the SDA were observed alongside significant reductions in resident BPSD. Though the precise mechanism underlying changes in staff job stress is uncertain, we speculate that reductions in staff stress were mediated by changes in staff perceptions of resident behaviour [22]. Moreover, in keeping with previous theoretical and empirical links between staff stress and resident BPSD [8, 9], results show that PND-specific training and clinical support are associated with measurable reductions in staff stress, which may in turn increase staff capacity to identify indicators of resident distress and respond accordingly [26].

While perhaps surprising, limited support for effects of the structured clinical protocol on BPSD in the RAC setting represents an important finding. While the absence of a statistically significant effect on BPSD may be at least partly related to the possibility that staff stress levels did not significantly change in the RAC [8, 26], site variation in BPSD outcomes should also be considered in light of organisational and workforce level barriers that may be unique to the RAC context. Firstly, due to the standardized nature of the clinical protocol and constraints on training resources, the number of staff receiving intensive clinical support (i.e., "behaviour champions") was limited to three per intervention setting. Since the RAC was a substantially larger facility both in terms of total staff and residents, the behaviour champion to staff ratio was substantially lower than in the SDA setting. Specifically, compared to the SDA setting in which the ratio of behaviour champions to staff was 1:3, the ratio of 1:15 in the RAC setting conferred considerably less opportunities for facility staff to observe and model behavioural support skills learnt by the behaviour champions. Similarly, compared to SDA where the ratio of behaviour champions to residents was 1:2, the lower behaviour champion to resident ratio in the RAC (i.e., 1:15) likely contributed to reduced opportunities for behaviour champions to deliver individualised behaviour support and facilitate a consistent approach to care. Taken together with the lower behaviour champion to staff ratio, the null results in the RAC are perhaps not surprising and underscore a need to consider these factors when implementing future RCTs in this population.

Secondly, to the best of our knowledge, this study represents the first to systematically measure baseline staff psychological characteristics, which may be another factor contributing to the observed differences in outcomes between sites. Interestingly, staff in RAC endorsed lower levels of motivation to engage in BPSD management at baseline. Though the correlates of reduced staff motivation cannot be established, we speculate that reduced staff motivation may be intimately associated with the organisational ethos of RAC, which focuses primarily on alleviating suffering and supporting the end of one's life [27], rather than engaging in more active management or neuro-rehabilitation approaches [23]. As such, in a residential facility where roles, policies, and procedures are situated within a more task-oriented framework, it is perhaps not surprising that staff would assign lesser value and endorse reduced motivation to engage in proactive, person-centred behaviour management approaches. In contrast, it is noteworthy that statistically significant effects were observed in the setting, where individually tailored, context-sensitive interventions are likely considered to align more closely to an organisational ethos centred on residents "living well" and retaining independence, where staff are encouraged to support resident participation and independence in daily activities.

Although speculative, the potential impact of these factors should prompt researchers to consider the influence of an organisation's clinical culture on intervention outcomes. To systematically address these factors in future research, targeted strategies and resources are needed to embed these principles into organisational procedures, thereby increasing the likelihood that staff will reconceptualise their clinical role and view behaviour management as a core component of their daily tasks and duties. Accordingly, adaptations to the current clinical protocol might involve embedding BSPD management principles into the general care regime at both intake and clinical handover (i.e., dedicated behaviour management component of clinical handover and mandatory behaviour charting). Based on anecdotal evidence from the current study, the success of these strategies will likely require top-down support from senior managers and staff who have capacity to lead, model, and embed these systemic changes into the general care regime. The allocation of appropriate resources (e.g., incentives/organisational recognition and higher staff:resident ratios) would also be required to make these feasible recommendations. These observations are in keeping with meta-analytic evidence that supportive workplace relations (e.g., support and incentive-based programs) are a key factor underlying the successful translation of skills into practice [28].

The current study did have several limitations. Since resource limitations precluded the possibility of extended follow-up, further studies are required to establish whether the observed gains are maintained over time. Furthermore, longitudinal studies of this nature are prone to sample attrition, reflected in the T2 follow-up rate of staff enrolled in the study. Despite this weakness, we collected detailed information on staff demographic and psychological variables, analyses of which revealed no significant differences between participating and nonparticipating groups at T2 follow-up.

A further caveat pertains to the intensity and duration of clinical support for behaviour champions. For instance, anecdotal evidence suggests that an extended period of clinical support (e.g., 12 months) with increased time between supervision sessions (e.g., monthly versus weekly sessions) may have been beneficial and provided additional scope to embed the structured clinical protocol into organisational policy and clinical procedures; an approach that would likely contribute to a more robust shift in organisational clinical culture.

Finally, since a large proportion of our sample comprised individuals living with multiple sclerosis (MS), the generalizability of our findings to lower prevalence PNDs (e.g., MND and PD) is somewhat limited. To account for potential variation in the behavioural profile and disease progression of MS and non-MS residents, data were reanalysed after excluding the non-MS residents. We found that exclusion of these residents did not significantly alter the results on any of the primary outcome measures. It is also important to note that despite the large proportion of residents with MS in this study, the composition of our sample is consistent with the higher population prevalence of multiple sclerosis, particularly among those living in residential care facilities housing individuals under the age of 65 years.

Despite the limitations of the study and the notable absence of significant reductions in BPSD at the RAC setting, it is noteworthy that training in the RAC was associated with significant increases in staff knowledge, skills, and confidence from pre- to posttraining. Taken together with evidence that reductions in staff ratings of job-related stress approached statistical significance (with a medium-to-large effect size), findings are in keeping with evidence linking increased knowledge, skills, and support to reduced likelihood of stress reactions and staff burnout, which may in turn have important implications for the frequency and severity of resident BPSD [6, 8].

5. Conclusions

To our knowledge, this study represents the first to evaluate the feasability and efficacy of a structured clinical protocol for managing BPSD in PNDs across two distinct residential accommodation settings. Our results suggest that PND-specific training and clinical support in patient-centred care are associated with benefits for both residents and staff in SDA. Importantly, while we found that the intervention was linked to significant reductions in staff job stress and resident BPSD in the SDA setting, these effects were not observed in the RAC. While the nonsignificant reduction in staff job stress may at least partly explain the null effect of the structured clinical protocol on BPSD in the RAC, site variation in BPSD outcomes may relate to organisational and workforce level barriers that may be unique to the RAC context and should be systematically addressed in future RCT studies of larger PND samples.

Ethical Approval

All work was conducted in accordance with the Declaration of Helsinki (1964). This research received ethics approval from the Calvary Health Care Bethlehem Ethics Committee and Melbourne Health Ethics Committee.

Acknowledgments

This study was supported by a grant from the IOOF Foundation and Perpetual Trustees.

References

[1] T. Pringsheim, K. Wiltshire, L. Day, J. Dykeman, T. Steeves, and N. Jette, "The incidence and prevalence of Huntington's disease: a systematic review and meta-analysis," *Movement Disorders*, vol. 27, no. 9, pp. 1083–1091, 2012.

[2] C. Ward, M. Phillips, A. Smith, and M. Moran, "Multidisciplinary approaches in progressive neurological disease: can we do better?," *Journal of Neurology, Neurosurgery & Psychiatry*, vol. 74, no. 90004, Supplement 4, pp. 8iv–812, 2003.

[3] S. Visser, M. McCabe, C. Hudgson, G. Buchanan, T. Davison, and K. George, "Managing behavioural symptoms of dementia: effectiveness of staff education and peer support," *Aging & Mental Health*, vol. 12, no. 1, pp. 47–55, 2008.

[4] D. Seitz, N. Purandare, and D. Conn, "Prevalence of psychiatric disorders among older adults in long-term care homes: a systematic review," *International Psychogeriatrics*, vol. 22, no. 07, pp. 1025–1039, 2010.

[5] R. Wetzels, S. Zuidema, I. Jansen, F. Verhey, and R. Koopmans, "Course of neuropsychiatric symptoms in residents with dementia in long-term care institutions: a systematic review," *International Psychogeriatrics*, vol. 22, no. 07, pp. 1040–1053, 2010.

[6] T. E. Davison, C. Hudgson, M. P. McCabe, K. George, and G. Buchanan, "An individualized psychosocial approach for "treatment resistant" behavioral symptoms of dementia among aged care residents," *International Psychogeriatrics*, vol. 19, no. 05, pp. 859–873, 2007.

[7] A.-K. Edberg, M. Bird, D. A. Richards, R. Woods, P. Keeley, and V. Davis-Quarrell, "Strain in nursing care of people with dementia: nurses' experience in Australia, Sweden and United Kingdom," *Aging & Mental Health*, vol. 12, no. 2, pp. 236–243, 2008.

[8] D. Edvardsson, P.-O. Sandman, R. Nay, and S. Karlsson, "Associations between the working characteristics of nursing staff and the prevalence of behavioral symptoms in people with dementia in residential care," *International Psychogeriatrics*, vol. 20, no. 4, pp. 764–776, 2008.

[9] A. Nazir, G. Arling, A. J. Perkins, and M. Boustani, "Monitoring quality of care for nursing home residents with behavioral and psychological symptoms related to dementia," *Journal of the American Medical Directors Association*, vol. 12, no. 9, pp. 660–667, 2011.

[10] B. Draper, S. Meares, and H. McIntosh, "A psychogeriatric outreach service to nursing homes in Sydney," *Australasian Journal on Ageing*, vol. 17, no. 4, pp. 184–186, 1998.

[11] G. Livingston, K. Johnston, C. Katona, J. Paton, C. G. Lyketsos, and Old Age Task Force of the World Federation of Biological Psychiatry, "Systematic review of psychological approaches to the management of neuropsychiatric symptoms of dementia," *The American Journal of Psychiatry*, vol. 162, no. 11, pp. 1996–2021, 2005.

[12] S. Turner, "Behavioural symptoms of dementia in residential settings: a selective review of non-pharmacological interventions," *Aging & Mental Health*, vol. 9, no. 2, pp. 93–104, 2005.

[13] I. P. Association, *Behavioral and Psychological Symptoms of Dementia (BPSD) Education Pack: Module 5: Non-pharmacological Management*, International Psychogeriatric Association, Skokie, IL, USA, 2002.

[14] M. McCabe, T. Davison, and K. George, "Effectiveness of staff training programs for behavioral problems among older people with dementia," *Aging & Mental Health*, vol. 11, no. 5, pp. 505–519, 2007.

[15] J. Cohen-Mansfield, "Measurement of inappropriate behavior associated with dementia," *Journal of Gerontological Nursing*, vol. 25, no. 2, pp. 42–51, 1999.

[16] I. R. Hallberg, A. K. Edberg, Å. Nordmark, K. Johnsson, and A. Norberg, "Daytime vocal activity in institutionalized severely demented patients identified as vocally disruptive by nurses," *International Journal of Geriatric Psychiatry*, vol. 8, no. 2, pp. 155–164, 1993.

[17] M. A. Rocca, M. P. Amato, N. De Stefano et al., "Clinical and imaging assessment of cognitive dysfunction in multiple sclerosis," *The Lancet Neurology*, vol. 14, no. 3, pp. 302–317, 2015.

[18] I. R. Hallberg, A. Norberg, and S. Erikson, "Functional impairment and behavioural disturibances in vocally disruptive patients in psychogeriatric wards compared with controls," *International Journal of Geriatric Psychiatry*, vol. 5, no. 1, pp. 53–61, 1990.

[19] S. Meares and B. Draper, "Treatment of vocally disruptive behaviour of multifactorial aetiology," *International Journal of Geriatric Psychiatry*, vol. 14, no. 4, pp. 285–290, 1999.

[20] M. Bird and A. Blair, "Clinical psychology and anxiety and depression in dementia: three case studies," *Nordic Psychology*, vol. 62, pp. 44–54, 2010.

[21] D. Brechin, G. Murphy, I. James, and J. Codner, "Briefing paper: alternatives to antipsychotic medication: psychological approaches in managing psychological and behavioural distress in people with dementia," *Leicester: The British Psychological Society*, 2013.

[22] M. P. McCabe, M. Bird, T. E. Davison et al., "An RCT to evaluate the utility of a clinical protocol for staff in the management of behavioral and psychological symptoms of dementia in residential aged-care settings," *Aging & Mental Health*, vol. 19, no. 9, pp. 799–807, 2015.

[23] G. Eva, J. Bayly, and E. D. Playford, "Neuropalliative rehabilitation–managing neurological disability in the context of a deteriorating illness," *Oxford Textbook of Neurorehabilitation*, vol. 1, pp. 341–351, 2015.

[24] J. L. Cummings, M. Mega, K. Gray, S. Rosenberg-Thompson, D. A. Carusi, and J. Gornbein, "The neuropsychiatric inventory: comprehensive assessment of psychopathology in dementia," *Neurology*, vol. 44, no. 12, pp. 2308–2308, 19942314, 1994.

[25] S. Wood, J. L. Cummings, M.-A. Hsu et al., "The use of the neuropsychiatric inventory in nursing home residents: characterization and measurement," *The American Journal of Geriatric Psychiatry*, vol. 8, pp. 75–83, 2001.

[26] D. Chrzescijanski, W. Moyle, and D. Creedy, "Reducing dementia-related aggression through a staff education intervention," *Dementia*, vol. 6, no. 2, pp. 271–286, 2007.

[27] R. S. Morrison, D. E. Meier, and C. Capello, "The place of love in the care of persons with advanced dementia," in *Geriatric Palliative Care*, pp. 30–36, Oxford University Press, New York, 1st edition, 2003.

[28] B. D. Blume, J. K. Ford, T. T. Baldwin, and J. L. Huang, "Transfer of training: a meta-analytic review," *Journal of Management*, vol. 36, no. 4, pp. 1065–1105, 2010.

5

The Effects of Transcranial Direct Current Stimulation on the Cognitive Functions in Older Adults with Mild Cognitive Impairment

Pablo Cruz Gonzalez,[1] Kenneth N. K. Fong,[1] and Ted Brown[2]

[1]*Department of Rehabilitation Sciences, The Hong Kong Polytechnic University, Hong Kong, Hong Kong*
[2]*Department of Occupational Therapy, Monash University, Melbourne, VIC, Australia*

Correspondence should be addressed to Kenneth N. K. Fong; rsnkfong@polyu.edu.hk

Academic Editor: Foteini Christidi

Objective. The aim of this pilot study was to investigate whether the use of anodal transcranial direct current stimulation (tDCS) on the left dorsolateral prefrontal cortex could boost the effects of a cognitive stimulation (CS) programme using a tablet on five older adults with mild cognitive impairment (MCI). *Method.* A single-subject study of A-B-C-A design was used. After the baseline with the administration of CS (phase A), a sham treatment with CS was applied (B). Following the withdrawal of sham treatment, tDCS was introduced in combination with CS (C). Finally, phase A was replicated a second time. *Results.* tDCS had a significant effect on processing speed, selective attention, and planning ability tasks in terms of performance and completion time. *Conclusion.* tDCS appears to have a positive impact on some cognitive components in CS in persons with MCI. Further study on its long-term effects and generalization of power to daily activities is warranted.

1. Introduction

Mild cognitive impairment (MCI) is a syndrome of cognitive decline below the typically expected age norm in an individual. It is commonly referred to as an intermediate phase between the expected cognitive decline of normal aging and the pathological cognitive decline linked to dementia and usually does not interfere with daily activities [1]. There is a difference between MCI and a formal diagnosis of dementia: the latter represents a more severe cognitive decline and has a substantial negative impact on daily functioning [2]. In some cases, MCI will revert to normal cognition or remain stable. Only an insignificant proportion of people presenting with known MCI, 12–15% per year, will gradually worsen and develop dementia, compared to 1-2% of the general population; approximately, 40–65% of patients with MCI will eventually progress to Alzheimer's disease (AD) [1].

Regarding possible interventions to tackle MCI, there is a lack of evidence for pharmacological interventions that can prevent cognitive decline or conversion to dementia. To date, drugs have proved to have no positive impact in MCI trials [3].

As a form of nonpharmacological intervention, cognitive rehabilitation is defined as "the therapeutic process of increasing or improving an individual's capacity to process and use incoming information so as to allow increased functioning in everyday life. This includes methods to train and restore cognitive function and compensatory techniques" [4].

One type of cognitive rehabilitation is cognitive stimulation (CS) which has been used as a potential intervention to slow down the deterioration of cognitive functions in people presenting with known MCI. According to the largest randomized controlled trial of cognitive intervention carried out with older adults to date, the experimental treatment approaches used in this study support the improvement of targeted cognitive areas in different groups in comparison to the control group, which did not receive any kind of intervention [5]. Contrary to conventional cognitive tasks that are performed with paper-and-pencil with a lack of simultaneous feedback, computerized cognitive stimulation is designed to be more enjoyable and engaging based on human-computer interaction [6, 7]. These cognitive stimulation strategies have also been shown to improve performance after repetition of computerized CT tasks in older adults presenting with known MCI [8].

A systematic review found evidence of memory and executive function enhancement while analyzing the effects of nonpharmacological interventions on cognitive functions in older people presenting with known MCI [9]. However, the appropriate protocol and optimal frequency for inducing benefits in the cognitive functioning of this population remain unknown.

Transcranial direct current stimulation (tDCS) is another type of nonpharmacological intervention that uses direct electrical currents to stimulate specific parts of the brain. It involves delivering a noninvasive weak direct current (1-2 mA) through at least two electrodes, at least one of which is placed on the scalp for a period of a few seconds to 20–30 minutes, which modulates neuronal activity. There are two types of stimulation: anodal stimulation acts to excite neuronal activity and cathodal stimulation has hyperpolarizing effects, inhibiting neuronal activity [10, 11]. As soon as tDCS is administered, the current travels in an anode-cathode circuit which is likely to cause neurons to fire in stimulated areas [10].

Priming is the change in repetitive behavior due to implicit learning based on previous stimuli [12], and it has recently been used for inducing neuroplasticity and enhancing the effects of conventional rehabilitation as combined approaches [13]. The excitability modulation induced by tDCS is considered a potential intervention to modulate the learning processes [14]. tDCS boosts subthreshold neuronal action potentials beyond their unaugmented state, thus, may achieve stronger firing patterns than would occur in the absence of tDCS. Although, repeated practice with cognitive stimuli in CS may elicit unintentional learning, mechanisms that circumvent cognitive impairments, targeting a neural circuit with tDCS whereas it is simultaneously engaged by a cognitive stimulation task, may produce better therapeutic effects than stimulating the same cortical area in the absence of cognitive stimuli [15, 16]. tDCS may augment the strength of transmission across synaptic circuits in pathways that are stimulated by cognitive practice, and thus it may also strengthen the circuits that are formed through unintentional, practice-related learning and maximize the possibility of enduring behavior change through such implicit learning. Given that CS and tDCS can enhance plastic changes, the combination of both techniques could cause a better synergistic positive effect on behavior [15, 17]. Indeed, it has been shown that anodal stimulation of the left dorsolateral prefrontal cortex (DLPFC) increases the performance of a sequential-letter working memory task in healthy young adults [18]. Recent research also indicates that healthy older adults can benefit from tDCS, enhancing retention skills of object-location learning a week after completion of the object-location task compared to participants who took part in a tDCS sham condition [19]. There is growing evidence that tDCS coupled with CS improves cognitive performance. After ten sessions of a working memory CS in combination with tDCS, healthy adults experience an enhanced effect and perform CS tasks more accurately than those who received sham tDCS [20].

The impact of tDCS has also been explored for AD, frontotemporal dementia, and mild vascular dementia. Positive effects were found in visual recognition memory tasks in persons with AD when applying anodal tDCS to the left temporal cortex [21]. Results after five consecutive sessions over five days in which anodal tDCS was applied over both hemispheres of the temporal cortex and an extracephalic cathodal tDCS (for a 30-minute period using 2 mA) showed significant improvement in the performance of a visual recognition memory test [22]. In a more recent study that involved participants presenting with mild vascular dementia, four consecutive day sessions of anodal tDCS (for a 20-minute period using 2 mA) on the left DLPFC generated positive additional effects on visual short-term memory, verbal working memory, and executive control [23].

The beneficial effects of tDCS on cognition in people presenting with known MCI have been demonstrated [24]; however, the literature on using tDCS on people presenting with known MCI is still very limited. The frequency and targeted areas are not the only significant issues that remain unknown. To optimize the positive and therapeutic benefits of noninvasive brain stimulation (NIBS), it is also worth investigating the uncertainty of combining tDCS with conventional behavioral treatments such as a CS that might also yield more information and understanding about the impact of tDCS effects for people at risk of MCI.

Based on the above background information, we considered the use of anodal tDCS on the left DLPFC (30 minutes 2 mA) with an extracephalic return electrode to be a promising and safe intervention approach to optimize the impact of CS on tablet PCs for older adults at risk of MCI. The current study aimed to compare the impact of anodal and sham tDCS applied to the left DLPFC on the cognitive performance of people at risk of MCI engaging in CS interventions on tablet PCs. We hypothesized that there would be a significant improvement in cognitive task performance after the use of tDCS, which would subsequently generalize to other cognitive domains—short-term memory, planning ability, working memory, attention, and processing speed skills. We also aim to determine the optimal frequency of tDCS application with the same dosage to improve the cognitive skills of older adults with MCI.

2. Materials and Methods

2.1. Participants. Five older adults with MCI were recruited by convenience sampling from community center groups in Hong Kong. The inclusion criteria followed the modified Petersen's criteria [25] (given by the MCI Working Group of the European Consortium on Alzheimer's Disease, Brescia Meeting, Italy, June 2005). Participants had to (a) be aged between 60 and 85; (b) obtain a score between 19 and 26 on the Montreal Cognitive Assessment Test (MoCA) [26]; (c) achieve a score of 0.5 or below on the clinical dementia rating (CDR) [27]; (d) self-report cognitive decline; (e) be

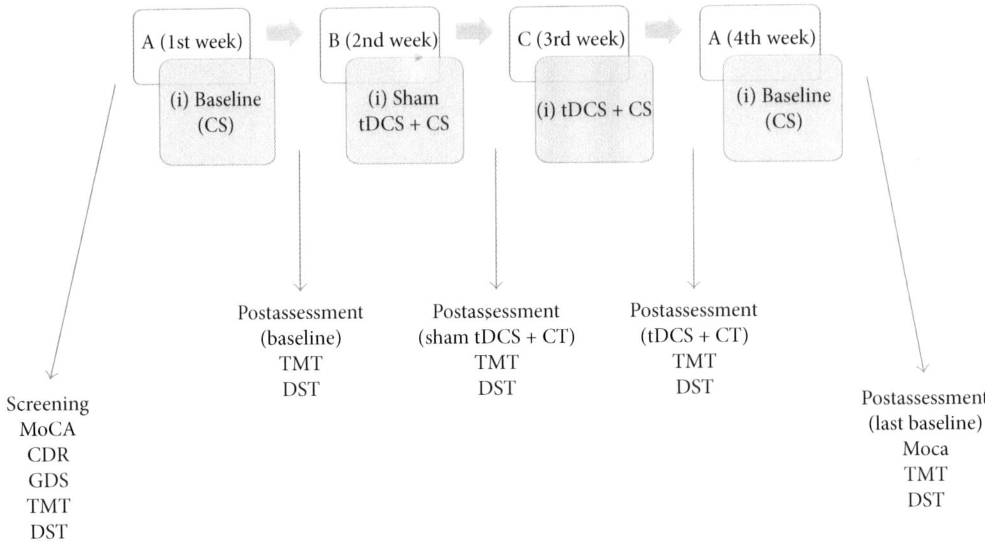

Figure 1: Intervention sequence. A-B-C-A design; MoCA: Montreal Cognitive Assessment; CDR: Clinical Dementia Rating; GDS: Geriatric Depression Scale; TMT: Trail Making Test; DST: digit span test. Phases. CS: cognitive stimulation; tDCS: transcranial direct current stimulation.

independent in daily living activities; and (f) have completed three or more years of primary education.

Regarding exclusion criteria, the following were excluded: (a) individuals presenting with a diagnosis of dementia or any other neurological disease and mental disorders; (b) individuals with depression, determined by a score of 5 or above on the Geriatric Depression Scale (GDS) [28]; and (c) individuals who had metallic fixtures around the cephalon.

The study was conducted in accordance with the Declaration of Helsinki and was approved by the human subject ethics committee of The Hong Kong Polytechnic University (ref. number: HSEARS20160415002). All participants gave informed written consent before the intervention began.

2.2. Design. This study utilized a prospective, single-subject design (SSD) with multiple nonconcurrent treatments—anodal tDCS + CS, sham tDCS + CS, and CS only. A four-phase A-B-C-A SSD was employed. After the baseline with the administration of CS (phase A), a sham tDCS with CS was applied (B). Following the withdrawal of this sham treatment, a tDCS treatment was introduced in combination with CS (C). Finally, phase A was replicated to provide the control needed to document the differences between the sham and tDCS phases (Figure 1).

In this design, it is assumed that both treatments—B and C—have differential and independent effects. Differences in the target responses are expected across the four phases of the study. The sham phase (B) was the first treatment intervention to be used to avoid possible carryover effects due to the tDCS stimulation treatment (i.e., phase C), thereby eliminating this potential treatment effect, which can be analyzed during the last baseline (A).

2.3. Cognitive Stimulation. "Neuron Up" was the CS administered to participants. It is a web platform (https://www.neuronup.com/) designed to serve as a fundamental support for professionals involved in cognitive rehabilitation and cognitive stimulation [29]. The display format was full screen in a 9.7-inch screen iPad situated on a desk approximately 35 centimeters in front of the participant.

Participants' individualized level was identified through two training sessions that were conducted for all the participants prior to the implementation. Five cognitive activities associated with different cognitive domains were selected:

(i) Sorting bugs: This task is associated with planning ability and divided attention. Participants are asked to move a bar located in the middle of the screen either to block the movement of bugs which are moving in different directions or to let them pass from one side to the other. The final goal is to keep the green bugs on the green side and the red bugs on the red side. Participants are allowed seven minutes to complete the task, and the completion time is measured. This task also trains sustained and selective attention.

(ii) The last light on: This task is associated with processing speed and selective attention. Participants are asked to pay attention to the windows in a building that light up. They have to touch the window which is the last to light up. This task is repeated five times per session, and the number of correct answers and completion time are measured.

(iii) Illuminated windows: This activity is associated with short-term memory. Participants are asked to remember which windows are illuminated in a building in an open memorization period. Then, all the lights are turned off and participants must identify the windows that had been lit. This activity is repeated five times. The number of correct answers, number of errors, memorization time, and completion time are measured.

(iv) Addition and subtraction questions. Both tasks are associated with calculation and working memory. Participants are given three addition operations involving four numbers of six digits each and six subtraction operations with two numbers of six digits each to solve. The number of errors and the completion time are measured.

These five cognitive activities were presented as a cognitive stimulation practice with one-to-one supervision from an occupational therapist in which all participants were exposed to repetitive testing via the computer system across sessions.

2.4. tDCS. The Soterix Medical 1×1 low-intensity tDCS stimulator was the device used to provide the stimulation. The two rubber electrodes employed for tDCS in this study were introduced in saline-soaked synthetic sponges (7×5 cm, 35 cm^2).

Anodal tDCS was delivered to the left DLPFC, and the cathode electrode was placed over the contralateral deltoid muscle as extracephalic cathode. The scalp electrode was positioned over F3 according to the 10–20 EEG international system. The left DLPFC was targeted as the stimulation site because of its role in high-order cognitive processes [30] and due to the existence of functional disconnection of the DLPFC in persons with MCI [31]. A constant current of 2 mA was applied for 30 minutes. For sham tDCS, the 2 mA intensity was only given for 30 seconds at the beginning and the end of the stimulation.

2.5. Experimental Protocol and Procedures. Each interval (A, B, C, and A) was staggered by a week at a time. During the baseline phases, three sessions of CS were implemented for all the participants. Both interventions, sham tDCS and anodal tDCS, were combined with the same CS that was performed for the baseline phases. However, the treatment phases varied from one to five sessions. The sessions per phase were distributed over five days. Participants were randomly assigned to combinations of intervention each of which had a different time span to compare the treatment frequency effect (Table 1).

The experimental sessions were 30 minutes in length. In this way, tDCS was administered for 30 minutes and the CS was begun five minutes after the tDCS began, thus running for 25 minutes. For the sham phase, the administration of the sham tDCS lasted 30 minutes too, with the difference that a ramping current of 2 mA was applied during the first and last 30 seconds. The participants remained blinded for both stimulation conditions.

2.6. Cognitive Measures. CS data were recorded for each task of each cognitive activity during the sessions. Data such as completion time and performance in terms of correct answers or number of errors were collected.

The standardized cognitive assessments used in this study for screening were the CDR (Hong Kong Version), and the scale was found to have good reliability with internal consistency ranging from 0.7 to 0.9 [32], the GDS-15 item (Hong Kong version) which has a satisfactory reliability with Cronbach alpha = 0.82 [33], and the MoCA (Hong Kong Version) with a sensitivity of 90% to detect MCI [26, 34].

The standardized cognitive measures to assess the study phases included the MoCA (Hong Kong version) [34], the digit span test (DST) [35], and the Trail Making Test ((TMT) Chinese version) which normative data has provided evidence that the part B (Chinese version) may be equivalent to the standard part B [36].

The participants were assessed in five phases: screening (pre-A), after baseline (post-A), after first intervention (post-B), after second intervention (post-C), and after final baseline (post-A).

To summarize, DST and TMT were conducted before the initial baseline and after each interval. However, the MoCA was only administered before the first baseline and after the last for a general comparison of the whole sequence and to avoid learning effect due to repeated testing (Figure 1).

2.7. Data Analysis. To study the effects of tDCS on the "Neuron Up" CS program across the design phases, visual analysis and two standard deviation procedures were used as analytical methods.

Visual analysis was based on observing the visual patterns presented in the graphs where the target parameter changed once the treatment was introduced or withdrawn. Difference in means among phases was also compared.

In the two standard deviation procedure, the levels of the baseline are compared to those of the intervention data points. The procedure assumes that if we are to extend the baseline, then ultimately 95 percent of our observations would be less than two standard deviations away from the baseline mean. The two standard deviations were calculated manually following the guidelines set out by Rubin and Babbie [37]. Data analyses of the cognitive assessments administered before the commencement of the baseline and after every single interval were compared.

3. Results

Although all five participants did well in the tDCS intervention, redness in the area was observed after removing the electrodes in one participant, and he also complained of having a mild headache a few hours after receiving the therapy. The remaining participants reported a tingling sensation in the DLPFC region during the stimulation phase which faded away after a few minutes of the onset of the stimulation. They completed all sessions as scheduled, with the exception of one participant who was not available to complete the last session of the last baseline.

3.1. Cognitive Stimulation Outcomes. The results are presented in graphs in the sequence in which the CS tasks were performed and following the order from fewer to more treatment sessions received. The *x*-axis corresponds to the observation points (the number of tasks) per day. The *y*-axis represents either the performance or the time taken to complete the task. The blue line is the measurement of the targeted problem across observation points. There were four intervals for each condition: (A) baseline, (B) sham tDCS

Table 1: Demographics, inclusion criteria scores, and number of sessions conducted in every interval by week.

Participant	Demographics			Inclusion assessment scores					Number of sessions conducted in every interval by week			
	Age	Gender	Medical history	MoCA preintervention	MoCA postintervention	MoCA gain (%)	CDR	GDS	1st week (A) CS alone	2nd week (B) sham tDCS + CS	3rd week (C) anodal tDCS + CS	4th week (A) CS alone
1	79	Female	Heart disease	24	26	6.66	0.5	3	3	1	1	3
2	68	Female	NA	24	25	3.33	0.5	1	3	2	2	3
3	67	Male	NA	24	29	16.6	0.5	1	3	3	3	3
4	69	Male	Diabetes	25	26	3.3	0.5	1	3	4	4	2
5	81	Male	Diabetes	26	27	3.3	0.5	2	3	5	5	3

MoCA: Montreal Cognitive Assessment; CDR: Clinical Dementia Rating; GDS: Geriatric Depression Scale; NA: not applicable; CS: cognitive stimulation; sham tDCS + CS: transcranial direct current stimulation + CS during the A, B, C, and A phases.

intervention, (C) tDCS intervention, and (A) baseline. Every single black line which crosses every interval is the mean of the performance, and the two standard deviations are marked by a black dotted line starting at the corresponding interval.

(i) Sorting bugs (Figure 2): All participants demonstrated fluctuating times of completion during the first baseline phase. There are positive effects for those subjects who received three or more tDCS sessions (participants 3, 4, and 5) with a general slight increase in time required to complete the task after withdrawal of the tDCS intervention, and a difference by more than two standard deviations was observed at the last baseline phase of participant 3.

(ii) The last light on (Figure 3): Figure 3 shows that there were differences by more than two standard deviations in participants 1, 3, and 5. With respect to the baselines and sham phases, all participants exhibited decreasing accuracy in the cognitive task in comparison with the experimental interval, except for participant 4, but no significant difference was found.

(iii) Illuminated windows (Figure 4): Despite all participants exhibiting similar outcomes in all phases, there is a slight general improvement in task performance across conditions, but no significant difference was found.

(iv) Additional question (Figure 5): Participants 1, 2, 3, and 4 demonstrated a clear intervention effect of tDCS administration, but no significant difference was found. Participants made fewer errors in operations when the tDCS was applied. However, participant 5 performed differently, reducing the number of errors after the sham tDCS intervention and especially achieved the best performance during the last baseline phase.

(v) Subtraction question (Figure 6): The outcomes of these operations were similar to the additional questions, but the change in level was not very pronounced. Participants 2, 3, and 5 were more accurate, solving the operations during the tDCS treatment, and the tendency during the baseline and sham phases was associated with a larger number of errors, but no significant difference was found. For participants 1 and 4, the results were almost identical across conditions.

3.2. Behavioral Assessment Outcomes

3.2.1. MoCA Test. All participants showed an improvement in MoCA scores. Participant 3 showed the largest improvement (Table 1).

3.2.2. Trail Making Test. Participants 1 and 4 demonstrated the greatest impact of the tDCS as revealed by the shortest completion time (parts A and B) right after the last session of the tDCS intervention. The negative ratio shown in Table 2 indicates a shorter time taken to complete the task after tDCS relative to sham tDCS. Participant 3 also improved during phase B and participant 5 during phase A (Table 2).

3.2.3. Digit Span Test. All participants improved in their digit span test scores when comparing the baseline to the last assessment. The trend shows that improvement follows a general and steady progressive pattern without obvious significant changes (Table 3).

4. Discussion

This pilot study combined anodal tDCS with CS to investigate their impact on the cognitive performance of older adults with MCI. The result shows that application of anodal tDCS to the left DLPFC and cathodal tDCS to the right deltoid muscle helps to enhance cognitive performance in processing speed, selective attention, and working memory activities, as well as the completion time in planning ability and divided attention tasks. One of the objectives of this study was to compare anodal tDCS and sham tDCS. Although the data generated with CS fluctuated and were variable, the participants did not show significantly better outcomes in the sham intervention than the baseline CS alone.

This was the first study of its kind to show mild benefits in multiple domains of cognition in older adults with MCI as other studies have focused on the possible benefits of tDCS in a single cognitive domain, usually working memory [13, 18, 38].

Placement of an anodal tDCS on the left DLPFC and a cathodal tDCS on the right deltoid muscle did not increase participants' performance in the short-term memory CS task. This agrees with previous studies that applied the same montage as the current study in combination with memory training in persons suffering from AD and which also observed no significant additional effect of tDCS on memory performance beyond that of sham tDCS with the same memory training [39].

Our study adopted extracephalic cathodal tDCS, which eliminated the confounding effect of a monocephalic cathode electrode placed on the scalp. Our findings are also in line with the study conducted by Boggio and colleagues [22] in which the return electrode was extracephalic and placed over the right deltoid muscle in people presenting with AD. The use of a monocephalic cathode setup has been controversial because "current flow direction/electrical field orientation relative to neuronal orientation might determine the effects of tDCS and it might be that the effects of an extracephalic electrode differs relevantly from that of a bipolar electrode arrangement" [40]. Monocephalic cathodes are also common in studies, but that does not mean that the return electrode is physiologically inert, since its positioning does have a critical impact on the electrical field orientation [13]. Notwithstanding, we are confident that the electrical current passes through the stimulated brain area—the left DLPFC—when

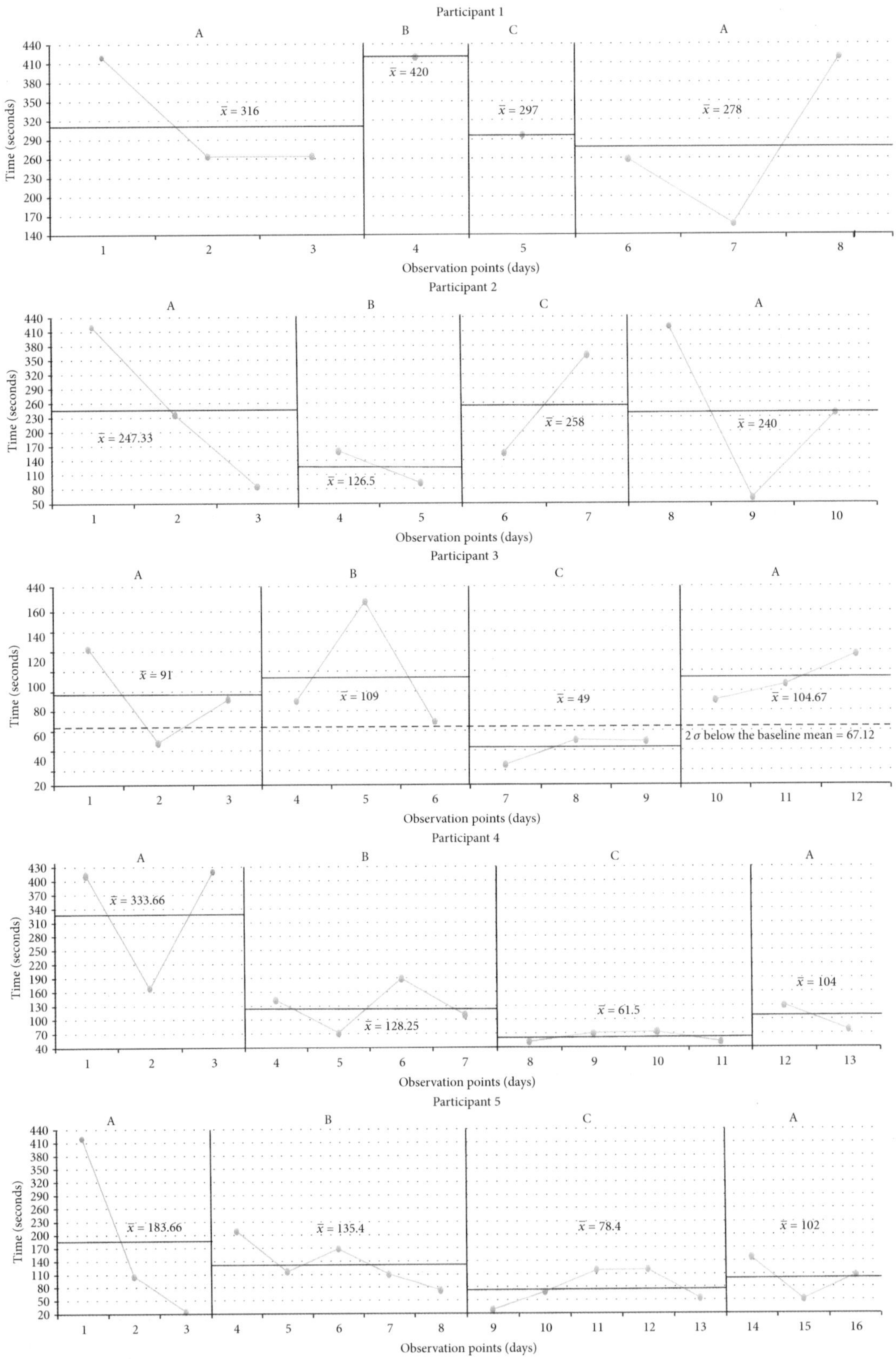

FIGURE 2: Sorting bugs. A: baseline; B: sham tDCS; C: tDCS; x-axis: observation points in days; y-axis: completion time in seconds. Scores are shown, along with black lines marking the average of each phase and with a black dotted line starting at the corresponding baseline marking 2-standard deviation (2 σ) when there is statistically significant difference (participant 3).

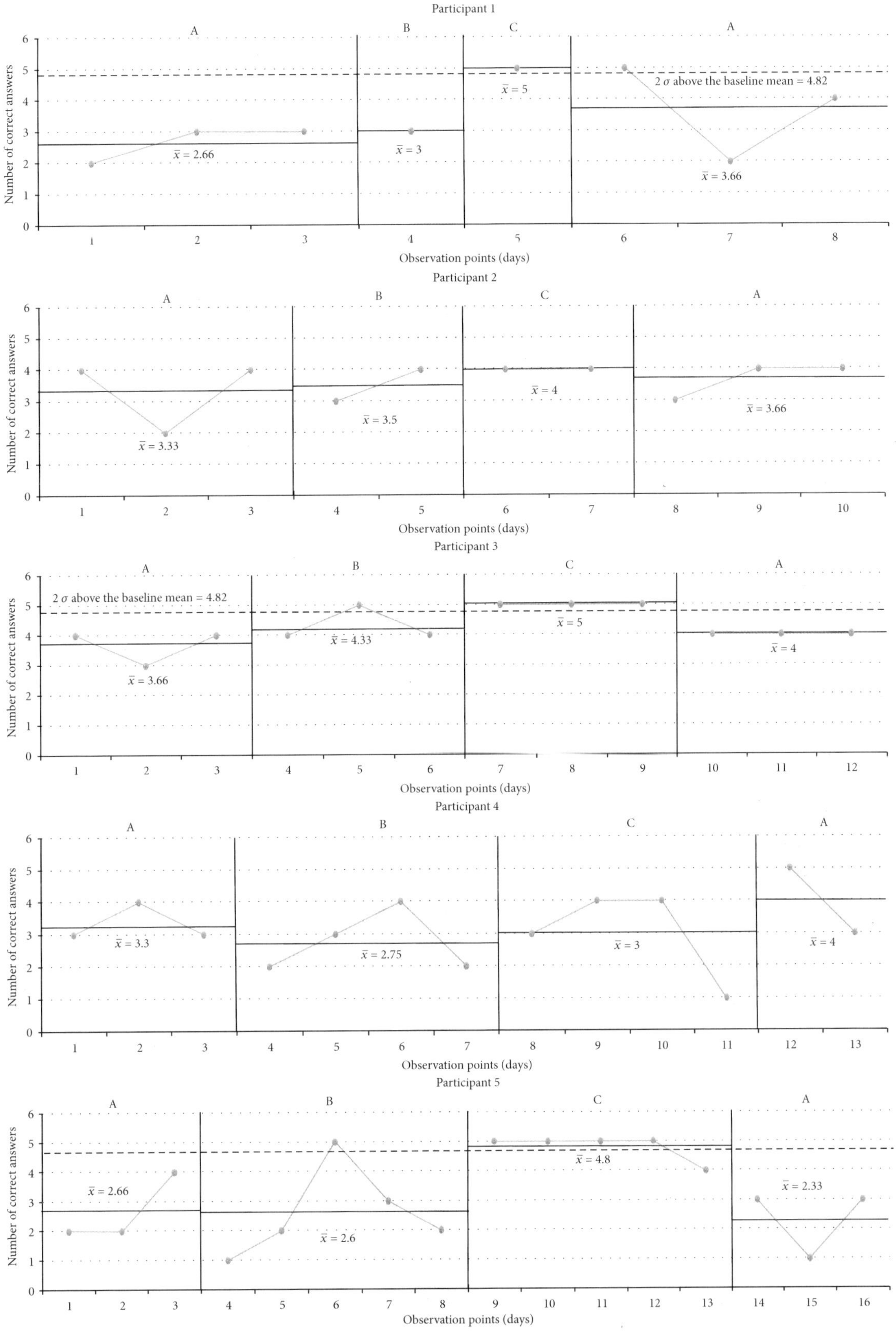

FIGURE 3: The last light on. A: baseline; B: sham tDCS; C: tDCS; x-axis: observation points in days; y-axis: number of correct answers. Scores are shown, along with black lines marking the average of each phase and with a black dotted line starting at the corresponding baseline marking 2-standard deviation (2σ) when there is statistically significant difference (participants 1, 3, and 5).

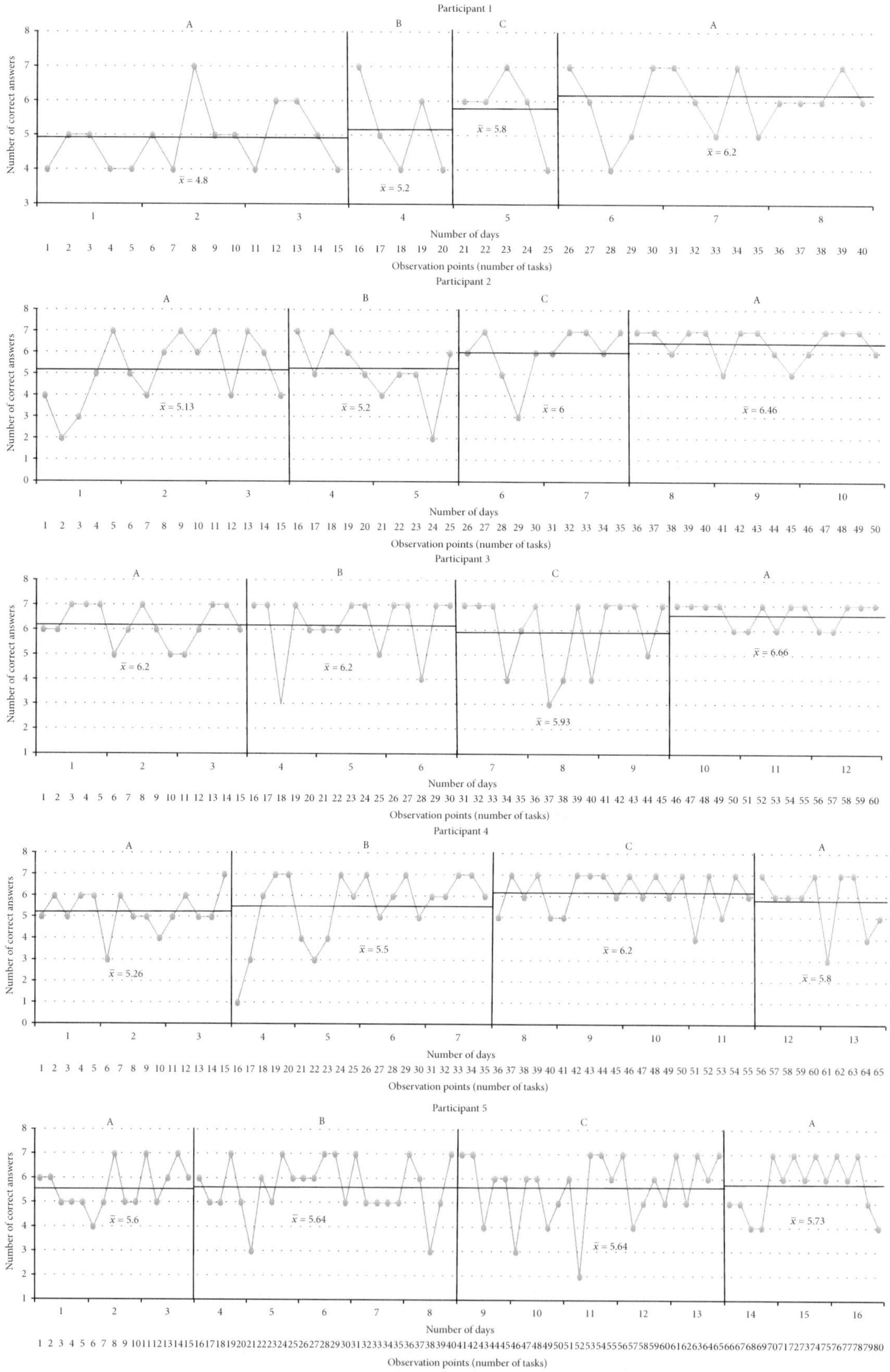

FIGURE 4: Illuminated windows. A: baseline; B: sham tDCS; C: tDCS; x-axis: observation points in number of tasks performed within days; y-axis: number of correct answers. Scores are shown, along with black lines marking the average of each phase.

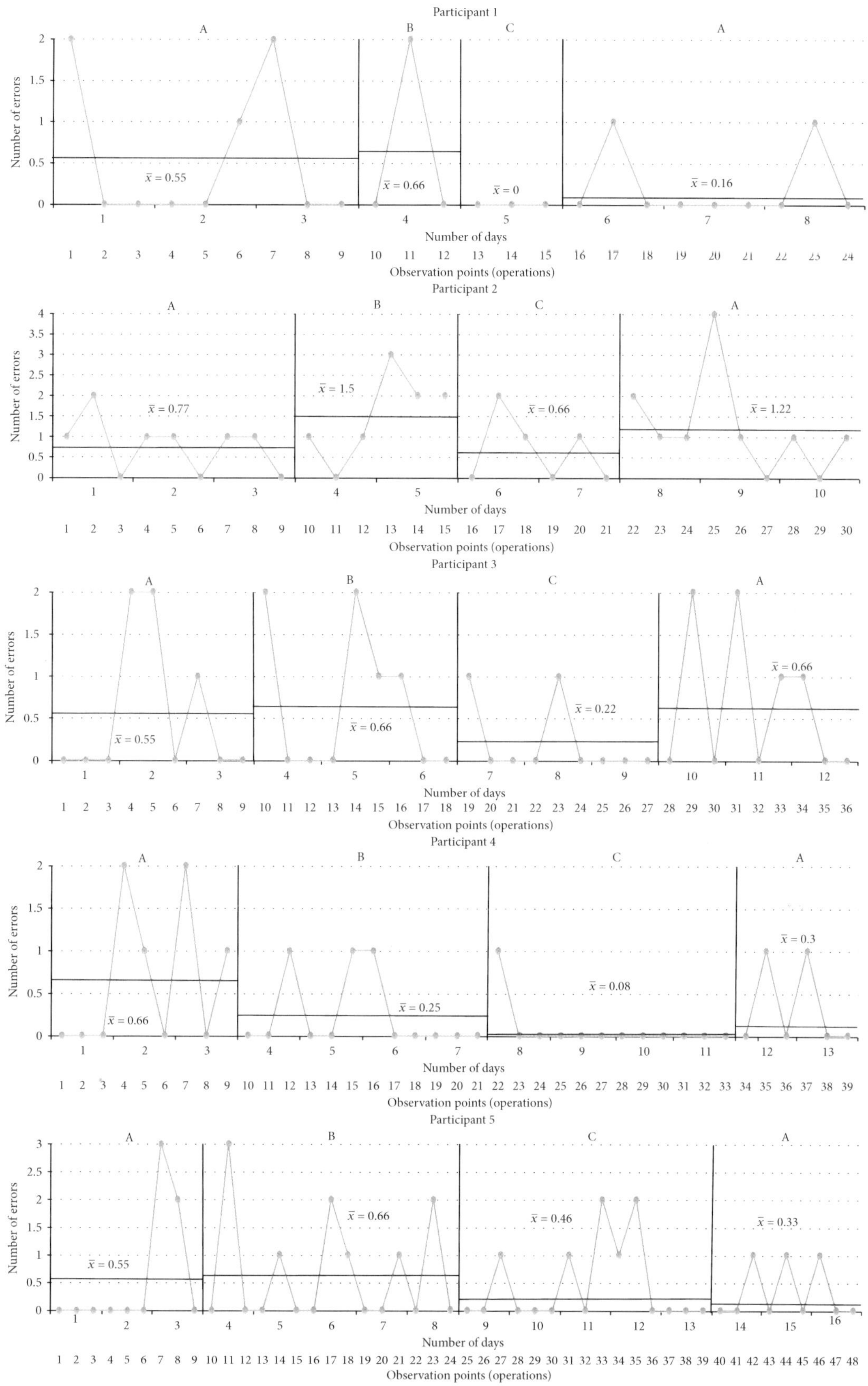

FIGURE 5: Additional question. A: baseline; B: sham tDCS; C: tDCS; x-axis: observation points in number of tasks performed within days; y-axis: number of errors. Scores are shown, along with black lines marking the average of each phase.

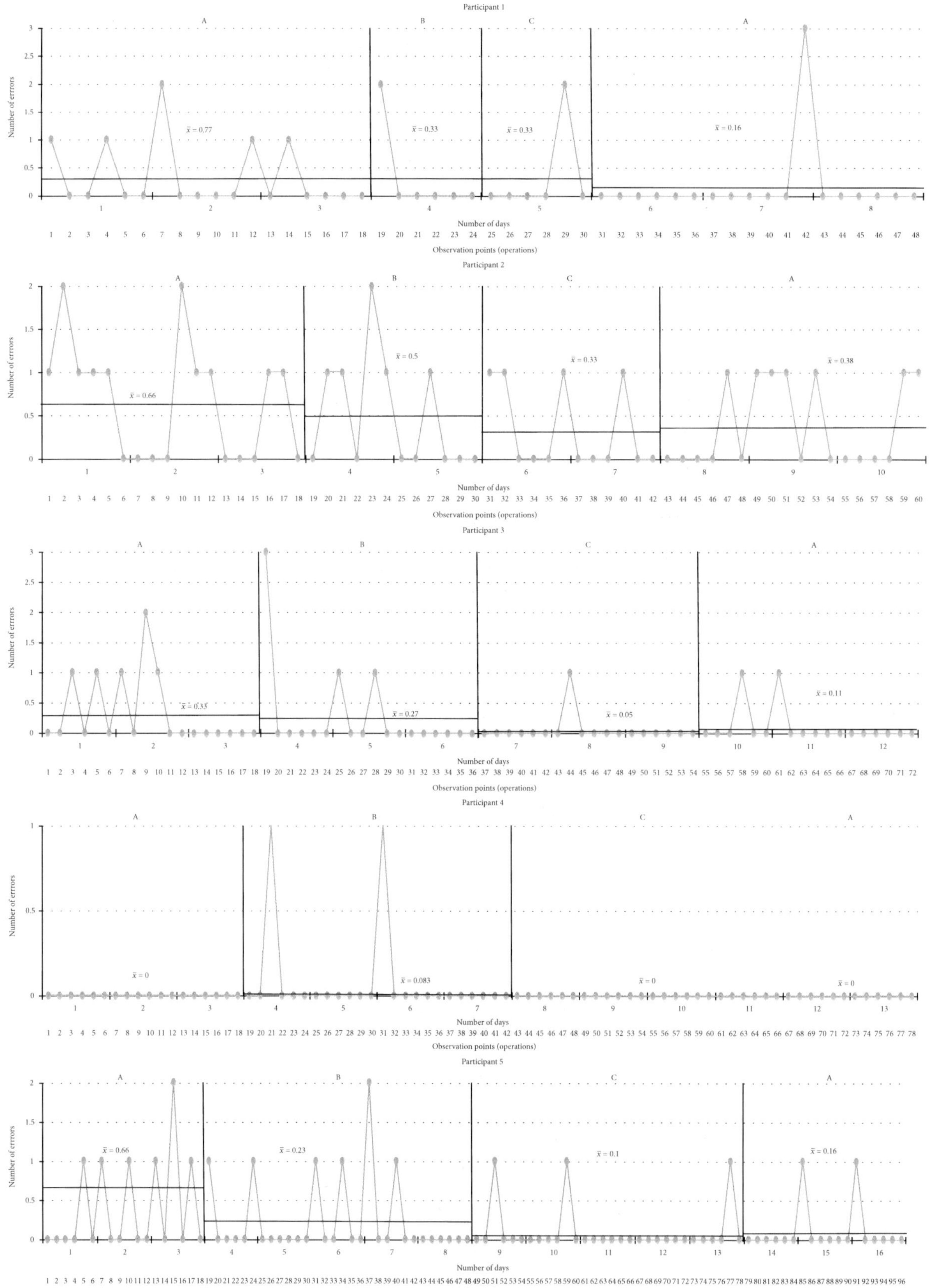

FIGURE 6: Subtraction question. A: baseline; B: sham tDCS; C: tDCS; x-axis: observation points in number of tasks performed within days; y-axis: number of errors. Scores are shown, along with black lines marking the average of each phase.

Table 2: Trail Making Test score.

Participant	Trail Making Test	Baseline	After first baseline (A1)	After sham tDCS (B)	After tDCS (C)	After last baseline (A2)	Immediate effect (seconds) (C versus baseline)	After-effect (seconds) (A2 versus C)	tDCS versus sham tDCS (seconds) (C versus B)
1	Part A	58.82	58.45	51.53	44.48	55.69	−14.34	10.81	−6.82
	Part B	109.74	87.22	67.7	60.52	67.45	−49.22	6.93	−7.18
2	Part A	38.46	38.4	32.92	41.34	28.03	2.88	−13.31	8.42
	Part B	55.45	83.04	75.73	56.55	64.77	1.1	8.22	−7.31
3	Part A	26.35	22.68	22.91	20.86	15.53	−5.49	−5.53	−2.05
	Part B	42	44.92	29.68	26.73	27.13	−15.87	0.4	−3.25
4	Part A	32.48	40.16	56.12	28.08	51.93	−4.4	23.85	−28.04
	Part B	51.6	56.23	51.5	42.35	56.74	−9.25	14.39	−9.15
5	Part A	37.58	50.4	43.76	38.48	46.55	−0.9	8.07	−5.28
	Part B	57.42	40.55	71.42	52.65	50.15	−4.77	−2.5	−18.77

Immediate effect (C versus baseline) is the gain in seconds after the application of tDCS compared with the baseline; after-effect (A2 versus C) is the maintenance or gain in seconds after tDCS withdrawal in phase C; tDCS versus sham tDCS (C versus B) is the comparison between tDCS and sham tDCS. A positive ratio implies decrement, a neutral ratio implies maintenance, and a negative ratio implies improvement in terms of time of completion.

Table 3: Digit span test score.

Participant	Digit span test	Baseline	After first baseline (A1)	After sham tDCS (B)	After tDCS (C)	After last baseline (A2)	Immediate effect (%) (C versus baseline)	After-effect (%) (A2 versus C)	tDCS versus sham tDCS (C versus B)
1	Forward score	15	16	16	15	16	0	3.33	−3.33
	Backward score	6	8	10	8	9	6.66	3.33	−6.66
	Total score	21	24	26	23	25	6.66	6.66	−9.99
2	Forward score	14	15	14	15	16	3.33	3.33	3.33
	Backward score	5	5	7	6	8	3.33	6.66	−3.33
	Total score	19	19	21	21	24	6.66	9.99	0
3	Forward score	14	16	16	16	16	6.66	0	0
	Backward score	9	9	9	9	13	0	13.32	0
	Total score	23	25	25	25	29	6.66	13.32	0
4	Forward score	16	16	16	16	16	0	0	0
	Backward score	7	8	5	8	8	3.33	0	9.99
	Total score	23	24	21	24	24	3.33	0	9.99
5	Forward score	13	16	16	16	16	9.99	0	0
	Backward score	4	4	5	7	5	9.99	−6.66	6.66
	Total score	17	20	21	23	22	19.98	−3.33	6.66

Immediate effect (C versus baseline) is the gain (%) after the application of tDCS compared with the baseline; after-effect (A2 versus C) is the maintenance or gain (%) after tDCS withdrawal in phase C; tDCS versus sham tDCS (C versus B) is the comparison in terms of gain (%) between tDCS and sham tDCS. A positive ratio implies improvement, a neutral ratio implies maintenance, and a negative ratio implies decrement in terms of accuracy.

applying tDCS. With the same cathode montage, both our study and that of Boggio and colleagues [22] indicate a significant improvement in visual recognition after the administration of multisession tDCS.

It is disappointing that all these positive CT findings are somewhat inconsistent with the results of standardized cognitive assessments, except for the TMT, in which most of the participants showed their best score of the tDCS intervention in all phases. Interestingly, TMT could be an indicator of processing speed [41] and visual selective attention domains [42], which might also correspond to the CS task improvement associated with these domains.

Despite our aim to determine the optimal frequency of tDCS application with the same dosage by modifying the number of sham tDCS and tDCS sessions among participants, the findings appear to be inconclusive. In some occasions, just one session of tDCS was sufficient to produce positive changes in performance while other participants who had up to five sessions of tDCS showed no evidence of benefiting from exposure to the tDCS intervention. Comparison of participants' individual performance of all the CS tasks indicates that the most beneficial dose of tDCS seems to be three sessions per week. However, conclusions cannot be gleaned from the session's variability due to the small sample of this study. This should be addressed in the future as it remains unclear.

Although this study has produced encouraging results, it also has several limitations. First, an A-B-C-A SSD was used without randomization among experimental conditions. The same order was used for all the participants because if tDCS was administered in phase B right after the baseline, then it could have affected the outcomes under the sham tDCS phase due to possible carryover effects of tDCS stimulation; therefore, it could have also disguised the sham effect we originally aimed to compare with real tDCS. This could have given rise to a second limitation during the last baseline A, either due to a training effect of the CS or a carryover effect of the tDCS administration in phase C, which cannot be separated for interpretation. This is a disadvantage of using an SSD in cognitive studies. We intended to monitor daily response in behavioral terms to different treatments, but the frequency of the application of CS in some of the participants in such a short period made it problematic to decouple what participants might have achieved by continued testing from what was changed by tDCS.

For the same reason, our original intention was to observe whether the CS outcomes could match the cognitive assessment score in every condition. To check this possibility, we administered a battery of assessments five times over a four-week interval, which might provide a learning effect and reduce overinterpreting the CS task outcomes by making a linkage with the standardized cognitive evaluations, and alternative forms of cognitive assessments to measure changes over time should be used.

Despite the limitations of this pilot study, it is essential to conduct pilot studies with NIBS techniques before the implementation of larger trials. The strength of this study allow us to monitor the daily cognitive response of single or coupling therapies gathering valuable data that can shape a future robust intervention. The ultimate purpose of using NIBS is to prove if it can be used as a feasible nonpharmacological therapy in couple with conventional treatment, in this case computer CS, for older adults with MCI. The emerging application of tDCS as a therapeutic intervention gives us the obligation of conducting studies to develop treatment programmes which can support evidence base and determine the future use of these innovative techniques in the field of cognitive rehabilitation.

5. Conclusion

The current study investigated the effects of anodal tDCS on CS in older adults with MCI and found mild beneficial effects on processing speed, selective attention, planning ability, and working memory which were better than those achieved by CS alone or by sham tDCS. The optimal frequency of tDCS administration remains unclear.

Further research is required to improve understanding of the neuromechanism and to determine the behavioral effects of tDCS on CS in a larger multicentered, randomized controlled study to determine the possibility of transferability to everyday cognition.

Acknowledgments

The authors thank Peggy Ma and Eileen Wang for their assessment of participants.

References

[1] R. C. Petersen, G. E. Smith, S. C. Waring, R. J. Ivnik, E. G. Tangalos, and E. Kokmen, "Mild cognitive impairment," *Archives of Neurology*, vol. 56, no. 3, pp. 303–308, 1999.

[2] S. Gauthier, B. Reisberg, M. Zaudig et al., "Mild cognitive impairment," *The Lancet*, vol. 367, no. 9518, pp. 1262–1270, 2006.

[3] K. M. Langa and D. A. Levine, "The diagnosis and management of mild cognitive impairment," *JAMA*, vol. 312, no. 23, pp. 2551–2561, 2014.

[4] M. M. Sohlberg and C. A. Mateer, "Training use of compensatory memory books: a three stage behavioral approach," *Journal of Clinical and Experimental Neuropsychology*, vol. 11, no. 6, pp. 871–891, 1989.

[5] K. Ball, D. B. Berch, K. F. Helmers et al., "Effects of cognitive training interventions with older adults," *JAMA*, vol. 288, no. 18, pp. 2271–2281, 2002.

[6] N. T. M. Hill, L. Mowszowski, S. L. Naismith, V. L. Chadwick, M. Valenzuela, and A. Lampit, "Computerized cognitive training in older adults with mild cognitive impairment or dementia: a systematic review and meta-analysis," *The American Journal of Psychiatry*, vol. 174, no. 4, pp. 329–340, 2017.

[7] A. L. Faria, A. Andrade, L. Soares, and S. B. i Badia, "Benefits of virtual reality based cognitive rehabilitation through simulated activities of daily living: a randomized controlled trial with stroke patients," *Journal of NeuroEngineering and Rehabilitation*, vol. 13, no. 1, p. 96, 2016.

[8] M. Finn and S. McDonald, "Computerised cognitive training for older persons with mild cognitive impairment: a pilot study using a randomised controlled trial design," *Brain Impairment*, vol. 12, no. 3, pp. 187–199, 2011.

[9] J. Olazarán, B. Reisberg, L. Clare et al., "Nonpharmacological therapies in Alzheimer's disease: a systematic review of efficacy," *Dementia and Geriatric Cognitive Disorders*, vol. 30, no. 2, pp. 161–178, 2010.

[10] M. A. Nitsche, L. G. Cohen, E. M. Wassermann et al., "Transcranial direct current stimulation: state of the art 2008," *Brain Stimulation*, vol. 1, no. 3, pp. 206–223, 2008.

[11] P. Nasseri, M. A. Nitsche, and H. Ekhtiari, "A framework for categorizing electrode montages in transcranial direct current stimulation," *Frontiers in Human Neuroscience*, vol. 9, p. 54, 2015.

[12] B. Hauptmann and A. Karni, "From primed to learn: the saturation of repetition priming and the induction of long-term memory," *Cognitive Brain Research*, vol. 13, no. 3, pp. 313–322, 2002.

[13] M. E. Stoykov and S. Madhavan, "Motor priming in neurorehabilitation," *Journal of Neurologic Physical Therapy*, vol. 39, no. 1, pp. 33–42, 2015.

[14] M. A. Nitsche, A. Antal, D. Liebetanz, N. Lang, F. Tergau, and W. Paulus, "Induction and modulation of neuroplasticity by

transcranial direct current stimulation," in *Transcranial Brain Stimulation for Treatment of Psychiatric Disorders*, M. A. Marcolin and F. Padberg, Eds., vol. 23, Karger, Basel, 2007.

[15] A. Birba, A. Ibáñez, L. Sedeño, J. Ferrari, A. M. García, and M. Zimerman, "Non-invasive brain stimulation: a new strategy in mild cognitive impairment?," *Frontiers in Aging Neuroscience*, vol. 9, p. 16, 2017.

[16] C. Miniussi, J. A. Harris, and M. Ruzzoli, "Modelling non-invasive brain stimulation in cognitive neuroscience," *Neuroscience & Biobehavioral Reviews*, vol. 37, no. 8, pp. 1702–1712, 2013.

[17] T. Ditye, L. Jacobson, V. Walsh, and M. Lavidor, "Modulating behavioral inhibition by tDCS combined with cognitive training," *Experimental Brain Research*, vol. 219, no. 3, pp. 363–368, 2012.

[18] F. Fregni, P. S. Boggio, M. Nitsche et al., "Anodal transcranial direct current stimulation of prefrontal cortex enhances working memory," *Experimental Brain Research*, vol. 166, no. 1, pp. 23–30, 2005.

[19] A. Flöel, W. Suttorp, O. Kohl et al., "Non-invasive brain stimulation improves object-location learning in the elderly," *Neurobiology of Aging*, vol. 33, no. 8, pp. 1682–1689, 2012.

[20] D. M. Martin, R. Liu, A. Alonzo et al., "Can transcranial direct current stimulation enhance outcomes from cognitive training? A randomized controlled trial in healthy participants," *International Journal of Neuropsychopharmacology*, vol. 16, no. 9, pp. 1927–1936, 2013.

[21] P. S. Boggio, L. P. Khoury, D. C. S. Martins, O. E. M. S. Martins, E. C. de Macedo, and F. Fregni, "Temporal cortex direct current stimulation enhances performance on a visual recognition memory task in Alzheimer disease," *Journal of Neurology, Neurosurgery & Psychiatry*, vol. 80, no. 4, pp. 444–447, 2009.

[22] P. S. Boggio, R. Ferrucci, F. Mameli et al., "Prolonged visual memory enhancement after direct current stimulation in Alzheimer's disease," *Brain Stimulation*, vol. 5, no. 3, pp. 223–230, 2012.

[23] S. André, S. Heinrich, F. Kayser et al., "At-home tDCS of the left dorsolateral prefrontal cortex improves visual short-term memory in mild vascular dementia," *Journal of the Neurological Sciences*, vol. 369, pp. 185–190, 2016.

[24] M. Meinzer, R. Lindenberg, M. T. Phan, L. Ulm, C. Volk, and A. Flöel, "Transcranial direct current stimulation in mild cognitive impairment: behavioral effects and neural mechanisms," *Alzheimer's & Dementia*, vol. 11, no. 9, pp. 1032–1040, 2015.

[25] F. Portet, P. Ousset, P. Visser, G. Frisoni, and the MCI Working Group of the European Consortium on Alzheimer's Disease (EADC), "Mild cognitive impairment (MCI) in medical practice: a critical review of the concept and new diagnostic procedure. Report of the MCI Working Group of the European Consortium on Alzheimer's Disease," *Journal of Neurology, Neurosurgery, and Psychiatry*, vol. 77, no. 6, pp. 714–718, 2006.

[26] Z. S. Nasreddine, N. A. Phillips, V. Bédirian et al., "The Montreal Cognitive Assessment, MoCA: a brief screening tool for mild cognitive impairment," *Journal of the American Geriatrics Society*, vol. 53, no. 4, pp. 695–699, 2005.

[27] J. Morris, "The Clinical Dementia Rating (CDR): current version and scoring rules," *Neurology*, vol. 43, no. 11, pp. 2412–2414, 1993.

[28] P. P. J. Lim, L. L. Ng, P. C. Chiam, P. S. Ong, F. T.-S. Ngui, and S. Sahadevan, "Validation and comparison of three brief depression scales in an elderly Chinese population," *International Journal of Geriatric Psychiatry*, vol. 15, no. 9, pp. 824–830, 2000.

[29] I. F. de Piérola, "Neuronup's next step: structured and clinically validated programs," *II International Workshop on Gamification in Health*, 2015, gHealth, http://ceur-ws.org/Vol-1547/paper5.pdf.

[30] S. Tremblay, J.-F. Lepage, A. Latulipe-Loiselle, F. Fregni, A. Pascual-Leone, and H. Théoret, "The uncertain outcome of prefrontal tDCS," *Brain Stimulation*, vol. 7, no. 6, pp. 773–783, 2014.

[31] P. Liang, Z. Wang, Y. Yang, X. Jia, and K. Li, "Functional disconnection and compensation in mild cognitive impairment: evidence from DLPFC connectivity using resting-state fMRI," *PLoS One*, vol. 6, no. 7, article e22153, 2011.

[32] A. S. Chan, A. Choi, H. Chiu, and L. Lam, "Clinical validity of the Chinese version of Mattis dementia rating scale in differentiating dementia of Alzheimer's type in Hong Kong," *Journal of the International Neuropsychological Society*, vol. 9, no. 1, pp. 45–55, 2003.

[33] A. Lam, C. W. Lam, and K. W. Boey, "The psychological well-being of elderly persons living in old urban areas of Hong Kong: a social perspective," *Citation Aging & Mental Health*, vol. 9, no. 2, pp. 162–166, 2005.

[34] A. Wong, Y. Y. Xiong, P. W. L. Kwan et al., "The validity, reliability and clinical utility of the Hong Kong Montreal cognitive assessment (HK-MoCA) in patients with cerebral small vessel disease," *Dementia and Geriatric Cognitive Disorders*, vol. 28, no. 1, pp. 81–87, 2009.

[35] D. Wechsler and M. De Lemos, *Wechsler Adult Intelligence Scale-Revised*, Australian Council for Educational Research Limited, Australia, 1981.

[36] L. Lu and E. D. Bigler, "Normative data on trail making test for neurologically normal, Chinese-speaking adults," *Applied Neuropsychology*, vol. 9, no. 4, pp. 219–225, 2002.

[37] A. Rubin and E. R. Babbie, *Research Methods for Social Work*, Brooks Cole Publishing Co., Pacific Grove, CA, USA, 2nd edition, 1993.

[38] S. H. Ohn, C.-I. Park, W.-K. Yoo et al., "Time-dependent effect of transcranial direct current stimulation on the enhancement of working memory," *NeuroReport*, vol. 19, no. 1, pp. 43–47, 2008.

[39] M. Cotelli, R. Manenti, M. Brambilla et al., "Anodal tDCS during face-name associations memory training in Alzheimer's patients," *Frontiers in Aging Neuroscience*, vol. 6, p. 38, 2014.

[40] A. R. Brunoni, M. A. Nitsche, N. Bolognini et al., "Clinical research with transcranial direct current stimulation (tDCS): challenges and future directions," *Brain Stimulation*, vol. 5, no. 3, pp. 175–195, 2012.

[41] T. A. Salthouse, "What cognitive abilities are involved in trail-making performance?," *Intelligence*, vol. 39, no. 4, pp. 222–232, 2011.

[42] J. M. Spikman, H. A. L. Kiers, B. G. Deelman, and A. H. van Zomeren, "Construct validity of concepts of attention in healthy controls and patients with CHI," *Brain and Cognition*, vol. 47, no. 3, pp. 446–460, 2001.

Biochanin A Reduces Inflammatory Injury and Neuronal Apoptosis following Subarachnoid Hemorrhage via Suppression of the TLRs/TIRAP/MyD88/NF-κB Pathway

Ling-yun Wu,[1] Zhen-nan Ye,[2,3] Zong Zhuang,[1] Yongyue Gao,[1] Chao Tang,[1] Chen-hui Zhou,[1] Chun-xi Wang,[1] Xiang-sheng Zhang,[1] Guang-bin Xie,[1] Jing-peng Liu,[3] Meng-liang Zhou,[1] Chun-hua Hang,[1,3] and Ji-xin Shi[1]

[1]*Department of Neurosurgery, Jinling Hospital, School of Medicine, Nanjing University, 305 East ZhongShan Road, Nanjing, Jiangsu Province 210002, China*
[2]*Department of Neurosurgery, the Second Affiliated Hospital of Guangzhou Medical University, Guangzhou, Guangdong Province 510260, China*
[3]*Department of Neurosurgery, Jinling Hospital, School of Medicine, Southern Medical University (Guangzhou), Nanjing, Jiangsu Province 210002, China*

Correspondence should be addressed to Chun-hua Hang; hang_neurosurgery@163.com and Ji-xin Shi; shijx52@hotmail.com

Academic Editor: Hailiang Tang

Inflammatory injury and neuronal apoptosis participate in the period of early brain injury (EBI) after subarachnoid hemorrhage (SAH). Suppression of inflammation has recently been shown to reduce neuronal death and neurobehavioral dysfunction post SAH. Biochanin A (BCA), a natural bioactive isoflavonoid, has been confirmed to emerge the anti-inflammatory pharmacological function. This original study was aimed at evaluating and identifying the neuroprotective role of BCA and the underlying molecular mechanism in an experimental Sprague-Dawley rat SAH model. Neurobehavioral function was evaluated via the modified water maze test and modified Garcia neurologic score system. Thus, we confirmed that BCA markedly decreased the activated level of TLRs/TIRAP/MyD88/NF-κB pathway and the production of cytokines. BCA also significantly ameliorated neuronal apoptosis which correlated with the improvement of neurobehavioral dysfunction post SAH. These results indicated that BCA may provide neuroprotection against EBI through the inhibition of inflammatory injury and neuronal apoptosis partially via the TLRs/TIRAP/MyD88/NF-κB signal pathway.

1. Introduction

Subarachnoid hemorrhage (SAH) is known as an acute catastrophic neurological disease with a high rate of perioperative mortality and permanent morbidity worldwide. Currently, at least a quarter of SAH patients pass away instantly and more than half of SAH survivors endure the pain of the severe long-term neurological deficits [1]. Recent basic and clinical studies have focused on the pathologic mechanism that occurs in the period from 0 h to 72 h post SAH, often known as early brain injury (EBI), the most crucial and etiological factor of poor clinical prognosis among SAH cases [2]. In recent years, excessive inflammatory activity and neuronal apoptosis post SAH have been found in clinical cases and animal experiments [3]. In addition, the degree of secondary inflammatory injury and severe neuronal apoptosis correlates with the progress of SAH, and many previous studies implicated that the uncontrolled inflammatory response and neuronal apoptosis may aggravate EBI post SAH [4].

Biochanin A (BCA), an organic isoflavone derived from natural plant sources, has been classified as a special phytoestrogen [5–7]. BCA has exhibited various beneficial bioactivities, such as antidiabetic, anticancer, antiallergic, and

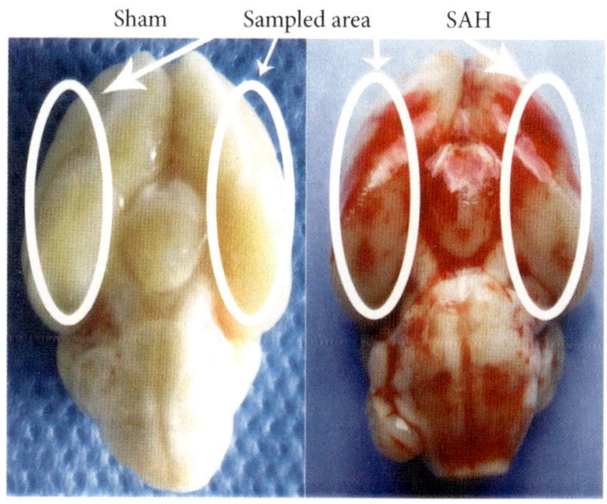

FIGURE 1: Sample collection location and rat SAH model.

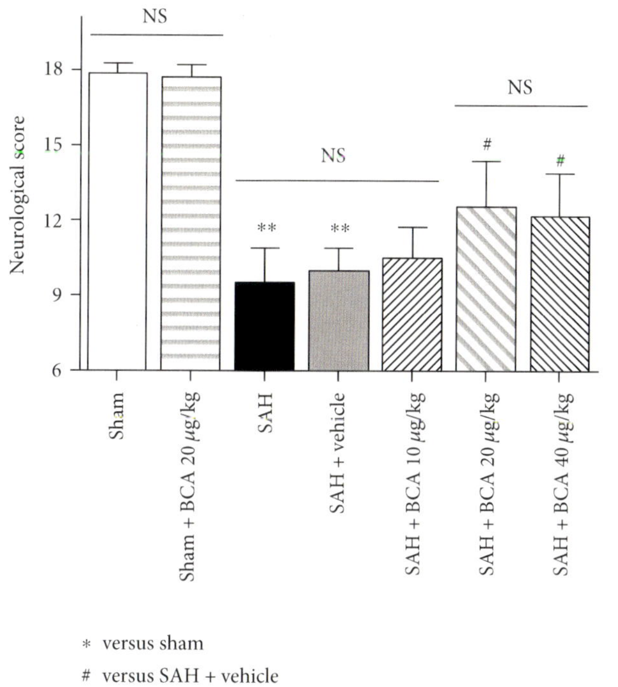

FIGURE 2: The effects of BCA on neurological function at 24-hour post-SAH rats and sham rats. ($n = 6$, each group; $^{**}P < 0.01$ versus sham; $^{\#}P < 0.05$ versus SAH + vehicle; $^{NS}P > 0.05$).

anti-inflammatory effects [8]. Recent studies demonstrated that BCA can provide affirmative neuroprotection against the cerebral ischemia/reperfusion-induced injury [9]. In addition, BCA attenuates lipopolysaccharide (a TLR-mediated pathway agonist, LPS)-induced inflammatory response and the transcription of NF-κB [10–14]. Moreover, we have previously found that TLR/NF-κB pathway-mediated inflammatory response and neuronal apoptosis participate in the EBI period post SAH [15, 16]. However, the neuroprotective role of BCA in EBI has not been studied so far. Above all, all these extend naturally to our hypothesis that BCA administration may provide neuroprotection via inhibiting the TLR/TIRAP/MyD88/NF-κB-related inflammation and reducing neuronal apoptosis after SAH in rats.

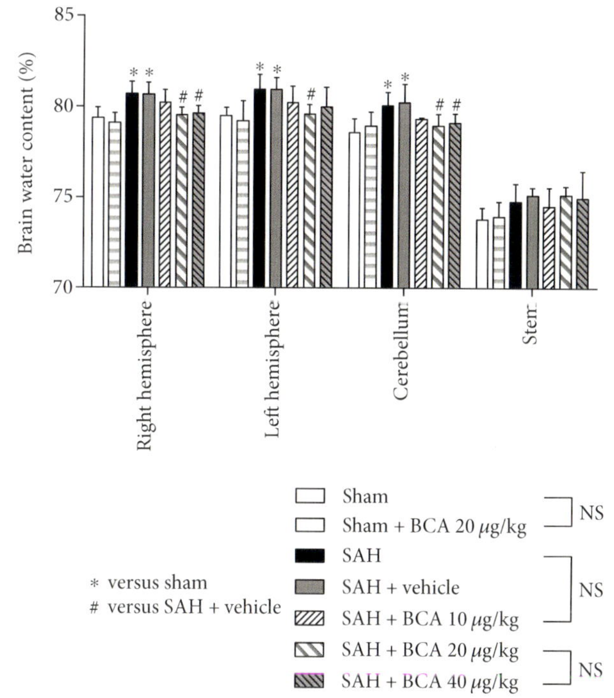

FIGURE 3: The effects of BCA on the brain water content levels in the left hemisphere, right hemisphere, cerebellum, and brain stem at 24 h post SAH ($n = 6$, each group; $^{*}P < 0.05$ versus sham; $^{\#}P < 0.05$ versus SAH + vehicle; $^{NS}P > 0.05$).

2. Methods

2.1. Experimental Sprague-Dawley Rats and BCA Administration. Experimental Sprague-Dawley rats (weighted 300 ± 20 g) were obtained from the experimental management animal center of Nanjing University, Jiangsu, China. All Sprague-Dawley rats were maintained under standard animal laboratory circumstances for one week before the experimental protocols. BCA powder reagent was obtained from Sigma Chemicals, USA, and dissolved in dimethyl sulfoxide (DMSO, as a vehicle, final concentration: 0.5% DMSO in 0.9% normal saline). BCA was given intracerebroventricular injection to rats at 1 h after the induction of SAH at a dosage of 10 μg/kg, 20 μg/kg, and 40 μg/kg.

All the experimental protocols including animal drug administration and animal surgical procedures were approved by the Institutional Animal Care and Use Committee of Nanjing University (Jinling Hospital) and were consistent with the guidelines for the Care and Use of Laboratory Animals by National Institutes of Health (China).

2.2. Rat SAH Model. We used prechiasmatic interspace injection (300 μl per rat) to build this rat SAH model according to our previous study [17]. In addition, 300 μl normal saline solution was given to the sham group. Rats that died during the experimental period were abandoned, and we wound repeated the surgery to make sure every group could get the planned sample size number.

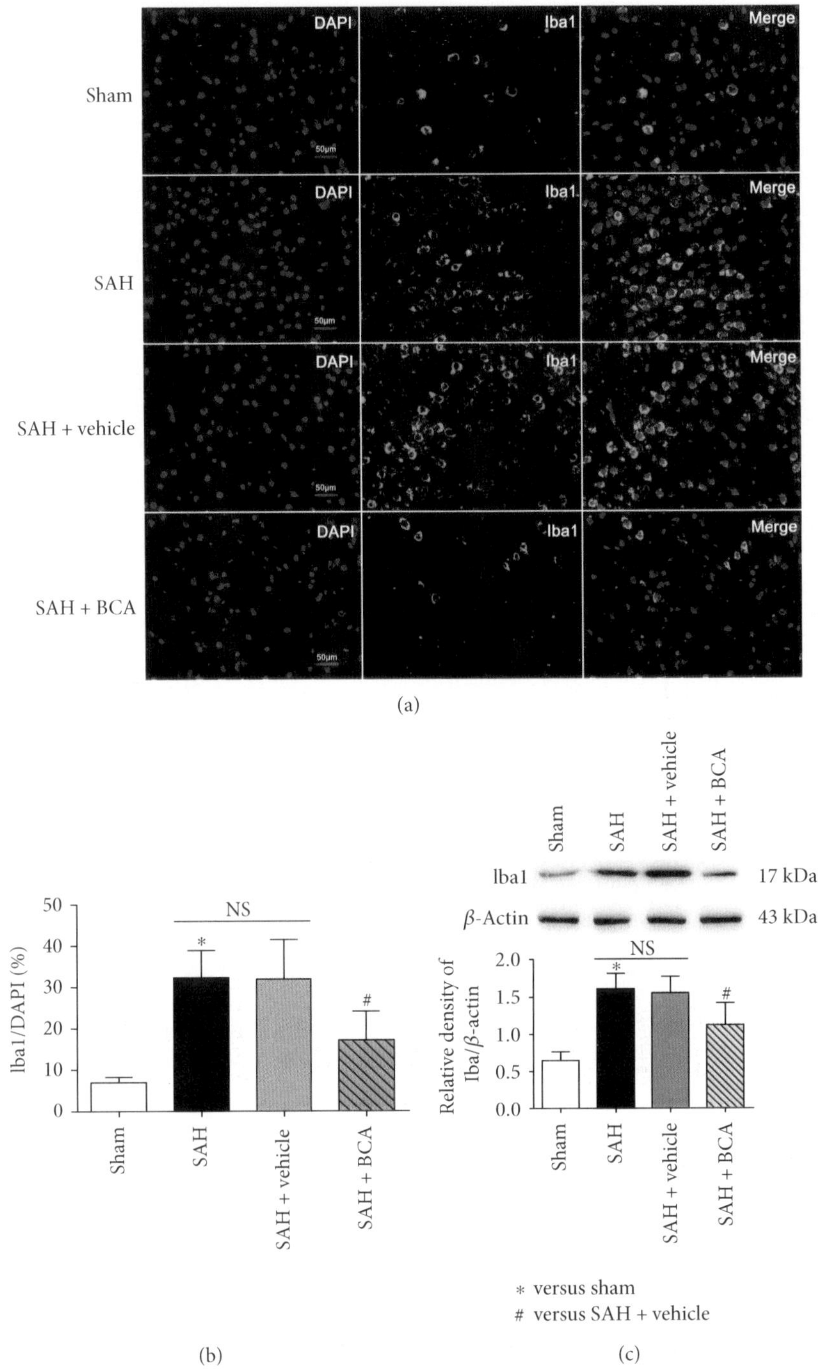

FIGURE 4: The effects of BCA on microglial activation at 24 h post SAH. (a, b) Immunofluorescence staining: Iba1 = green, DAPI = blue, scale bars = 50 μm. (c) Western blot analysis.($n = 6$, each group; $^{*}P < 0.05$, versus sham; $^{\#}P < 0.05$ versus SAH + vehicle; $^{NS}P > 0.05$).

2.3. Experimental Design and Tissue Preparation Time Point. A total 172 of rats were divided into 7 groups randomly as follows: sham group ($n = 32$), sham + BCA 20 μg/kg group ($n = 20$), SAH group ($n = 32$), SAH + vehicle group ($n = 32$), SAH + BCA 10 μg/kg group ($n = 12$), SAH + BCA 20 μg/kg group ($n = 32$), and SAH + BCA 40 μg/kg group ($n = 12$). According to the results from previous studies on SAH-induced inflammation and neuronal apoptosis, we choose the 24 h after SAH for sample collection [18, 19]. Respectively, 132 rats in the abovementioned groups were euthanized for sample tissue preparation, sample obtained location, and tissue preparation method according to our previous study [16] (Figure 1). The left rats in part of groups were prepared to do the modified water maze test.

2.4. Brain Water Content. Left hemisphere brain tissue, right hemisphere brain tissue, cerebellum tissue, and brain stem tissue from rat brain tissue were dried in 100°C for three days to get the brain dry weight data after weighing for wet data. [16].

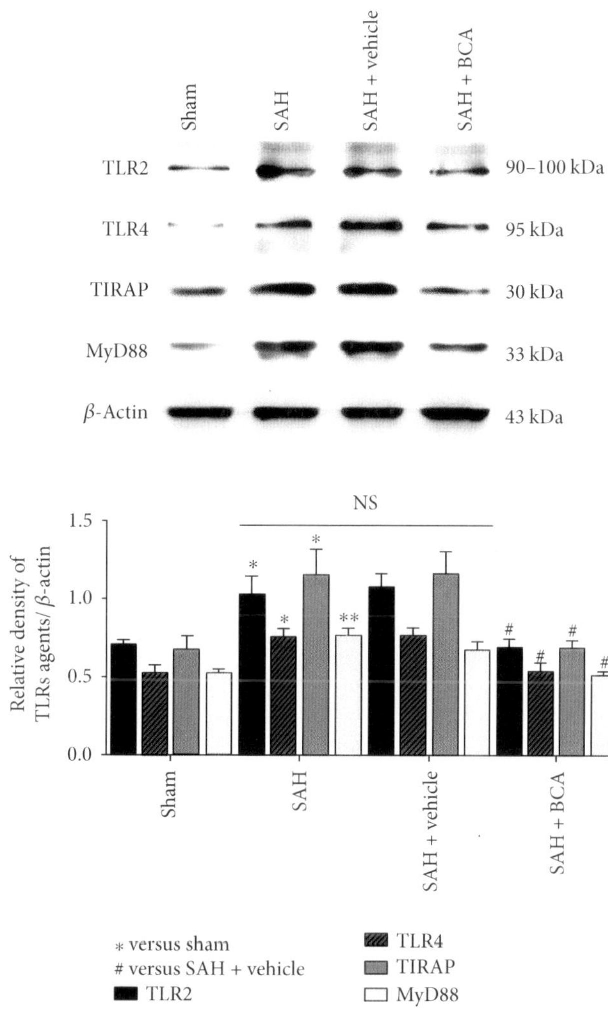

FIGURE 5: The effects of BCA on TLR2/TLR4/TIRAP/Myd88 signal protein expression at 24 hours post SAH ($n = 6$, each group; $^{*}P < 0.05$ and $^{**}P < 0.01$ versus sham; $^{\#}P < 0.05$ versus SAH + vehicle; $^{NS}P > 0.05$).

2.5. Western Blot Reagent. Primary antibodies were as follows: myeloid differentiation factor 88 (MyD88, Santa Cruz, USA, 1 : 200–1 : 400), TIR domain-containing adaptor protein (TIRAP, Abcam, USA, 1 : 1000), TLR4 (Santa Cruz, USA, 1 : 200–1 : 400), TLR2 (Santa Cruz, USA, 1 : 200–1 : 400), Iba1 (anti-IBA, ab15690, Abcam, USA, 1 : 500, active microglial marker), NF-κB P65 (Santa Cruz, USA, 1 : 200–1 : 400), Bax (Santa Cruz, USA, 1 : 200–1 : 400), Bcl-2 (Santa Cruz, USA, 1 : 200–1 : 400), caspase-3 (Bioss, Beijing, China, 1 : 100–1 : 500). Histone 3 (anti-H3, ab1791, Abcam, USA, 1 : 1000, nuclear loading control) and β-actin (1 : 5000, Bioworld Technology, USA) were used as a loading control in nuclear protein and total protein. After conjunction with the HRP-secondary antibody (1 : 1000, Bioworld Technology, USA), the target protein bands were visualized and recorded by Tanon-5200 Chemiluminescent Imaging System [20].

2.6. Enzyme-Linked Immunosorbent Assay (ELISA) and Electrophoretic Mobility Shift Assay (EMSA). The ELISA assay kit system for rats (Affymetrix eBioscience, Santa Clara, USA) was used to evaluate the concentration of TLR downstream productive cytokines in a total protein sample [16]. The EMSA Assay kit System (Affymetrix eBioscience, Santa Clara, USA) was used to evaluate the degree of NF-κB/DNA-combining activity [16].

2.7. TUNEL Immunofluorescence Staining. Immunofluorescence (IF) staining was operated to detect the TUNEL-positive neurons (anti-NeuN, Alexa Fluor® 488 conjugated, Millipore, USA, 1 : 100) and the immunoreactivity of Iba1 (anti-IBA, ab15690, Abcam, USA, 1 : 100, active microglial marker) [21]. Apoptosis was determined by TUNEL detection kit (TMR red immunofluorescence staining kit from Sigma-Aldrich, MO, USA). Positive-cell counting and statistical analysis were restricted to our previous study [22]. The percentage of TUNEL-positive cells was calculated as follows: (number of TUNEL − positive neurons/total number of neurons) × 100%.

2.8. Neurologic Scoring and Spatial Learning and Cognitive Memory Testing. We used the modified Garcia score system to assess the rats' neurological changes according to our previous study [23]. Spatial learning and cognitive memory ability were assessed via a modified water maze test

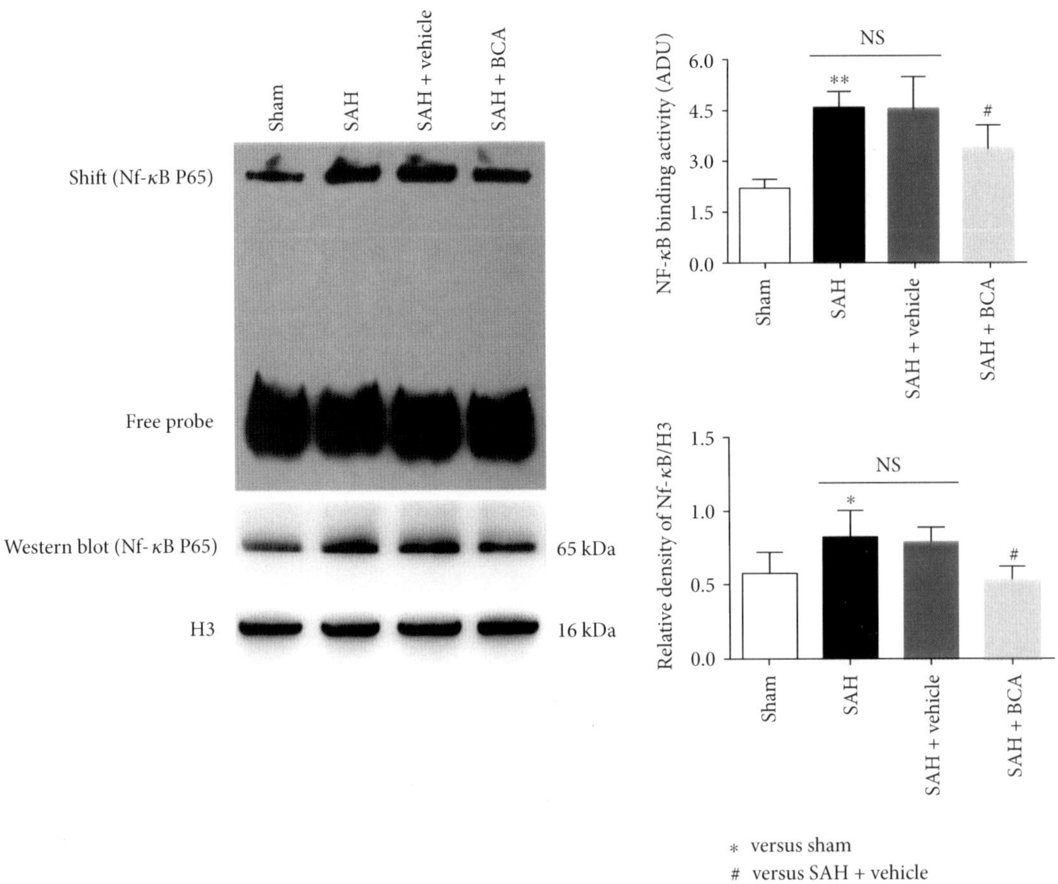

FIGURE 6: BCA administration suppressed NF-κB/DNA-combining activation and the nuclear level of NF-κB p65 at 24 hours post SAH ($n = 6$, each group; $^{*}P < 0.05$ versus sham; $^{**}P < 0.01$ versus sham; $^{\#}P < 0.05$ versus SAH + vehicle; $^{NS}P > 0.05$).

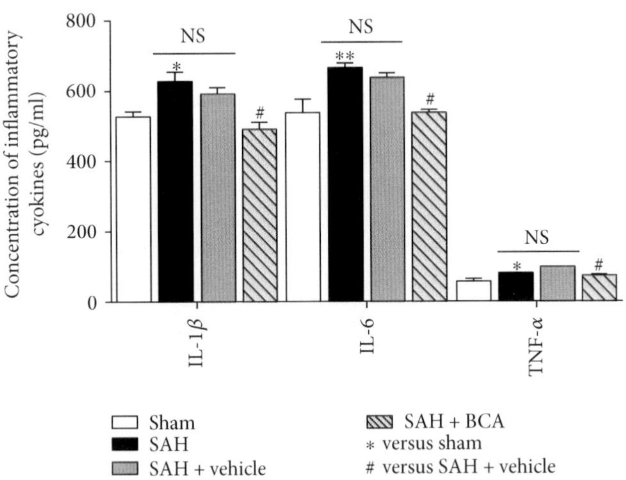

FIGURE 7: The effects of BCA on the concentrations of inflammatory cytokines at 24 hours post SAH ($n = 6$, each group; $^{*}P < 0.05$ and $^{**}P < 0.01$ versus sham; $^{\#}P < 0.05$ versus SAH + vehicle; $^{NS}P > 0.05$).

[16]. Data from the modified water maze test were as follows: escape latencies (s, time data and average data) and swimming distance (cm, distance data and average data) in every test trail for the rats to get on the hidden platform in the water maze [24].

2.9. Statistical Analysis. All the experimental data in this study was presented as mean value ± SD score. SPSS 19.0 was used for statistical analysis and calculation. All the data was subjected to one-way ANOVA comparison test. Values of $^{*}p$ and $^{\#}p < 0.05$ were considered data statistically significant.

3. Results

3.1. General Mortality and Sample Collection Location. The total rate of mortality in the sham group was 0% (0/32 rats), that in the sham + BCA group was 0% (0/20), and that in the SAH-processed group was 21.57% (33/153 rats). As shown in Figure 1, we collected samples at the locations shown in Figure 1 in each group at 24 h after the establishment of SAH for the further bimolecular analyses performed.

3.2. BCA Improves the Rats' Neurological Score and Reduces Cerebral Hemisphere and Cerebellum Edema at 24 h Post SAH. In this part, modified Garcia score and rats' right and left hemisphere, cerebellum, and stem water content were recorded and evaluated. As shown in Figures 2 and 3, treatment with BCA at 20 μg/kg and 40 μg/kg both improved the modified Garcia score and reduced cerebral hemisphere and cerebellum edema at 24 hours post SAH. However, the higher dose (40 μg/kg) did not bring a better therapeutic effect than the dose at 20 μg/kg did. Meanwhile, BCA at

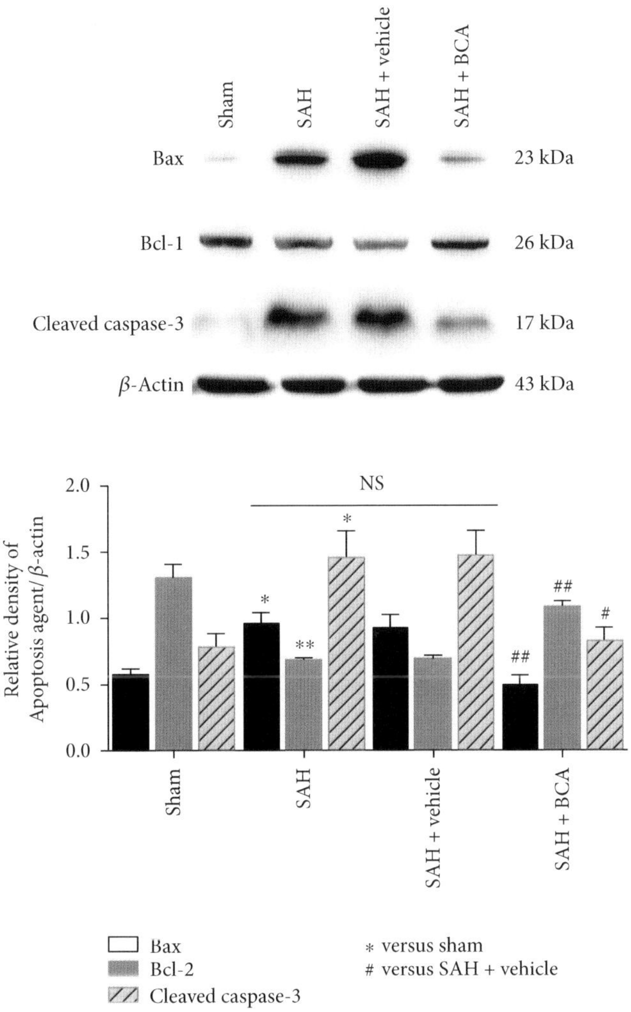

FIGURE 8: BCA administration suppressed the apoptotic process at 24 hours post SAH ($n = 6$, each group; $^{*}P < 0.05$ and $^{**}P < 0.01$ versus sham; $^{\#}P < 0.05$ and $^{\#\#}P < 0.01$ versus SAH + vehicle; $^{NS}P > 0.05$).

20 μg/kg did not produce the side effect of neurological toxicity on sham rats. Therefore, 20 μg/kg was selected as the best treatment dose for the further mechanism study and spatial learning/cognitive memory test.

3.3. BCA Reduced the Cell Number of Active Microglia at 24 Hours Post SAH. We use the ionized calcium-binding adaptor molecule 1 (Iba-1) as the marker of activated microglia; the percent of Iba-1-positive microglia increased after the SAH operative process. BCA administration at 20 μg/kg reduced the percentage of active microglia which demonstrated its potential anti-inflammatory effects in this SAH model study. The percentage was calculated as follows: (number of Iba1 − positive microglia/total number of DAPI) × 100% (Figure 4).

3.4. BCA Suppressed the Levels of TLR2/TLR4/TIRAP/MyD88 Pathway Protein and NF-κB/DNA-Combining Activity at 24 Hours Post SAH. The pathway-related proteins were suppressed via the administration of BCA versus vehicle treatment rats at 24 hours post SAH (Figure 5, Western blot). Lower DNA-combining activity and lower nuclear transfer of NF-κB were found in the SAH + BCA group versus vehicle treatment rats at 24 hours post SAH (Figure 6, EMSA).

3.5. BCA Decreases the Cytokine Release in Rats' Brain at 24 Hours Post SAH. According to the results of ELISA, with the administration of BCA, the concentrations of inflammation-related cytokines in rats' brain tissue were lower than in the vehicle treatment group in this study. This is obviously the certain consequence of inhibition of NF-κB transcription-related cytokine release (Figure 7).

3.6. BCA Modulated the Apoptosis-Related Functional Proteins and Reduced the Percent of Neuronal Apoptotic Death at 24 Hours Post SAH. BCA treatment downregulated the levels of Bax (proapoptosis) and cleaved caspase-3 (proapoptosis) and upregulated the expression of Bcl-2 (antiapoptosis) versus the vehicle treatment group (Figure 8). As a consequence, the percentage of TUNEL (red)-positive neurons (green) in the BCA treatment group reduced to less than 40% versus more than 40% in vehicle treatment rats (Figure 9).

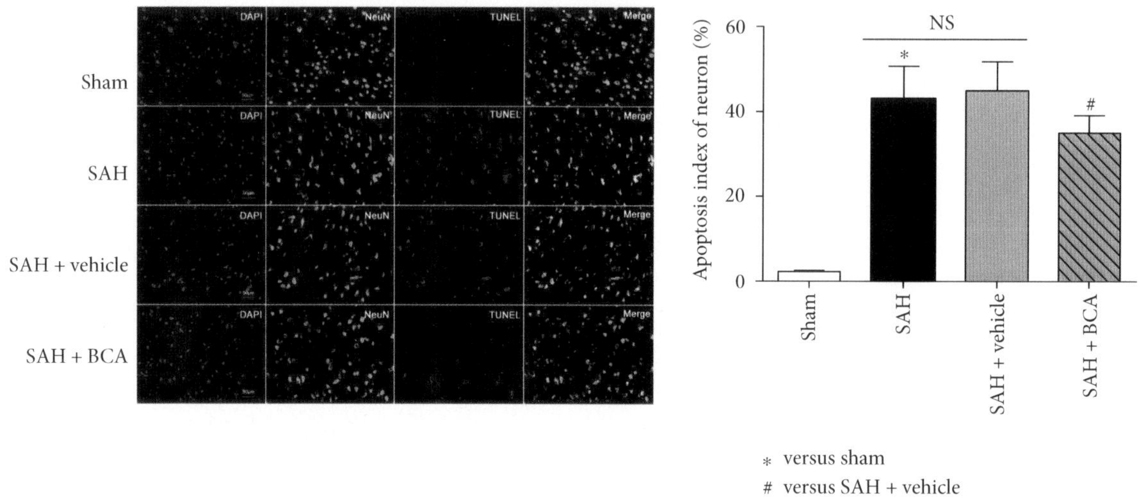

FIGURE 9: BCA attenuates the level of TUNEL-positive neurons at 24 hours post SAH. (TUNEL = red, NeuN = green, DAPI = blue, scale bars 50 μm $n = 6$, each group; $^{*}P < 0.05$ versus sham; $^{\#}P < 0.05$ versus SAH + vehicle; $^{NS}P > 0.05$).

3.7. BCA Improved SAH Rats' Spatial Learning and Cognitive Memory Dysfunction. In the Morris water maze test, each rat was tested for 4 trials/day from day 2 to day 5 after the induction of SAH (Figures 10(a)–10(d)). Data analysis indicated that SAH rats exhibited severe spatial learning and cognitive memory dysfunction; many experiment objects in the SAH group showed a blind search movement during the 4-day test. What is surprising is that BCA treatment facilitated SAH rats to get the hidden platform in a shorter time period and path distance versus the vehicle group (Figures 10(a) and 10(c)). The averaged data showed the same phenomenon of improvement (Figures 10(b) and 10(d)) via BCA treatment versus the vehicle treatment group. In summary, BCA improved rats' spatial learning and cognitive memory dysfunction after SAH and exhibited no side effects on sham rats.

4. Discussion

BCA has been considered an anti-inflammatory, antioxidative, and antiproliferative compound in many previous studies [5, 25–27]. According to our results, we found that the dosage at 20 μg/kg and 40 μg/kg BCA improved the neurological dysfunction and ameliorated cerebral edema post SAH. A further increase in the dosage may exceed the ability of the cerebrospinal fluid to deliver the drug, which led to no better therapeutic effect at a higher dosage (40 μg/kg). Therefore, we selected 20 μg/kg as the best effective therapeutic concentration in CSF for treatment. A more reasonable route of administration and time window for treatment is still worthy of further exploration. In addition, BCA at 20 μg/kg did not have an effect on sham rats in brain water content, neurological function scores, and spatial learning and cognitive memory ability. These data suggested that BCA might serve as one ideal therapeutic medicine for SAH treatment without apparent side effects.

The toll-like receptor (TLR) family owns the responsibility of initiating innate immunity response including inflammatory response in the stress status [28]. In addition, MyD88 and TIRAP act as binding proteins among TLR-mediated immunity response activity cases [29–31]. TLRs, MyD88, and TIRAP form a complex network structure of the TLR-mediated inflammatory cascade. When SAH occurred and blood flowed into the subarachnoid space, the cleavage products released from cracked blood cells (especially red blood cells) could lead to the activation of a TLR/MyD88/TIRAP signal complex so-called pathogens, which could initiate inflammatory cascade response and then damage neurons and other functional cells [32, 33]. In addition, the nuclear factor NF-κB, as the most important downstream transcription factor following the TLR-mediated signal complex, was closely associated with the release of cytokines [34]. Moreover, in inflammatory injury cases, an acute excess production or release of inflammatory cytokines could exert potential harmful effects on the tissue system [35]. According to our previous studies, inhibiting the TLR/NF-κB cascade pathway could show therapeutic effects on EBI following SAH, which means that the TLR4/NF-κB pathway could be an important therapeutic target in SAH treatment [36]. In this SAH model research, we confirmed our hypothesis that BCA inhibited the expression of TLR2/4/MyD88/TIRAP/NF-κB signal axis protein and reduced the production and release of cytokines post SAH. It is noteworthy that the inhibitory effect of BCA on the TLR/NF-κB pathway is consistent with its antineuronal apoptosis and anti-TLR-mediated-inflammatory effect and therapeutic effect on neurological dysfunction. Furthermore, BCA relieved the severity of brain edema, rendering that the role of BCA in blood-brain barrier functional protection is worthy of further study. Our study results revealed that BCA inhibited the TLR/MyD88/TIRAP/NF-κB-signaling pathway while alleviating EBI, suggesting that suppression of the TLR/MyD88/TIRAP/NF-κB-signaling pathway at least may be one of the mechanisms under its therapeutic effect.

According to published clinical research, nearly more than half of SAH survivors have suffered cognitive awareness dysfunction and neurological disorder [37]. In the present study, rats suffering experimental SAH showed apparent

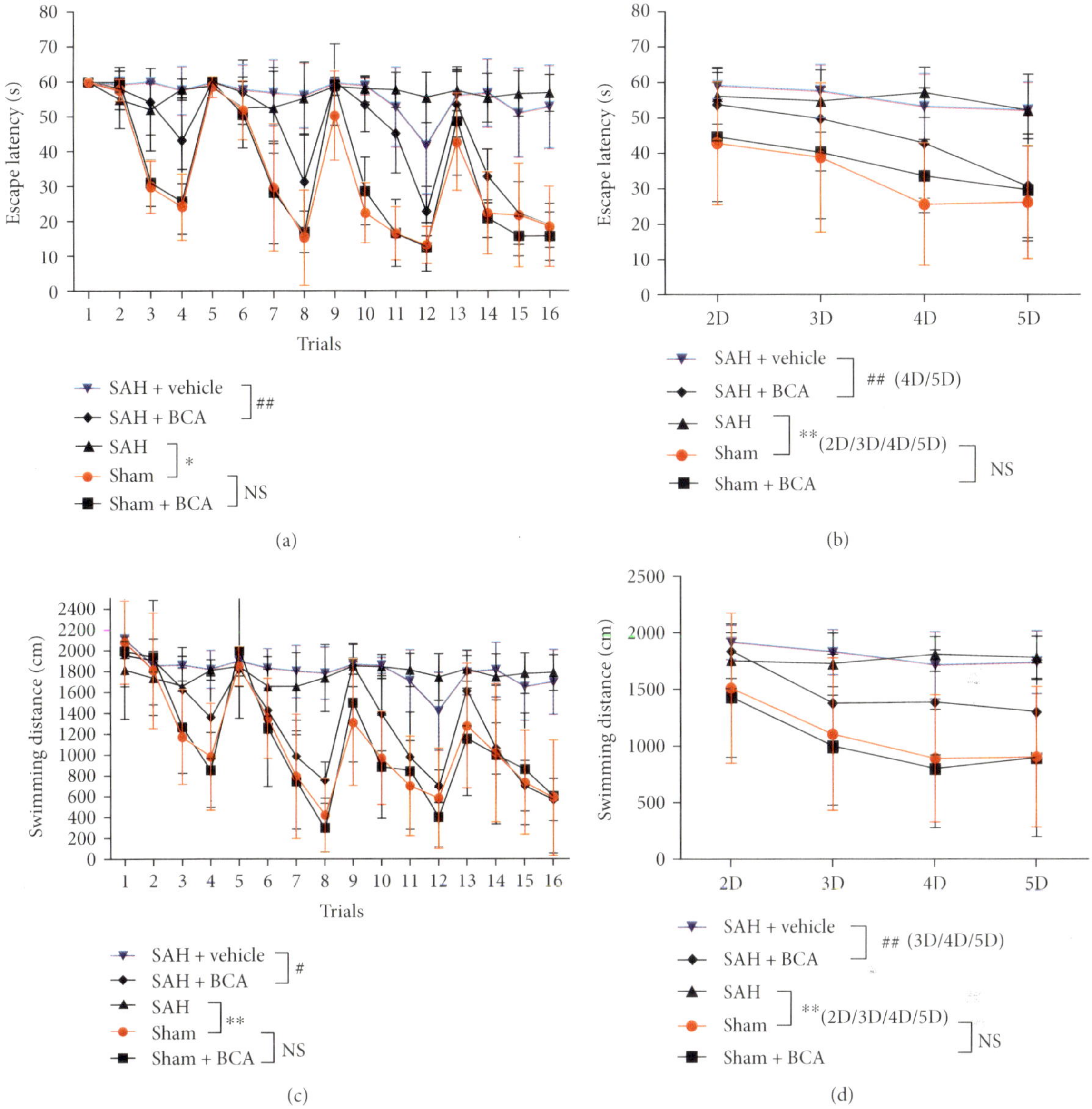

FIGURE 10: BCA reduced the escape latency (a, $n = 8$, $^{*}P < 0.05$ and $^{\#\#}P < 0.01$, one-way ANOVA) and traveled distance (c, $n = 8$, $^{**}P < 0.01$ and $^{\#}P < 0.05$) in 16 trials post SAH. In addition, the averaged data showed significantly shorter escape latency (b, $n = 8$, $^{**}P < 0.01$ and $^{\#\#}P < 0.01$, one-way ANOVA) on day 4 and day 5 and traveled distance (d, $n = 8$, $^{**}P < 0.01$ and $^{\#\#}P < 0.01$, one-way ANOVA) on day 3, day 4, and day 5 in the BCA treatment group.

spatial learning and cognitive memory deficits, which were visualized and investigated in the modified Morris water maze test [37]. Moreover, one recent study found that BCA improves cognitive deficit in the ischemic stroke mice model [38]. We are pleased to verify the same therapeutic effect of BCA on rats' spatial learning and memory deficits in this model of SAH, along with the downregulation of the apoptotic process and inflammatory response. In summary, BCA may exhibit a great potential in understanding and treating cognitive or neurobehavioral deficits post SAH due to its anti-TLR/NF-κB-mediated inflammatory and antineuronal apoptotic effects.

In this study, we speculated that BCA could alleviate the inflammatory responses contributing to EBI post SAH. However, the signal network of inflammation-related injury and neuronal apoptosis in EBI post SAH is very complicated and intricate. Multiple independent proteins and intricate signaling pathways may participate in the therapeutic effects of BCA. In this study, we cannot exclude the possibilities that BCA may protect against EBI via some other inflammatory signal pathway. Hence, further studies are warranted to address these issues. We hope our current research will help to further demonstrate the role and value of BCA in cerebrovascular disease, especially in SAH study.

5. Conclusions

In conclusion, our present data indicate that BCA provides neuroprotection against EBI possibly via suppressing TLR/NF-κB pathway-mediated inflammatory agents and suppressing excessive neuronal apoptosis post SAH. Consequently, BCA further supports its protective role as a potential pharmacological reagent to reduce EBI post SAH.

Authors' Contributions

Ling-yun Wu and Zhen-nan Ye contributed equally to this work.

Acknowledgments

The authors acknowledge the support for this research by grants from the National Natural Science Foundation of China (no. 81271297 for Ji-xin Shi, no. 81371294 for Chun-hua Hang, no. 81400980 for Zong Zhuang, no. 81571162 for Meng-liang Zhou, and no. 81501022 for Xiang-sheng Zhang).

References

[1] E. S. Connolly, A. A. Rabinstein, J. R. Carhuapoma et al., "Guidelines for the management of aneurysmal subarachnoid hemorrhage: a guideline for healthcare professionals from the American Heart Association/American Stroke Association," *Stroke*, vol. 43, no. 6, pp. 1711–1737, 2012.

[2] S. Chen, H. Feng, P. Sherchan et al., "Controversies and evolving new mechanisms in subarachnoid hemorrhage," *Progress in Neurobiology*, vol. 115, pp. 64–91, 2014.

[3] C. Gao, X. Liu, H. Shi et al., "Relationship between sympathetic nervous activity and inflammatory response after subarachnoid hemorrhage in a perforating canine model," *Autonomic Neuroscience*, vol. 147, no. 1-2, pp. 70–74, 2009.

[4] W. Zhong, Z. Zhang, P. Zhao et al., "The impact of initial systemic inflammatory response after aneurysmal subarachnoid hemorrhage," *Turkish Neurosurgery*, vol. 27, no. 3, 2016.

[5] L. Kole, B. Giri, S. K. Manna, B. Pal, and S. Ghosh, "Biochanin-A, an isoflavon, showed anti-proliferative and anti-inflammatory activities through the inhibition of iNOS expression, p38-MAPK and ATF-2 phosphorylation and blocking NFκB nuclear translocation," *European Journal of Pharmacology*, vol. 653, no. 1–3, pp. 8–15, 2011.

[6] M. M. Youssef, M. F. Tolba, N. N. Badawy et al., "Novel combination of sorafenib and biochanin-A synergistically enhances the anti-proliferative and pro-apoptotic effects on hepatocellular carcinoma cells," *Scientific Reports*, vol. 6, no. 1, article 30717, 2016.

[7] J. Chen, B. Ge, Y. Wang, Y. Ye, S. Zeng, and Z. Huang, "Biochanin A promotes proliferation that involves a feedback loop of microRNA-375 and estrogen receptor alpha in breast cancer cells," *Cellular Physiology and Biochemistry*, vol. 35, no. 2, pp. 639–646, 2015.

[8] A. M. Jalaludeen, W. Y. Lee, J. H. Kim et al., "Therapeutic efficacy of biochanin A against arsenic-induced renal and cardiac damage in rats," *Environmental Toxicology and Pharmacology*, vol. 39, no. 3, pp. 1221–1231, 2015.

[9] W. Wang, L. Tang, Y. Li, and Y. Wang, "Biochanin A protects against focal cerebral ischemia/reperfusion in rats via inhibition of p38-mediated inflammatory responses," *Journal of the Neurological Sciences*, vol. 348, no. 1-2, pp. 121–125, 2015.

[10] J.-S. Oh, I. A. Cho, K. R. Kang et al., "Biochanin-A antagonizes the interleukin-1β-induced catabolic inflammation through the modulation of NFκB cellular signaling in primary rat chondrocytes," *Biochemical and Biophysical Research Communications*, vol. 477, no. 4, pp. 723–730, 2016.

[11] S. Piegholdt, K. Pallauf, T. Esatbeyoglu et al., "Biochanin A and prunetin improve epithelial barrier function in intestinal CaCo-2 cells via downregulation of ERK, NF-κB, and tyrosine phosphorylation," *Free Radical Biology & Medicine*, vol. 70, pp. 255–264, 2014.

[12] J. Wang, W. Y. Wu, H. Huang, W. Z. Li, H. Q. Chen, and Y. Y. Yin, "Biochanin A protects against lipopolysaccharide-induced damage of dopaminergic neurons both in vivo and in vitro via inhibition of microglial activation," *Neurotoxicity Research*, vol. 30, no. 3, pp. 486–498, 2016.

[13] X. Ming, M. Ding, B. Zhai, L. Xiao, T. Piao, and M. Liu, "Biochanin A inhibits lipopolysaccharide-induced inflammation in human umbilical vein endothelial cells," *Life Sciences*, vol. 136, pp. 36–41, 2015.

[14] W. Y. Wu, Y. Y. Wu, H. Huang et al., "Biochanin A attenuates LPS-induced pro-inflammatory responses and inhibits the activation of the MAPK pathway in BV2 microglial cells," *International Journal of Molecular Medicine*, vol. 35, no. 2, pp. 391–398, 2015.

[15] C.-H. Zhou, C.-X. Wang, G.-B. Xie et al., "Fisetin alleviates early brain injury following experimental subarachnoid hemorrhage in rats possibly by suppressing TLR 4/NF-κB signaling pathway," *Brain Research*, vol. 1629, pp. 250–259, 2015.

[16] Z. Wang, L. Wu, W. You, C. Ji, and G. Chen, "Melatonin alleviates secondary brain damage and neurobehavioral dysfunction after experimental subarachnoid hemorrhage: possible involvement of TLR4-mediated inflammatory pathway," *Journal of Pineal Research*, vol. 55, no. 4, pp. 399–408, 2013.

[17] H. Li, J. S. Yu, D. D. Zhang et al., "Inhibition of the receptor for advanced glycation end-products (RAGE) attenuates neuroinflammation while sensitizing cortical neurons towards death in experimental subarachnoid hemorrhage," *Molecular Neurobiology*, vol. 54, no. 1, pp. 755–767, 2017.

[18] C. Zhou, G. Xie, C. Wang et al., "Decreased progranulin levels in patients and rats with subarachnoid hemorrhage: a potential role in inhibiting inflammation by suppressing neutrophil recruitment," *Journal of Neuroinflammation*, vol. 12, no. 1, p. 200, 2015.

[19] Z. Guo, Q. Hu, L. Xu et al., "Lipoxin A4 reduces inflammation through formyl peptide receptor 2/p38 MAPK signaling pathway in subarachnoid hemorrhage rats," *Stroke*, vol. 47, no. 2, pp. 490–497, 2016.

[20] H. Li, W. Wu, Q. Sun et al., "Expression and cell distribution of receptor for advanced glycation end-products in the rat cortex following experimental subarachnoid hemorrhage," *Brain Research*, vol. 1543, pp. 315–323, 2014.

[21] W. Li, H. P. Ling, W. C. You et al., "Elevated cerebral cortical CD24 levels in patients and mice with traumatic brain injury: a potential negative role in nuclear factor kappa B/

inflammatory factor pathway," *Molecular Neurobiology*, vol. 49, no. 1, pp. 187–198, 2014.

[22] L.-Y. Wu, Z.-N. Ye, C.-H. Zhou et al., "Roles of pannexin-1 channels in inflammatory response through the TLRs/NF-kappa B signaling pathway following experimental subarachnoid hemorrhage in rats," *Frontiers in Molecular Neuroscience*, vol. 10, p. 175, 2017.

[23] T. Sugawara, R. Ayer, V. Jadhav, and J. H. Zhang, "A new grading system evaluating bleeding scale in filament perforation subarachnoid hemorrhage rat model," *Journal of Neuroscience Methods*, vol. 167, no. 2, pp. 327–334, 2008.

[24] J. Szyndler, A. Piechal, K. Blecharz-Klin et al., "Effect of kindled seizures on rat behavior in water Morris maze test and amino acid concentrations in brain structures," *Pharmacological Reports*, vol. 58, no. 1, pp. 75–82, 2006.

[25] P. Mishra, R. K. Kale, and A. Kar, "Chemoprevention of mammary tumorigenesis and chemomodulation of the antioxidative enzymes and peroxidative damage in prepubertal Sprague Dawley rats by Biochanin A," *Molecular and Cellular Biochemistry*, vol. 312, no. 1-2, pp. 1–9, 2008.

[26] A. Jain, J. C. K. Lai, and A. Bhushan, "Biochanin A inhibits endothelial cell functions and proangiogenic pathways: implications in glioma therapy," *Anti-Cancer Drugs*, vol. 26, no. 3, pp. 323–330, 2015.

[27] K.-H. Lee and E.-M. Choi, "Biochanin A stimulates osteoblastic differentiation and inhibits hydrogen peroxide-induced production of inflammatory mediators in MC3T3-E1 cells," *Biological and Pharmaceutical Bulletin*, vol. 28, no. 10, pp. 1948–1953, 2005.

[28] K. Fadakar, S. Dadkhahfar, A. Esmaeili, and N. Rezaei, "The role of toll-like receptors (TLRs) in stroke," *Reviews in the Neurosciences*, vol. 25, no. 5, pp. 699–712, 2014.

[29] H. S. Zhang, H. Li, D. D. Zhang et al., "Inhibition of myeloid differentiation factor 88(MyD88) by ST2825 provides neuroprotection after experimental traumatic brain injury in mice," *Brain Research*, vol. 1643, pp. 130–139, 2016.

[30] A. Castoldi, T. T. Braga, M. Correa-Costa et al., "TLR2, TLR4 and the MYD88 signaling pathway are crucial for neutrophil migration in acute kidney injury induced by sepsis," *PLoS One*, vol. 7, no. 5, article e37584, 2012.

[31] P. Gray, A. Dunne, C. Brikos, C. A. Jefferies, S. L. Doyle, and L. A. J. O'Neill, "MyD88 adapter-like (Mal) is phosphorylated by Bruton's tyrosine kinase during TLR2 and TLR4 signal transduction," *Journal of Biological Chemistry*, vol. 281, no. 15, pp. 10489–10495, 2006.

[32] P. Ascenzi, A. Bocedi, P. Visca et al., "Hemoglobin and heme scavenging," *IUBMB Life*, vol. 57, no. 11, pp. 749–759, 2005.

[33] G. Pradilla, K. L. Chaichana, S. Hoang, J. Huang, and R. J. Tamargo, "Inflammation and cerebral vasospasm after subarachnoid hemorrhage," *Neurosurgery Clinics of North America*, vol. 21, no. 2, pp. 365–379, 2010.

[34] T. Lawrence, "The nuclear factor NF-κB pathway in inflammation," *Cold Spring Harbor Perspectives in Biology*, vol. 1, no. 6, article a001651, 2009.

[35] R. Sercombe, Y. R. Tran Dinh, and P. Gomis, "Cerebrovascular inflammation following subarachnoid hemorrhage," *The Japanese Journal of Pharmacology*, vol. 88, no. 3, pp. 227–249, 2002.

[36] C. X. Wang, G. B. Xie, C. H. Zhou et al., "Baincalein alleviates early brain injury after experimental subarachnoid hemorrhage in rats: possible involvement of TLR4/NF-κB-mediated inflammatory pathway," *Brain Research*, vol. 1594, pp. 245–255, 2015.

[37] H. Jeon, J. Ai, M. Sabri, A. Tariq, and R. L. Macdonald, "Learning deficits after experimental subarachnoid hemorrhage in rats," *Neuroscience*, vol. 169, no. 4, pp. 1805–1814, 2010.

[38] S. M. Biradar, H. Joshi, and T. K. Chheda, "Biochanin-A ameliorates behavioural and neurochemical derangements in cognitive-deficit mice for the betterment of Alzheimer's disease," *Human & Experimental Toxicology*, vol. 33, no. 4, pp. 369–382, 2014.

7

Scoping Review of the Driving Behaviour of and Driver Training Programs for People on the Autism Spectrum

Nathan J. Wilson,[1] Hoe C. Lee,[2] Sharmila Vaz,[2] Priscilla Vindin,[2] and Reinie Cordier[2]

[1]*School of Nursing and Midwifery, Western Sydney University, Hawkesbury Campus, Locked Bag 3, Richmond, NSW 2753, Australia*
[2]*School of Occupational Therapy Social Work and Speech Pathology, Faculty of Health Sciences, Curtin University, GPO Box U1987, Perth, WA 6845, Australia*

Correspondence should be addressed to Hoe C. Lee; hoe.lee@curtin.edu.au

Academic Editor: Veit Roessner

Gaining a driver's licence represents increased independence and can lead to improved quality of life for individuals and their families. Learning to drive a motor vehicle and maintaining safe on-road skills are often more difficult for people on the autism spectrum. Many countries currently have no autism-specific licencing requirements for learner drivers, and there is a general lack of ASD-specific support and training packages for individuals, their families, and driving instructors. This review synthesises the peer-reviewed literature about the driving characteristics of drivers on the spectrum and driver training available for the cohort. The evidence in this review showed that individuals on the autism spectrum drive differently from their neurotypical counterparts. There are shortcomings in tactical skills of drivers on the autism spectrum, but the extent to which this affects their own safety or the safety of other road users is unclear. Tactical skills can be improved through training programs. There are few autism spectrum-specific learner training programs available. Development of an effective training program will benefit individuals on the spectrum to learn to drive, be independent, and be safe on the road.

1. Introduction

People on the autism spectrum experience problems with social and communication skills that are associated with executive function deficits affecting working memory, motor coordination, attention, planning, mental flexibility, and visual perception [1, 2]. This means that learning to drive a motor vehicle and maintaining safe on-road skills are often more difficult for people on the autism spectrum. Many people on the autism spectrum face barriers to community inclusion, which can create lifelong obstacles to experiencing individual independence. In most countries, gaining a driver's licence represents increased independence and can lead to improved quality of life for individuals and their families [3]. In fact, a recent retrospective longitudinal study showed that fewer people on the autism spectrum had a licence and generally, they obtained their licence later when compared to their peers [4]. Although recent estimates suggest that prevalences of people on the autism spectrum in Western countries range from 0.6% to 2.2% [5–7]; as far as we are aware, in the Australian context, there are currently no evidence-based autism-specific driving interventions available to people on the spectrum to help counter community mobility limitations that affect social and community participation. This review synthesises the peer-reviewed literature about the driving characteristics of drivers on the spectrum and driver training available for the cohort.

Driving plays a critical developmental role during the transition to adulthood and is associated with greater chances of securing paid employment, accessing education, training and services, and maintaining social relationships [8, 9]. Learner drivers on the autism spectrum demonstrate problems with driving skill acquisition and performance and typically require more, and longer, driving lessons and need to take the practical driving test more often when compared to their neurotypical peers [2, 3]. Further, research shows that people on the autism spectrum are also at greater risk of being involved in motor vehicle accidents, which poses risks not only for them but also for other road users in the community [10, 11].

Driving requires higher-order executive function mechanisms to work in a coordinated fashion to respond to, manage, and cope with multiple demands and unexpected and unpredictable driving situations [10]. Research has shown that people on the autism spectrum may experience executive function deficits [2, 9], which will directly impact on their ability to develop driving skills and drive safely. Research investigating the driving behaviour of people on the autism spectrum found that they notice driving hazards but they displayed a delay in response to social hazards that required interactions with other road users, such as failing to give way to pedestrians who show clear intent to cross the road [12–14]. This is thought to be related to a combination of reduced processing of social stimuli and attention deficits, which is very problematic when learning to drive a motor vehicle—a process which requires collaborative problem-solving skills [3]. These challenges are further confounded by research supporting the notion that people on the autism spectrum have atypical eye-gaze patterns, such as prolonged fixation of the speedometer to check the car speed and scanning repeatedly on traffic-irrelevant roadside objects such as advertisement billboards [2].

Three reviews of the literature covering various aspects of driving and use of public transportation in people on the autism spectrum have been published. The first review by Classen and Monahan [15] presented an overview of evidence-based intervention and predictor studies of driving performance in young people with attention deficit hyperactivity disorder (ADHD) or autism spectrum disorder (ASD). A total of ten papers, published between 1995 and 2011, met the criteria for inclusion in this review with nine of the ten papers focussing on driving in people with ADHD. Only one observational case-control study included ASD participants and focussed on hazard recognition in young people with and without ASD, using a virtual reality video display interface [14]. Thus, this first review highlighted the paucity of studies in the area and the urgent need for more empirical studies. The second review focussed on barriers and facilitators associated with driving and public transportation in people with ASD [9]. The review included 14 studies and narratively summarised findings related to (1) difficulties faced in obtaining a driver's licence (e.g., handling unexpected changes, sustaining attention for long drives, merging into traffic, and limited ability to read facial expressions and gestures), (2) driver confidence (e.g., due to lower reaction time and anxiety), (3) driving behaviours (e.g., avoiding heavy traffic or highways or driving at night, adherence to speed regulation, and lane maintenance), and (4) strategies advocated to improve driving skills in ASD (e.g., direct communication, minimal verbal correction, and-short duration lessons; introduction to driving in low noise density/quiet areas; and strategies to address anxiety). A third review focussed on the likely effects that ASD has on driving abilities in young people [16]. The authors reported that drivers on the autism spectrum (1) were less likely to identify social hazards (i.e., males with ASD), (2) had increased reaction times, (3) had more tactical driving difficulties, (4) reported more traffic crashes, citations, and intentional driving violations, and (5) had poorer situational awareness skills than drivers without autism. A major implication of this review was the need for strategic and systematic approaches to train people on the autism spectrum to drive.

In summary, the body of knowledge on driving and ASD needs further consolidation. A comprehensive review of both empirical and grey literatures that focuses on barriers and enablers to obtaining a licence that are related to (a) people on the autism spectrum (skills, behaviours), (b) the learning environment (policy, driver-training practice, instructor, and physical/built environments), and (c) within-the-person-environment context is needed to guide the design of a training intervention on the person with autism spectrum disorder, as well as their driving instructors [1, 9]. Many countries currently have no autism-specific licencing requirements for learner drivers and there is a general lack of ASD-specific support and training packages for individuals, their families, and driving instructors [3, 4, 17].

2. Methodology

2.1. Aim. The aim of this scoping review was to synthesise the current peer-reviewed research literature about the driving behaviours of individuals on the autism spectrum and explore the available training programs for this cohort with a view to suggest future research that promotes better training outcomes for learner drivers on the autism spectrum.

2.2. Design. A scoping review of contemporary peer-reviewed research articles published in English between 2000 and August 2017 was undertaken. Seven databases were searched: PubMed, Scopus, ProQuest, Embase, Medline, CINAHL, and TRID.

2.3. Search Strategy. The following search terms were used as appropriate, for each database: "Child development disorders, pervasive" OR "child developmental disorder*" OR "pervasive developmental disorder*" OR autism OR Asperger OR "autism spectrum disorder*" OR "autistic disorder*" OR "Developmental disabil*" AND "Automobile Driving" OR driving or "driv* training" OR "driver behaviour" OR "driver performance" OR "driver characteristic" OR "driv* education" OR "driv* testing" OR "driv* procedures" OR "driving hazard*" OR "car driv*"OR "automobile driv*" OR "driv*packages".

2.4. Study Selection. The search yielded 1389 results from all seven databases. After removing 609 duplicates, a total of 780 articles were screened at an abstract level for inclusion. Studies were excluded if they did not involve people with ASD and if they did not focus on an aspect of driver training or driving skill development. After two authors reviewed the abstracts, 56 articles were deemed to be suitable for review at full-text level. Of the 56 studies reviewed at full-text level, 28 were excluded based on the following exclusion criteria: (1) not peer-reviewed article, (2) no full text available, (3) focus on other disabilities (not ASD), and (4) focus on transportation rather than independent driving. This resulted in a total of 28 studies for analysis; Figure 1 provides an illustration of the review process.

3. Results

All articles were grouped into four broad categories based on all author-agreed interpretation of each study's findings. These categories included (1) on-road driving behaviours and transport statistics reports on drivers on the spectrum ($n = 7$), (2) performance in driving simulators ($n = 9$), (3) performance in virtual reality driving ($n = 9$), and (4) barriers to obtaining a licence and training of drivers on the spectrum ($n = 3$). Although driving simulators represent a virtual reality context, the simulator category differs from the virtual reality driving category as the context of the latter was using devices such as a desktop computer, rather than a fully functional simulator. Between the two assessment regimes, the low-cost computer-based driving simulator has a better face validity in observing driving behaviours. Descriptive information was extracted from all articles and included the authors, year of publication, study design, objectives, population, and key findings. Study designs were described using the decision matrix recommended by the Centre for Evidence-Based Medicine [18]. This information is summarised in Table 1.

There was not a wide distribution of empirical studies from around the globe, with over 70% of the studies from the USA ($n = 20$), followed by Australia ($n = 3$), the UK ($n = 3$), Canada ($n = 1$), and Sweden ($n = 1$). Research on the topic area was mainly conducted in high-income countries. A total of 1481 participants on the autism spectrum were included across all 28 studies, with 79% of those participants being male. In terms of research designs, there were a total of 23 observational studies, two case studies, two review articles, and one driving simulator study with a quasi-experimental design. The published case study [19] used the same single male subject on the autism spectrum that was used in a comparison with a neurotypical male peer of the same age [20]. In the quasi-experimental study, the intervention group consisted of novice drivers on the autism spectrum ($n = 51$) and the comparison group ($n = 333$) was experienced licenced drivers without autism aged over 25 years [21].

4. Key Categories

4.1. On-Road Driving Behaviours and Transport Statistics Reports on Drivers on the Spectrum. Drivers on the autism spectrum were reported to have proportionally more traffic offences than their neurotypical counterparts ($p < 0.05$) [22]. This study also reported that drivers on the autism spectrum obtained their licence later than other drivers and self-rated their driving skills on a 10-point Likert scale as lower. Cox et al. [21] reported on a greater proportion of traffic offences in drivers on the autism spectrum. Other studies reported that drivers on the autism spectrum demonstrated decreased manoeuvring ability, particularly in left- and right-hand turns and an increased response time to traffic hazards, particularly in circumstances that required interaction with other road users (e.g., being hesitant to merge into another lane when other drivers had already gestured and reduced speed to allow the manoeuvre to happen) [14, 23]. Chee et al. [23] also found that drivers on the autism spectrum performed better than neurotypical drivers in rule-following aspects of driving, such as using the indicator and checking for traffic when approaching an intersection.

Performing complex driving functions that required multitasking skills (e.g., merging and using roundabouts) were often more difficult for the person on the autism spectrum [23, 24]. Driving tasks, or situations, that were sometimes difficult for drivers on the autism spectrum included driving in heavy traffic, night driving, maintaining the correct speed, lane maintenance, judging distance, and undertaking long journeys. In particular, drivers on the autism spectrum sometimes struggled to interpret the driving actions of other road users and found slight deviations from traffic rules of other drivers—a challenge and anxiety provoking [23].

4.2. Performance in Driving Simulators. All of the studies in this category used a comparison group of drivers not on the autism spectrum, except for one study by Monahan et al. [19]. Bishop et al. [12] and Brooks et al. [1] reported that in comparing drivers on the spectrum and the drivers in the control groups, there were no between-group differences in reaction time to hazard perception and motor response time during predriving assessments. In Brooks et al.'s [1] driving simulator study, when compared with the neurotypical controls, participants on the autism spectrum required an additional 30–35 minutes to complete 18 rounds of steering and pedal skill exercises.

Other driving simulator studies reported no between-group differences in (1) errors of maintenance of lane position and speed, (2) adjustment to distractions and poorer right-sided visual acuity [10], (3) response time in braking and overall driving ability [2], and (4) interpreting the gap between the front car, the speed, and the traffic flow of specific traffic scenarios [19]. Reimer et al. [25] also reported that participants on the autism spectrum showed different eye-gaze patterns. When responding to added cognitive demands, they positioned their vertical gaze higher and toward distant objects with more visual diversion. This can reduce the detection of hazards on the peripheral visual field of the individuals. The only quasi-experimental study included in the review used a driving simulator to training drivers on the spectrum [21]. The study showed that drivers on the autism spectrum had poorer baseline executive function and underperformed in tactical skills during simulated scenarios of unanticipated traffic demands [21]. Participants were trained in stages using a driving simulator program during one-hour training sessions across 10–12 weeks, focusing on alternated training of executive functions and tactical driving skills in driving. Outcome measures from the study showed that the training program significantly improved both executive function and driving skills.

4.3. Performance in Virtual Reality Driving. These studies all used some form of a desktop computer and screen as the

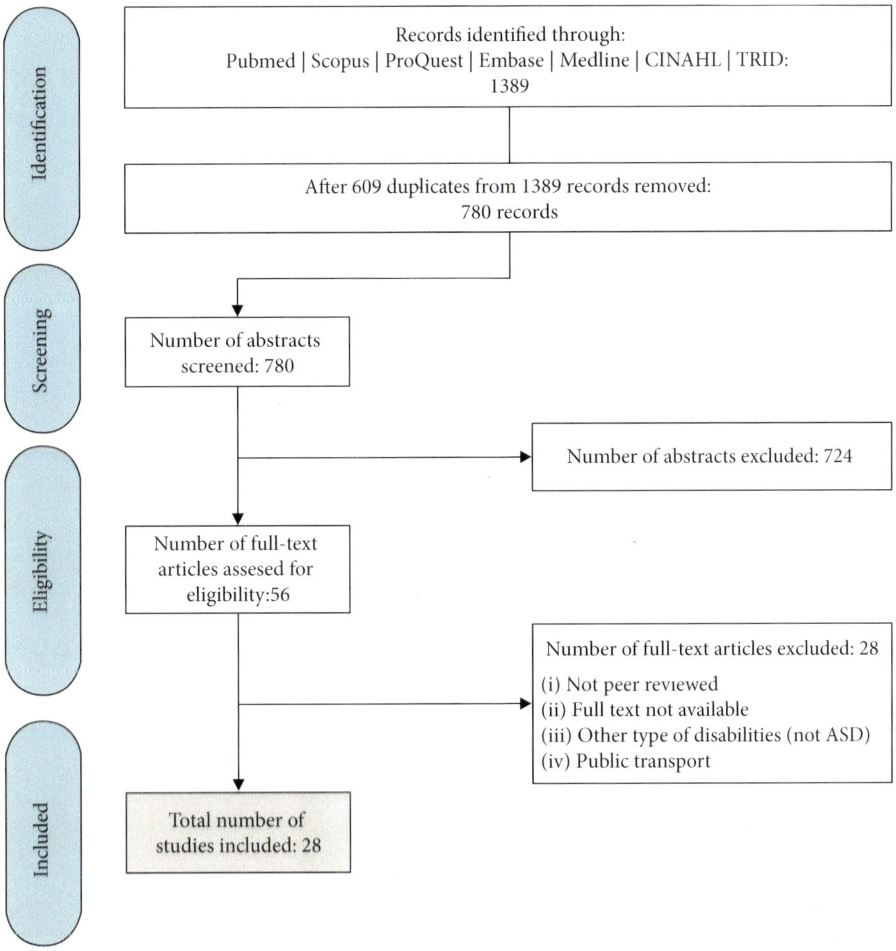

FIGURE 1: Flowchart of included studies.

basis of the virtual reality driving experience with driving-styled consoles (e.g., Logitech™ steering wheel) attached, to enable the participant to mimic driving. Six of the seven studies were led by various members from the same US Electrical Engineering and Computer Science research team. Many were proof of concept studies to determine whether the various data collection methods and tools can be augmented with a virtual reality program to detect between subject differences in areas, for example, such as eye gaze, EEG data, and physiological responses. The seventh study was from a team of UK researchers and reported that participants on the autism spectrum did not detect the time to arrival of two moving cars on a straight road as accurately as the comparison group [26]. Although this study used a virtual reality driving program, none of the participants were actual drivers and so the ability to draw real-life conclusions is limited.

4.4. Barriers to Obtaining a Licence and Training of Drivers on the Spectrum. Both drivers with ASD (learners and with a licence) experienced greater problems with driving and require more lessons and more tests than neurotypical drivers. Learning to drive was sometimes more difficult for the person on the autism spectrum as the process of reading, understanding, and converting driving theory into driving practice was demanding [3]. Unexpected changes to the usual routine or driving norms—where other drivers did not obey the traffic rules—were problematic for people on the autism spectrum [3]. Other reported problems included a lack of confidence, overconfidence, sensory overload, anxiety, poorer concentration, and greater distractibility.

Although all the research studies in this category were either observational or literature reviews that focussed on barriers, there were a few suggestions of potential ways to overcome these barriers. These included strategies to assist driving instructors, such as using direct communication and concrete instructions, providing shorter driving lessons, to commence each lesson in a quiet neighbourhood, and only giving the minimum amount of required information at a time [9]. There was a broad suggestion to use strategies to address anxiety; however, these would need to be individualised to the person on the autism spectrum. In Tyler's [17] four case studies with young adult males on the autism spectrum, some of these individualised strategies included using parent/learner/instructor communication logbooks to enhance consistency, structured language, tasks analysis, and breakdown, using a range of "what if" scenarios to increase insight into unpredictable driving and traffic situations and using visual markers to aid with judging distance.

TABLE 1

Authors, year (country)	Type of study (study design)	Objective	Population	Key findings	Study limitations
On-road driving behaviours and transport statistics reports on drivers on the spectrum ($n = 7$)					
Chee et al. 2015 (Australia) [28]	Cross-sectional study	To understand people with ASD's viewpoints on driving using Q-methodology (e.g., whether or not they are confident and prefer driving than other transportation).	$n = 100$ 50 with ASD (MA = 21.8 years; 82% male) 57 young adults without ASD (MA = 23.6 years; 72% male)	(i) Some young adults with ASD perceived themselves as confident and independent drivers. (ii) Some preferred to use public transportation or walk; anxiety was a barrier to driving for some. (iii) 34% with ASD had a driver licence compared to 68% of typical developing.	Diagnosis of ASD based on self-report Underrepresentation of nondrivers in the control group.
Chee et al. 2017 (Australia) [23]	Cross-sectional study	(i) To assess and compare the driving performance of drivers with and without ASD in suburban traffic environment (ii) To explore how the symptomatology of ASD hinders or facilitates the on-road driving performance	$n = 37$ 16 with ASD (MA = 25.43 years; 86% male) 21 TD (MA = 27 years; 93% male)	(i) Drivers with ASD underperformed in vehicle manoeuvring, especially at left turns, right turns (hesitant and slower), and pedestrian crossings. (ii) Drivers with ASD outperformed the TD group in rule-following aspects such as using the indicator at roundabouts and checking for cross-traffic when approaching intersections.	Being small in sample size, the participants of this study may not be representative of the broader population and can impact on the generalisability of the results. Assessor bias—not blinded to diagnosis of participants or the purpose of the study No use of independent assessor or interrater reliability checks Impact of environmental factors, such as time of day and weather conditions on driving performance, cannot be disregarded. Driving route is developed by a researcher using the route of convenience for experimentation purposes; whether it mimics traffic demands on a normal road is questionable.
Cox et al. 2012 (USA) [24]	Cross-sectional study	An online survey to understand driving and ASD by surveying parents/caregivers of adolescents and young adults with ASD, who had driving licence or were in the process of learning to drive	$n = 123$ parents/caregivers (mother 81%, father 13%, and caregiver 6%) The mean age of their child with ASD was 19 years, 73% male; 83% Asperger's/high-function ASD, 9% PDD-NOS, 3% autistic disorder, and 5% others	(i) Parents were active in the teaching process (mother 81%; father 62%). (ii) 48% had a driver's licence, 29% possessed a learner's permit, and 70% of the parents stated that ASD affected driving ability. (iii) Particular challenges for people with ASD are complex driving demands (e.g., merging into traffic, traffic awareness, multitasking, handling	Diagnosis of ASD is not confirmed through review of medical records Confounding impact of comorbidity is not accounted. Respondent bias (use of caregivers other than the person on the spectrum) limits validity. Use of a sample that was nonrepresentative; data collection is limited to internet survey.

Table 1: Continued.

Authors, year (country)	Type of study (study design)	Objective	Population	Key findings	Study limitations
				unexpected changes, and sustaining attention on a long drive) (iv) Other difficulties include interpreting the actions of other drivers (e.g. reading their nonverbal social cues when in ambiguous situations).	
Daly et al. 2014 (USA) [22]	Cross-sectional study	An online survey using a modified version of the Driver Behaviour Questionnaire to determine whether differences exist between adult drivers with ASD and non-ASD adult drivers in terms of (i) driving history and driving behaviours, (ii) the rates of reporting violations/mistakes/driving slips as defined by DBQ, and (iii) the relative risk of such behaviours as quantified by the DBQ.	$n = 172$ 78 licenced drivers with ASD (MA = 32.9 years; 56% male, 98.7% autism/Asperger's, and 1.3% PDD-NOS) 94 non-ASD drivers (MA = 35.5 years; 31% male)	(i) Drivers with ASD obtained their driver's licence approximately 2 years later that non-ASD drivers. (ii) Drivers with ASD drove less days per week and had significantly lower ratings of their driving ability and a higher number of traffic violations. (iii) Drivers with ASD were also more likely to place voluntary restrictions on driving.	The pilot study relied on anonymous self-report. Participants, due to poor insight or difficulty in comparing their own driving behaviour with other drivers, may underreport their symptoms and overrate their driving ability. Report of driving behaviours through the use of standardized self-report measures would have improved the study rigor. Only the use of internet outlets for data collection may limit sample representativeness. Impact of comorbidity cannot be disregarded.
* Deka et al. 2016 (USA) [31]	Cross-sectional study	An online survey to learn about the travel patterns, needs, and barriers people with ASD encounter regarding the use of different transportation modes.	$n = 703$ Male : female = 3 : 16	(i) Only 9.3% of the adults with ASD had a driver's licence and many are using it as identity card rather than a licence to drive. (ii) 55.3% of the drivers with ASD ($n = 47$) had difficulty dealing with traffic, 34% mentioned difficulty caused by distractions near roads; 27.7% mentioned difficulty judging distance, and 27.7% had difficulty with parking. (iii) Because of these difficulties, 26.1% did not drive at all.	Low representation of views of ASD adults who had a driving licence and that have driven a car regularly
Huang et al. 2012 (USA) [32]	Cross-sectional study	An online survey to compare the characteristics of age-eligible driving and nondriving teens and explore the driving outcomes for teens with higher	$n = 235$ (MA = 16.39 years; 83%; 24.7% autistic disorder, 14.5% PDD-NOS, 1.5% ASD,	(i) 63% of teens currently drive or plan to drive. (ii) 29% who are eligible to drive currently drive.	Respondent bias (use of caregivers other than the person on the spectrum) limits validity. Selection bias leading to

Table 1: Continued.

Authors, year (country)	Type of study (study design)	Objective	Population	Key findings	Study limitations
		functioning autism spectrum disorders	46.4% Asperger's, and 4.7% others)	(iii) Driving predictors included individualised education plans with driving goals, indicators of functional status, and parent experience with teaching teens to drive. (iv) 12% of teens received driving citations, and 12% of teens had been involved in a motor vehicle crash.	nonrepresentative samples: families of teens who currently drive or plan to drive are more likely to participate in this study
Sheppard et al. 2017 (UK) [33]	Case control study	Videos of 20 different driving situations with inbuilt hazards to (i) compare the ability of identifying the driving hazards by stopping the video and pointing to the hazard between people with ASD and without ASD and (ii) define whether people with ASD have difficulty in responding to hazards or orienting to them.	$n = 35$ 18 ASD males (MA = 18.79 years) 17 TD males (MA = 18.19 years)	(i) Although nonsignificant, participants with ASD showed a slower fixation on the hazard source and a slower orientation to the hazards. (ii) Greater attentional capture in the time preceding the hazards' onset was associated with lower verbal IQ. (iii), Suggesting individuals with ASD may distribute or direct their attention differently when identifying driving hazards.	The study is limited to young male ASD adults with no specific training or driving experience. Results cannot be generalised to ASD drivers with a licence or of different age ranges or females with ASD.
Performance in driving simulators ($n = 9$)					
Bishop et al. 2017 (USA) [12]	Cross-sectional study	To investigate how drivers with ASD respond to social and nonsocial hazards in a driving simulator compared to typically developing drivers using a driving simulator	$n = 32$ 16 ASD drivers (MA = 23.88 years; 15% male) 16 TD drivers (MA = 22.94 years; 15% male)	(i) There was no difference in reaction time to social versus nonsocial hazards for drivers with ASD. (ii) Typically developing drivers reacted more quickly to social hazards as compared to nonsocial hazards.	Small sample size and underpowered Low scores on ASD symptomatology: ASD Social Responsive Scale. Unclear of any real-life translation of the simulated driving assessment
Brooks et al. 2016 (USA) [1]	Cross-sectional study	To investigate the utility of using a driving simulator and interactive exercises (steering and pedal tasks) to address the motor aspects of predriving skills of young adults with ASD	$n = 41$ 10 ASD (MA = 15.9 years; 10 male) 31 TD (MA = 16.7 years; males = 18)	(i) Minimal performance differences were observed between the two groups in terms of the motor aspects of predriving skills. (ii) Participants with ASD needed more time (30–35 minutes) to complete the 18 interactive steering and pedal exercises. (iii) The interactive exercises and the process used worked well to	Small sample size and underpowered Females are excluded in the ASD group. Unclear of any real-life translation: interactive exercises do not include any road scenes that help to eliminate the sensory overload, anxiety, and stress that participants might experience in naturalistic driving environments

TABLE 1: Continued.

Authors, year (country)	Type of study (study design)	Objective	Population	Key findings	Study limitations
				address motor-related aspects of predriving skills in young adults with ASD.	
Classen and Monahan 2013 (USA) [15]	Literature review	To conduct an evidence-based review of intervention studies and predictor studies related to driving outcomes in teens with ADHD or ASD	$n = 10$ intervention studies (2 RCT, 7 quasi-experiments, and 1 prospective observational study) Quasi-experimental studies: 7 on ADHD and 1 on ASD	(i) The ASD group perceives driving hazards via video clips but has difficulty in perceiving hazards if the task also requires processing of social information. (ii) The ASD group responds slower to hazard perceptions compared to controls. (iii) An instrumented vehicle, simulator training, and parent involvement invention had positive effect for speeding and hard braking for teens with ADHD. (iv) Male drivers with ADHD improved in hazard perception response times following training with hazard videos.	Heterogeneity among the studies: variability in age Inclusion criteria restricted to articles published in English and male participants Using different driving simulators, driving scenarios, outcome measures of assessment, failure to control for any prior rehabilitation, or clinical interventions lessened the methodological rigour of the studies. Grey literature is not included in the search.
Classen et al. 2013 (USA) [8]	Observational study	Using a driving simulator to examine the demographic, clinical, and simulated driving (type and number of driving errors) differences between teens with ADHD-ASD, healthy controls (HCs).	$n = 44$ 22 ADHD-ASD (MA = 15.05 years; 17% male) 22 healthy controls (MA = 14.32 years; 59% male)	(i) Teens with ADHD-ASD performed more poorly on right eye visual acuity, selective attention, visual motor integration, cognition, and motor performance. (ii) Teens with ADHD-ASD made more errors on the driving simulator regarding visual scanning, speed regulation, lane maintenance, adjustment to stimuli, and total number of driving errors. (iii) Compared with HC teens, teens with ADHD-ASD may have more predriving skill deficits.	Sample of convenience: a Caucasian sample is not representative of the population of interest. Small sample size: underpowered study Selection bias: more concerned parents and teens with better insight enrolled in the study Berkson's bias: test taking and driving behaviours could be influenced by the evaluator's sitting next to the client. Hawthorne bias: the test-taking and driving behaviours are influenced by the testing site and social conditions. Did not control for medication effects on driving Simulator study: questionable of real-life driving equivalence

TABLE 1: Continued.

Authors, year (country)	Type of study (study design)	Objective	Population	Key findings	Study limitations
Cox et al. 2016 (USA) [2]	Cross-sectional study	To examine the relationship between driving performance and executive functioning for novice drivers, with and without ASD, using a driving simulator	$n = 44$ males 17 ASD (MA = 18.28 years) 27 healthy controls (MA = 16.59 years)	(i) ASD drivers had significantly slower reaction times during steering but not braking. (ii) ASD drivers demonstrated impaired working memory functioning, such that adding working memory demands resulted in a significant decrement in their driving performance relative to control drivers. (iii) ASD drivers demonstrated poorer overall driving ability than the control drivers.	Simulator study—questionable real-life equivalence Diagnosis based on parent report: medical records/doctors not consulted Cognitive measure is not used to assess intellectual functioning. Equivalence of comparison groups questionable: the control group was younger licenced drivers, whereas the ASD group had learner's permits. Previous driving experience was not accounted for in both groups.
Cox et al. 2017 (USA) [21]	Pre- and post-quasi-experimental studies	Using a virtual reality driving simulator to investigate how novice drivers with ASD differ from experienced drivers and whether virtual reality driving simulation training (VRDST) improves ASD driving performance	51 novice ASD drivers (MA = 17.96 years; 78% male) 23 in routine training (RT) 14 in standard VRDST 14 in automated VRDST 18 in eye-tracking VRDST only 333 normative licenced comparison group (MA = 40 years; 73% male)	(i) ASD drivers showed worse baseline executive function (EF) and driving skills than experienced drivers. (ii) ASD drivers performed worse than normative drivers on general tactical driving (iii) Both standard and automated VRDST significantly improved driving (e.g., better steering and speed control) and EF performance compared to RT. (iv) Eye-tracking VRDST did not significantly improve tactical performance relative to RT.	No random assignment of subjects to groups Small sample size: the study can be under powered
Monahan et al. 2012 (USA) [19]	Single subject case study	To illustrate the predriving skills of a teen with ADHD/ASD using a driving simulator	1 male with ASD/ADHD, 15 years old	(i) Demonstrated significant impairments related to visual motor integration and attention shift (ii) Did not perform visual scanning for traffic at cross streets and during lane changes (iii) Approached all interactions with excessive speed (iv) Poor understanding of traffic flow (v) Made gap acceptance error related to being overcautious	Single case study design: inherently faces the lack of representativeness of general population

Table 1: Continued.

Authors, year (country)	Type of study (study design)	Objective	Population	Key findings	Study limitations
Monahan et al. 2013 (USA) [20]	Cross-sectional study	Using a driving simulator to compare the predriving skills of a teen with ADHD/ASD to an age- and gender-matched healthy control.	1 male with ADHD/ASD, 15 years old 1 youth without ADHD/ASD, 15 years old	(i) Youth with ADHD/ASD demonstrated impairments in the ability to shift attention, perform simple sequential tasks, integrate visual-motor responses, and coordinate motor responses (ii) Youth without ADHD/ASD demonstrated intact skills in these abilities. (iii) Youth with ADHD/ASD made 44 driving error, while the youth without ADHD/ASD made 17 during the driving. (iv) Youth with ADHD/ASD had more lane maintenance, visual scanning, and speeding errors compared to the youth without ADHD/ASD.	Single participant in each comparison group
Reimer et al. 2013 (USA) [25]	Cross-sectional study	Using a driving simulator to explore driving behaviour and visual attention in young adult drivers with high-function (HF) ASD in comparison with a community sample of nonaffected individuals matched for age and sex	$n = 20$ 10 male with HF-ASD (MA = 20.2 years) 10 matched controls (MA = 20.7 years)	(i) Youth with HF-ASD performed comparable to controls in terms of the frequency of simulated crashes and vehicle control. (ii) Youth with HF-ASD displayed a nominally higher and unvaried heart rate compared to controls. (iii) Youth with HF-ASD showed a gaze pattern suggestive of a diversion of visual attention away from high-stimulus areas of the roadway when responding to increased cognitive demands (cell phone task; continuous performance task). (iv) Youth with HF-ASD tended to position their vertical gaze higher and away from nearer objects and more toward the distance than controls.	Sample of convenience—Caucasian comparison groups are not representative of the population of interest—limits generalisability of results. Small sample size: underpowered study Without screening on age and cognitive functions, a convenient sample from the community as the control group Assessment of intellectual functioning or ASD was not obtained. Degree to which outcome measures relate to other covariates such as driving frequency and exposure is not reported.

Table 1: Continued.

Authors, year (country)	Type of study (study design)	Objective	Population	Key findings	Study limitations
Performance in virtual reality driving ($n = 9$)					
Bian et al. 2016 (USA) [34]	Study one: descriptive study Study two: case control experimental design, random allocation of members to comparison groups	To assess the feasibility of outcome measures for and responsiveness of virtual reality driving package	4 teenagers with ASD—3 male and one female 2 in the performance-sensitive system (PS) group (degree of difficulty changed based on performance only) 2 in the engagement-sensitive system (ES) group (degree of difficulty changed based on performance and engagement)	(i) All participants reported that they "enjoyed the game" and noticed the changes in task difficulty. (ii) The physiological data was successfully used to assess the user's engagement level and performance enabling the dynamic adjustment of the driving difficulty level.	Small sample size: underpowered study Equivalence of groups was questionable: effects of neither age nor driving experience are sufficiently controlled for the studies Study design does not take into account the possibility of comorbidity of ADHD in the sample group. Unclear of any real-life translation of the driving simulator study.
Fan et al. 2018 (USA) [35]	Descriptive study	To generate proof of concept data to determine if EEG data is useful in ASD driving interventions	20 ASD (MA = 15.29 years; 19 males and 1 female)	(i) EEG-based group level classification models are feasible for recognizing affect and workload recognition in individuals with ASD in the context of using a desktop virtual reality driving program. (ii) Although promising, the applicability of this approach to collecting outcome data in other interventions requires further development.	Small sample size of the neurotypical comparison group Limits with interpreting EEG data of virtual reality environments as in real-life contexts
Sheppard et al. 2010 (UK) [14]	Cross-sectional study	To compare the ability of identifying 10 different driving hazards by stopping the video and pointing to the hazard between people with ASD and without ASD	$n = 44$ 23 males with ASD (MA = 18.55 years; 30% ASD and 70% Asperger's) 21 males without ASD (MA = 18.83 years)	(i) Participants with ASD identified fewer social hazards (those that involved people like pedestrians, cyclists), but not nonsocial hazards (e.g., cars). (ii) Participants with ASD were slower to respond than those without ASD.	Participants of the study are likely to have strategies prior to the experience to identify and respond to both types of hazard. Limited to only male participants Results cannot be generalised to ASD drivers with a licence or of different age ranges or females with ASD.
Sheppard et al. 2016 (UK) [26]	Cross-sectional study	To investigate whether individuals with ASD have difficulty judging the location of moving objects in a driving context using a time-to-arrival task on a desktop virtual reality program	$n = 44$ 23 males with ASD (MA = 18.55 years; 7 with Autism and 16 with Asperger's) 21 males in comparison group (MA = 18.83 years)	(i) Participants with ASD were less accurate at predicting which of the two cars in the virtual reality program would arrive first at an intersection on a straight road. (ii) There were no differences between participants with ASD and the comparison group when the simulation was along a curved road.	Participants were all nondrivers so generalisability to drivers is not possible. Unclear of any real-life translation

Table 1: Continued.

Authors, year (country)	Type of study (study design)	Objective	Population	Key findings	Study limitations
Sheppard et al. 2017 (UK) [33]	Case control study	Videos of 20 different driving situations with inbuilt hazards to (i) compare the ability of identifying the driving hazards by stopping the video and pointing to the hazard between people with ASD and without ASD and (ii) define whether people with ASD have difficulty in responding to hazards or orienting to them.	$n = 35$ 18 ASD males (MA = 18.79 years) 17 TD males (MA = 18.19 years)	(i) Although nonsignificant, participants with ASD showed a slower fixation on the hazard source and a slower orientation to the hazards. (ii) Greater attentional capture in the time preceding the hazards onset was associated with lower verbal IQ, suggesting that individuals with ASD may distribute or direct their attention differently when identifying driving hazards.	Limited to male young adults with ASD, but with no specific training or driving experience Results cannot be generalised to ASD drivers or of different age ranges or females with ASD.
Wade et al. 2014 (USA) [36]	Cross-sectional study	To determine if a novel virtual reality driving environment can detect between-group differences	$n = 8$ 4 males with ASD (MA = 16.87 years) 4 TD controls (MA = 15.34 years; 3 males and 1 female)	(i) The ASD group experiencing a higher number of simulated driving failures (ii) Participants with ASD had a vertically higher and horizontally right visual gaze. (iii) The ASD group had a significantly higher skin conduction level and skin conductance response rate suggesting that participants with ASD may have greater anxiety.	Small sample size: underpowered study Unclear of any real-life translation
Wade et al. 2015 (USA) [11]	Cross-sectional study	To compare the effects on driving performance and gaze patterns using the gaze-contingent system and the gaze-insensitive, performance-based system	$n = 18$ 12 males with ASD in the gaze-contingent group (MA = 14.65 years) 6 in the performance-based group (MA = 15.93 years)	(i) The performance-based group showed a significantly higher mean vertical and right-sided gaze component when compared to the gaze-contingent group. (ii) The performance-based group showed a decrease in trial failures from pre- to post-post.	Small sample size: underpowered study. Equivalence of groups was questionable.
Zhang et al. 2015 (USA) [37]	Descriptive study	To evaluate the feasibility of combining psychophysiological data collection with performance based data using a virtual reality program	10 with ASD (age range = 13 to 17 years)	(i) The best accuracy to assess cognitive load was by combining eye gaze and EEG data in a hybrid data analysis model.	Small sample size: underpowered study Applicability to real-life situations was questionable.
Zhang et al. 2014 (USA) [38]	Descriptive study	To determine if performance data and affective data can be combined to predict the optimum driving difficulty level of a virtual reality program	7 with ASD (age range = 13 to 17 years)	(i) Combining performance and affective state data was better at predicting the difficulty level when compared to separating the data. (ii) The number of driving performance failures and the	Small sample size: underpowered study

Table 1: Continued.

Authors, year (country)	Type of study (study design)	Objective	Population	Key findings	Study limitations
				enjoyment level had a strong relationship with the difficulty level.	
Barriers to obtaining a licence and training on drivers of the spectrum ($n = 3$)					
Almberg et al. 2017 (Sweden) [3]	Descriptive study	Questionnaires with open and closed questions to explore the facilitators or barriers in driving education experienced by individuals with ASD or ADHD who obtained a learner's permit, from the perspective of the learner drivers and their driving instructors	$n = 33$ 14 male ADHD 19 ASD (MA = 20.7 years; 16 males and 3 females) 9 driving instructors (4 with ADHD learner drivers and 5 with ASD learner drivers)	(i) Participants with ASD required twice as many driving lessons and more on-road test than those with ADHD. (ii) Reading difficulties meant converting theory into practice was difficult. (iii) Adjusting to on-road situations that were unfamiliar of deviated from the "textbook" script was challenging. (iv) Paying attention to other road users and road signs was reported to be a problem. (v) Hazard perception and the ability to regulate the driving according to the traffic conditions were difficult for ASD participants.	Small sample size: underpowered study Use of nonvalidated outcome measures Did not consider comorbidity as a confounder Did not consider impact of prior familiarity and experience in working with people with ASD and ADHD in measuring outcomes
*Lindsay 2017 (Canada) [9]	Systematic literature review	To systematically review the literature on factors (e.g., barriers and facilitators) affecting driving and motor vehicle transportation experiences of people with ASD	22 studies from eight databases with 2919 participants (mean age 17.3 years 364 individuals with ASD 2555 parents of youth with ASD	13 studies focused on factors affecting driving including the following: (i) Challenges in obtaining a licence (e.g., handling unexpected changes, sustaining attention for long drives, merging into traffic, and limited ability to read facial expressions and gestures) (ii) Driving confidence (not confident in reaction time, much resulted from experiences of anxiety) (iii) Driving behaviours (e.g., avoiding heavy traffic or highways, driving at night, adhering to speed regulation, and lane maintenance) (iv) Strategies to improving driving skills (e.g., direct communication, providing lessons in short intervals, starting off in quiet	Research conducted on March 2015 Inclusion restricted to articles published in English Grey literature not included

Table 1: Continued.

Authors, year (country)	Type of study (study design)	Objective	Population	Key findings	Study limitations
				areas, not giving too much information or verbal correction, and address anxiety).	
Tyler 2013 (Australia) [17]	Case study	To examine the problems faced by supervisors and instructors during training and the strategies that can be implemented to decrease the risks associated for drivers with Asperger's syndrome	Four case studies on the following: (i) 20-year-old male with Asperger's/ADHD (ii) 26-year-old male, with Asperger's/anxiety/depression (iii) 20-year-old male with Asperger's/ADHD/ (iv) 18-year-old male with Asperger's/dyspraxia	(i) Problems included being easily distracted during driving, poor concentration, anxiety, and sensory overload (ii) Strategies included are as follows: (a) Communication book for parents/learners/instructors to reinforce the sequence of tasks using a consistent approach are provided. (b) Regular lessons were conducted. (c) The use of keywords and structured language in instructions for consistency reduced confusion and anxiety. (d) Reduce discussions on topic of interest to increase focus on the driving task. (e) Break tasks down and working through smaller components in sequence to reduce anxiety. (f) Instructors used "what if" scenarios to broaden participant's understanding of unpredictable drivers and pedestrians. (g) Instructors used visual markers for judgement of distance, crash avoidance space, and indicator distance rules.	Interpretation of results of the study dependent on the sensitivity and integrity of the investigator Case study design: inherently faces the lack of representativeness of general population Efforts undertaken to ensure trustworthiness, credibility, transferability, dependability, confirmability, and rigour of the study were not reported.

*Study included the collection of both driving and public transport data, with sufficient data about driving to be included in this review.

5. Discussion

There is inconsistent evidence on the driving ability of people on the autism spectrum. For example, some studies reported that there is no difference between drivers on the autism spectrum and neurotypical counterparts in the maintenance of lane position and speed [8], response time in braking, and overall driving ability [2]. These studies were conducted either in simulated driving or in virtual reality environments generated by computer desktops. Conversely, when the ability of drivers was assessed in naturalistic on-road driving environments, drivers on the autism spectrum experience difficulty in complex traffic scenarios, especially driving tasks that required nonverbal communications with other drivers [23]. In addition, when compared with neurotypical controls, drivers on the autism spectrum had difficulty in multitasking and performing complex driving tasks and consistently maintaining a safe speed. They were also observed to have decreased manoeuvring ability and increased in response time to traffic hazards [23]. Unexpected changes to the usual driving routine or driving norms from other drivers distracted the attention of drivers on the autism spectrum and induced performance anxiety. When responding to added cognitive demands, drivers on the autism spectrum had poorer baseline executive function and performed worse on general and tactical driving [23].

Similarly, discrepancies were found by Cox et al. [21] who reported a greater proportion of traffic offences in drivers on the autism spectrum, whereas Chee et al. [23] found that drivers on the autism spectrum performed better than neurotypical drivers in rule-following aspects of driving. A possible explanation for these discrepancies is that the Cox et al. [21] study observed drivers on the autism spectrum using a driving simulator assessment, which is an artificial context. Consequentially, the real-life behaviour changes of drivers on the autism spectrum in responding to high-demand traffic scenarios were not known. This notion is supported in a validity study using driving simulators to assess driving behaviours of older drivers. Lee et al. [27] reported that only 67% of driving behaviours observed in a driving simulator was transferable to an on-road driving environment. Simulated driving environments might not be sensitive enough to detect changes of the driving performance. On-road driving is the gold standard to assess and observe ability of drivers. Drivers on the autism spectrum underperform in some aspects of driving or drive differently in naturalistic environments, but there is insufficient evidence to support the notion that drivers on the spectrum are more at risk of being involved in an accident than their neurotypical counterparts [28].

The observational studies [8, 26] using cross-sectional designs reported drivers on the autism spectrum to have difficulty in interpreting the driving actions of other road users. The eye-gaze patterns of drivers on the autism spectrum demonstrated an increased response time in detecting hazards, especially those associated with ineffective interpretation of the intentions of other drivers by means of body gesture and social clues. Insufficient attention to the traffic events detected on the peripheral visual fields can be hazardous and unsafe on road [26].

Individuals on the autism spectrum appear to have decreased ability to multitask and manoeuvre through complex traffic scenarios. To accomplish these tasks, drivers on the autism spectrum require training on the tactical level skills of the Michon's model of driving [29]. Tactical behaviour in driving involves striking a balance between the demands of driving and the driver's ability to drive safely in accordance to the road rules [30]. Successful acquisition of the tactical skills may allow drivers on the autism spectrum to reserve their cognitive capacity to cope with tasks with high number of executive functions and decision-making demands.

In identifying the training of the individuals on the spectrum, there is no experimental study aimed at testing novel ways to train individuals on the autism spectrum to obtain their driver's licence. In the current review, most observational studies described the barrier individuals on the autism spectrum experience in getting a driver's licence. None of them focussed on investigating the best strategies to help individuals on the spectrum to obtain their driver's licence.

5.1. Future Research. The current literature reviewed provides a preliminary driving profile of individuals on the autism spectrum in simulated contexts or during on-road assessments with predetermined routes. Given that individuals on the autism spectrum are susceptible to stress and anxiety, their driving experience is very likely to deteriorate in a test environment. For this particular cohort, research into the individuals in naturalistic driving environments will generate a more comprehensive driver profile. Driving is essential for individuals on the spectrum, but they showed a relatively low take-up rate of formal driving licence. There is limited research on how to effectively train individuals on the autism spectrum to drive independently and safely. Future research should focus on identifying strategies and the best practice of training to support individuals on the autism spectrum to get their licences.

5.2. Limitations. Most of the studies included in this review used to establish a profile of drivers on the spectrum were based on observations in driving simulator and/or virtual reality settings. This is a major limitation, given the low transferability of observations from a driving simulator environment to real-life on-road driving [27]. Findings from this scoping review should be interpreted with caution, as we only included studies published in English; grey literature, books, and theses were outside the scope of our review. Further, there are eight studies that employed self-report methodology to collect information from individuals on the autism spectrum on their ability to drive. Although there is no incentive for the participants to have falsely reported their driving ability, their reporting may have inflated their ability to drive and may have been influenced by recall bias.

6. Conclusion

Synthesis of the evidence in this review showed that individuals on the autism spectrum drive differently from their neurotypical counterparts. There are shortcomings in tactical skills of the drivers on the autism spectrum, but the extent to which this affects their own safety or the safety of other road users is not yet clear. Tactical skills can be improved through targeted training programs, specifically designed to accommodate the driving characteristics of the autism population. There are few autism spectrum-specific learner training programs available. Development of an effective training program will benefit the individuals on the spectrum to learn to drive, be independent, and be safe on the road.

Acknowledgments

The authors acknowledge the financial support of the Cooperative Research Centre for Living with Autism Spectrum Disorders (Autism CRC), established and supported under the Australian Government's Cooperative Research Centres Program. They also acknowledge Ms. Zhen Lin from Western Sydney University and Dr. Elinda Lee from Curtin University who were employed as Research Assistants to support the conduct of the literature search.

References

[1] J. Brooks, J. Kellett, J. Seeanner et al., "Training the motor aspects of pre-driving skills of young adults with and without autism spectrum disorder," *Journal of Autism and Developmental Disorders*, vol. 46, no. 7, pp. 2408–2426, 2016.

[2] S. M. Cox, D. J. Cox, M. J. Kofler et al., "Driving simulator performance in novice drivers with autism spectrum disorder: the role of executive functions and basic motor skills," *Journal of Autism and Developmental Disorders*, vol. 46, no. 4, pp. 1379–1391, 2016.

[3] M. Almberg, H. Selander, M. Falkmer, S. Vaz, M. Ciccarelli, and T. Falkmer, "Experiences of facilitators or barriers in driving education from learner and novice drivers with ADHD or ASD and their driving instructors," *Developmental Neurorehabilitation*, vol. 20, no. 2, pp. 59–67, 2017.

[4] A. E. Curry, B. E. Yerys, P. Huang, and K. B. Metzger, "Longitudinal study of driver licensing rates among adolescents and young adults with autism spectrum disorder," *Autism*, vol. 22, no. 4, pp. 479–488, 2017.

[5] Australian Bureau of Statistics, *Autism in Australia 2012*, Australian Bureau of Statistics, Canberra, ACT, Australia, 2014.

[6] S. Baron-Cohen, F. J. Scott, C. Allison et al., "Prevalence of autism-spectrum conditions: UK School-Based Population Study," *The British Journal of Psychiatry*, vol. 194, no. 6, pp. 500–509, 2009.

[7] M. Elsabbagh, G. Divan, Y. J. Koh et al., "Global prevalence of autism and other pervasive developmental disorders," *Autism Research*, vol. 5, no. 3, pp. 160–179, 2012.

[8] S. Classen, M. Monahan, and Y. Wang, "Driving characteristics of teens with attention deficit hyperactivity and autism spectrum disorder," *American Journal of Occupational Therapy*, vol. 67, no. 6, pp. 664–673, 2013.

[9] S. Lindsay, "Systematic review of factors affecting driving and motor vehicle transportation among people with autism spectrum disorder," *Disability and Rehabilitation*, vol. 39, no. 9, pp. 837–846, 2017.

[10] S. Classen, M. Monahan, K. E. Brown, and S. Hernandez, "Driving indicators in teens with attention deficit hyperactivity and/or autism spectrum disorder: indicateurs de la conduite automobile chez les jeunes ayant un déficit de l'attention avec hyperactivité ou un trouble du spectre autistique," *Canadian Journal of Occupational Therapy*, vol. 80, no. 5, pp. 274–283, 2013.

[11] J. Wade, D. Bian, J. Fan et al., "A virtual reality driving environment for training safe gaze patterns: application in individuals with ASD," in *International Conference on Universal Access in Human-Computer Interaction*, pp. 689–697, Los Angeles, CA, USA, 2015, Springer.

[12] H. J. Bishop, F. J. Biasini, and D. Stavrinos, "Social and non-social hazard response in drivers with autism spectrum disorder," *Journal of Autism and Developmental Disorders*, vol. 47, no. 4, pp. 905–917, 2017.

[13] M. Chita-Tegmark, "Social attention in ASD: a review and meta-analysis of eye-tracking studies," *Research in Developmental Disabilities*, vol. 48, pp. 79–93, 2016.

[14] E. Sheppard, D. Ropar, G. Underwood, and E. van Loon, "Brief report: driving hazard perception in autism," *Journal of Autism and Developmental Disorders*, vol. 40, no. 4, pp. 504–508, 2010.

[15] S. Classen and M. Monahan, "Evidence-based review on interventions and determinants of driving performance in teens with attention deficit hyperactivity disorder or autism spectrum disorder," *Traffic Injury Prevention*, vol. 14, no. 2, pp. 188–193, 2013.

[16] C. Silvi, B. Scott-Parker, and C. Jones, "A literature review of the likely effects of autism spectrum disorder on adolescent driving abilities," in *Adolescent Research Review*, pp. 1–17, Springer, 2017.

[17] S. Tyler, "Asperger's syndrome: the implications for driver training methods and road safety," *Journal of the Australasian College of Road Safety*, vol. 24, no. 1, pp. 55–63, 2013.

[18] D. A. Grimes and K. F. Schulz, "An overview of clinical research: the lay of the land," *The Lancet*, vol. 359, no. 9300, pp. 57–61, 2002.

[19] M. Monahan, S. Classen, and P. Helsel, "Pre-driving skills of a teen with attention deficit hyperactivity and autism spectrum disorder," *Developmental Disabilities Special Interest Section Quarterly*, vol. 35, no. 4, pp. 1–4, 2012.

[20] M. Monahan, S. Classen, and P. V. Helsel, "Pre-driving evaluation of a teen with attention deficit hyperactivity disorder and autism spectrum disorder," *Canadian Journal of Occupational Therapy*, vol. 80, no. 1, pp. 35–41, 2013.

[21] D. J. Cox, T. Brown, V. Ross et al., "Can youth with autism spectrum disorder use virtual reality driving simulation training to evaluate and improve driving performance? An exploratory study," *Journal of Autism and Developmental Disorders*, vol. 47, no. 8, pp. 2544–2555, 2017.

[22] B. P. Daly, E. G. Nicholls, K. E. Patrick, D. D. Brinckman, and M. T. Schultheis, "Driving behaviors in adults with autism spectrum disorders," *Journal of Autism and Developmental Disorders*, vol. 44, no. 12, pp. 3119–3128, 2014.

[23] D. Y. Chee, H. C. Lee, A.-H. Patomella, and T. Falkmer, "Driving behaviour profile of drivers with autism spectrum disorder (ASD)," *Journal of Autism and Developmental Disorders*, vol. 47, no. 9, pp. 2658–2670, 2017.

[24] N. B. Cox, R. E. Reeve, S. M. Cox, and D. J. Cox, "Brief report: driving and young adults with ASD: parents' experiences," *Journal of Autism and Developmental Disorders*, vol. 42, no. 10, pp. 2257–2262, 2012.

[25] B. Reimer, R. Fried, B. Mehler et al., "Brief report: examining driving behavior in young adults with high functioning autism spectrum disorders: a pilot study using a driving simulation paradigm," *Journal of Autism and Developmental Disorders*, vol. 43, no. 9, pp. 2211–2217, 2013.

[26] E. Sheppard, E. van Loon, G. Underwood, and D. Ropar, "Difficulties predicting time-to-arrival in individuals with autism spectrum disorders," *Research in Autism Spectrum Disorders*, vol. 28, pp. 17–23, 2016.

[27] H. C. Lee, D. Cameron, and A. H. Lee, "Assessing the driving performance of older adult drivers: on-road versus simulated driving," *Accident Analysis and Prevention*, vol. 35, no. 5, pp. 797–803, 2003.

[28] D. Y.-T. Chee, H. C.-Y. Lee, M. Falkmer et al., "Viewpoints on driving of individuals with and without autism spectrum disorder," *Developmental Neurorehabilitation*, vol. 18, no. 1, pp. 26–36, 2015.

[29] J. A. Michon, "A critical view of driver behavior models: what do we know, what should we do?," in *Human Behavior and Traffic Safety*, pp. 485–524, Springer, 1985.

[30] W. Macdonald, J. M. Pellerito, and M. Di Stefano, "Introduction to driver rehabilitation and community mobility," in *Driver Rehabilitation and Community Mobility: Principles and Practice*, K. Falk, Ed., pp. 3–22, Elsevier Mosby, St. Louis, MO, USA, 2006.

[31] D. Deka, C. Feeley, and A. Lubin, "Travel patterns, needs, and barriers of adults with autism spectrum disorder: report from a survey," *Transportation Research Record: Journal of the Transportation Research Board*, vol. 2542, no. 2542, pp. 9–16, 2016.

[32] P. Huang, T. Kao, A. E. Curry, and D. R. Durbin, "Factors associated with driving in teens with autism spectrum disorders," *Journal of Developmental & Behavioral Pediatrics*, vol. 33, no. 1, pp. 70–74, 2012.

[33] E. Sheppard, E. van Loon, G. Underwood, and D. Ropar, "Attentional differences in a driving hazard perception task in adults with autism spectrum disorders," *Journal of Autism and Developmental Disorders*, vol. 47, no. 2, pp. 405–414, 2017.

[34] D. Bian, J. Wade, Z. Warren, and N. Sarkar, "Online engagement detection and task adaptation in a virtual reality based driving simulator for autism intervention," in *International Conference on Universal Access in Human-Computer Interaction*, pp. 538–547, Toronto, ON, Canada, 2016, Springer.

[35] J. Fan, J. W. Wade, A. P. Key, Z. E. Warren, and N. Sarkar, "EEG-based affect and workload recognition in a virtual driving environment for ASD intervention," *IEEE Transactions on Biomedical Engineering*, vol. 65, no. 1, pp. 43–51, 2018.

[36] J. Wade, D. Bian, L. Zhang et al., "Design of a virtual reality driving environment to assess performance of teenagers with ASD," in *International Conference on Universal Access in Human-Computer Interaction*, pp. 466–474, Heraklion, Crete, Greece, 2014, Springer.

[37] L. Zhang, J. Wade, D. Bian et al., "Multimodal fusion for cognitive load measurement in an adaptive virtual reality driving task for autism intervention," in *International Conference on Universal Access in Human-Computer Interaction*, pp. 709–720, Los Angeles, CA, USA, 2015, Springer.

[38] L. Zhang, J. W. Wade, D. Bian, A. Swanson, Z. Warren, and N. Sarkar, "Data fusion for difficulty adjustment in an adaptive virtual reality game system for autism intervention," in *International Conference on Human-Computer Interaction*, pp. 648–652, Heraklion, Crete, Greece, 2014, Springer.

8

Neurohealth Properties of *Hericium erinaceus* Mycelia Enriched with Erinacines

I-Chen Li,[1] Li-Ya Lee,[1] Tsai-Teng Tzeng,[2] Wan-Ping Chen,[1] Yen-Po Chen,[1] Young-Ju Shiao,[2] and Chin-Chu Chen[1,3,4,5]

[1] *Grape King Bio Ltd, Zhong-Li Dist., Taoyuan City, Taiwan*
[2] *Institute of Biopharmaceutical Sciences, National Yang-Ming University, Taipei City, Taiwan*
[3] *Institute of Food Science and Technology, National Taiwan University, Taipei City, Taiwan*
[4] *Department of Food Science, Nutrition and Nutraceutical Biotechnology, Shih Chien University, Taipei City, Taiwan*
[5] *Institute of Biotechnology, National Changhua University of Education, Changhua, Taiwan*

Correspondence should be addressed to Chin-Chu Chen; gkbioeng@grapeking.com.tw

Academic Editor: Cheng-Yu Wei

Hericium erinaceus, an ideal culinary-medicinal mushroom, has become a well-established candidate in promoting positive brain and nerve health-related activities by inducing the nerve growth factor from its bioactive ingredient. Among its active compounds, only erinacine A has confirmed pharmacological actions in the central nervous system in rats. Hence, this review has summarized the available information on the neurohealth properties of *H. erinaceus* mycelia enriched with erinacines, which may contribute to further research on the therapeutic roles of these mycelia. The safety of this mushroom has also been discussed. Although it has been difficult to extrapolate the *in vivo* studies to clinical situations, preclinical studies have shown that there can be improvements in ischemic stroke, Parkinson's disease, Alzheimer's disease, and depression if *H. erinaceus* mycelia enriched with erinacines are included in daily meals.

1. Introduction

Diseases of the aging nervous system, such as Parkinson's disease, Alzheimer's disease, and stroke, are serious global public health crises as there is no cure for them currently. These lucrative markets have thus attracted the interest of a majority of large pharmaceutical companies which have put a tremendous effort into seeking medications to relieve the symptoms. However, despite successful preclinical testing, clinical trials for novel drugs have a poor track record of success.

In stroke and traumatic brain injuries, a variety of N-methyl-D-aspartate receptor antagonists have halted the progression of secondary damages in rodent models [1, 2], yet they have failed in human clinical trials due to unwanted side effects of the drugs [3, 4]. Likewise, levodopa is the primary treatment for Parkinson's disease that passes through the blood-brain barrier and gets converted into dopamine, but its long-term use can elicit additional clinical symptoms such as psychosis, mood fluctuations, increased cognitive impairment, or drug-induced dyskinesias [5]. Similarly, despite one new drug out of 244 compounds tested in 413 Alzheimer's disease clinical trials between 2002 and 2012 being approved for use, it cannot stop Alzheimer's from progressing [6]. Even though several other studies are underway, huge disappointment from the largest pharmaceutical companies, such as Axovant Sciences Ltd., Merck & Co Inc., Biogen Inc., Prana Biotechnology Ltd., and Pfizer Inc., was observed during recent times [7]. With a significant number of failed clinical trials and without a clear understanding of the potential mechanism of these diseases, dementia specialists have therefore turned their focus from treatment to prevention to stop further disease progression [8].

It is time to stop dementia before it starts. Recently, the search for small preventative neurotrophic compounds that can cross the brain-blood and are responsible for the maintenance, survival, and regeneration of neurons has attracted much attention [9]. In particular, compounds derived from natural sources with fewer side effects that can be part of everyday nutrition may help with dementia prevention. Mushrooms, which are considered nutritionally functional foods and sources of physiologically beneficial medicines, can be excellent candidates for this cause.

Among all culinary mushrooms, *Hericium erinaceus* (most commonly known as lion's mane) has been widely reported to have therapeutic activities related to the promotion of nerve and brain health. Different compounds isolated from this mushroom inducing the expression of neurotrophic factors such as nerve growth factors (NGF) have been actively studied and reported [10–15]. Hericenones were typically found in the fruiting bodies while erinacines were derived from the mycelia of the mushroom (Figure 1).

A previous double-blinded clinical study has shown that oral administration of *H. erinaceus* fruiting body was effective in improving mild cognitive impairment in 50- to 80-year-old Japanese patients [16]. However, when examining the constituents of this effect, hericenones failed to stimulate NGF gene expression in primary cultured rat astroglial cells and 1321N1 human astrocytoma cells [17], suggesting that hericenones were not the key components responsible for the neuroprotective activities of this mushroom. On the other hand, the prominent beneficial effect of erinacine A was confirmed in the central nervous system in rats [18]. It is essential to know the concentrations of the bioactive compounds present in the functional ingredients to better assess their effects on the quality and bioactivity. For food industries, it is even critical that strict specifications of their ingredients are complied with. Therefore, this review will summarize the recent advances on the neurohealth properties of *H. erinaceus* mycelia enriched with erinacines (≥3 mg/g) and discuss the potential mechanisms of action responsible for these medicinal properties.

2. Erinacines

Erinacines are groups of cyathin diterpenoids that show biological activities as stimulators of NGF synthesis and could be useful as a treatment for neurodegenerative disorders and peripheral neuropathy [19]. To date, 15 erinacines (erinacines A–K and P–S) have been identified (Figure 2) and further investigations have demonstrated that eight of them have various neuroprotective properties, such as enhancing NGF release (erinacines A–I), reducing amyloid-β deposition, increasing insulin-degrading enzyme (IDE) expression (erinacines A and S), or managing neuropathic pain (erinacine E), while others are either being currently discovered or have other pharmacological activities (Table 1). However, no direct evidence has yet shown that these compounds could pass through the blood-brain barrier. While other bioactive agents are still being explored, erinacine A has currently been the only one designed specifically to correlate results from *in vitro* studies with outcomes observed from *in vivo* studies [18], which could bring

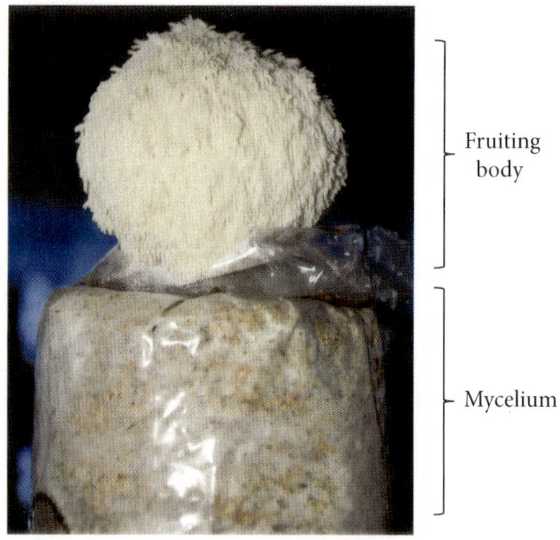

Figure 1: Fruiting body and mycelium of *H. erinaceus*.

scientists a step closer to developing a better treatment option for neurodegenerative disorders.

2.1. Erinacine A. Erinacine A, the main representative of the erinacine group, not only has an enhancing effect on NGF synthesis *in vitro* [12] but also can increase NGF and catecholamine content in the locus coeruleus and hippocampus of rats after administration (8 mg/kg body weight) [18]. This enhanced amount of NGF appears to markedly increase neuronal survival in different brain areas and substantially improve behavioral outcomes in various animal models. In the experimental model of stroke, 1 mg/kg erinacine A administered intraperitoneally in rats for 90 min significantly increased cell survival, attenuated the expression of proinflammatory mediators, and reduced infarct volume after transient focal cerebral ischemia [24]. In another study, it was shown that oral treatment with erinacine A could reduce amyloid-β plaque burden by increasing $A\beta$ degradation by elevating the level of IDE in 5-month-old APPswe/PS1ΔE9 double transgenic mice [20]. These preclinical studies are very encouraging and suggest that erinacine A is effective in reducing neurodegenerative disease-induced cell death. However, no studies have shown that erinacine A could be absorbed into the blood capillaries, cross the blood-brain barrier, and be localized in the brain. Hence, future studies measuring the concentration of erinacine A in the brain and blood could be performed to clarify these mechanisms in detail.

Interestingly, neuroprotective compounds may also be effective in cancer therapy. Given the increasing evidence showing that genes are upregulated in central nervous system disorders and downregulated in cancers and *vice versa* [25], it suggests a bright future for developing common therapeutic approaches in the treatment of these diseases. In line with this finding, treatments with erinacine A have been found to inhibit the proliferation of DLD-1 colorectal adenocarcinoma cells *in vitro* as well as the growth of DLD-1 tumors *in vivo* [21] (Table 1). Despite the promising results, erinacines in *H. erinaceus* mycelia are usually present in microquantities and minor variations in the environment can

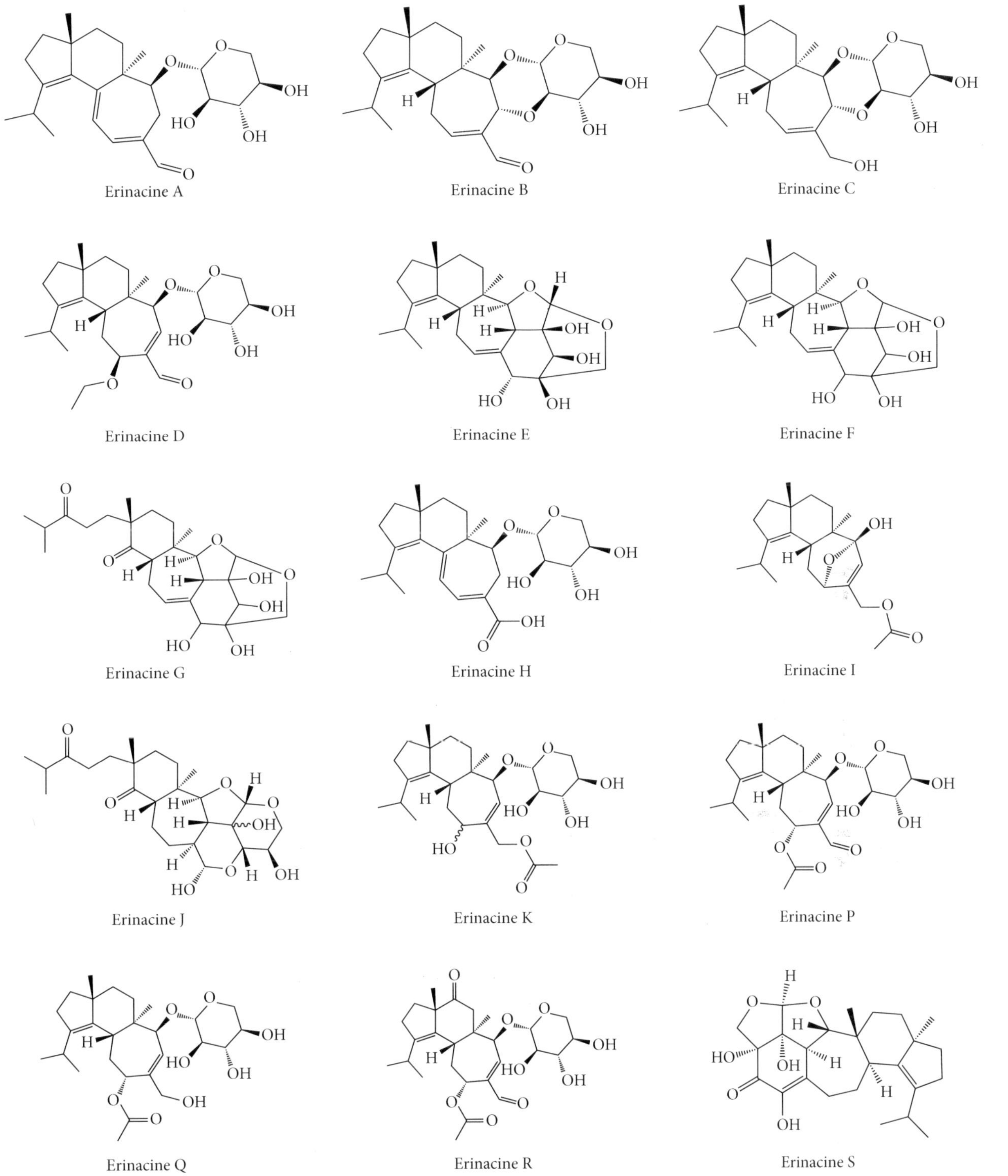

FIGURE 2: Chemical structures of 15 erinacines.

have huge impacts on the quantity, quality, and diversity of the metabolic products.

3. Production of Erinacines

As the fruiting body was reported to contain no erinacines [26], the best option would be to enhance erinacine production in *H. erinaceus* mycelia via submerged fermentation under constantly controlled culture parameters. Although chemical syntheses of cyathane-type diterpenoids are not impossible, they are complex, multistep processes that result in low yields and low purity levels [27]. Therefore, it seems highly desirable to biosynthesize erinacines using bioreactors to obtain a high yield of mycelia with high

TABLE 1: Erinacines with biological activities demonstrated *in vitro* and *in vivo*.

Erinacines	Tests	Concentration	Biological activities	Reference
Erinacine A	*In vitro*	1 mM	Induced 250.1 ± 36.2 pg/ml NGF synthesis	[12]
	In vivo	30 mg/kg body weight/day	(1) Reduced amyloid burden by 38.1 ± 19.7% (2) Increased IDE levels by 141.1 ± 63.7%	[20]
	In vivo	1 mg/kg body weight/day	Inhibited DLD-1 tumor growth by 66%	[21]
	In vivo	30 mg/kg body weight/day	(1) Reduced both the size and number of amyloid plaques (2) Increased IDE levels by 303.5% (3) Recovered from impairments in burrowing, nesting, and Morris water maze tasks	[22]
Erinacine B	*In vitro*	1 mM	Induced 129.7 ± 6.5 pg/ml NGF synthesis	[12]
Erinacine C	*In vitro*	1 mM	Induced 299.1 ± 59.6 pg/ml NGF synthesis	[12]
Erinacine D	*In vitro*	1.67 mM	Induced 141.5 ± 18.2 pg/ml NGF synthesis	[14]
Erinacine E	*In vitro*	5 mM	Induced 105.0 ± 5.2 pg/ml NGF synthesis	[13]
	In vitro	IC_{50}	Binding inhibitor for κ-opioid receptor at 0.8 μM	[23]
Erinacine F	*In vitro*	5 mM	Induced 175.0 ± 5.2 pg/ml NGF synthesis	[13]
Erinacine H	*In vitro*	70.8 mM	Induced 31.5 ± 1.7 pg/ml NGF synthesis	[15]
Erinacine S	*In vivo*	30 mg/kg body weight/day	(1) Reduced amyloid burden by 40.2 ± 15.2% (2) Increased IDE levels by 130.5 ± 68.9%	[20]
	In vivo	30 mg/kg body weight/day	(1) Reduced the size of amyloid plaques (2) Increased IDE levels by 269.8% (3) Recovered from impairments in burrowing, nesting, and Morris water maze tasks	[22]

concentrations of bioactive metabolites, which can expand mushroom potentialities for the development of functional foods, nutraceuticals, and novel drugs [28].

While there may have been various strategies developed over the past few decades for erinacine accumulation, it appeared, however, that only three reports concerning erinacines A and C have been published. In a 10 l bioreactor, a medium comprised of glucose 69.87 g/l, casein peptone 11.17 g/l, NaCl 1.45 g/l, $ZnSO_4$ 55.24 mg/l, and KH_2PO_4 1.0 g/l with a pH of 4.5 has produced 192 ± 42 mg/l of erinacine A after 8 days of cultivation [29]. With the monitoring of the temperature and ventilation during the processing, the highest yield of 206 ± 7 mg/l (17.34 mg/g) of erinacine A could be obtained after 14 days of cultivation using a 100 l bioreactor with the medium containing 0.5% yeast extract, 4% glucose, 0.5% soybean powder, 0.25% peptone, 1% oat, and 0.05% KH_2PO_4 at pH 5 [30]. These results suggest that a carbon-to-nitrogen (C/N) ratio of 6 and a pH value of 4 to 5 in a medium may be important parameters in promoting the biosynthesis of erinacine A in *H. erinaceus* mycelia.

Scale-up of pilot plant fermentors to large-scale bioreactors to enhance the biomass as well as erinacine production could also be an attractive proposal. Although various factors such as improper distribution of oxygen, uneven distribution of the media, or insufficient agitation environment could cause negative impacts on product formation and quality at a higher scale of operation [31], there has been one successful example of commercial exploitation. In this case, the medium was optimized for a C/N ratio of 10, temperature of 26°C, pH of 4.5, and agitation of 120 rpm. The highest accumulation of erinacine A (5 mg/g) was observed with 20-ton fermentors after 12 days [32]. This preliminary result was satisfactory, showing that implementation and successful commercial exploitation of research results in large-scale bioreactors are possible.

For erinacine C production, the optimal medium was found to include 5 g/l oatmeal, 1.5 g/l calcium carbonate, and 0.5 g/l Edamin® K at pH 7.5, which can generate concentrations up to 2.73 g/l after six days of cultivation [33]. However, it is noteworthy that this process was accomplished in a two-step course. The fungal pellets were concentrated by centrifugation to remove preculture medium components before inoculation of the main culture. Although an inoculation ratio of 5 : 10 volume/volume (*v*/*v*) is beneficial in producing erinacine C, it is only reproducible at a small laboratory scale and not feasible in industrial operations as the concentrated biomass is not easily adapted for the aseptic handling of large volumes.

These findings are extremely important as they could be used as references to enhance the production of useful secondary metabolites for industrial applications. Moreover, it should be noted that the presence of erinacines in *H. erinaceus* mycelia can also achieve pharmacological benefits. In this regard, isolation of erinacines from *H. erinaceus* mycelia is particularly important, as they could serve as quality controls in assuring the efficacy, quality, and safety of this mushroom in future markets.

4. *In Vivo* Preclinical Studies of *Hericium erinaceus* Mycelia Enriched with Erinacines

While 1/5 of dementia cases can be reversible in some cases when caused by drugs, alcohol, hormone imbalances, or depression, a significant proportion of individuals suffer

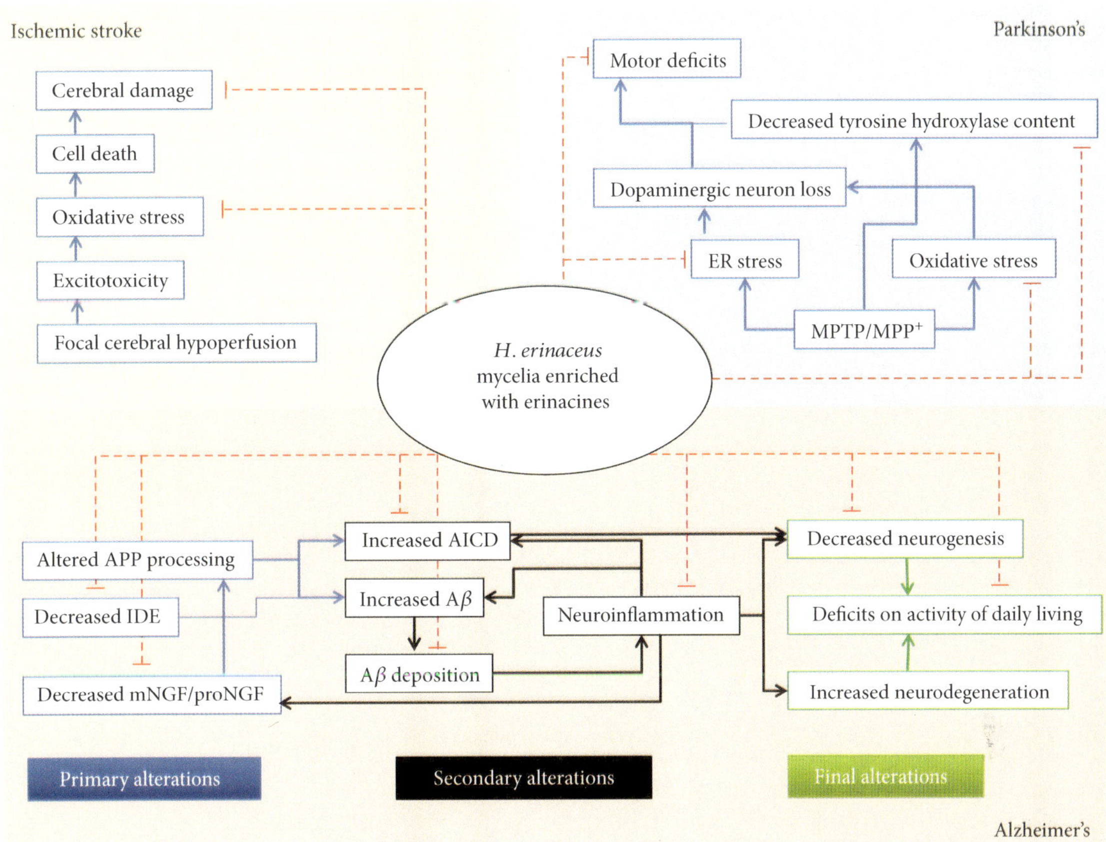

FIGURE 3: Summary of mechanisms of action of *H. erinaceus* mycelia enriched with erinacines in dementia. Primary alterations are possible contributors and drivers in the pathogenesis of Alzheimer's disease. Secondary alterations include increased amyloid precursor protein intracellular domain (AICD) and accumulation of $A\beta$, leading to neuroinflammation. Finally, decreased neurogenesis and increased neurodegeneration can cause deficits in activities of daily living. The red dashed lines indicate potential mechanisms of *H. erinaceus* mycelia-attenuated pathological and behavioral changes in stroke, Parkinson's disease, and Alzheimer's disease.

from dementias that are irreversible [34]. The most common irreversible dementia types include Alzheimer's disease, vascular dementia, Lewy body dementia, Parkinson's disease, and frontotemporal dementia [35]. Luckily, growing preclinical studies have demonstrated that the risk of dementia and cognitive impairment could be reduced in the early stages by erinacine-enriched *H. erinaceus* mycelium consumption. Figure 3 illustrates the overall therapeutic mechanism of action of *H. erinaceus* mycelia enriched with erinacine in dementia.

4.1. Protection against Ischemic Stroke. In a rat model of transient focal cerebral ischemia via the middle cerebral artery occlusion method, pretreatment with 3 mg/g erinacine A-enriched *H. erinaceus* mycelia orally at concentrations of 50 and 300 mg/kg for 5 days could reduce the total infarcted volumes by 22% and 44%, respectively [24]. Moreover, immunohistochemistry for neuronal nuclei (NeuN) revealed the presence of significantly more neurons after brain injuries in rats which were treated with erinacine A-enriched *H. erinaceus* mycelia. Excessive reactive oxygen species and oxidative stress have been strongly implicated in the pathogenesis of ischemic brain injury [36]. Decreased levels of proinflammatory cytokines and inducible NO synthase (iNOS), however, have been detected in ischemic neurons after mycelia exposure. These findings suggested that erinacine A-enriched *H. erinaceus* mycelia may be a promising agent for stroke injury as these have the ability to decrease neuronal apoptosis and reduce stroke cavity size in the rat brains by targeting iNOS/reactive nitrogen species (RNS) and p38 mitogen-activated protein kinase (MAPK)/CCAAT enhancer-binding protein homologous protein (CHOP) pathways.

4.2. Protection against Parkinson's Disease. Parkinson's disease (PD) is the second most common neurodegenerative disorder that is characterized by the progressive loss of dopaminergic cells in the substantia nigra pars compacta region of the brain, which results in motor problems including resting tremor, rigidity, bradykinesia, and postural instability [37]. Among models of PD, the involvement of the drug 1-methyl-4-phenyl-1,2,3,6-tetrahydropyridine (MPTP) is most widely used. Once inside the brain, MPTP is metabolized into the toxic cation 1-methyl-4-phenylpyridinium (MPP^+) by the enzyme monoamine oxidase B, resulting in nigral dopaminergic neuronal death and mitochondrial damage, which can mimic the clinical and pathological features of PD [38]. In one study, the neuroprotective effect of erinacine

A-enriched *H. erinaceus* mycelia was assessed in the MPTP-induced PD model. Results showed that dopaminergic lesions and oxidative stress in the stratum and substantia nigra were significantly improved after pretreatment with 3 mg/g erinacine A-enriched *H. erinaceus* mycelia for 25 days [39]. Furthermore, the mycelia could reverse MPTP-associated motor deficits, as revealed by the analysis of the rotarod assessment. The mechanisms underlying the neuroprotective effect of erinacine A-enriched *H. erinaceus* mycelia were associated with the inhibition on the endoplasmic reticulum stress by lowering the expression of Fas and Bax via inositol-requiring enzyme 1α (IRE1α)/tumor necrosis factor receptor-associated factor 2 (TRAF2) complex formation and phosphorylation of c-Jun N-terminal protein kinase (JNK) 1/2, p38 and nuclear factor kappa light chain enhancer of activated B cell (NF-κB) pathways. Taken together, these results have demonstrated that erinacine A-enriched *H. erinaceus* mycelia have the potential to be a new therapeutic agent for the prevention and treatment of PD.

4.3. Protection against Alzheimer's Disease. There has been growing evidence which suggested that Alzheimer's disease progression becomes a runaway chain reaction after a certain point. In the presence of amyloid-β plaques, secondary injuries such as inflammation, excitotoxicity, and apoptosis may trigger the deposition of hyperphosphorylated tau proteins [40]. Once the process starts, the tau tangles are unabated even after the removal of amyloid-β plaques. Moreover, studies in transgenic amyloid precursor protein (APP) mice have shown that therapies are most effective when administered before plaque formation [41, 42]. Therefore, amyloid-β has become an ideal therapeutic target for primary prevention.

In one study, APPswe/PS1dE9 transgenic mice were utilized to evaluate the therapeutic effect of *H. erinaceus* mycelia containing 19 mg/g erinacine A on Alzheimer's disease. After 30 days of oral administration to 5-month-old transgenic mice, these mycelia were able to attenuate cerebral Aβ plaque burden, prevent recruitment and activation of plaque-associated microglia and astrocytes, promote the expression of IDE, increase the NGF-to-NGF precursor (proNGF) ratio, and enhance the proliferation of neuron progenitors and the number of newly born neurons in the dentate gyrus region [43]. Additionally, improvements in the impairment of other multiple brain regions were also shown when APP/PS1 transgenic mice treated with *H. erinaceus* mycelia could recover behavioral deficits after 81 days of administration. Collectively, these findings raise the possibility that prevention with erinacine A-enriched *H. erinaceus* mycelia could be an effective therapeutic strategy for managing Alzheimer's disease.

4.4. Protection against Depressive Symptoms. Depression is the most frequently occurring psychiatric comorbidity, with prevalence in Alzheimer's, Parkinson's, and stroke as high as 87%, 75%, and 79%, respectively [44]. Prior data has shown that levels of NGF are significantly lower in patients with major depressive disorder than in healthy subjects [45]. *H. erinaceus* mycelia enriched with erinacines, which are involved in the creation of the neurotrophic factors, are thereby hypothesized to play a role in depression.

In animal models, chronic restraint stress is known to cause decreased BDNF expression in the hippocampus and depression-like behaviors [46]. Hence, alleviation of *H. erinaceus* mycelia enriched with erinacines in animals subjected to repeated chronic stress was examined [47]. Two weeks of treatment with *H. erinaceus* mycelia have reduced the immobility time in the tail suspension test and forced swimming test as well as decreased the number of entries and the time spent in the open arm. In addition, restraint-induced low levels of norepinephrine, dopamine, serotonin, high interleukin-6, and tumor necrosis factor-α in the hippocampus were completely reversed by *H. erinaceus* mycelium administration. Furthermore, *H. erinaceus* mycelium was shown to activate the BDNF pathways and block NF-κB signals in mice. Hence, these results indicate that *H. erinaceus* mycelia could be an attractive agent for the treatment of depressive disorders through the modulation of monoamine neurotransmitters and proinflammatory cytokines as well as the regulation of brain-derived neurotrophic factor (BDNF) pathways.

4.5. Protection against Neuropathic Pain. Currently, there is a growing realization that lesions to the peripheral or central nervous system could lead to neuropathic pain [48]. Currently, both ionotropic P2X receptors and metabotropic P2Y receptors have been identified as key receptors in mediating neuropathic pain [49]. As *H. erinaceus* mycelium has a crucial role in nerve regeneration via the stimulation of neurotrophic factors, the analgesic potential of this mycelium using both a P2 purinergic receptor-coupled Ca^{2+} signaling platform and an *in vivo* model was investigated. The results indicated that the extracts of *H. erinaceus* mycelium could completely block ATP-induced Ca^{2+} signaling in human HOS cells, suggesting its inhibitory potential as a modulator of pain-related P2X receptors [50]. In addition, administration of the extracts of *H. erinaceus* mycelium in heat-induced mice could significantly postpone the tail-flick response to heat stimulation as well as the paw-lifting response to a hot plate, indicating that it has an excellent potential for pain relief.

4.6. Protection against Presbycusis. Recent research has highlighted that presbycusis may precede the onset of clinical dementia and may present as an early manifestation of probable Alzheimer's disease [51]. Exogenous application of NGF has been the first to promote nerve fiber regrowth or sprouting in deafened guinea pigs caused by neomycin [52]. Moreover, clinical studies in patients with sensorineural hearing defects have revealed that the amount of circulating NGF is relatively lower compared to the level found in normal patients [53]. Therefore, the otoprotective effect of *H. erinaceus* mycelia enriched with erinacines in rapidly aging mice has been observed [54]. The results indicated that the *H. erinaceus* mycelium-treated group had significantly lower hearing thresholds according to auditory brainstem responses measured using click sounds and 8 kHz and 16 kHz tone burst sound stimulation when compared with the control group. These findings suggested that *H. erinaceus*

Table 2: The beneficial activities of *H. erinaceus* mycelium and its active components on age-associated cognitive change and early dementia.

Material studied (dose used)	*In vivo* models	Effects	Reference
Erinacine A	Normal Wistar rats	Enhanced NGF and catecholamine secretion in the LC and hippocampus after intragastric dosing erinacine A at 8 mg/kg body weight	[18]
Erinacine A-enriched mycelia and erinacine A	Ischemic stroke in Sprague-Dawley rats	(1) Mycelia at 50 and 300 mg/kg body weight reduced infarcted volume in cortex and subcortex of transient stroke rats (2) Erinacine A at 1, 5, and 10 mg/kg body weight reduced levels of proinflammatory cytokines such as iNOS, IL-1β, IL-6, and TNF-α in the serum of transient stroke rats	[24]
Erinacine A-enriched mycelia	APPswe/PS1dE9 transgenic mice	(1) Mycelia at 300 mg/kg body weight reduced amyloid plaque burden in the area including the cerebral cortex and hippocampus (2) Increased NGF/proNGF ratio and promoted hippocampal neurogenesis (3) Restored nesting behavior	[43]
Erinacine A Erinacine S	APPswe/PS1dE9 transgenic mice	(1) Both compounds at 30 mg/kg body weight reduced amyloid plaque burden in the cerebral cortex (2) Increased the level of IDE in the cortex by 130.5 ± 68.9% and 141.1 ± 63.7%, respectively	[20]
Erinacine A-enriched mycelia	MPTP-induced neurotoxicity in C57BL/6 mice	(1) Treatment at 10.76 and 21.52 mg/day elevated dopamine, NGF, and GSH levels (2) Reduced motor dysfunction (3) Reduced dopaminergic neurons apoptosis in the striatum and substantia nigra	[39]
Mycelia ethanolic extract	C57BL/6 mice	(1) Treatment at 2000 mg/kg body weight blocked the rise in [Ca^{2+}] induced by ATP (2) Increased the latency in tail-flick and paw-lifting times exposed to a thermal stimulus	[50]
Erinacine A-enriched mycelium	Restraint stress induced depression in ICR mice	(1) Treatment at 200 and 400 mg/kg body weight increased dopamine and serotonin levels (2) Increased BDNF, TrκB, and PI3K expressions in the hippocampus (3) Reduced IL-6 and TNF-α levels (4) Reduced the immobility time in the tail suspension test and forced swimming test, as well as decreased the number of entries and the time spent in the open arm	[47]

mycelium diet supplementation was effective in slowing hearing threshold deterioration.

The beneficial activities of *H. erinaceus* mycelia on age-associated cognitive change and early dementia are summarized in Table 2. Given the fact that all seven of these studies have provided very encouraging findings, it is also of paramount importance that the daily intake of *H. erinaceus* mycelia in the context of the entire diet is established before the treatment is administered.

5. Toxicology Studies

To date, all experimental studies have suggested that *H. erinaceus* mycelium is safe and devoid of adverse effects (Table 3). In an animal study, the acute oral LD_{50} of *H. erinaceus* mycelia enriched with its active compounds was found to be higher than 5 g/kg in rats [55], indicating that the mycelium is reasonably safe in cases of overdose. Repeated daily doses of *H. erinaceus* mycelium enriched with its active compounds up to 3 g/kg have also been used without any adverse effects in rats [32]. Moreover, *H. erinaceus* mycelium was found not to be mutagenic in the bacterial reverse mutation test (Ames test), *in vitro* chromosome aberration test, and *in vivo* erythrocyte micronucleus test, with and without metabolic activation [56]. Further investigations also showed that erinacine-enriched *H. erinaceus* mycelium was not teratogenic in Sprague-Dawley rats with doses up to 2625 mg/kg [55]. In a well-designed clinical trial, erinacine-enriched *H. erinaceus* mycelia demonstrated significant clinical efficacy and had good safety and tolerability in 36 patients with Alzheimer's disease (unpublished data).

6. Conclusion

The evidence so far has shown that *H. erinaceus* mycelium enriched with its active compounds is capable of delaying neuronal cell death in rats with neurodegenerative diseases, such as ischemic stroke, Parkinson's disease, Alzheimer's disease, and depression. Moreover, results have indicated that administration of *H. erinaceus* mycelia enriched with its active compounds can promote functional recovery and enhance nerve regeneration in rats with neuropathic pain or presbycusis. Despite that more clinical research is needed to fully understand the potential applications of erinacine-

Table 3: The safety of *H. erinaceus* mycelia.

Material studied (dose used)	*In vivo* models	Effects	Reference
Erinacine A-enriched mycelia	Normal ICR mice	No adverse effects in (1) Bacterial reverse mutation test (Ames test) up to 5 mg/plate (2) *In vitro* chromosome aberration test up to 2.5 mg/ml (3) *In vivo* erythrocyte micronucleus test up to 5 mg/kg body weight	[56]
Erinacine A-enriched mycelia	Normal Sprague-Dawley rats	(1) Ethanolic extract induced neuritogenesis in postnatal cortical neurons (2) No adverse effect up to 5 g/kg body weight/day after acute exposure (3) No adverse effect up to 2625 mg/kg body weight/day for prenatal developmental study	[55]
Erinacine A-enriched mycelia	Normal Sprague-Dawley rats	No adverse effect up to 3 g/kg body weight/day for 28 days	[32]

Based on these results, the toxicity profile of *H. erinaceus* mycelium enriched with its active compound is extremely low and therefore has the potential to be developed into a functional ingredient or food associated with improved brain and nerve health. With this idea in mind, the first erinacine A-enriched *H. erinaceus* mycelium product was introduced to the market in 2015 in Taiwan [57].

enriched *Hericium erinaceus* mycelium, the majority of preclinical data strongly suggests that it is safe and offers much-needed neuroprotective applications.

Abbreviations

AICD: Amyloid precursor protein intracellular domain
APP: Amyloid precursor protein
BDNF: Brain-derived neurotrophic factor
CHOP: CCAAT enhancer-binding protein homologous protein
C/N: Carbon to nitrogen
ERK: Extracellular-signal-regulated kinase
IDE: Insulin-degrading enzyme
iNOS: Inducible NO synthase
IRE1α: Inositol-requiring enzyme 1α
JNK: c-Jun N-terminal protein kinase
MAPK: Mitogen-activated protein kinase
MPTP: 1-Methyl-4-phenyl-1,2,3,6-tetrahydropyridine
MPP^+: 1-Methyl-4-phenylpyridinium
NeuN: Neuronal nuclei
NF-κB: Nuclear factor kappa light chain enhancer of activated B cells
NGF: Nerve growth factor
PD: Parkinson's disease
proNGF: NGF precursor
RNS: Reactive nitrogen species
TRAF2: Tumor necrosis factor receptor-associated factor 2
v/*v*: Volume/volume.

Acknowledgments

The authors thank Hsin-Yun Yang for editing the manuscript.

References

[1] J.-M. Lee, G. J. Zipfel, and D. W. Choi, "The changing landscape of ischaemic brain injury mechanisms," *Nature*, vol. 399, 6738 Supplement, pp. A7–A14, 1999.

[2] B. Meldrum, "Protection against ischaemic neuronal damage by drugs acting on excitatory neurotransmission," *Cerebrovascular and Brain Metabolism Reviews*, vol. 2, no. 1, pp. 27–57, 1990.

[3] G. F. Morris, R. Bullock, S. B. Marshall et al., "Failure of the competitive *N*-methyl-D-aspartate antagonist Selfotel (CGS 19755) in the treatment of severe head injury: results of two Phase III clinical trials," *Journal of Neurosurgery*, vol. 91, no. 5, pp. 737–743, 1999.

[4] S. M. Davis, K. R. Lees, G. W. Albers et al., "Selfotel in acute ischemic stroke : possible neurotoxic effects of an NMDA antagonist," *Stroke*, vol. 31, no. 2, pp. 347–354, 2000.

[5] T. Hershey, K. J. Black, J. L. Carl, L. McGee-Minnich, A. Z. Snyder, and J. S. Perlmutter, "Long term treatment and disease severity change brain responses to levodopa in Parkinson's disease," *Journal of Neurology, Neurosurgery & Psychiatry*, vol. 74, no. 7, pp. 844–851, 2003.

[6] J. L. Cummings, T. Morstorf, and K. Zhong, "Alzheimer's disease drug-development pipeline: few candidates, frequent failures," *Alzheimer's Research & Therapy*, vol. 6, no. 4, pp. 37–37, 2014.

[7] J. Cummings, G. Lee, T. Mortsdorf, A. Ritter, and K. Zhong, "Alzheimer's disease drug development pipeline: 2017," *Alzheimer's & Dementia: Translational Research & Clinical Interventions*, vol. 3, no. 3, pp. 367–384, 2017.

[8] L. Robinson, E. Tang, and J.-P. Taylor, "Dementia: timely diagnosis and early intervention," *British Medical Journal*, vol. 350, article h3029, 2015.

[9] M. R. Castellanos-Ortega, R. Cruz-Aguado, and L. Martinez-Marti, "Nerve growth factor: possibilities and limitations of its clinical application," *Revista de Neurologia*, vol. 29, no. 5, pp. 439–447, 1999.

[10] H. Kawagishi, M. Ando, H. Sakamoto et al., "Hericenones C, D and E, stimulators of nerve growth factor (NGF)-synthesis, from the mushroom *Hericium erinaceum*," *Tetrahedron Letters*, vol. 32, no. 35, pp. 4561–4564, 1991.

[11] H. Kawagishi, M. Ando, K. Shinba et al., "Chromans, hericenones F, G and H from the mushroom Hericium erinaceum," *Phytochemistry*, vol. 32, no. 1, pp. 175–178, 1992.

[12] H. Kawagishi, A. Shimada, R. Shirai et al., "Erinacines A, B and C, strong stimulators of nerve growth factor (NGF)-synthesis, from the mycelia of *Hericium erinaceum*," *Tetrahedron Letters*, vol. 35, no. 10, pp. 1569–1572, 1994.

[13] H. Kawagishi, A. Shimada, S. Hosokawa et al., "Erinacines E, F, and G, stimulators of nerve growth factor (NGF)-synthesis, from the mycelia of *Hericium erinaceum*," *Tetrahedron Letters*, vol. 37, no. 41, pp. 7399–7402, 1996.

[14] H. Kawagishi, A. Simada, K. Shizuki et al., "Erinacine D, a stimulator of NGF-synthesis, from the mycelia of *Hericium erinaceum*," *Heterocyclic Communications*, vol. 2, no. 1, 1996.

[15] E. W. Lee, K. Shizuki, S. Hosokawa et al., "Two novel diterpenoids, erinacines H and I from the mycelia of *Hericium erinaceum*," *Bioscience, Biotechnology, and Biochemistry*, vol. 64, no. 11, pp. 2402–2405, 2000.

[16] K. Mori, S. Inatomi, K. Ouchi, Y. Azumi, and T. Tuchida, "Improving effects of the mushroom Yamabushitake (*Hericium erinaceus*) on mild cognitive impairment: a double-blind placebo-controlled clinical trial," *Phytotherapy Research*, vol. 23, no. 3, pp. 367–372, 2009.

[17] K. Mori, Y. Obara, M. Hirota et al., "Nerve growth factor-inducing activity of *Hericium erinaceus* in 1321N1 human astrocytoma cells," *Biological & Pharmaceutical Bulletin*, vol. 31, no. 9, pp. 1727–1732, 2008.

[18] M. Shimbo, H. Kawagishi, and H. Yokogoshi, "Erinacine A increases catecholamine and nerve growth factor content in the central nervous system of rats," *Nutrition Research*, vol. 25, no. 6, pp. 617–623, 2005.

[19] S. C. Apfel and J. A. Kessler, "Neurotrophic factors in the treatment of peripheral neuropathy," *Growth Factors as Drugs for Neurological and Sensory Disorders*, vol. 196, pp. 98–108, 1996.

[20] C.-C. Chen, T. T. Tzeng, C. C. Chen et al., "Erinacine S, a rare sesterterpene from the mycelia of *Hericium erinaceus*," *Journal of Natural Products*, vol. 79, no. 2, pp. 438–441, 2016.

[21] C.-C. Lu, W. S. Huang, K. F. Lee et al., "Inhibitory effect of erinacines A on the growth of DLD-1 colorectal cancer cells is induced by generation of reactive oxygen species and activation of p70S6K and p21," *Journal of Functional Foods*, vol. 21, pp. 474–484, 2016.

[22] T. T. Tzeng, C. C. Chen, C. C. Chen et al., "The cyanthin diterpenoid and sesterterpene constituents of *Hericium erinaceus* mycelium ameliorate Alzheimer's disease-related pathologies in APP/PS1 transgenic mice," *International Journal of Molecular Sciences*, vol. 19, no. 2, 2018.

[23] T. Saito, F. Aoki, H. Hirai et al., "Erinacine E as a kappa opioid receptor agonist and its new analogs from a basidiomycete, *Hericium ramosum*," *The Journal of Antibiotics*, vol. 51, no. 11, pp. 983–990, 1998.

[24] K. F. Lee, J. H. Chen, C. C. Teng et al., "Protective effects of *Hericium erinaceus* mycelium and its isolated erinacine A against ischemia-injury-induced neuronal cell death via the inhibition of iNOS/p38 MAPK and nitrotyrosine," *International Journal of Molecular Sciences*, vol. 15, no. 9, pp. 15073–15089, 2014.

[25] K. Ibáñez, C. Boullosa, R. Tabarés-Seisdedos, A. Baudot, and A. Valencia, "Molecular evidence for the inverse comorbidity between central nervous system disorders and cancers detected by transcriptomic meta-analyses," *PLoS Genetics*, vol. 10, no. 2, article e1004173, 2014.

[26] B. J. Ma, J. W. Shen, H. Y. Yu, Y. Ruan, T. T. Wu, and X. Zhao, "Hericenones and erinacines: stimulators of nerve growth factor (NGF) biosynthesis in *Hericium erinaceus*," *Mycology*, vol. 1, no. 2, pp. 92–98, 2010.

[27] B. B. Snider, N. H. Vo, S. V. O'Nei, and B. M. Foxman, "Synthesis of (±)-allocyathin B2 and (+)-erinacine A," *Journal of the American Chemical Society*, vol. 118, no. 32, pp. 7644-7645, 1996.

[28] V. Elisashvili, "Submerged cultivation of medicinal mushrooms: bioprocesses and products (review)," *International Journal of Medicinal Mushrooms*, vol. 14, no. 3, pp. 211–239, 2012.

[29] W. Krzyczkowski, E. Malinowska, and F. Herold, "Erinacine A biosynthesis in submerged cultivation of *Hericium erinaceum*: quantification and improved cultivation," *Engineering in Life Sciences*, vol. 10, no. 5, pp. 446–457, 2010.

[30] C. C. Chen, S. C. Hsu, L. Y. Lee, and W. P. Chen, *Cultivation Method for Preventing Rapid Degradation of Erinacine A during Fermentation of Hericium erinaceus Mycelium*, G.K.B. Inc, Taiwan, 2016.

[31] T. L. da Silva and A. Reis, "Scale-up problems for the large scale production of algae," in *Algal Biorefinery: An Integrated Approach*, D. Das, Ed., pp. 125–149, Springer International Publishing: Cham, 2015.

[32] I. C. Li, Y. L. Chen, L. Y. Lee et al., "Evaluation of the toxicological safety of erinacine A-enriched *Hericium erinaceus* in a 28-day oral feeding study in Sprague-Dawley rats," *Food and Chemical Toxicology*, vol. 70, pp. 61–67, 2014.

[33] N. Wolters, G. Schembecker, and J. Merz, "Erinacine C: a novel approach to produce the secondary metabolite by submerged cultivation of *Hericium erinaceus*," *Fungal Biology*, vol. 119, no. 12, pp. 1334–1344, 2015.

[34] V. M. E. Bello and R. R. Schultz, "Prevalence of treatable and reversible dementias: a study in a dementia outpatient clinic," *Dementia & Neuropsychologia*, vol. 5, no. 1, pp. 44–47, 2011.

[35] P. Carr, "Types of dementia: an introduction," *British Journal of Healthcare Assistants*, vol. 11, no. 3, pp. 132–135, 2017.

[36] C. L. Allen and U. Bayraktutan, "Oxidative stress and its role in the pathogenesis of ischaemic stroke," *International Journal of Stroke*, vol. 4, no. 6, pp. 461–470, 2009.

[37] T. R. Mhyre, J. T. Boyd, R. W. Hamill, and K. A. Maguire-Zeiss, "Parkinson's disease," *Subcellular Biochemistry*, vol. 65, pp. 389–455, 2012.

[38] G. E. Meredith and D. J. Rademacher, "MPTP mouse models of Parkinson's disease: an update," *Journal of Parkinson's Disease*, vol. 1, no. 1, pp. 19–33, 2011.

[39] H. C. Kuo, C. C. Lu, C. H. Shen et al., "*Hericium erinaceus* mycelium and its isolated erinacine A protection from MPTP-induced neurotoxicity through the ER stress, triggering an apoptosis cascade," *Journal of Translational Medicine*, vol. 14, no. 1, p. 78, 2016.

[40] L. Wang, T. L. Benzinger, Y. Su et al., "Evaluation of tau imaging in staging Alzheimer disease and revealing interactions between β-amyloid and tauopathy," *JAMA Neurology*, vol. 73, no. 9, pp. 1070–1077, 2016.

[41] P. Das, C. Verbeeck, L. Minter et al., "Transient pharmacologic lowering of $A\beta$ production prior to deposition results in sustained reduction of amyloid plaque pathology," *Molecular Neurodegeneration*, vol. 7, no. 1, p. 39, 2012.

[42] R. B. DeMattos, J. Lu, Y. Tang et al., "A plaque-specific antibody clears existing β-amyloid plaques in Alzheimer's disease mice," *Neuron*, vol. 76, no. 5, pp. 908–920, 2012.

[43] T. Tsai-Teng, C. Chin-Chu, L. Li-Ya et al., "Erinacine A-enriched *Hericium erinaceus* mycelium ameliorates Alzheimer's disease-related pathologies in APPswe/PS1dE9 transgenic mice," *Journal of Biomedical Science*, vol. 23, no. 1, p. 49, 2016.

[44] L. B. Strober and P. A. Arnett, "Assessment of depression in three medically ill, elderly populations: Alzheimer's disease, Parkinson's disease, and stroke," *The Clinical Neuropsychologist*, vol. 23, no. 2, pp. 205–230, 2009.

[45] Y.-W. Chen, P. Y. Lin, K. Y. Tu, Y. S. Cheng, C. K. Wu, and P. T. Tseng, "Significantly lower nerve growth factor levels in patients with major depressive disorder than in healthy subjects: a meta-analysis and systematic review," *Neuropsychiatric Disease and Treatment*, vol. 11, pp. 925–933, 2015.

[46] X. Chu, Y. Zhou, Z. Hu et al., "24-Hour-restraint stress induces long-term depressive-like phenotypes in mice," *Scientific Reports*, vol. 6, no. 1, article 32935, 2016.

[47] C.-H. Chiu, C. C. Chyau, C. C. Chen et al., "Erinacine A-enriched *Hericium erinaceus* mycelium produces antidepressant-like effects through modulating BDNF/PI3K/Akt/GSK-3β signaling in mice," *International Journal of Molecular Sciences*, vol. 19, no. 2, p. 341, 2018.

[48] M. de Tommaso, L. Arendt-Nielsen, R. Defrin, M. Kunz, G. Pickering, and M. Valeriani, "Pain in neurodegenerative disease: current knowledge and future perspectives," *Behavioural Neurology*, vol. 2016, Article ID 7576292, 14 pages, 2016.

[49] G. Burnstock, "Purinergic mechanisms and pain," *Advances in Pharmacology*, vol. 75, pp. 91–137, 2016.

[50] P. S. Liu, S. H. Chueh, C. C. Chen, L. Y. Lee, and L. Y. Shiu, "Lion's mane medicinal mushroom, *Hericium erinaceus* (Agaricomycetes), modulates purinoceptor-coupled calcium signaling and murine nociceptive behavior," *International Journal of Medicinal Mushrooms*, vol. 19, no. 6, pp. 499–507, 2017.

[51] G. A. Gates, M. L. Anderson, M. P. Feeney, S. M. McCurry, and E. B. Larson, "Central auditory dysfunction in older persons with memory impairment or Alzheimer dementia," *Archives of Otolaryngology–Head & Neck Surgery*, vol. 134, no. 7, pp. 771–777, 2008.

[52] S. B. Shah, H. B. Gladstone, H. Williams, G. T. Hradek, and R. A. Schindler, "An extended study: protective effects of nerve growth factor in neomycin-induced auditory neural degeneration," *The American Journal of Otology*, vol. 16, no. 3, pp. 310–314, 1995.

[53] F. Salvinelli, M. Casale, F. Greco et al., "Nerve growth factor serum level is reduced in patients with sensorineural hearing impairment: possible clinical implications," *Journal of Biological Regulators and Homeostatic Agents*, vol. 16, no. 3, pp. 176–180, 2002.

[54] Y. C. Chan, C. C. Chen, L. Y. Lee, and W. P. Chen, *Active Substances for Preventing Hearing Deterioration, the Composition Containing the Active Substances, and the Preparation Method There of*, G.K.B. LTD, Taiwan, 2017.

[55] I. C. Li, W. P. Chen, Y. P. Chen, L. Y. Lee, Y. T. Tsai, and C. C. Chen, "Acute and developmental toxicity assessment of erincine A-enriched *Hericium erinaceus* mycelia in Sprague-Dawley rats," *Drug and Chemical Toxicology*, pp. 1–6, 2018.

[56] I. C. Li, Y. L. Chen, W. P. Chen et al., "Genotoxicity profile of erinacine A-enriched *Hericium erinaceus* mycelium," *Toxicology Reports*, vol. 1, pp. 1195–1201, 2014.

[57] C.-C. Chen, "Neurohealth manifestations rendered by erinacine-A enriched *Hericium erinaceus* mycelia," in *In the 14th Asian Consortium for the Conservation and Sustainable Use of Microbial Resources*, National Taiwan University Hospital International Convention Center, 2017.

9

Risk Factors for the Progression of Mild Cognitive Impairment in Different Types of Neurodegenerative Disorders

Pei-Hao Chen,[1,2,3] Shih-Jung Cheng,[1,2,4] Hui-Chi Lin,[1] Chuo-Yu Lee,[1,2,5] and Chih-Ho Chou[6,7]

[1]*Department of Neurology, MacKay Memorial Hospital, Taipei, Taiwan*
[2]*Department of Medicine, Mackay Medical College, New Taipei City, Taiwan*
[3]*Graduate Institute of Mechanical and Electrical Engineering, National Taipei University of Technology, Taipei, Taiwan*
[4]*Department of Physical Therapy and Assistive Technology, National Yang-Ming University, Taipei, Taiwan*
[5]*Graduate Institute of Chemistry, Tamkang University, New Taipei City, Taiwan*
[6]*Department of Neurology, Chi-Mei Medical Center, Tainan, Taiwan*
[7]*Chia Nan University of Pharmacy and Science, Tainan, Taiwan*

Correspondence should be addressed to Chih-Ho Chou; d940397@mail.chimei.org.tw

Academic Editor: Woon-Man Kung

Objective. Mild cognitive impairment (MCI) is a transitional state between normal aging and early dementia. It has a heterogeneous etiology and clinical course. This study aimed to examine the factors associated with the progression of MCI in different types of dementia disorders. *Method.* A retrospective, longitudinal, observational study of outpatients with MCI was conducted at a medical center in northern Taiwan. Patient medical records were reviewed, and risk factors were analyzed by multivariate analysis. *Results.* Among 279 patients with MCI, 163 (58.4%), 68 (24.4%), and 48 (17.2%) were diagnosed with Alzheimer's disease, vascular cognitive impairment, and Lewy body diseases, respectively. During the observation period, 37.2% of patients progressed to dementia. Older age and a higher Clinical Dementia Rating Scale-Sum of Boxes were associated with the risk of progression. Hyperlipidemia was associated with a decreased risk. Converters were more likely to receive an antidementia prescription. *Conclusion.* Our study suggests the importance of comprehensive clinical profiling, risk factor assessment, and detailed drug history evaluations in improving our understanding and management of dementia subtypes.

1. Introduction

Dementia can result from several underlying diseases, including Alzheimer's disease (AD), cerebrovascular disease, Lewy body diseases (LBD), frontotemporal dementia, and other less common disorders such as Huntington's disease, supranuclear palsy, and others. Mild cognitive impairment (MCI) is considered an intermediate state between normal cognitive aging and very early dementia. Individuals diagnosed with MCI may remain stable, return to normal (14.4–55.6% of patients), or progress to dementia [1]. There is extensive literature on MCI in AD but limited to other types of dementia. Many epidemiological studies have reported that the presence of vascular risk factors (i.e., hypertension, diabetes, cerebrovascular disease, and hyperlipidemia) in midlife is associated with an increased risk of cognitive impairment and dementia, particularly AD and vascular dementia (VaD) [2, 3]. Previous studies have reported older age, lower education status, prestroke cognitive and functional status, and history of diseases as risk factors for poststroke dementia [4]. However, cardiovascular risk factors in the midlife increase the risk of dementia, but their roles in the late-life are less clear [5]. Apart from vascular risk factors, other clinical conditions have been reported to show associations with MCI and dementia, including chronic obstructive pulmonary disease [6], chronic heart disease [7], cirrhosis [8], and chronic kidney disease [9]. By contrast, there has been a limited focus on whether chronic comorbid illnesses exhibit differential associations for different types of dementia. Cognitive impairment, seen with both delirium and dementia, has been associated with polypharmacy. Inappropriate use of benzodiazepine (BZD) in the elderly is also a major public health problem. The consequences of inappropriate BZD use include falls, delirium, other cognitive dysfunction, acute respiratory failure, car accidents, dependence, and withdrawal symptoms [10]. Studies on associations between sedative hypnotics and cognitive decline in elderly patients have yielded mixed findings [11]. Previous studies cannot yet determine whether the observed epidemiological association is a causal effect or the result of unmeasured confounding variables.

It is important to understand which clinical and medical factors might be associated with cognitive decline. Identifying these risk factors that hasten the onset of dementia is crucial for timely medical intervention and predicting prognoses. Improved knowledge of comorbidities in patients with MCI would facilitate the development of preventive strategies aimed at slowing rapid clinical and functional deterioration. This study aimed to examine the association between common clinical and neuropsychological factors in later life at the MCI stage and the risk of converting to dementia, with a particular focus on specific dementia disorders.

1.1. Specific

1.1.1. Study Design. This was a retrospective, longitudinal, observational study that used an unselected sample to test for associations between comorbidities in patients with MCI and the rate of cognitive decline or dementia.

1.1.2. Setting. Data used for this present study were obtained from a dementia care database from January 2014 to June 2017.

1.1.3. Participants. Patients were enrolled and studied at the neurological department of the MacKay Memorial Hospital (Taiwan). We recruited patients by reviewing electronic medical records and documenting information related to clinical measurements, diagnoses, comorbidities, neuroimaging reports, biochemical tests, and neuropsychological assessments at the first visit. The medical records were reevaluated by a dementia expert who was not involved in the assessments of the patients. The rate of decline in cognition was measured based on changes in the Mini-Mental Status Exam (MMSE) scores [12] and Clinical Dementia Rating Scale-Sum of Boxes (CDR-SB) [13]. A previous study reported that the conversion to dementia from MCI stages could be predicted by MMSE changes over time instead of single measurements [14]. This approach is useful for the detection of AD and other dementias in people with MCI. The Clinical Dementia Rating Scale (CDR) was initially designed to stage clinical dementia in older persons [15]. It yields both a global score and CDR-SB score. The global score is used to stage dementia severity, whereas the CDR-SB score is a more detailed quantitative version of that scale [16]. Progression of MCI to dementia (converter) was defined as a change in the overall CDR score from 0.5 to ≥1.0. The inclusion criteria were as follows: (1) cognitive complaints not normal for the age of the individual, (2) no dementia (cut-off MMSE score > 23 in persons with at least 6 years of education or >13 in persons with less than 6 years of education and CDR = 0.5), (3) cognitive decline, and (4) essentially normal functional activities in everyday life at the first visit [17]. All participants were evaluated from the first visit and followed up at regular intervals for at least one year until a clinical diagnosis of specific dementia (converter) or MCI (nonconverter) was reached. We included patients who had received regular ambulatory care for 12 months or longer. The intervals between two cognitive assessments were greater than six months. Exclusion criteria were as follows: (1) inability to establish a definite diagnosis for converters at the end of the study; (2) clinical suspicion of frontotemporal dementia, corticobasal degeneration, progressive supranuclear palsy, or other rare types of dementia; and (3) mixed dementia or mixed neurodegenerative diagnoses. In cases of atypical clinical manifestations, one optimal diagnosis for each patient was made under the consensus of neurologists. We excluded patients with uncertain dementia syndromes. Figure 1 provides a flowchart of the inclusion/exclusion criteria.

1.1.4. Classification of Dementia Syndromes. Diagnoses of dementia syndromes were confirmed by two study clinicians who reviewed clinical, neuropsychological, and brain imaging data and biochemical tests. Comprehensive neuropsychological testing was performed by an experienced clinical psychologist. Dementia subtypes were classified using international consensus clinical criteria. Dementia due to AD was diagnosed in patients who fulfilled the National Institute of Neurological and Communicative Disorders and Stroke and the Alzheimer's Disease and Related Disorders Association criteria for probable AD [18]. Dementia or MCI due to vascular disease was diagnosed in patients who fulfilled the American Heart Association/American Stroke Association Statement on Vascular Contributions to Cognitive Impairment and Dementia criteria [19]. LBD is an umbrella term for two closely related clinical diagnoses: Parkinson's disease dementia (PDD) and dementia with Lewy bodies (DLB). The third report of the DLB Consortium was used for probable DLB diagnoses [20]. The diagnosis of PDD was made based on recommendations of the movement disorder society task force [21]. The onset age of dementia was defined as the date on which the clinical symptoms and neuropsychological tests first allowed the diagnosis to be made. For nonconverters, MCI due to AD was diagnosed based on the National Institute on Aging and the Alzheimer's Association work group criteria [22]. Neuroimaging criteria for vascular cognitive disorders were based on the 2014 International Society for Vascular Behavioral and Cognitive Disorders (VASCOG) statement [23]. Diagnostic criteria for MCI due to Parkinson's disease or DLB are based on international consensus clinical criteria [24, 25].

1.1.5. Comorbidities and Medication History. Comorbidities, including diabetes mellitus, hypertension, hypercholesterolemia, heart disease (history of coronary artery disease,

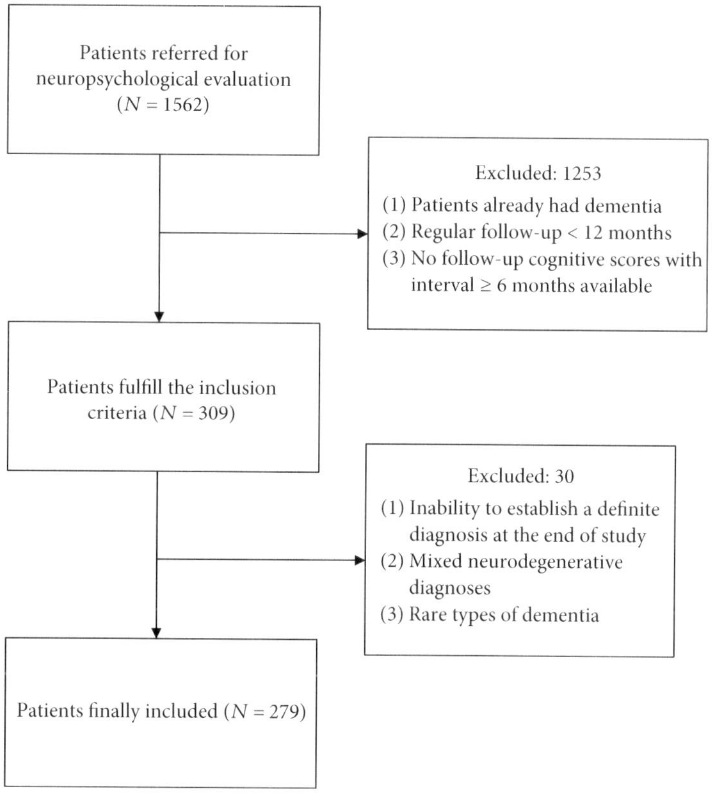

Figure 1: Flow diagram showing the patient exclusion criteria.

atrial fibrillations, heart failure, or valvular heart disease), gastrointestinal disorder, chronic kidney disease, liver function impairment, anemia, and depression, were documented by reviewing the medical records and laboratory documents in the hospital. Medication history of using antidementia agents (cholinesterase inhibitors or memantine) and hypnotic agents, including BZD or nonbenzodiazepine hypnotic agents ("Z drugs") during observational periods, were identified from the medical records and/or medical history interviews. Taking five or more regular medications prescribed >30 days at the time of diagnosis was defined as polypharmacy in our study.

1.1.6. Statistical Methods. We used a stepwise multiple logistic regression model to analyze the data. Each categorical variable was examined using χ^2 tests. The Student t-test was used to analyze continuous variables. Variables with a p value ≤ 0.1 were included in the multiple regression model. The effects of each variable were represented by odds ratios and corresponding 95% confidence intervals (CIs), which were calculated based on the exponential coefficient of the multiple logistic regression model. We also analyzed these factors in different etiologic subgroups. All statistical analyses were performed using R version 3.4.2 (2017-09-28).

1.1.7. Ethical Review. This present study was reviewed and approved by the MacKay Memorial Hospital Institutional Review Board (number 18MMHIS037).

2. Results

We recruited 279 patients with MCI from the database. A total of 163 patients were diagnosed with AD (female 64.4%), 68 had vascular cognitive impairment (female 30.9%), and 48 had Lewy body diseases (LBD) (female 45.8%). The distributions of age did not differ significantly among these groups. In this patient cohort, 58.7%, 31.8%, and 46.5% had hypertension, diabetes, and hypercholesterolemia, respectively, while 19.2% diagnosed as having depressive disorders. Additionally, 37.4% of our MCI patients progressed to dementia with a mean follow-up period of 27.09 ± 15.09 months. The proportion of conversion in the three dementia syndromes was 39.9% in AD, 38.2% in VaD, and 27.1% in LBD ($p = 0.2683$) (Figure 2). Univariate tests showed that the ages of onset, CDR-SB, and baseline MMSE were significant between stable MCI and converters (Table 1). Converters were more likely to receive antidementia agents (66.3% versus 34.9%, $p < 0.001$). The MMSE scores could be divided into subscores for orientation, memory, calculation, language, and perceptual motor function. The subscores of orientation were significantly different between MCI converters and nonconverters.

A multiple logistic regression model revealed that older age at onset, female sex, and a greater CDR-SB were significantly associated with a higher risk of converting from MCI to dementia. Receiving antidementia agents was strongly associated with a higher probability of this conversion

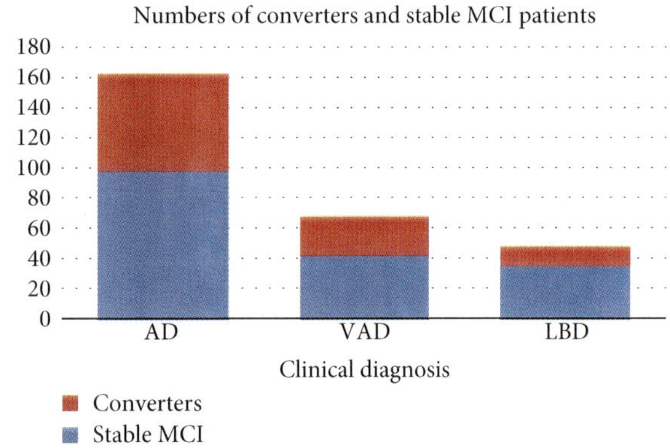

FIGURE 2: Proportions of conversion to dementia in patients with different clinical diagnoses. AD: Alzheimer's disease; VaD: vascular dementia; LBD: Lewy body diseases.

TABLE 1: Univariate analysis of clinical characteristics in 279 MCI patients who remained stationary course or progressed to dementia.

	Stable MCI $N = 175$ (percentage)	Dementia $N = 104$ (percentage)	p value
	AD 98 (56)	AD 65 (62.5)	
Etiology	VaD 42 (24)	VaD 26 (25)	0.268
	LBD 35 (20)	LBD 13 (12.5)	
Age of onset	70.9	74.7	<0.001
Female	100 (57.1)	48 (46.2)	0.098
Education	6.9	7.3	0.425
CDR-SB	2.20	2.96	<0.001
MMSE	24.5	23.3	0.004
Hypertension	101 (57.7)	63 (60.6)	0.954
DM	51 (29.1)	38 (36.5)	0.373
Dyslipidemia	90 (51.4)	39 (37.5)	0.021
Liver disease	24 (13.7)	19 (18.3)	0.279
Renal disease	20 (11.4)	14 (13.5)	0.844
Gastrointestinal disease	82 (46.9)	50 (48.1)	0.942
Anemia	10 (5.7)	7 (6.7)	0.918
Heart disease	73 (41.7)	47 (45.2)	0.894
Stroke	43 (24.6)	25 (24)	1.000
Depression	26 (14.9)	25 (24)	0.065
Antidementia agents	61 (34.9)	69 (66.3)	<0.001
Hypnotic agents	61 (34.9)	49 (47.1)	0.064
Polypharmacy	103 (58.9)	69 (67.0)	0.314

AD: Alzheimer's disease; VaD: vascular dementia; LBD: Lewy body diseases; MMSE: Mini-Mental State Examination; CDR-SB: Clinical Dementia Rating-Sum of Boxes; DM: diabetes mellitus. Remark: antidementia agents: acetylcholinesterase inhibitors and memantine. Hypnotic agents: benzodiazepines and nonbenzodiazepine hypnotics.

(Table 2). Hyperlipidemia was associated with a decreased risk of conversion. The interaction between hyperlipidemia and etiologies was nonsignificant. We also evaluated baseline MMSE scores (substituting CDR-SB in the model), and the

TABLE 2: Logistic regression model of variables associated with conversion to dementia in the MCI cohort.

	OR	2.50%	97.50%	p value
(Intercept)	0.0014	$1.00E-04$	0.029	<0.001
VaD	2.082	0.910	4.909	0.089
LBD	0.536	0.225	1.223	0.146
Age	1.071	1.032	1.113	<0.001
Gender	0.540	0.293	0.980	0.044
CDR-SB	1.553	1.221	2.008	<0.001
Hyperlipidemia	0.554	0.310	0.980	0.044
Depression	1.624	0.730	3.623	0.233
Antidementia agents	5.162	2.663	10.522	<0.001
Hypnotic agents	1.346	0.719	2.517	0.352

VaD: vascular dementia; LBD: Lewy body diseases; CDR-SB: Clinical Dementia Rating-Sum of Boxes. Remark: antidementia agents: acetylcholinesterase inhibitors and memantine. Hypnotic agents: benzodiazepines and nonbenzodiazepine hypnotic agents.

results of the other risk factors were unaltered. We tested four interactions between etiologies and each one of DM, hypertension, stroke, and heart disease, respectively, in the multiple logistic regression model, and all were nonsignificant. These interactions were not reported. Selection of risk factors in the model was based on the previous studies and aforementioned statistical criteria.

We performed a subgroup analysis from the MCI cohort according to the etiology. Age of onset was a significant risk factor in AD and VaD. Female was associated with an increased risk in AD. CDR-SB was associated with higher risk in AD and VaD. Receiving antidementia agents was significantly associated with conversion in AD. The trend was mostly consistent with the finding in the main cohort (Table 3). The LBD and AD subgroups had very similar risk factor profiles of conversion from MCI to dementia.

3. Discussion

MCI is heterogeneous in its etiology and clinical course. Older age and higher CDR-SB are major important markers for the identification of patients at a higher risk of progression. In our present study, we found that CDR-SB is highly indicative both in the whole cohort and different subgroup analyses. Because of the scoring rule, a CDR global score of 0.5 was unable to detect the cognitive categories that were affected (i.e., memory, orientation, judgment/problem solving, community affairs, hobbies, and personal care). In contrast, CDR-SB includes all categories, and the sensitivity might differ from the CDR global score.

Cholesterol has been recently shown to be important for synaptic transmission, and many neurodegenerative diseases, including AD and PD, are characterized by impaired cholesterol turnover in the brain [26]. A population-based prospective cohort study from Denmark showed that subjects with objective cognitive impairment who were most likely to progress were older, physically inactive, had a higher level of total cholesterol, and had a history of depression [27]. Reviews and meta-analyses revealed that midlife high total serum

TABLE 3: Logistic regression model of variables associated with conversion to dementia in the AD (a), LBD (b), and VaD (c) cases of the MCI cohort.

(a) Subgroup of AD

	OR	2.50%	97.50%	p value
(Intercept)	0.008	1.00E − 04	0.309	0.013
Age	1.058	1.010	1.112	0.021
Gender	0.424	0.202	0.874	0.021
CDR-SB	1.395	1.030	1.913	0.034
Hyperlipidemia	0.761	0.364	1.569	0.462
Depression	1.124	0.419	2.985	0.814
Antidementia agents	3.411	1.572	7.789	0.003
Hypnotic agents	1.800	0.808	4.051	0.151

(b) Subgroup of LBD

	OR	2.5%	97.50%	p value
(Intercept)	0	0	0.529	0.067
Age	1.186	1.021	1.446	0.051
Gender	0.143	0.012	1.009	0.080
CDR-SB	1.079	0.486	2.358	0.845
Dyslipidemia	0.321	0.045	1.825	0.218
Depression	7.221	0.720	106.364	0.109
Antidementia agents	66.025	7.839	1340.956	0.001
Hypnotic agents	0.410	0.057	2.3819	0.337

(c) Subgroup of VaD

	OR	2.50%	97.5%	p value
(Intercept)	0.000	0.000	0.068	0.009
Age	1.106	1.030	1.203	0.010
Gender	0.563	0.129	2.233	0.421
CDR-SB	2.172	1.229	4.309	0.015
Hyperlipidemia	0.459	0.131	1.550	0.211
Depression	8.786	1.059	101.545	0.057
Hypnotic agents	0.820	0.216	2.934	0.762

AD: Alzheimer's disease; VaD: vascular dementia; LBD: Lewy body diseases; CDR-SB: Clinical Dementia Rating-Sum of Boxes. Remark: hypnotic agents indicate benzodiazepines and nonbenzodiazepine hypnotic agents. Antidementia agents were not reimbursed for VaD patients in Taiwan health insurance system. They were not analyzed in the model due to sparsity.

cholesterol was associated with an increased risk of MCI, AD, and cognitive decline in late-life; however, high cholesterol in late-life was not associated with MCI, AD, VaD, any dementia, or cognitive decline [28]. Patients with late-life cardiovascular factors, including body mass index, atrial fibrillation, hypertension, hyperlipidemia, and diabetes, were more likely to have a diagnosis of VaD than the normal populations. However, there were no associations between AD and DLB with hypertension, hyperlipidemia, or diabetes [5]. In our study, we found that hypercholesterolemia was not a risk factor but had a nonsignificant protective effect on the progression of MCI. More than 70% of our patients used statins during the study period. However, we were not sure based on the prescription pattern, whether these patients received treatment from other hospitals or clinics. A previous study concluded that statins may slow the rate of cognitive decline and delay the onset of AD and all-cause dementia in cognitively healthy elderly individuals, whereas individuals with MCI may not have comparable cognitive protection from these agents [29]. A meta-analysis of two large trials, including a total of 26,340 patients aged ≥ 40 years with cardiovascular risk factors, reported that statins administered in later life do not prevent cognitive decline or dementia [30].

In Taiwan, cholinesterase inhibitors and memantine can be provided by the health insurance system under the following rules. AD or PDD was diagnosed by a neurologist or psychiatrist using the clinical diagnostic criteria. They had the latest MMSE scores of 10–26 and did not have contraindications. The authority required annual reevaluations of the initial prescription, and the reimbursement would be discontinued in case there is too much deterioration in MMSE scores or CDR. In our study, 45.5% of patients received antidementia agents during the observation period. Prescribing these medicines was associated with the likelihood of converting to dementia. However, those who received antidementia treatments also had higher CDR-SB (significant) and lower baseline MMSE scores (not significant). A possible explanation is that the physicians more likely prescribed antidementia agents to improve the cognitive functions in patients who they found were more severe at baseline. The results did not imply that the clinical courses in MCI patients were changed by these treatments.

Risks of cognitive decline and delirium were known to be associated with polypharmacy. In a prospective cohort study of 294 elderly patients, 22% taking five or fewer medications were found to have impaired cognition when compared with 33% of patients taking 6–9 medications and 54% in patients taking 10 or more medications [31]. A previous study of patients with cognitive impairment found that 70.4% were on multiple medications and 42% took BZD [32]. In our study, 61.5% of patients took more than five types of medications and almost 40% of patients were prescribed sedative/hypnotic drugs for at least 30 days during the study. In a large cohort of postmenopausal women, all types of antidepressant use and different levels of depression severity were associated with subsequent cognitive impairment [33]. By contrast, MCI has reported being a risk factor for depressive and anxiety disorders, suggesting common pathological pathways for cognitive and psychiatric outcomes [34]. A recently published article found that executive dysfunction in elderly people with depression may be associated with the age effect [35]. The reciprocal effects of depression and MCI were inconclusive. Our data revealed a nonsignificant trend ($p = 0.06$) supporting a link between depression and cognitive decline.

The effects of hypnotic agents and risk of dementia remained a subject of debate. A recent study based on longitudinal data found a slight association, but no dose-effect, in elderly nondemented individuals [36]. We found that hypnotic agents were very commonly used in depressed patients in our cohort. Neither depression nor hypnotics use was associated with conversion from MCI to dementia. These findings are consistent with a recent study performed in Taiwan [37].

3.1. Limitations. In our study, the diagnosis of dementia syndromes was justified by two clinicians who were experienced in dementia care. Comprehensive neuropsychological testing was performed by an experienced clinical psychologist. We excluded MCI of uncertain etiology and mixed neurodegenerative diagnoses. Lack of pathological confirmation was a weakness of our study, similar to the majority of the previously published articles. The primary clinical etiologic diagnosis remained stable in more than 90% of our patients. Previous results from a multicenter longitudinal database suggested that hospital-based studies were more accurate in categorizing dementia subtypes because they involve a multidisciplinary diagnostic approach and an adequate diagnostic infrastructure compared with community-based studies [38]. Due to the Personal Data Protection Act of 2010 of Taiwan, medication history may not be perfectly completed. The small case numbers limited our capacity to analyze whether there were any differences among different dementia syndromes.

4. Conclusions

Our retrospective, longitudinal, observational study showed the distribution of dementia subtypes from MCI and described the clinical progression, comorbidity, and medication history associated with dementia subtypes. We believe that comprehensive clinical profiling, assessments of risk factors, and detailed drug history evaluations are helpful to better understand and manage dementia subtypes. Our study suggests the importance of early detection of individuals with MCI. In the future, prospective studies should establish which of these factors are the most influential to aid the development of treatment and prevention strategies. Polypharmacy and hypnotic sedatives should be avoided if they are not essential, especially in elderly patients with MCI.

References

[1] R. C. Petersen, O. Lopez, M. J. Armstrong et al., "Practice guideline update summary: mild cognitive impairment: report of the guideline development, dissemination, and implementation subcommittee of the American Academy of Neurology," *Neurology*, vol. 90, no. 3, pp. 126–135, 2018.

[2] M. Baumgart, H. M. Snyder, M. C. Carrillo, S. Fazio, H. Kim, and H. Johns, "Summary of the evidence on modifiable risk factors for cognitive decline and dementia: a population-based perspective," *Alzheimer's & Dementia*, vol. 11, no. 6, pp. 718–726, 2015.

[3] Y. D. Reijmer, E. Berg, J. M. Dekker et al., "Development of vascular risk factors over 15 years in relation to cognition: the Hoorn study," *Journal of the American Geriatrics Society*, vol. 60, no. 8, pp. 1426–1433, 2012.

[4] G.-C. Hu and Y.-M. Chen, "Post-stroke dementia: epidemiology, mechanisms and management," *International Journal of Gerontology*, vol. 11, no. 4, pp. 210–214, 2017.

[5] B. N. Dugger, M. Malek-Ahmadi, S. E. Monsell et al., "A cross-sectional analysis of late-life cardiovascular factors and their relation to clinically defined neurodegenerative diseases," *Alzheimer Disease & Associated Disorders*, vol. 30, no. 3, pp. 223–229, 2016.

[6] K. Kakkera, K. P. Padala, M. Kodali, and P. R. Padala, "Association of chronic obstructive pulmonary disease with mild cognitive impairment and dementia," *Current Opinion in Pulmonary Medicine*, vol. 24, no. 2, pp. 173–178, 2017.

[7] J. W. Sacre, J. Ball, C. Wong et al., "Mild cognitive impairment is associated with subclinical diastolic dysfunction in patients with chronic heart disease," *European Heart Journal - Cardiovascular Imaging*, vol. 19, no. 3, pp. 285–292, 2018.

[8] T. B. Chen, S. Y. Yiao, Y. Sun et al., "Comorbidity and dementia: a nationwide survey in Taiwan," *PLoS One*, vol. 12, no. 4, article e0175475, 2017.

[9] A. R. Zammit, M. J. Katz, M. Bitzer, and R. B. Lipton, "Cognitive impairment and dementia in older adults with chronic kidney disease: a review," *Alzheimer Disease & Associated Disorders*, vol. 30, no. 4, pp. 357–366, 2016.

[10] G. Airagnes, A. Pelissolo, M. Lavallée, M. Flament, and F. Limosin, "Benzodiazepine misuse in the elderly: risk factors, consequences, and management," *Current Psychiatry Reports*, vol. 18, no. 10, p. 89, 2016.

[11] J. D. Picton, A. B. Marino, and K. L. Nealy, "Benzodiazepine use and cognitive decline in the elderly," *American Journal of Health-System Pharmacy*, vol. 75, no. 1, pp. e6–e12, 2018.

[12] M. F. Folstein, S. E. Folstein, and P. R. McHugh, ""Mini-mental state". A practical method for grading the cognitive state of patients for the clinician," *Journal of Psychiatric Research*, vol. 12, no. 3, pp. 189–198, 1975.

[13] S. E. O'Bryant, S. C. Waring, C. M. Cullum et al., "Staging dementia using Clinical Dementia Rating Scale Sum of Boxes scores: a Texas Alzheimer's research consortium study," *Archives of Neurology*, vol. 65, no. 8, pp. 1091–1095, 2008.

[14] I. Arevalo-Rodriguez, N. Smailagic, M. Roqué i Figuls et al., "Mini-Mental State Examination (MMSE) for the detection of Alzheimer's disease and other dementias in people with mild cognitive impairment (MCI)," *Cochrane Database of Systematic Reviews*, no. 3, article Cd010783, 2015.

[15] C. P. Hughes, L. Berg, W. L. Danziger, L. A. Coben, and R. L. Martin, "A new clinical scale for the staging of dementia," *The British Journal of Psychiatry*, vol. 140, no. 6, pp. 566–572, 1982.

[16] C. A. Lynch, C. Walsh, A. Blanco et al., "The clinical dementia rating sum of box score in mild dementia," *Dementia and Geriatric Cognitive Disorders*, vol. 21, no. 1, pp. 40–43, 2006.

[17] R. C. Petersen, "Mild cognitive impairment," *CONTINUUM: Lifelong Learning in Neurology*, vol. 22, no. 2, Dementia, pp. 404–418, 2016.

[18] G. M. McKhann, D. S. Knopman, H. Chertkow et al., "The diagnosis of dementia due to Alzheimer's disease: recommendations from the National Institute on Aging-Alzheimer's Association workgroups on diagnostic guidelines for Alzheimer's disease," *Alzheimer's & Dementia*, vol. 7, no. 3, pp. 263–269, 2011.

[19] P. B. Gorelick, A. Scuteri, S. E. Black et al., "Vascular contributions to cognitive impairment and dementia: a statement for healthcare professionals from the American Heart Association/American Stroke Association," *Stroke*, vol. 42, no. 9, pp. 2672–2713, 2011.

[20] I. G. McKeith, D. W. Dickson, J. Lowe et al., "Diagnosis and management of dementia with Lewy bodies: third report of the DLB Consortium," *Neurology*, vol. 65, no. 12, pp. 1863–1872, 2005.

[21] B. Dubois, D. Burn, C. Goetz et al., "Diagnostic procedures for Parkinson's disease dementia: recommendations from the movement disorder society task force," *Movement Disorders*, vol. 22, no. 16, pp. 2314–2324, 2007.

[22] M. S. Albert, S. T. DeKosky, D. Dickson et al., "The diagnosis of mild cognitive impairment due to Alzheimer's disease: recommendations from the National Institute on Aging-Alzheimer's Association workgroups on diagnostic guidelines for Alzheimer's disease," *Alzheimer's & Dementia*, vol. 7, no. 3, pp. 270–279, 2011.

[23] P. Sachdev, R. Kalaria, J. O'Brien et al., "Diagnostic criteria for vascular cognitive disorders: a VASCOG statement," *Alzheimer Disease & Associated Disorders*, vol. 28, no. 3, pp. 206–218, 2014.

[24] I. Litvan, J. G. Goldman, A. I. Tröster et al., "Diagnostic criteria for mild cognitive impairment in Parkinson's disease: *Movement* Disorder Society Task Force guidelines," *Movement Disorders*, vol. 27, no. 3, pp. 349–356, 2012.

[25] American Psychiatric Association, *Diagnostic and Statistical Manual of Mental Disorders*, iGroup Press Co., LTd., Washington, DC, USA, 5th edition, 2013.

[26] A. M. Petrov, M. R. Kasimov, and A. L. Zefirov, "Brain cholesterol metabolism and its defects: linkage to neurodegenerative diseases and synaptic dysfunction," *Acta Naturae*, vol. 8, no. 1, pp. 58–73, 2016.

[27] J. Skov Neergaard, K. Dragsbæk, C. Christiansen, M. Asser Karsdal, S. Brix, and K. Henriksen, "Objective cognitive impairment and progression to dementia in women: the prospective epidemiological risk factor study," *The Journal of Prevention of Alzheimer's Disease*, vol. 4, no. 3, pp. 194–200, 2017.

[28] K. J. Anstey, K. Ashby-Mitchell, and R. Peters, "Updating the evidence on the association between serum cholesterol and risk of late-life dementia: review and meta-analysis," *Journal of Alzheimer's Disease*, vol. 56, no. 1, pp. 215–228, 2017.

[29] K. Bettermann, A. M. Arnold, J. Williamson et al., "Statins, risk of dementia, and cognitive function: secondary analysis of the ginkgo evaluation of memory study," *Journal of Stroke & Cerebrovascular Diseases*, vol. 21, no. 6, pp. 436–444, 2012.

[30] B. McGuinness, D. Craig, R. Bullock, P. Passmore, and Cochrane Dementia and Cognitive Improvement Group, "Statins for the prevention of dementia," *Cochrane Database of Systematic Reviews*, no. 1, article Cd003160, 2016.

[31] J. Jyrkkä, H. Enlund, P. Lavikainen, R. Sulkava, and S. Hartikainen, "Association of polypharmacy with nutritional status, functional ability and cognitive capacity over a three-year period in an elderly population," *Pharmacoepidemiology & Drug Safety*, vol. 20, no. 5, pp. 514–522, 2011.

[32] A. Robles Bayon and F. Gude Sampedro, "Inappropriate treatments for patients with cognitive decline," *Neurología*, vol. 29, no. 9, pp. 523–532, 2014.

[33] J. S. Goveas, P. E. Hogan, J. M. Kotchen et al., "Depressive symptoms, antidepressant use, and future cognitive health in postmenopausal women: the Women's Health Initiative Memory Study," *International Psychogeriatrics*, vol. 24, no. 08, pp. 1252–1264, 2012.

[34] S. S. Mirza, M. A. Ikram, D. Bos, R. Mihaescu, A. Hofman, and H. Tiemeier, "Mild cognitive impairment and risk of depression and anxiety: a population-based study," *Alzheimer's & Dementia*, vol. 13, no. 2, pp. 130–139, 2017.

[35] K.-C. Wang, P. K. Yip, Y. Y. Lu, and Z. T. Yeh, "Depression in older adults among community: the role of executive function," *International Journal of Gerontology*, vol. 11, no. 4, pp. 230–234, 2017.

[36] S. L. Gray, S. Dublin, O. Yu et al., "Benzodiazepine use and risk of incident dementia or cognitive decline: prospective population based study," *BMJ*, vol. 352, article i90, 2016.

[37] H. I. Shih, C. C. Lin, Y. F. Tu et al., "An increased risk of reversible dementia may occur after zolpidem derivative use in the elderly population: a population-based case-control study," *Medicine*, vol. 94, no. 17, p. e809, 2015.

10

Mining EEG with SVM for Understanding Cognitive Underpinnings of Math Problem Solving Strategies

Paul Bosch, [1] **Mauricio Herrera**, [1] **Julio López**, [2] **and Sebastián Maldonado** [3]

[1]*Facultad de Ingeníera, Universidad del Desarrollo, Av. Plaza 700, Las Condes, Santiago, Chile*
[2]*Facultad de Ingeniería y Ciencias, Universidad Diego Portales, Ejército 441, Santiago, Chile*
[3]*Facultad de Ingeniería y Ciencias Aplicadas, Universidad de los Andes, Monseñor Álvaro del Portillo 12455, Las Condes, Santiago, Chile*

Correspondence should be addressed to Sebastián Maldonado; smaldonado@uandes.cl

Academic Editor: Guido Rubboli

We have developed a new methodology for examining and extracting patterns from brain electric activity by using data mining and machine learning techniques. Data was collected from experiments focused on the study of cognitive processes that might evoke different specific strategies in the resolution of math problems. A binary classification problem was constructed using correlations and phase synchronization between different electroencephalographic channels as characteristics and, as labels or classes, the math performances of individuals participating in specially designed experiments. The proposed methodology is based on using well-established procedures of feature selection, which were used to determine a suitable brain functional network size related to math problem solving strategies and also to discover the most relevant links in this network without including noisy connections or excluding significant connections.

1. Introduction

Recently, there has been an outburst in the number of investigations related to the applications of data mining tools to neuroscience [1, 2]. Data mining in this domain is usually related, on one hand, to processing/analyzing three-dimensional images from different medical imaging modalities that capture structural (e.g., MRI, CT, and histology) and functional/physiological (e.g., PET, fMRI, and SPECT) information about the human brain [3, 4]. On the other hand, some tools and approaches have been specifically tailored to grasp the complexity of brain electric activity through the analysis of electroencephalographic (EEG) signals [5]. However, the vast majority of these studies commonly seek to discover patterns in electrophysiological signals and images correlated with the diagnosis, prognosis, and evolution of a particular pathology or brain disorder and with the image analysis of normal/disease resting state fMRI [6, 7]. Comparatively, only very few works in this area use machine learning techniques for studying normal brain cognitive high level functions; probably because in these cases, the interpretation of the effects of single brain regions or connections between these regions on the separation of *pattern classes* is more complicated, given that discriminative brain pattern is a description of the cumulative contributions of many features that contribute to cognitive underpinning of brain high-level functions.

In this work, we use machine learning techniques to discover patterns of synchrony in functional brain networks, constructed from the EEG registers of a group of healthy individuals while they were solving specially designed math problems. The problems were devised specifically to detect and measure analytic processing. An intuitive resolution could lead to a quick and simple but incorrect response that should be overridden analytically. This study aims to correlate types of responses (correct or incorrect) with specific patterns of neural synchronization. The primary finding is that classification of these patterns using data mining tools on datasets from complex cognitive processes related to math performance is achievable. For each pair of EEG channels, corresponding to time windows associated with correct and incorrect answers given by the participants, correlations and phase synchrony were calculated. With these measures as entries, we construct connectivity (synchronization) networks as proxies of functional brain networks. A novel feature selection methodology that identifies the most relevant connections in these networks is proposed by using a nonlinear SVM-based classifier. This methodology allows us to determine not only a suitable network size but also the most relevant connections in the network, reducing the complexity and, therefore, facilitating the interpretation of mined patterns.

1.1. Synchronization/Correlation Networks of Normal Brain Cognitive High-Level Functions Used in Resolution of Math Problems. Lately, investigations have shifted from the study of local activation of large groups of neurons to the analysis of integration patterns among these groups. It is thought that the physiological bases of information processing and mental representation are provided by functional networks [8]. In fact, there is a great deal of current interest in the recent development of different techniques to extract large-scale functional and anatomical brain connectivity networks based on methods for creating correlation networks [9–11].

Researchers have developed a widely used method for creating correlation networks by using neural synchronization. Neural synchronization is a fundamental process in cortical computation which is believed to play an important role in information processing in the brain at both cellular and macroscopic levels [12, 13]. Brain oscillations that are ubiquitous phenomena in all brain areas become synchronized and consequently allow an implementation of the whole range of brain functions [12]. In particular, in our work, we use neural synchronization to measure the integrated activity of the functional brain network responsible for different math performances. Specifically, we use linear correlation and phase synchronization as measures for neural synchronization.

The correlation coefficient estimates linear coupling among signals of EEG channels, and its values are distributed over the unit interval. But the assumption that only linear interdependencies are relevant is actually not correct. Strictly speaking, linear correlation analysis based on Pearson's correlation coefficient and its derivatives can potentially miss important features of any dynamic system, particularly when we study brain functional network integration dynamics. Thus, in addition to linear correlation, we use phase synchronization between distant brain oscillating foci [14–18].

Phase synchrony in EEG channels assesses the stability of differences between phases of EEG signals at equivalent frequencies taken simultaneously by different electrodes. More simply stated, it is a measure of how the relative phase is distributed over the unit circle. If the two signals are phase synchronized, the relative phase will occupy a small portion of the circle, and the mean phase coherence is high. Phase synchronization has previously been considered to be a very good indicator of the functional coupling of neural activity in distant brain areas [19, 20]. To our knowledge, to date, phase synchrony in EEG channels has not been used to study brain networks involved in mathematical activities. So, using it creates a relevant contribution to understanding the collaborative and integrative nature of neural functioning in mathematics.

The large-scale functional integration of different brain zones is a relevant aspect of understanding the neural mechanisms responsible for the use of diverse problem-solving strategies in mathematics. The cognitive underpinnings of several mathematical activities have previously been related to a widely distributed brain network that includes parietal, temporal, and frontal structures as their main nodes [21–23]. Our research uses electroencephalographic (EEG) analysis [18] for the study of the whole-brain connectivity network and shows how mathematical cognition depends upon the integration of activities from distributed brain regions.

Some researches on EEG analysis have shown that specific aspects of mathematical reasoning could be related to different features of electric activity in some frequency bands (see, e.g., [24, 25]). In [25], for example, it is shown that incorrect performance in simple mathematical tasks is preceded by higher delta activity (signal frequencies < 4 Hz) in the lateral and medial areas of the right prefrontal cortex and by higher theta activity (4–8 Hz) bilaterally in the medial frontal zones. These slow wave patterns precede the subject's erroneous performance and show inhibited activity of the error-monitoring areas during erroneous mathematical calculations (i.e., these areas were simply not recruited). Therefore, a failure in the functional integration of these zones during problem resolution would be responsible for the subject's erroneous mathematical performance. On the other hand, correct answers were preceded by alpha activity (8–12 Hz) in the right posterior parietal area, a zone previously linked to mathematics. These early findings suggest that the size and integration of the functional network of different brain zones entailed in the resolution of problems are a relevant issue for understanding the neural mechanisms underlying math performance.

1.2. Graph Theoretical (Network) Approaches and SVM Working Together. Network theory is helpful in characterizing the interdependencies of various brain zones. However, graph theoretical (network) approaches in the study of brain functional networks suffer from some important methodological difficulties [26, 27]. For example, graph measures are strongly dependent on the network size (number of nodes), network density (percentage of links present), and degree (number of connections per vertex). This makes comparing results from different studies, which generally use distinct criteria to build functional networks, very difficult. Indeed, to construct unweighed networks, one has to apply a threshold on the connectivity values of the original weighted network. This results in scaling of the network properties as a function of the threshold [26]. The threshold can be chosen in a variety of ways, for example, based on an arbitrary choice, or using statistical criteria of connectivity strength, based on the average degree, or based on the density of the network. Fixing a standard number of vertices and the average degree could solve these size effects but could also introduce spurious connections or ignore strong connections in the network [27].

Recently, the use of a minimum spanning tree (a subnetwork of the original weighted network that connects all vertices in the network without forming loops and has the minimum total weight of all possible spanning trees), see [28], has been proposed to solve many of these methodological difficulties.

1.3. Top-Down Approach and Main Motivations for This Study. Students often arrive at universities without a well-formed background in abstract reasoning and with limited experience in the application of mathematical strategies. They lack proper understanding of some mathematical topics and often use inappropriate associations of different facts while trying to solve mathematical problems. These associations are fast internal reactions to external stimuli and appear to be related to the way in which the mind processes information.

Many authors in educational research have pointed out the persistence of student errors and misconceptions with respect to specific topics and tasks. For example, in [29], the authors observed that students react in a similar way to a wide variety of conceptually nonrelated problems that share some external common features. This fact led them to suggest that many responses described in the literature as alternative conceptions (misconceptions) could be better explained as evolving from a few common intuitive rules such as *More of A—More of B, Same A—Same B, Everything can be divided,* and *Over-generalized linearity.*

The present work applies a dual-process model of cognitive processing to these kinds of problems, testing the hypothesis that relative amounts of intuitive/analytic processing by the brain promote different strategies in the resolution of mathematical problems, leading to accurate or faulty solutions.

This work aims to solve these methodological difficulties by using some advanced tools from data mining. Specifically, the main methodological contribution is twofold: First, we extend the ξ-SOCP method [30], originally developed for linear binary classification, to nonlinear modeling thanks to the use of kernel functions. This model proposes a robust setting based on second-order cone programming, in which the traditional maximum margin approach for SVM is adapted by replacing the reduced convex hulls by ellipsoids [31], leading to a potentially superior classification performance [30, 31]. Additionally, we propose a novel feature selection methodology that identifies the most relevant connections in the network of interest while constructing the classifier using the ξ-SOCP method [30].

The rest of this article is structured as follows: Section 2 presents the methodology for capturing the data used in the modelling process. Section 3 provides a brief description of developments for feature selection and SVM, in which our ξ-SOCP method and the novel-embedded feature selection strategy is highlighted. Section 4 describes our results using neural synchronization datasets collected for this study. A summary of this paper can be found in Section 5, where we provide the main conclusions of this study and address future developments.

2. Materials and Methods: Cognitive Neuroscience

2.1. The Dual Process Theory. As our theoretical framework, we use the dual process theory (DPT) [32, 33]. According to DPT, our cognition and behavior operate in parallel with two quite different modes, called system 1 (S1) and system 2 (S2), roughly corresponding to our commonly held notions of intuitive and analytical thinking. The S1 and S2 modes are activated by different parts of the brain and have different evolutionary origins (S2 being more recent evolutionary and, in fact, largely reflecting cultural evolution). Like perception, S1 processes are characterized by being fast, automatic, effortless, unconscious, and inflexible (hard to change or overcome). Unlike perception, S1 processes can be language-mediated and relate to events not in the here-and-now (i.e., events in faraway locations and in the past or future). In contrast, S2 processes are slow, conscious, effortful, and relatively flexible. The two systems differ mainly along the dimension of accessibility: how fast and how easily things come to mind. Although both systems can at times run in parallel, S2 often overrides the input of S1 when analytic tendencies are activated and cognitive resources are available. For example, it is known that in geometry-related math problems, students tend to handle attributes of the problems such as distance, size, and similarity that are automatically registered by S1 quickly and spontaneously. We used this fact to design tests with some salient stimuli in such a way that each alternative for answering the problem would clearly indicate whether the participant took an intuitive/wrong strategy or an analytic/correct one.

The use of S2, consciously accessed, analytical processes trigger global and large-scale patterns of integrated neural activity. This fact appears as a variation on the global amount of synchrony between different brain areas. A greater proportion of S2 processes will appear as a greater amount of global synchrony. On the other hand, typical math errors due to semiautomatic use of heuristics will appear neurally as a reduced coupling of central work space neurons. Central work space neurons are thought to be particularly dense in the parietal, prefrontal, and cingulate cortices [21].

2.2. Test Designing Based on Cognitive Neuroscience. DPT enables understanding diverse phenomena because it predicts different judgments qualitatively depending on which reasoning system is used. DPT has been applied successfully to diverse domains and phenomena across a wide range of fields. While heuristic processing may render some manageable mathematics problems (by reducing the number of consciously driven operations), on some occasions, it can lead to errors and bias, reducing the effectiveness of a strategic plan of resolution. Available evidence and theory suggest that a converging suite of intuitive cognitive processes facilitates and supports some common rule-based flaw strategies in the resolution of math problems, which is a central aspect of deficient mathematical performance. In this way, stereotyped errors come from the semiautomatic and insufficiently evaluated application of highly repeated S1 system heuristics for solving problems. Under most circumstances, S1 procedures lead to correct answers (e.g., linearity is a common property of many, but not to all, mathematical operations) but in certain cases, it can lead to mistakes. To avoid these errors, the subjects must inhibit their semiautomatic responses to allow proper, conscious evaluation of the problem [34]. Some neuroscience researches have linked response inhibition to prefrontal activity, especially in its medial zones [35]; error monitoring in general (see [36], for detailed review) and mathematical error monitoring in particular [22] have been linked to the frontal lobes, mainly to their medial structures.

However, individual differences in the tendency to override initially flawed intuitions in reasoning analytically could be associated with different mathematical performances. In fact, elaborative processing must entail a deeper level of consciously controlled stimulus analysis. This processing is assumed to involve more effortful, analytical thought and is less likely to lead to errors and biases, although sometimes it may prove to be dysfunctional due to effects such as *paralysis by analysis*—the tendency to become overwhelmed by too much information processing.

Some attributes of the problem denominated in DPT as *natural assessments* could lead to wrong strategies and answers, because students could ignore other, less accessible, attributes of the problem, or some instructions that should be considered in the resolution.

Another possible source of errors is called *attribute substitution*. According to [32], when people try to solve a complex problem, they often substitute attributes. That is to say, an individual assesses a specific real attribute of the problem heuristically by means of another attribute, which comes to mind more easily. The real attribute is less accessible, and another, related attribute which is more available replaces the first one. This substitution is so fast that S2 monitoring functions cannot be activated. The individual does not notice that he/she is really answering another question.

The math tasks in our experiments were designed to highlight different problem resolution strategies. An intuitive approach, for example, will produce a quick and easy, yet incorrect, answer that must be analytically overridden to be correct. In every case, participants choosing different resolution strategies will at the same time choose different alternatives to answer the math problem. Appendix B presents three of the math problems for illustrative purposes. The complete list of the 20 math problems can be found as supplementary material (available here).

2.3. Preprocessing the Dataset from EEG Recording. The raw data for the training and test subsets (see the next sections) were extracted from the EEGs of a group of engineering students that were recorded while each one of them was solving a set of 20 math problems. The relevant metadata for the various participants is presented in Appendix A. These EEGs (10–10 position convention) were registered in a semidark room with a low level of environmental noise while each student was sitting in a comfortable chair. The data were recorded with the 64-channel Geodesic Sensor Net (EGI, USA) at the sampling frequency of 1000 Hz.

Since the sensors in the outer ring of the net were excluded from the analysis, because of low-quality signals, only 61 sensors were used for computations. The data were previously filtered (FIR, band-pass of 1–100 Hz), rereferenced against the common average reference, and segmented into nonoverlapping 1-s epochs using NS3 software.

As preliminary work for cleaning the dataset, we separated the oscillatory EEG-evoked electric activity from the induced one [37]. To do this, the EEG-evoked activity for each subject and his/her specific math problem was measured and averaged. This evoked activity was then subtracted from the total EEG activity through tests, subjects, and electrodes. The resulting EEG subtraction signal was analyzed with a fast Fourier transform on mobile overlapping and longtime windows between 5 and 10 seconds, because we did not know a priori what the interesting cognitive events to measure would be.

The measurement for each subject-math problem was segmented into time intervals ranging from −0.1 s to 61 s. In $t = 0$, the math problem is presented, while at $t = 60$ s, the question mark appears. The value −500 ms is considered to be the baseline of before the occurrence of the problem.

2.4. Constructing the Correlation and Synchronization Matrices from the Raw Dataset. As will be shown in the following sections, a new method for feature extraction from EEG signals was developed by choosing elements of the correlation or synchronization matrices. The EEG time series recorded for each participant/math problem were used to construct the correlation and synchronization matrices of the functional brain networks with rows and columns representing sensors. These matrices contain information about (linear) interdependence and long-range synchronies between EEG channels. Both types of information would be used for classification purposes. Moreover, in the case of the synchronization matrix, we would also manage information about frequency bands.

The correlation coefficient $r_{x,y}$ is perhaps one of the most well-known measures for (linear) interdependence between two signals x and y:

$$r_{x,y} = \frac{1}{N}\sum_{k=1}^{N}\frac{(x(k)-\bar{x})(y(k)-\bar{y})}{\sigma_x\sigma_y}, \quad (1)$$

where N is the length of the signals, $\bar{x}$ and $\bar{y}$ are the (sample) means of x and y, respectively, and σ_x^2 and σ_y^2 are the (sample) variances of x and y, respectively.

The correlation coefficient $r_{x,y}$ quantifies the linear correlation between x and y. If x and y are not linearly correlated, $r_{x,y}$ is close to zero; on the other hand, if both signals are identical, then $r_{x,y} = 1$.

Every correlation coefficient $r_{i,j}$ is a bivariate measure that serves as a coupling coefficient that links the electrode nodes i and j. With these coefficients as entries, we construct a connectivity matrix (adjacency matrix) **Corr**, representing

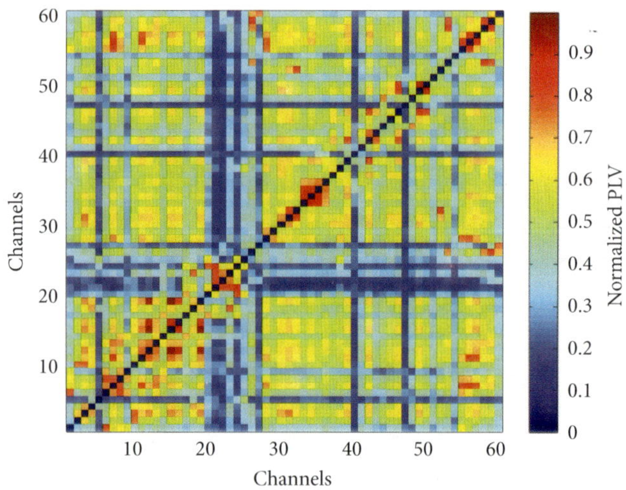

FIGURE 1: An example of the synchronization matrix for an individual and specific mathematics problem, in this case, corresponding to the beta (14–30 Hz) band. The colors indicate the extent to which two sensor locations are synchronized, which are quantified by the normalized PLV between every two EEG-recording sites i and j with $i, j = 1, \ldots, 61$.

a functional brain network. Thus, we have a connectivity matrix 61×61 composed of undirected and weighted edges consistent with the correlation coefficients. The matrix **Corr** is symmetric, so it has $N(N-1)/2 = 1830$ independent elements. Zeros are placed in diagonal elements.

In order to discover to what extent two sensor locations were synchronized, we also used the phase locking value (PLV) [18, 19]. Sample PLV is one of the most widely used measures of brain synchronization. It quantifies the phase relationship between two signals with high temporal resolution without making any statistical assumptions on the data.

Given two time series of signals $x(t)$ and $y(t)$ and a frequency of interest f, the procedure computes a measure of phase locking between the components of $x(t)$ and $y(t)$ for each latency at frequency f. This requires the extraction of the instantaneous phase of every signal at the target frequency. The phases are calculated by convolving each signal with a complex wavelet function:

$$\Psi(t) = e^{-(t^2/2\sigma_t^2)} e^{2i\pi f t}, \quad (2)$$

that is,

$$W_x(t) = (\Psi \circ x)_t = \int \Psi(t') x(t' - t) dt' = A_x^W(t) e^{i\Phi_x^W(t)}, \quad (3)$$

where $A_x^W(t)$ represents the signal amplitude. Following [19], we take $\sigma_t = 7/f$ and we define $W_y(t)$ in the same way as $y(t)$. Next, we can calculate the phase differences $\Phi_{x,y}^W(t) = \Phi_x^W(t) - \Phi_y^W(t)$. The phase locking value is then defined at time t, as the average value:

$$\text{PLV}_{x,y}(t) = \frac{1}{N} \left| \sum_{n=1}^{N} e^{i\Phi_{x,y}^W(t,n)} \right|, \quad (4)$$

for all time-bins t and trial $n \in \{1, \ldots, N\}$.

In our experiments, PLV measures were normalized relative to a baseline [38]. Specifically, this was done by using the 500 ms baseline before the onset of the math problem. The normalized signal was obtained by subtracting the average activity of the baseline from the raw signal and then dividing by the standard deviation of the baseline in a frequency-by-frequency manner.

By construction, PLV will be zero if the phases are not synchronized at all and will be one when the phase difference is in perfect, constant synchronization. The key feature of PLV is that it is only sensitive to phases, irrespective of the amplitude of each signal.

From the $N = 61$ EEG channels, we computed a symmetric 61×61 synchronization matrix **S** for each participant and for each math problem within a specific frequency band. Each element $\mathbf{S}_{i,j}$ of the matrix **S** corresponds to the PLV computed for the electrode pair i and $j\text{PLV}_{i,j}(t)$. The matrix **S** is also symmetric, so it has $N(N-1)/2 = 1830$ independent elements and, as before, zeros are placed in diagonal elements.

Each matrix element of **S** is the PLV computed for the corresponding pair of sensors. An illustrative example of the synchronization matrix is presented in Figure 1.

*2.5. From the Correlation (**Corr**) and Synchronization (**S**) Matrices to a Binary Classification Problem.* For classification purposes, we prepared two datasets using the correlation **Corr** and synchronization **S** matrices separately. Each data point corresponds to an answer of a participant to a specific mathematics problem. The participant could answer the math problem in a correct way $(y = +1)$ or incorrectly $(y = -1)$.

With the help of these matrices, we further constructed feature vectors **x** of size $N(N-1)/2$, whose components are in one case the elements of the matrix **Corr**, and in other cases elements of the matrix **S**. Here, N is the number of EEG sensors used in signal recordings, and we also used the fact that both matrices **Corr** and **S** are symmetric.

This way, the datasets for the learning machine are given by the set:

$$\left(\mathbf{x}_1^{(a)}, y_1\right), \ldots, \left(\mathbf{x}_l^{(a)}, y_l\right), \quad (5)$$

with characteristic vectors $\mathbf{x}^{(a)} \in \Re^{N(N-1)/2}$, $a = \{\mathbf{Corr}, \mathbf{S}\}$ corresponding to **Corr** or **S** matrix entries, respectively, and the output label $y_l \in \{-1, +1\}$, where the subindex l denotes the number of participants multiplied by the number of math problems given to each participant.

Thus, with the previously preprocessed dataset collected from 14 participants, with a 61-channel $(N = 61)$ EEG Geodesic Sensor Net (EGI) and with 20 math problems for each of them, we have $l = 14 \times 20 = 280$ sample vectors of dimension $N(N-1)/2 = 1830$ to train SVM models and make a preliminary classification for each **Corr** and **S** cases.

For the case of synchronization matrix **S**, we further developed the datasets considering the analysis for frequencies in three distinct domains, which we have called as follows: *Low*, corresponding to δ (<4 Hz) and θ (4–8 Hz) bands; *Medium*, corresponding to the α (8–12 Hz) and β (14–30 Hz) bands; and *High*, corresponding to γ (30–80 Hz) bands. In the case of the *Medium* frequency domain, we also studied the β band in a separate way. A classification study is performed using each frequency domain for synchrony detection in order to find the one that lead to the best classification.

3. Materials and Methods: Support Vector Machines and Feature Selection

Among the existing machine learning methods, SVM has demonstrated superior performance in several domains and, in particular, in neuroscience [39]. Its appealing characteristics, such as the absence of local minima and an adequate generalization of new samples, thanks to the *structural risk minimization* principle [40], made SVM one of the preferred classification approaches among researchers and practitioners [41].

Feature selection is a very important topic in high-dimensional applications, and, in particular, in neurology [1]. Finding the adequate subset of relevant variables for a given data mining task reduces the risk of overfitting, improving the model's predictive performance, and provides important insight into the process that generates the data, enhancing the interpretability of the model [42]. Support Vector Machine, however, cannot derive the feature's importance within the respective model, and therefore variable selection methods need to be used in order to reduce the level of noise in high-dimensional datasets [43].

In this section, the traditional SVM model developed for binary classification by [44] is presented in both linear- and kernel-based versions. Subsequently, two recently developed extensions are discussed, namely, the twin SVM method [45, 46] and the SVM method based on second-order cone programming presented in [30] (ξ-SOCP). Finally, two feature selection approaches used to address the issue of high dimensionality are described: the Fisher score and RFE-SVM method.

Among all SVM variations, we chose Twin SVM and SOCP SVM due to their superior performance we observed in previous studies (see e.g., [30, 47]). Twin SVM has shown positive empirical performance compared with the standard SVM formulation, being also computationally more efficient since the construction of these classifiers can be done by splitting the optimization problem into two smaller subproblems [45, 46]. Regarding ξ-SOCP, it is based on robust optimization, considering the worst-case setting for the class conditional densities related to the two training patterns in binary classification. In machine learning, robustness is a valuable property since it reduces the risk of overfitting, guaranteeing that the test performance does not deteriorate too much compared to the training performance when slight changes in the data distribution occur [30, 47].

3.1. Soft-Margin SVM. Let $\{(\mathbf{x}_i, y_i)\}_{i=1}^{m}$ be a set of examples $\mathbf{x}_i \in \Re^n$ with labels $y_i \in \{-1, +1\}$, $i = 1, \dots, m$. The traditional soft-margin SVM formulation [44] finds a classifier of the form $\mathbf{w}^T\mathbf{x} + \mathbf{b} = 0$ by solving the following model:

$$\begin{aligned} \min_{\mathbf{w},\mathbf{b},\xi} \quad & \frac{1}{2}\|\mathbf{w}\|^2 + C\sum_{i=1}^{m}\xi_i \\ \text{s.t.} \quad & y_i\left(\mathbf{w}^T\mathbf{x}_i + \mathbf{b}\right) \geq 1 - \xi_i, \\ & \xi_i \geq 0, \\ & i = 1, \dots, m. \end{aligned} \tag{6}$$

For each training example, a slack variable ξ_i is introduced, while C is a positive parameter that controls the trade-off between margin maximization and model fit.

A nonlinear decision surface can be obtained by using a kernel function [48]. A maximum margin classifier is constructed in a higher dimensional space by computing the dual of Formulation 4 and applying the kernel trick, leading to the following problem:

$$\begin{aligned} \min_{\alpha} \quad & \frac{1}{2}\sum_{i,s=1}^{m}\alpha_i\alpha_s y_i y_s K(\mathbf{x}_i, \mathbf{x}_s) - \sum_{i=1}^{m}\alpha_i \\ \text{s.t.} \quad & \sum_{i=1}^{m}\alpha_i y_i = 0, \quad 0 \leq \alpha_i \leq C, \quad i = 1, \dots, m, \end{aligned} \tag{7}$$

where α is a vector in $\Re^m$ of the dual variables corresponding to the constraints in 4 and $K : \Re^n \times \Re^n \to \Re$ is a kernel function. A typical choice of kernel is the *Gaussian kernel*, which usually leads to better results [43]. This kernel is as follows:

$$K(\mathbf{x}_i, \mathbf{x}_s) = \exp\left(-\frac{\|\mathbf{x}_i - \mathbf{x}_s\|^2}{2\sigma^2}\right), \tag{8}$$

where $\sigma > 0$ is the kernel width parameter [46].

3.2. Twin Support Vector Machine. The twin SVM method [45] constructs two nonparallel hyperplanes instead of the single classifier used in the soft-margin SVM formulation. Formally, two hyperplanes of the form $\mathbf{w}_1^T\mathbf{x} + \mathbf{b}_1 = 0$, $\mathbf{w}_2^T\mathbf{x} + \mathbf{b}_2 = 0$ are obtained in such a way that each of the functions is closer to the samples of one of the two labels and, at the same time, is as far as possible from those points of the other class. The following two problems are solved in order to find the following hyperplanes:

$$\begin{aligned} \min_{\mathbf{w}_1,\mathbf{b}_1,\xi_2} \quad & \frac{1}{2}\|\mathbf{A}\mathbf{w}_1 + \mathbf{e}_1\mathbf{b}_1\|^2 + \frac{c_3}{2}\left(\|\mathbf{w}_1\|^2 + \mathbf{b}_1^2\right) + c_1\mathbf{e}_2^T\xi_2 \\ \text{s.t.} \quad & -\left(\mathbf{B}\mathbf{w}_1 + \mathbf{e}_2\mathbf{b}_1\right) \geq \mathbf{e}_2 - \xi_2, \quad \xi_2 \geq 0, \\ \min_{\mathbf{w}_2,\mathbf{b}_2,\xi_1} \quad & \frac{1}{2}\|\mathbf{B}\mathbf{w}_2 + \mathbf{e}_2\mathbf{b}_2\|^2 + \frac{c_4}{2}\left(\|\mathbf{w}_2\|^2 + \mathbf{b}_2^2\right) + c_2\mathbf{e}_1^T\xi_1 \\ \text{s.t.} \quad & \left(\mathbf{A}\mathbf{w}_2 + \mathbf{e}_1\mathbf{b}_2\right) \geq \mathbf{e}_1 - \xi_1, \quad \xi_1 \geq 0, \end{aligned} \tag{9}$$

where **A** and **B** are the data matrix for the positive and negative class, respectively, c_i are trade-off positive parameters ($i = \{1, 2, 3, 4\}$), and $\mathbf{e}_1$ and $\mathbf{e}_2$ are vectors of one's appropriate dimension. Previous formulation is known as twin-bounded SVM (TB-SVM) [46], which is similar compared to the twin SVM (TW-SVM) method proposed by Jayadeva et al. [45] when setting $c_1 = c_2 = \varepsilon$.

Similarly to the soft-margin formulation, a nonlinear decision surface can be obtained by applying the kernel trick. The kernel-based twin SVM method solves the following two problems:

$$\begin{aligned} \min_{\mathbf{u}_1,\mathbf{b}_1,\xi_2} \quad & \frac{1}{2}\left\|K\left(\mathbf{A}^T,\mathbb{X}\right)\mathbf{u}_1+\mathbf{e}_1\mathbf{b}_1\right\|^2+\frac{c_3}{2}\left(\|\mathbf{u}_1\|^2+\mathbf{b}_1^2\right)+c_1\mathbf{e}_2^T\xi_2 \\ \text{s.t.} \quad & -\left(K\left(\mathbf{B}^T,\mathbb{X}\right)\mathbf{u}_1+\mathbf{e}_2\mathbf{b}_1\right)\geq\mathbf{e}_2-\xi_2, \quad \xi_2\geq 0, \end{aligned} \tag{10}$$

$$\begin{aligned} \min_{\mathbf{u}_2,\mathbf{b}_2,\xi_1} \quad & \frac{1}{2}\left\|K\left(\mathbf{B}^T,\mathbb{X}\right)\mathbf{u}_2+\mathbf{e}_2\mathbf{b}_2\right\|^2+\frac{c_4}{2}\left(\|\mathbf{u}_2\|^2+\mathbf{b}_2^2\right)+c_2\mathbf{e}_1^T\xi_1 \\ \text{s.t.} \quad & \left(K\left(\mathbf{A}^T,\mathbb{X}\right)\mathbf{u}_2+\mathbf{e}_1\mathbf{b}_2\right)\geq\mathbf{e}_1-\xi_1, \quad \xi_1\geq 0, \end{aligned} \tag{11}$$

where $\mathbb{X} = [\mathbf{A}^T \ \mathbf{B}^T]$ is the matrix of both training patterns (sorted by class) and $K : \Re^n \times \Re^n \rightarrow \Re$ is the kernel function.

Finally, a new data point is assigned to label +1 ($k = 1$) or −1 ($k = 2$) according to its proximity to the two hyperplanes. That is, $\mathbf{x} \in \Re^n$ belongs to the label k^* iff

$$k^* = \operatorname*{argmin}_{k=1,2}\left\{\frac{|\mathbf{w}_k^T\mathbf{x}+b_k|}{\|\mathbf{w}_k\|}\right\}. \tag{12}$$

The twin SVM method has been recently applied in neuroscience [49] and, in particular, in pattern analysis with EEG signal data [50, 51].

3.3. ξ-Second-Order Cone Programming SVM. In this study, we also used the robust SVM version based on second-order cones presented by [30]. For instance, if we suppose that $\mathbf{X}_1$ and $\mathbf{X}_2$ are random vector variables that generate samples of positive class (brain synchrony pattern of a participant that made a good resolution of the math problem) and negative class (brain synchrony pattern of participant that made an incorrect resolution of the math problem), respectively, we should construct a maximum margin linear classifier such that the false-negative and false-positive error rates do not exceed $\eta_1 \in (0, 1]$ and $\eta_2 \in (0, 1]$, respectively, in the following Quadratic Chance-Constrained Programming (QCCP) problem:

$$\begin{aligned} \min_{\mathbf{w},\mathbf{b},\xi} \quad & \frac{1}{2}\|\mathbf{w}\|^2+C\xi \\ \text{s.t.} \quad & \Pr\left\{\mathbf{w}^T\mathbf{X}_1+\mathbf{b}\geq 1-\xi\right\}\geq\eta_1, \\ & \Pr\left\{\mathbf{w}^T\mathbf{X}_2+\mathbf{b}\leq -1+\xi\right\}\geq\eta_2, \\ & \xi\geq 0. \end{aligned} \tag{13}$$

False negative could appear, for example, due to not completely reliable math assessment. In this case, there is a possibility of correct answers to a math problem, despite that it is registered as a pattern of low synchronization in the brain activity, that is, when a student correctly solves the problem without performing a deep analytical thinking.

The proposed robust setting suggests classifying each label correctly, up to the rate η_k, even for the worst data distribution. Thanks to Chebyshev's inequality [52, Lemma 1], this approach leads to the following deterministic problem:

$$\begin{aligned} \min_{\mathbf{w},\mathbf{b},\xi} \quad & \frac{1}{2}\|\mathbf{w}\|^2+C\xi \\ \text{s.t.} \quad & \mathbf{w}^T\boldsymbol{\mu}_1+\mathbf{b}\geq 1-\xi+\kappa_1\sqrt{\mathbf{w}^T\Sigma_1\mathbf{w}}, \\ & -\left(\mathbf{w}^T\boldsymbol{\mu}_2+\mathbf{b}\right)\geq 1-\xi+\kappa_2\sqrt{\mathbf{w}^T\Sigma_2\mathbf{w}}, \quad \xi\geq 0, \end{aligned} \tag{14}$$

where $\boldsymbol{\mu}_k$ and Σ_k are the means and covariance matrices for each class $k = 1, 2$ and $\kappa_k = \sqrt{\eta_k/1-\eta_k}$, and $C > 0$ is a tradeoff parameter. The constraints appearing in the previous problem are called second-order cone constraints [53]. Thus, we refer to this problem as the ξ-SOCP formulation.

Similar to [54], a nonlinear version can be also derived for ξ-SOCP via the kernel trick. The kernel-based ξ-SOCP method is as follows:

$$\begin{aligned} \min_{s,\mathbf{b},\xi} \quad & \frac{1}{2}\mathbf{s}^T\mathbf{K}s+C\xi \\ \text{s.t.} \quad & \mathbf{s}^T\mathbf{g}_1+\mathbf{b}\geq 1-\xi+\kappa_1\sqrt{\mathbf{s}^T\Xi_1\mathbf{s}}, \\ & -\left(\mathbf{s}^T\mathbf{g}_2+\mathbf{b}\right)\geq 1-\xi+\kappa_2\sqrt{\mathbf{s}^T\Xi_2\mathbf{s}}, \quad \xi\geq 0, \end{aligned} \tag{15}$$

where $\mathbf{K} = [\mathbf{K}_{11}, \mathbf{K}_{12}; \mathbf{K}_{21}, \mathbf{K}_{22}] \in \Re^{m\times m}$, with $\mathbf{K}_{11} = AA^T$, $\mathbf{K}_{12} = \mathbf{K}_{21}^T = BA^T$, $\mathbf{K}_{22} = BB^T$ and

$$\begin{aligned} \mathbf{g}_k &= \frac{1}{m_k}\begin{bmatrix}\mathbf{K}_{1k}e_k \\ \mathbf{K}_{2k}e_k\end{bmatrix}, \\ \Xi_k &= \frac{1}{m_k}\begin{bmatrix}\mathbf{K}_{1k} \\ \mathbf{K}_{2k}\end{bmatrix}\left(I_{m_k}-\left(\frac{1}{m_k}\right)e_ke_k^T\right)\left[\mathbf{K}_{1k}^T \ \mathbf{K}_{2k}^T\right]. \end{aligned} \tag{16}$$

3.4. Feature Selection for SVM. In this work, two feature selection strategies that have been used frequently for binary classification with SVM are considered: the Fisher score and RFE-SVM [42]. The first technique assesses variable relevance before applying SVM, constructing a ranking of attributes that can be used as input for the SVM model. This ranking is based on the distance between μ_j^+ and μ_j^-, the means for the jth attribute in the positive and negative labels are as follows:

$$F(j) = \left|\frac{\mu_j^+-\mu_j^-}{\left(\sigma_j^+\right)^2+\left(\sigma_j^-\right)^2}\right|, \tag{17}$$

where σ_j^+ (σ_j^-) is the standard deviation for the positive (negative) label. RFE-SVM, in contrast, performs a feature selection process embedded in the model, eliminating those variables that have the lowest contribution iteratively [42]. The variable contribution (the SVM margin when removing a given attribute) can be written in terms of the dual variables as follows:

$$W^2(\boldsymbol{\alpha}) = \sum_{i,s=1}^{N} \alpha_i \alpha_s y_i y_s K(\mathbf{x}_i, \mathbf{x}_s). \quad (18)$$

The RFE-SVM algorithm was successfully applied to linear Twin SVM in [55]. However, the RFE algorithm has not been extended before to ξ-SOCP, to the best of our knowledge. In this work, we implement the RFE algorithm for the ξ-SOCP method. This strategy together with the kernel-based ξ-SOCP formulation is a novel methodological contribution of this work. We should note that the characteristics of feature vectors $\mathbf{x}$ are elements of the synchronization matrices, which represent the weights of network edges. So, this procedure determines the most significant features or, in other words, the most noticeable network edges that make the difference in separation of the strategies used in the resolution of mathematical problems, in a correct or incorrect way.

4. Results and Discussion

We applied the classification and feature selection approaches described in the previous section on five different datasets corresponding to correlation data **Corr** and to synchronization data **S** which comprise three frequency domains (*Low*, *Medium*, and *High*) and the β frequency band. Each of the datasets has 280 samples (100 right answers and 180 wrong answers) described by 1830 variables.

For model evaluation, we chose a nested cross-validation (CV) strategy: training and test subsets were obtained using a 10-fold CV (outer loop), and the training subset was further split in training and validation subsets in order to find the right hyperparameter setting. The final feature ranking and classification were then performed with the full training subset from the outer loop for the best combination of hyperparameters, and the classification performance was computed by averaging the test results. This way, the test subsets from the outer loop remain unseen during the hyperparameter selection procedure. The following values for the hyperparameters were studied: C, c_i and $\sigma \in \{2^{-7}, \ldots, 2^{7}\}$ and $\eta_k \in \{0.2, 0.4, 0.6, 0.8\}$.

All experiments were performed on an HP Envy dv6 with 16 GB RAM, 750 GB SSD, an Intel Core Processor i7-2620 M (2.70 GHz), and using Microsoft Windows 8.1 OS (64 bits). The toolbox LibSVM [56] was used for standard SVM approaches, while the SeDuMi Matlab Toolbox [57] and the codes provided by Shao et al., the author of Twin-Bounded SVM [46] (publicly available in http://www.optimal-group.org/), were used for ξ-SOCP and TB-SVM, respectively.

Table 1 presents the best performance of the model selection procedure for all classification methods (standard SVM, TB-SVM, and ξ-SOCP in their linear and nonlinear versions) and for all five datasets without performing feature selection. The average performance among all techniques for each data is also reported. The two best performances among all methods are highlighted in bold type.

From Table 1, we observe that *Medium* and **Corr** are the ones with better average performance among the five different datasets. For the remaining analysis, we focus on these two datasets.

TABLE 1: Performance summary for different classification approaches. All datasets.

	High	*Medium*	*Low*	**Corr**	Beta
SVM_l	64.6	68.6	67.9	67.9	65.0
SVM_{nl}	67.5	67.9	67.9	66.1	65.0
TB-SVM	66.1	66.8	67.5	66.4	64.6
$TB\text{-}SVM_{nl}$	65.0	66.5	65.7	67.1	61.8
ξ-SOCP	58.6	63.2	63.9	65.7	65.3
$\xi\text{-}SOCP_{nl}$	65.7	67.1	64.3	66.1	63.6
Average	64.6	**66.7**	66.2	**66.5**	64.2

TABLE 2: Performance summary for different feature selection approaches. *Medium* and **Corr** datasets.

	Medium	*n*	**Corr**	*n*
Fisher + SVM_l	66.8	50	67.9	50
Fisher + SVM_{nl}	67.1	1000	67.5	50
Fisher + TB-SVM	68.2	500	67.1	50
Fisher + $TB\text{-}SVM_{nl}$	67.5	1000	67.9	500
Fisher+ξ-SOCP	67.1	250	68.2	250
Fisher+$\xi\text{-}SOCP_{nl}$	66.4	500	**68.6**	100
RFE + SVM_l	**68.2**	20	68.2	10
RFE + SVM_{nl}	68.2	250	67.5	20
RFE + TB-SVM	67.5	500	67.1	20
RFE+ξ-SOCP	65.4	1000	68.2	10

Next, we studied both feature selection approaches (Fisher score and recursive feature elimination) with the following number of selected attributes: 10, 20, 50, 100, 250, 500, 1000, and 1830 (i.e., with no features removed). The nested cross-validation strategy was performed for each subset of features, and the best performance is reported in Table 2, indicating the optimal number of selected variables for each case. The best performance among all methods is highlighted in bold type for each dataset.

In Table 2, we first observe that feature selection can improve predictive performance compared to a case with all available information, confirming what the specialized literature on this topic suggests [42]. In our case, an improvement of around 2% is achieved by eliminating those attributes that introduce noise in the modelling process. The best strategies are ξ-SOCP in its kernel-based version in combination with Fisher score and standard linear SVM in combination with RFE for the **Corr** and *Medium* datasets, respectively. Notice that the best approach is the one with fewer selected attributes in case of ties in accuracy.

Next, we construct the accuracy curves for the different subsets of selected variables, based on the four best methods presented in Table 2. For both frequency domains, we plot the classification performance of the four selected strategies

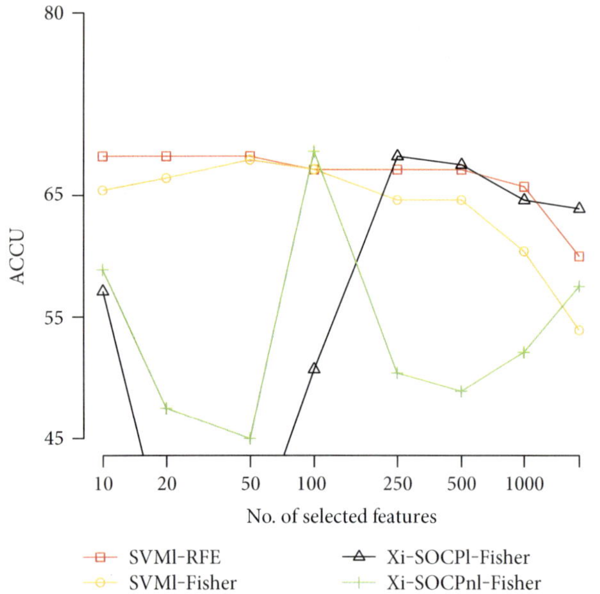

FIGURE 2: Accuracy versus the number of selected variables for **Corr** dataset.

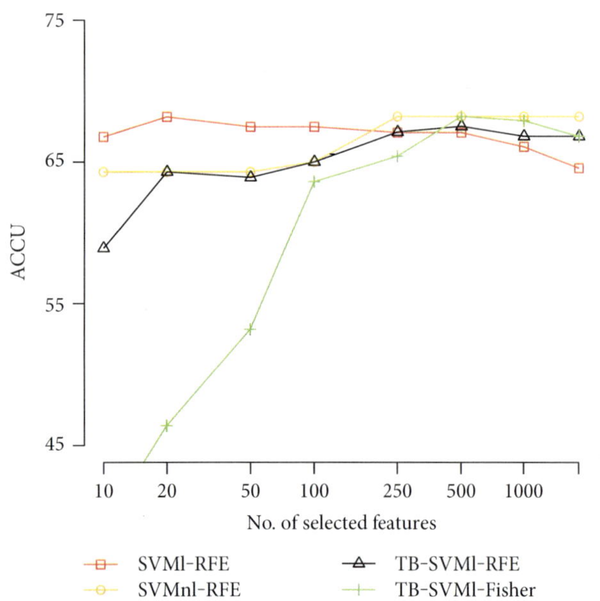

FIGURE 3: Accuracy versus the number of selected variables for *Medium* dataset.

to assess stability and overall predictive power. These results are presented in Figures 2 and 3.

In Figures 2 and 3, we first observe that no method outperformed others, and a reasonably broad range of classifiers is needed to define a good classifier adequately. The overall best performance is achieved with ξ-SOCP as the classification method and using Fisher score for feature ranking, although the most stable strategy corresponds to standard SVM with linear kernel, and the RFE algorithm for variable elimination. Notice also that the best performance is usually achieved between 10 and 100 attributes, discarding more than 90% of the available information.

Finally, we select the most relevant variables for each dataset. This is performed by combining the two best ranking strategies, namely, Fisher score and standard linear SVM in combination with RFE, and selecting the common variables (notice that each of these variables means a link between two EEG channels) that appear in both rankings (those with the highest importance).

Figures 4(a) and 4(b) show resulting networks constructed with statistically significant connections for the best classification methods and the set of connections that best discriminates the two classes of correct and incorrect answers during solving of math problems for correlation **Corr** and synchronization **S** matrices, respectively.

5. Conclusions

The discriminative brain pattern is a description of the cumulative contributions of many features. Therefore, the interpretation of the effects of single brain regions or connections between regions on the separation of the pattern classes is a complicated matter. However, some marked contributions aimed to solve this problem are present in this study.

It is well known that neural synchrony, which is involved in the large-scale transient integration of functional areas widely distributed over the brain, is required for normal cognitive operations [18]. Figure 4(a) shows precisely how the correlation can and should be used to measure this integration of different functional areas in normal processes related with math problem resolution.

Despite the apparent differences in patterns of connections (that were obtained by different methodologies), there are nodes that are common to both figures: AF4, F1, Fz, FT7, CF3, C1, C5, C6, P3, P7, and O1. These nodes precisely correspond to a widely distributed brain network previously identified as related to several mathematical activities [21–23].

The most discriminative connections (selected features) for the **S** case happen in the *Medium* range of frequencies from 8 to 30 Hz. Interestingly, these relevant connections are present in both the α and β bands. The α frequency band is widely associated with attention processes [58–62], and there is a large consensus that under conditions of inattention, some stimuli fail to be seen because the subject's attention is occupied with a different task and/or with another salient stimulus [63–65]. In such cases, perceptual, lexical, and/or semantic processing of the math problems could occur in the absence of conscious perception. As a result, stronger nonconscious effects are observed that may lead to erroneous mathematical performance.

In [66], it was suggested that focused attention elicits α large phase locking during the processing of a target stimulus. This phase response can be interpreted as reflecting temporal attention. Thus, the α phase should also play a crucial role in the attentional blink phenomenon, which represents reduced ability to report a second target after identifying the first target in visual stimuli. The explanations of the phenomenon proposed so far have focused primarily on some cognitive

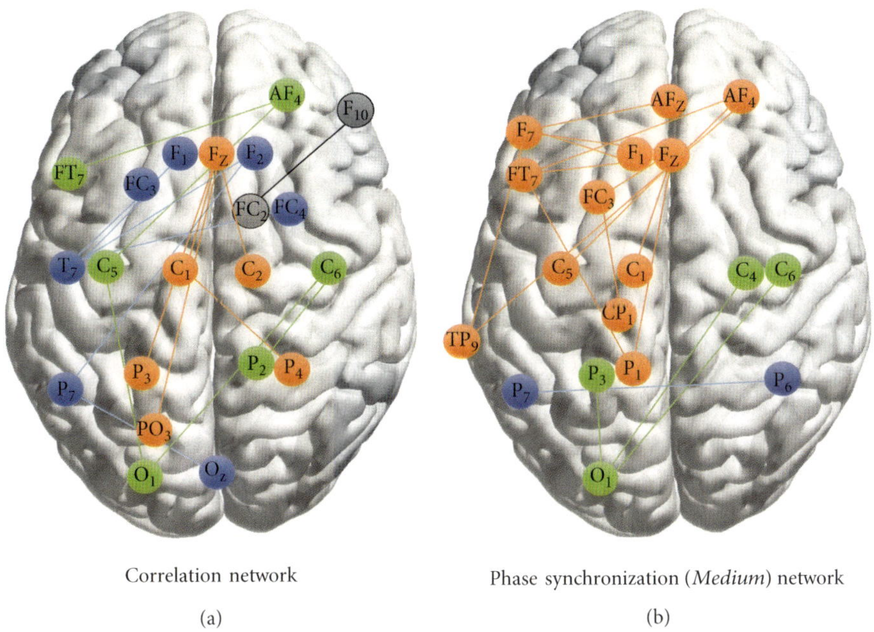

FIGURE 4: Graphic representation in which the vertices indicate EEG sensor locations (according to 10–10 position convention), and the edges represent the most significant features in the SVM classification and feature selection procedure. The colors represent different disconnected network components. BrainNet Viewer software [75] was used for the graph visualization.

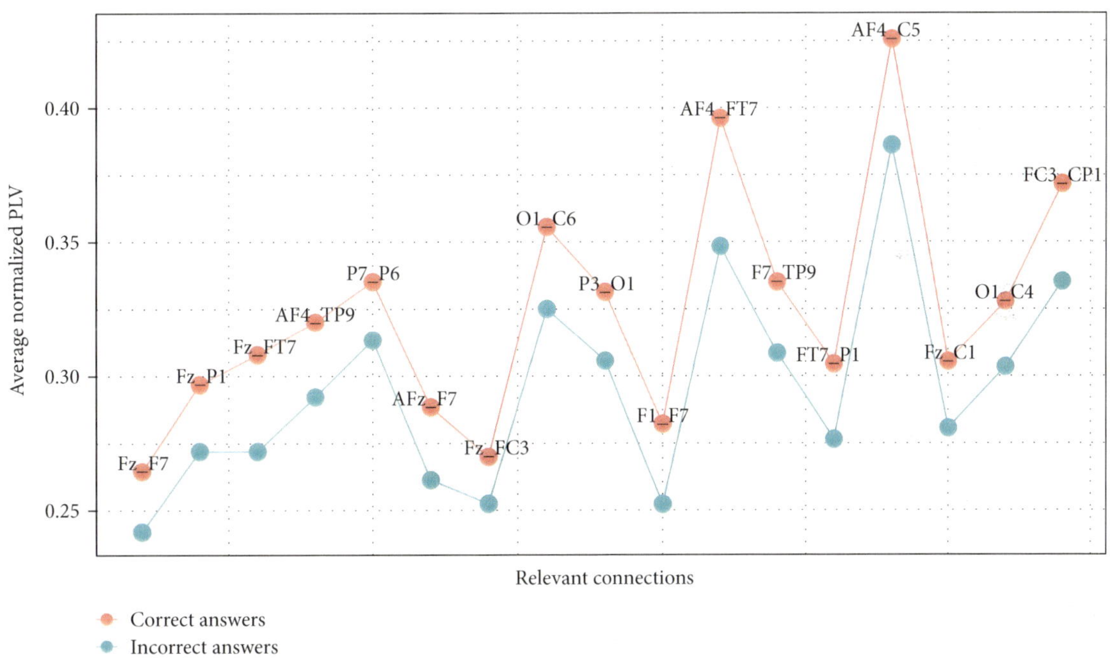

FIGURE 5: Average synchrony for relevant connections in the case of *Medium* dataset. Note that for every relevant connection, the average PLV is higher for correct answers than for incorrect ones.

aspects, such as attentional filters, capacity limitation, and retrieval failure processes [67, 68].

Figure 5 shows the average PLV calculated for relevant connections that were determined by the procedure of feature selection explained in Section 3.4. This average was taken for all measurements made for both classes of mathematical problems, that is, the ones that were answered properly and the ones that were answered incorrectly.

Figure 5 depicts two important results. First, the measures of the synchronization in the relevant connections indicate two types of different behaviors in regard to the cases of correct responses and incorrect responses. In the first case, synchronization is consistently higher than in the case of incorrect responses, indicating a different kind of resolution strategy whose neurological correlate shows a coordinated integration of different brain areas.

Secondly, synchronization measured by PLV values is not excessively high. The interpretation of this fact is interesting. It indicates that by building a proxy of a functional brain network, using synchronization networks able for distinguishing underlying normal cognitive processes in solving complex problems, the crucial point is not the detection of a high level of synchronization but rather the determination of which areas or groups are integrated with a stable synchronization. Traditional methods based on the choice of a threshold value in correlation/synchronization networks (e.g., using a threshold value greater than 0.5) would exclude much of the analysis described in this paper, which inevitably cause the loss of relevant information related to the neurological correlates that support the cognitive processes studied.

The primary finding of this study is that classification using automated SVM of datasets from complex cognitive processes related to math performance is feasible. Moreover, feature selection is a valuable procedure for reducing the complexity and, therefore, facilitating the interpretation of the mined patterns.

The observed differences in the math performance of participants and the success of SVM classification with a reasonable statistical significance suggest the potential use of this methodology as a novel approach to study patterns of connectivity in functional brain networks related to normal cognitive processes beneath the execution of complex tasks.

A still unsolved problem in graph theoretical approach for studying brain functional network integration is that network threshold can be chosen in a variety of ways based on an arbitrary choice or using statistical criteria of connectivity strength, based on the average degree or based on the network density. Particularly, when the threshold is based on a fixed number of connections in the network, this choice may result in either inclusion of spurious or noisy connections in networks (for too high density values or too high average degree) or the exclusion of relevant connections in networks (for too low density values or too low average degree) [27]. The procedure proposed here, based on feature selection tools, allows to determine not only a suitable network size by decreasing the size of feature vector but also the most relevant connections in network, that is, the ones that contribute most to the classification. As was shown in Table 2, feature selection improves predictive performance, which means that the optimal choices of the numbers of significant variables (connections) happen without including noisy connections or exclusion of significant connections.

There are some limitations to our study. First, the present analysis was performed on EEG data in sensor space, which contains some inherent spurious correlations because volume conduction causes the signal at each sensor to be a mixture of blurred activity from different inner cortical sources. More accurate inferences about anatomical locations need a source reconstruction of the activity in the cortex [69]. Second, in pattern classification, there are always uncertainties, for example, training datasets may contain incomplete information, there is input noise, there is noise in measurements, or underlying process is stochastic. As a result of such a probabilistic setting, uncertainties arise in learning from data. In order to get more reliable and reproducible results, we constructed a classifier whose misclassification rate does not exceed a defined maximum tolerable limit. For this, we presented in Section 3.3 a methodology for classification with uncertainties using SVM. However, general approaches of chance-constrained problems require the use of more suitable numerical methods for solving problems with linear constraints of probability to get computationally tractable approximations.

Table 3: Metadata for all participants.

Subject	Gender	Age	Correct answers	% C.A	Incorrect answers	% I.A	RT (ms)
1	Male	21	7	35	13	65	Null
2	Male	22	4	20	16	80	Null
3	Female	20	5	25	15	75	Null
—	—	—	—	—	—	—	—
4	Male	20	9	45	11	55	33091.80
5	Male	20	9	45	11	55	50645.45
6	Male	21	6	30	14	70	38395.85
7	Male	24	10	50	10	50	46157.05
8	Female	21	8	40	12	60	36193.85
9	Male	19	4	20	16	80	43862.60
10	Male	22	4	20	16	80	40500.10
11	Male	20	6	30	14	70	36475.95
12	Female	20	4	20	16	80	32184.35
13	Male	23	6	30	14	70	37211.10
14	Male	23	7	35	13	65	39002.50
15	Male	22	6	30	14	70	36721.80
16	Male	20	15	75	5	25	42437.95
17	Female	23	6	30	14	70	32250.65
Ave.	—	21.24	7	36	13	64	38938.00

Appendix

A. Basic and Behavioral Data

The subjects in the experiment were first-year engineering students enrolled in calculus and algebra courses. All participants were right-handed, healthy individuals, without any known neurological disorder, and with an average age of 21.24 ± 1.43. The basic metadata is presented in Table 3.

B. Mathematical Problems

Example 1 (attribute substitution). According to Kahneman et al. [32], attribute substitution often occurs when people try to solve a complex problem. This happens when an individual heuristically assesses a specific real attribute of the problem by means of another attribute, which comes easier to the mind. The real attribute is less accessible, and another related attribute, which is more available, replaces the first one. This substitution occurs so fast thatthe S2 monitoring functions cannot be activated, so it happens in a practically unconscious way. In geometry problem resolution, for example, students quickly handle attributes such as distance, dimensions, and similarity that are automatically/unconsciously recorded. These attributes are called "natural assessments." Managing these estimators can lead to errors, essentially because students ignore less accessible attributes that are critical to successfully solve the problem. We used this fact in Problem 1. In the resolution of this problem, some students ignored the values of angles and seem to have in mind the idea that the square has twice the area of the triangle. The average score obtained by students in this problem was 1.26 of a maximum of 4, showing that this was a fairly common error.

Problem 1. In the figure, the area of the triangle BCE is S. The area of the square ABCD is as follows:

(a) $2S$.

(b) $2\sqrt{3}S$. ✓

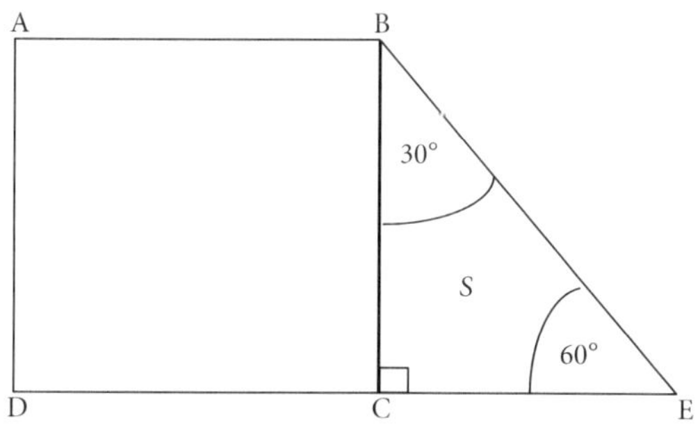

Example 2 (intuitive rules). In [29, 70, 71], the authors observed that students react in a similar way to a wide variety of conceptually nonrelated problems but share some common features. This fact allowed them to suggest that many misconceptions described by educational research literature could be explained as consequences of some few common intuitive rules, such as "More of A—More of B," "Same A—Same B," "Everything can be divided," and "Overgeneralized linearity." The fundamental contribution of the intuitive rules is the observation that human response is often determined by irrelevant externalities of the tasks and not by the really important concepts and ideas. Intuitive rules showed that subjects during the resolution of a problem, under certain circumstances, can completely ignore some important data to save the immediacy. Using this fact, Problem 3 and Problem 4 were constructed. Problem 3 is intuitive and evident; the score obtained in this problem was the maximum possible: 4.0. However, equal areas do not necessarily imply equal volumes, and this mistake led to an average score 1.89 from a maximum of 4.0 for Problem 4. Problem 2 was also constructed by following intuitive rules, in particular, "Same A—Same B" [29].

Problem 2

(a) Angle 2 is greater than angle 1. ✓

(b) Angle 1 is equal to angle 2.

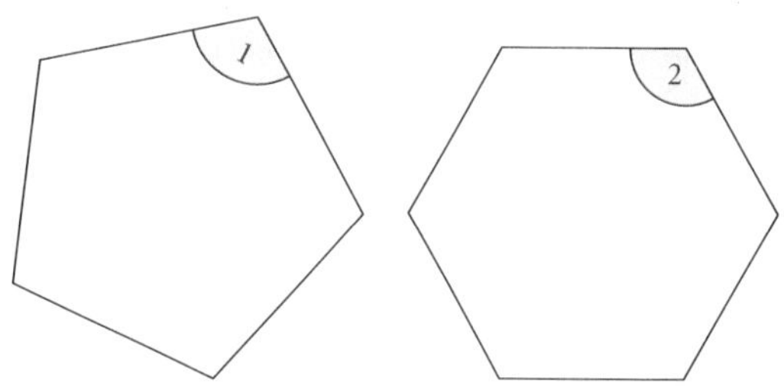

Problem 3. The rectangle A_1 is rotated 90° to obtain the rectangle A_2.

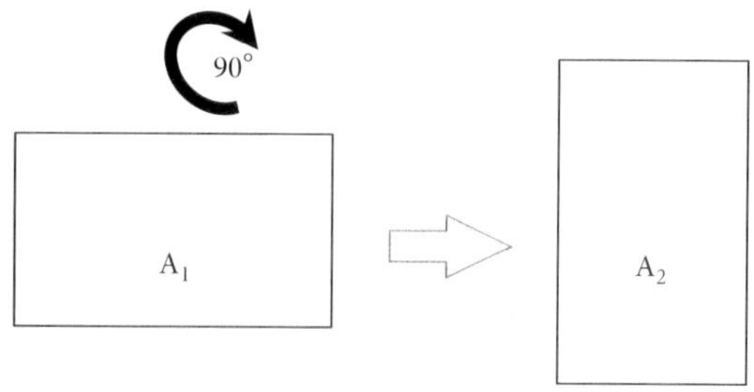

Indicate the correct alternative:

(a) The area of rectangle A_1 is different from the area of triangle A_2.

(b) The areas of both rectangles are equal. ✓

Problem 4. The rectangle A is wound in the ways indicated in the figures to construct the cylinders B and C.

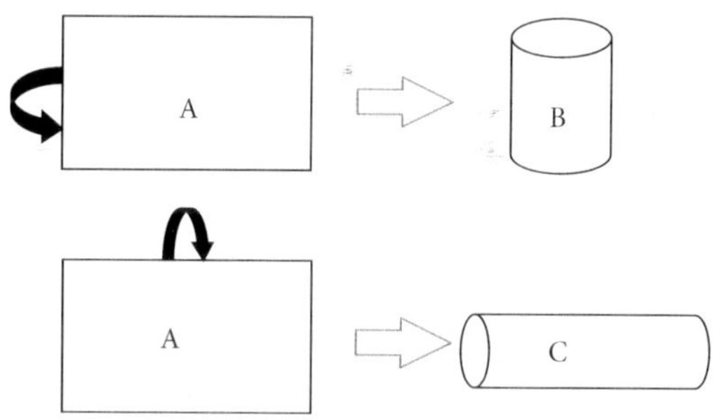

Indicate the correct alternative:

(a) The volume of cylinder C is different from the volume of cylinder B.

(b) The volumes of both cylinders are equal.

Example 3 (mathematical sets and conceptual metaphors). Lakoff and Nunez [72] stated that the concept of mathematical set is internalized using the image-schema CONTAINER [73]. The container is the source domain, whereas the mathematical set is the target domain of a conceptual metaphor. The various properties of the set are conceptualized through the metaphor "sets are containers." Thus, for example, "an element belongs to the set" is conceptualized as "the element is inside the container," and "A is a subset of B" is conceptualized as "The container A is inside the container B." In contrast, Fischbein and Baltsan [74] postulated that the mathematical set is conceptualized as an image-schema COLLECTION. Although Fischbein does not use the term metaphor, using *tacit model* instead, there are no major differences if we assume "sets are collections" as a new metaphor about the mathematical sets. We focus on common mistakes to detect the use of this type of conceptualizations. For this, we build Problem 6 to Problem 10 (see the supplementary material). In Problem 5, for example, the conceptualization of mathematical sets as collections was difficult in practice. It is counterintuitive to think of a collection of elements without any elements. For this reason, we should expect incorrect answers in cases of conceptualizations through collections. The average score on this problem was 0.42 out of a maximum of 4.0.

Problem 5. Given the proposition,

$P =$ "with the solutions of the system of equations

$$4x + 3y = 2,$$
$$4x + 3y = -2, \tag{B.1}$$

it is possible to build a set," indicate the correct alternative:

(a) p is false.

(b) p is true. ✓

Acknowledgments

This research was partially supported by CONICYT, FONDECYT Projects 1160894 (Paul Bosch and Julio López) and 1160738 (Sebastián Maldonado), and the Universidad del Desarrollo Institutional Projects 20141013112757683278 (Paul Bosch) and 20111016102627393115 (Mauricio Herrera). This work was funded by the Complex Engineering Systems Institute (CONICYT-PIA FB0816).

References

[1] P. Battista, C. Salvatore, and I. Castiglioni, "Optimizing neuropsychological assessments for cognitive, behavioral, and functional impairment classification: a machine learning study," *Behavioural Neurology*, vol. 2017, Article ID 1850909, 19 pages, 2017.

[2] L. Squarcina, U. Castellani, M. Bellani et al., "Classification of first-episode psychosis in a large cohort of patients using support vector machine and multiple kernel learning techniques," *NeuroImage*, vol. 145, pp. 238–245, 2017.

[3] Y. Chen, J. Storrs, L. Tan, L. Mazlack, J.-H. Lee, and L. Lua, "Detecting brain structural changes as biomarker from magnetic resonance images using a local feature based SVM approach," *Journal of Neuroscience Methods*, vol. 221, pp. 22–31, 2014.

[4] B. S. C. Wade, S. H. Joshi, B. Gutman, and P. Thompson, "Machine learning on high dimensional shape data from subcortical brain surfaces: a comparison of feature selection and classification methods," *Pattern Recognition*, vol. 63, pp. 731–739, 2017.

[5] L. Vezard, P. Legrand, M. Chavent, F. Faita-Ainseba, and L. Trujillo, "EEG classification for the detection of mental states," *Applied Soft Computing*, vol. 32, pp. 113–131, 2015.

[6] S. Hojjati, A. Ebrahimzadeh, A. Khazaee, and A. Babajani-Feremi, "Predicting conversion from MCI to AD using resting-state fmri, graph theoretical approach and SVM," *Journal of Neuroscience Methods*, vol. 282, pp. 69–80, 2017.

[7] B. Rashid, M. Arbabshirani, E. Damaraju et al., "Classification of schizophrenia and bipolar patients using static and dynamic resting-state fMRI brain connectivity," *NeuroImage*, vol. 134, pp. 645–657, 2016.

[8] S. L. Bressler, "Large-scale cortical networks and cognition," *Brain Research Review*, vol. 20, no. 3, pp. 288–304, 1995.

[9] M. Rubinov and O. Sporns, "Complex network measures of brain connectivity: uses and interpretations," *NeuroImage*, vol. 52, no. 3, pp. 1059–1069, 2010.

[10] O. Sporns, "Structure and function of complex brain networks," *Dialogues in Clinical Neuroscience*, vol. 15, pp. 247–262, 2013.

[11] O. Sporns, "Contributions and challenges for network models in cognitive neuroscience," *Nature Neuroscience*, vol. 17, no. 5, pp. 652–660, 2014.

[12] G. Buzsaki, *Rhythms of the Brain*, Oxford University Press, New York, NY, USA, _rst edition edition, 2006.

[13] P. Uhlhaas and W. Singer, "Neural synchrony in brain disorders: relevance for cognitive dysfunctions and pathophysiology," *Neuron*, vol. 52, no. 1, pp. 155–168, 2006.

[14] S. Doesburg, A. Roggeveen, K. Kitajo, and L. Ward, "Large-scale gamma-band phase synchronization and selective attention," *Cerebral Cortex*, vol. 18, no. 2, pp. 386–396, 2008.

[15] J.-P. Lachaux, E. Rodriguez, L. Michel, L. Antoine, J. Martinerie, and J. Francisco, "Studying single-trials of phase synchronous activity in the brain," *International Journal of Bifurcation and Chaos*, vol. 10, no. 10, pp. 2429–2439, 2000.

[16] F. Mormann, K. Lehnertz, P. David, and C. EElger, "Mean phase coherence as a measure for phase synchronization and its application to the EEG of epilepsy patients," *Physica D*, vol. 144, pp. 358–369, 2000.

[17] A. Ossadtchi, R. Greenblatt, V. Towle, M. Kohrman, and K. Kamada, "Inferring spatiotemporal network patterns from intracranial EEG data," *Clinical Neurophysiology*, vol. 121, pp. 823–835, 2010.

[18] F. Varela, E. J-P Lachaux, E. Rodriguez, and J. Martinerie, "The brain web: phase synchronization and large-scale integration," *Nature Reviews Neuroscience*, vol. 2, no. 4, pp. 229–239, 2001.

[19] J.-P. Lachaux, E. Rodriguez, J. Martinerie, and F. Varela, "Measuring phase synchrony in brain signals," *Human Brain Mapping*, vol. 8, no. 4, pp. 194–208, 1999.

[20] P. Uhlhaas, G. Pipa, B. Lima et al., "Neural synchrony in cortical networks: history, concept and current status," *Frontiers in Integrative Neuroscience*, vol. 17, no. 3, 2009.

[21] J. Danker and J. Anderson, "The roles of prefrontal and posterior parietal cortex in algebra problem solving: a case of using cognitive modeling to inform neuroimaging data," *NeuroImage*, vol. 35, pp. 1365–1377, 2007.

[22] V. Menon, K. Mackenzie, S. Rivera, and A. Reiss, "Pre-frontal cortex involvement in processing incorrect arithmetic equations: evidence from event-related fMRI," *Human Brain Mapping*, vol. 16, no. 2, pp. 119–130, 2002.

[23] L. Zago, L. Petit, M. Turbelin, F. Andersson, M. Vigneau, and N. Tzourio-Mazoyer, "How verbal and spatial manipulation networks contribute to calculation: an fMRI study," *Neuropsychologia*, vol. 49, no. 9, pp. 2403–2414, 2008.

[24] T. Fernandez, T. Harmony, M. Rodriguez et al., "EEG activation patterns during the performance of tasks involving different components of mental calculation," *Electroencephalography and Clinical Neurophysiology*, vol. 94, no. 3, pp. 175–182, 1995.

[25] T. Fernandez, T. Harmony, J. Silva-Pereyra et al., "Specific EEG frequencies at specific brain areas and performance," *Neuroreport*, vol. 11, no. 12, pp. 2663–2668, 2000.

[26] A. Fornito, A. Zalesky, and E. T. Bullmore, "Network scaling effects in graph analytic studies of human resting-state fMRI data," *Frontiers in Systems Neuroscience*, vol. 4, no. 22, 2010.

[27] B. C. van Wijk, C. J. Stam, and A. Daffertshofer, "Comparing brain networks of different size and connectivity density using graph theory," *PLoS One*, vol. 5, no. 10, article e13701, 2010.

[28] P. Tewarie, E. van Dellen, A. Hillebrand, and C. J. Stam, "The minimum spanning tree: an unbiased method for brain network analysis," *NeuroImage*, vol. 104, pp. 177–188, 2014.

[29] D. Tirosh and R. Stavy, "Intuitive rules: a way to explain and predict students' reasoning," *Educational Studies in Mathematics*, vol. 38, pp. 51–66, 1999.

[30] S. Maldonado and J. Lopez, "Alternative second-order cone programming formulations for support vector classification," *Information Sciences*, vol. 268, pp. 328–341, 2014.

[31] S. Nath and C. Bhattacharyya, "Maximum margin classifiers with specified false positive and false negative error rates," *Proceedings of the SIAM International Conference on Data mining*, 2007.

[32] D. Kahneman and A. Tversky, "Extensional vs. intuitive reasoning: the conjunction fallacy in probability judgement," *Psychological Review*, vol. 90, no. 4, pp. 293–315, 1983.

[33] K. E. Stanovich and R. F. West, "Individual differences in reasoning: implications for the rationality debate?," *Behavioural and Brain Sciences*, vol. 23, no. 5, pp. 645–665, 2000.

[34] R. West, M. Toplak, and K. Stanovich, "Heuristics and biases as measures of critical thinking: associations with cognitive ability and thinking dispositions," *Journal of Educational Psychology*, vol. 100, no. 4, pp. 930–941, 2008.

[35] D. Sharp, V. Bonnelle, X. . De Boissezon et al., "Distinct frontal systems for response inhibition, attentional capture, and error processing," *Proceedings of the National Academy of Sciences of the United States of America*, vol. 107, no. 13, pp. 6106–6111, 2010.

[36] S. Taylor, E. Stern, and W. Gehring, "Neural systems for error monitoring," *The Neuroscientist*, vol. 13, no. 2, pp. 160–172, 2007.

[37] C. Tallon-Baudry and O. Bertrand, "Oscillatory gamma activity in humans and its role in object representation," *Trends in Cognitive Sciences*, vol. 3, no. 4, pp. 151–162, 1999.

[38] S. Makeig, S. Debener, J. Onton, and A. Delorme, "Mining event-related brain dynamics," *Trends in Cognitive Sciences*, vol. 8, no. 5, pp. 204–210, 2004.

[39] A. Cerasa, I. Castiglioni, C. Salvatore et al., "Biomarkers of eating disorders using support vector machine analysis of structural neuroimaging data: preliminary results," *Behavioural Neurology*, vol. 2015, Article ID 924814, 10 pages, 2015.

[40] V. Vapnik, *Statistical Learning Theory*, John Wiley and Sons, 1998.

[41] S. Wang, W. Jiang, and K.-L. Tsui, "Adjusted support vector machines based on a new loss function," *Annals of Operations Research*, vol. 174, no. 1, pp. 83–101, 2010.

[42] I. Guyon, S. Gunn, M. Nikravesh, and L. A. Zadeh, *Feature Extraction, Foundations and Applications*, Springer, Berlin, 2006.

[43] S. Maldonado, R. Weber, and J. Basak, "Kernel-penalized SVM for feature selection," *Information Sciences*, vol. 181, no. 1, pp. 115–128, 2011.

[44] C. Cortes and V. Vapnik, "Support-vector networks," *Machine Learning*, vol. 20, pp. 273–297, 1995.

[45] R. Jayadeva, R. Khemchandani, and S. Chandra, "Twin support vector machines for pattern classification," *IEEE Transactions on Pattern Analysis and Machine Intelligence*, vol. 29, no. 5, pp. 905–910, 2007.

[46] Y. H. Shao, C. H. Zhang, X. B. Wang, and N. Y. Deng, "Improvements on twin support vector machines," *IEEE Transactions on Neural Networks*, vol. 22, no. 6, pp. 962–968, 2011.

[47] S. Maldonado and J. Lopez, "Synchronized feature selection for support vector machines with twin hyperplanes," *Knowledge-Based Systems*, vol. 132C, pp. 119–128, 2017.

[48] B. Scholkopf and A. J. Smola, *Learning with Kernels*, MIT Press, 2002.

[49] S. Wang, M. Chen, Y. Li, Y. Shao, Y. Zhang, and S. Du, "Morphological analysis of dendrites and spines by hybridization of ridge detection with twin support vector machine," *PeerJ*, vol. 4, article e2207, 2016.

[50] Q. She, Y. Ma, M. Meng, and Z. Luo, "Multiclass posterior probability twin svm for motor imagery EEG classification," *Computational Intelligence and Neuroscience*, vol. 2015, Article ID 251945, 9 pages, 2015.

[51] S. Soman and Jayadeva, "High performance EEG signal classification using classifiability and the twin SVM," *Applied Soft Computing*, vol. 30, pp. 305–318, 2015.

[52] G. Lanckriet, L. E. Ghaoui, C. Bhattacharyya, and M. Jordan, "A robust minimax approach to classification," *Journal of Machine Learning Research*, vol. 3, pp. 555–582, 2003.

[53] F. Alizadeh and D. Goldfarb, "Second-order cone programming," *Mathematical Programming*, vol. 95, no. 1, pp. 3–51, 2003.

[54] P. Bosch, J. Lopez, H. Ramirez, and H. Robotham, "Support vector machine under uncertainty: an application for hydroacoustic classification of fish-schools in chile," *Expert Systems with Applications*, vol. 40, no. 10, pp. 4029–4034, 2013.

[55] Z.-M. Yang, J.-Y. He, and Y. Shao, "Feature selection based on linear twin support vector machines," *Procedia Computer Science*, vol. 17, pp. 1039–1046, 2013.

[56] C.-C. Chang and C.-J. Lin, "LIBSVM: a library for support vector machines," *ACM Transactions on Intelligent Systems and Technology*, vol. 2, no. 3, pp. 1–27, 2011.

[57] J. F. Sturm, "Using sedumi 1.02, a matlab toolbox for optimization over symmetric cones," *Optimization Methods and Software*, vol. 11, no. 12, pp. 625–653, 1999, Special issue on Interior Point Methods (CD supplement with software).

[58] C. H. Brunia, "Waiting in readiness: gating in attention and motor preparation," *Psychophysiology*, vol. 30, no. 4, pp. 327–339, 1993.

[59] J. J. Foxe, G. V. Simpson, and S. P. Ahlfors, "Parieto-occipital ~1 0Hz activity reflects anticipatory state of visual attention mechanisms," *Neuroreport*, vol. 9, no. 17, pp. 3929–3933, 1998.

[60] W. Klimesch, M. Doppelmayr, H. Russegger, T. Pachinger, and J. Schwaiger, "Induced alpha band power changes in the human EEG and attention," *Neuroscience Letters*, vol. 244, no. 2, pp. 73–76, 1998.

[61] F. Lopes da Silva, "Neural mechanisms underlying brain waves: from neural membranes to networks," *Electroencephalography and Clinical Neurophysiology*, vol. 79, pp. 81–93, 1991.

[62] M. Steriade, P. Gloor, R. R. Llinas, F. H. L. Dasilva, and M. M. Mesulam, "Basic mechanism of cerebral rhythm activities," *Electroencephalography and Clinical Neurophysiology*, vol. 76, no. 6, pp. 481–508, 1990.

[63] S. Dehaene and J.-P. Changeux, "Neural mechanisms for access to consciousness," in *The Cognitive Neurosciences III*, M. Gazzaniga, Ed., pp. 1145–1157, MIT Press, 2003.

[64] S. Dehaene and L. Naccache, "Towards a cognitive neuroscience of consciousness: basic evidence and a workspace framework," *Cognition*, vol. 79, no. 1-2, pp. 1–37, 2001.

[65] S. Kouider and S. Dehaene, "Levels of processing during nonconscious perception: a critical review of visual masking," *Philosophical Transactions of the Royal Society of London B Biological Sciences*, vol. 362, no. 1481, pp. 857–875, 2007.

[66] S. Hanslmayr, A. Aslan, T. Staudigl, W. Klimesch, C. S. Herrmann, and K. H. Bauml, "Prestimulus oscillations predict visual perception performance between and within subjects," *NeuroImage*, vol. 37, no. 4, pp. 1465–1473, 2007.

[67] E. W. Martin, J. T. Enns, and K. L. Shapiro, "Turning the attentional blink on and off: opposing effects of spatial and temporal noise," *Psychonomic Bulletin and Review*, vol. 18, no. 2, pp. 295–301, 2011.

[68] K. L. Shapiro, J. E. Raymond, and K. M. Arnell, "The attentional blink," *Trends in Cognitive Sciences*, vol. 1, no. 8, pp. 291–296, 1997.

[69] M. Chavez, M. Valencia, V. Latora, and J. Martinerie, "Complex networks: new trends for the analysis of brain connectivity," *International Journal of Bifurcation and Chaos*, vol. 20, no. 6, pp. 1677–1686, 2010.

[70] P. Tsamir, "When intuition beats logic: prospective teachers' awareness of their same sides-same angles solutions," *Educational Studies in Mathematics*, vol. 65, no. 3, pp. 255–279, 2007.

[71] P. Tsamir and D. Tirosh, "Summing up and looking ahead: a personal perspective on infinite sets," in *Proceedings 30th Conference of the International Group for the Psychology of Mathematics Education*, vol. 1, pp. 49–63, 2006.

[72] G. Lakoff and R. Nunez, *Where Mathematics Comes from: How the Embodied Mind Brings Mathematics into Being*, Basic Books, New York, NY, USA, 2000.

[73] T. Oakley, *The Oxford Handbook of Cognitive Linguistics, Chapter Image schemas*, Oxford University Press, New York, NY, USA, 2007.

[74] E. Fischbein and M. Baltsan, "The mathematical concept of set and collection' model," *Educational Studies in Mathematics*, vol. 37, pp. 1–22, 1999.

[75] M. Xia, J. Wang, and Y. He, "Brainnet viewer: a network visualization tool for human brain connectomics," *PLoS One*, vol. 8, no. 7, article e68910, 2013.

11

Social Cognition Dysfunctions in Neurodegenerative Diseases: Neuroanatomical Correlates and Clinical Implications

Foteini Christidi,[1] Raffaella Migliaccio,[2] Hernando Santamaría-García,[3] Gabriella Santangelo,[4] and Francesca Trojsi[5]

[1] *First Department of Neurology, Aeginition Hospital, Medical School, National and Kapodistrian University of Athens, Athens, Greece*
[2] *INSERM U 1127, CNRS UMR 7225, Sorbonne Universités, and Université Pierre et Marie Curie-Paris 6, UMRS 1127, Institut du Cerveau et de la Moelle Épinière (ICM), 75013 Paris, France*
[3] *Pontificia Universidad Javeriana Bogotá, Colombia, Centro de Memoria y Cognición Intellectus Hospital Universitario San Ignacio, Bogotá, Colombia*
[4] *Department of Psychology, University of Campania "Luigi Vanvitelli", Caserta, Italy*
[5] *Department of Medical, Surgical, Neurological, Metabolic, and Aging Sciences, University of Campania "Luigi Vanvitelli", Naples, Italy*

Correspondence should be addressed to Francesca Trojsi; francesca.trojsi@unicampania.it

Academic Editor: Péter Klivényi

Social cognitive function, involved in the perception, processing, and interpretation of social information, has been shown to be crucial for successful communication and interpersonal relationships, thereby significantly impacting mental health, well-being, and quality of life. In this regard, assessment of social cognition, mainly focusing on four key domains, such as theory of mind (ToM), emotional empathy, and social perception and behavior, has been increasingly evaluated in clinical settings, given the potential implications of impairments of these skills for therapeutic decision-making. With regard to neurodegenerative diseases (NDs), most disorders, characterized by variable disease phenotypes and progression, although similar for the unfavorable prognosis, are associated to impairments of social cognitive function, with consequent negative effects on patients' management. Specifically, in some NDs these deficits may represent core diagnostic criteria, such as for behavioral variant frontotemporal dementia (bvFTD), or may emerge during the disease course as critical aspects, such as for Parkinson's and Alzheimer's diseases. On this background, we aimed to revise the most updated evidence on the neurobiological hypotheses derived from network-based approaches, clinical manifestations, and assessment tools of social cognitive dysfunctions in NDs, also prospecting potential benefits on patients' well-being, quality of life, and outcome derived from potential therapeutic perspectives of these deficits.

1. Introduction

Social cognition refers to a wide range of cognitive capacities elicited by, about, and directed towards other people [1]. In particular, these skills allow humans to both understand themselves and interact with and understand others, engaging in appropriate goal-directed behaviors [1]. Given that social cognition may play a prominent role in clinical care of most psychiatric and neurological illnesses [2], including neurodegenerative conditions, an emerging literature addresses the study of the neurobiological processes underlying social interactions and the behavioral correlates of the breakdown of these processes. In particular, growing evidence suggests that neurodegenerative diseases (NDs) are associated with some level of social cognitive impairment that has the potential to disrupt interpersonal relationships, thereby eliminating the benefits that social interactions may have for patients with other neurocognitive impairments. However, the frequency, extent, and clinical correlates of these abnormalities are not fully established.

This review aims to summarize some of the basic components of social cognition, also referring recent hypotheses derived from network-based approaches, and to discuss clinical manifestations of social cognitive dysfunctions in most NDs, addressing the pertinent literature published in the last 10 years.

1.1. Social Cognition, Social Behavior, and Social Functioning. The term "social" implies that the processing demands are related to specific classes of stimuli, such as emotional expressions on a face, in the voice, or from body posture, also including higher-order functions, such as making inferences about other people's mental states (e.g., theory of mind (ToM)), making moral decisions, regulating emotions and feelings, and experiencing and expressing empathy [1, 3, 4]. Moreover, at the outset, it is useful to clarify the significance of social behavior, cognition, and functioning, which are substantially related to one another.

"Social cognition" refers to any cognitive processing (e.g., perception, reasoning, memory, attention, motivation, and decision-making) that appears to be relatively specialized for the social domain. It causes "social behavior" that comprises the readily observable interactions between an individual and other people, while "social functioning" is broader than social behavior in that it consists in the long-term and contextualized ability of an individual to interact with others (i.e., social behavior when integrated over time and context) [5]. Finally, the "social brain" historically refers to a number of brain structures, some of which, when damaged, may be involved in the impairment of social cognition and behavior (i.e., ventromedial and dorsomedial prefrontal cortex, temporoparietal junction and superior temporal cortex, insula, and fusiform gyrus) [3], while others have been found activated in healthy brains when people perform social tasks in a magnetic resonance scanner by using functional magnetic resonance imaging (fMRI) [1, 3, 6]. Furthermore, considering that no social process can be attributed to a single structure alone, the recent network-based approach to brain function, principally related to the growing implementation of resting state fMRI (rs-fMRI) studies, allowed the identification of a distributed network supporting social function, which included regions from the original social brain [1, 6, 7].

1.2. Network-Based Approach to Social Cognition. A core social cognition network is centered on the amygdala which has been proven to play a pivotal role in emotion processing, from triggering emotional responses to detecting socially salient stimuli and performing social affiliative behaviors [4, 8, 9], and to be connected to multiple brain regions involved in emotion circuits [10, 11]. Abnormalities within this network, comprising most components of the social brain (i.e., medial prefrontal cortex, orbitofrontal cortex (OFC), anterior cingulate cortex, temporoparietal junction, inferior frontal gyrus, and superior temporal sulcus), have been revealed in patients affected by schizophrenia [12, 13], frontotemporal lobar degeneration (FTLD) [14, 15], and autism spectrum disorder [16-18]. In particular, activation in the OFC and ventromedial prefrontal cortex has been shown to be not essential for affective responses, but critical for the attribution of meaning to an affective stimulus [19], while activation in the lateral part of the prefrontal region has been found to be associated with a feeling of displeasure and inhibits behavior [20]. Therefore, alterations in these areas may lead to inappropriate social behaviors [21, 22].

A second network involved in social cognition is the so-called "mentalizing" network, which includes the right temporoparietal junction as a key region [23], found to be activated when a subject spontaneously tracks others' mental states [24, 25] and when mentalizing is required as part of another judgment, such as in the case of moral judgments [26] or even when a subject observes a scenario in which a protagonist holds a false belief [27, 28, 29]. In this regard, while ToM refers to the cognitive ability to infer and reason about our own and other people's beliefs, intentions, or emotions, empathy consists in a basic perceptual capacity of understanding others' feelings and subjective psychological states [30], motivating prosocial behaviors [31]. The empathy network, the third circuit implicated in social cognition, includes cingulo-insular structures [32] and has been shown to be impaired in several neuropsychiatric conditions [33, 34]. Finally, of interest for social interactions is also the so-called "mirror neuron system", mainly involving the inferior frontal gyrus, the inferior parietal lobule, the fusiform face area, and the superior temporal sulcus [35, 36], activated during the observation of the actions of others, including emotion recognition [37, 38], and, therefore, typically impaired in autism [39-41].

1.3. Clinical Assessment of Social Cognition. From a clinical point of view, failures of social cognition, most often characterized by impairment of one or more of the four networks cited above, have been assessed using more specific tools useful to investigate the four different domains. Evidence underlined the need for introducing validated tasks of social cognition in the assessment of patients with neurodegenerative diseases [42-44]. In particular, some neurological disorders, characterized by the neurodegeneration of frontomedian areas, such as the behavioral variant frontotemporal dementia (bvFTD), need more specific neuropsychological testing of social cognition for assessing frontomedian cortex functions, in contrast to the well-known sensitivity of executive tests mainly for the frontolateral cortex [45].

With regard to social cognitive measures designed to detect abnormal social behaviors, a range of informant-rated measures (i.e., patients' self-report data might be distorted because of the lack of emotional insight), such as those derived from the Frontal Systems Behavior Scale (FrSBe) [46] and Frontal Behavioral Inventory (FBI) [47], both exploring changes in personality and behavior that are associated with frontoexecutive dysfunction, and from Socioemotional Dysfunction Scale (SDS) [48], Social Inappropriateness Scale [49], and Social Impairment Rating Scale (SIRS) [50], focused on the detection of interpersonal phenomena and social impairment.

With regard to assessing ToM abilities, several tools allow exploring a patient's ability to infer what others are thinking and feeling, and to reason about how their thoughts and feelings will influence their behavior. False-belief tasks [51] are extensively validated measures of ToM that assess the ability to disregard one's own knowledge about the world and consider that someone else might have a different, erroneous belief.

Measures that assess social inference, such as the ability to detect sarcasm, also provide insight into the potential difficulties related to social interaction, such as The Awareness of Social Inference Test (TASIT) [52] that allows the detection of sincerity. ToM alterations can also be assessed with the Strange Stories test [53], in which patients are asked to demonstrate their understanding of stories in which characters' behavior can be best understood by attributing to him/her a specific underlying mental state. The Faux-Pas Test [54] also involves a series of written stories, but patients are asked to detect the *faux pas* and to understand beliefs, intentions, and inappropriateness. Finally, the Reading the Mind in the Eyes Test (RMET) [55] explores the ability to make inferences on the basis of observable features, such as facial expression and eye gaze, asking participants to infer the mental state of a person on the basis of a photograph of their eyes and the surrounding area.

To provide potential insights into empathic disturbances, valuable information may be derived from self-rated and informant-rated measures of affective empathy, such as the Empathic Concern subscale of the Interpersonal Reactivity Inventory (IRI-EC) [56], which investigates the feelings of warmth, compassion, and concern for others; the Perspective-Taking subscale of the IRI (IRI-PT), which allows distinguishing between affective abnormalities that reflect a lack of caring and those that reflect a lack of understanding; and the Empathy Quotient (EQ) [57], which measures the ability of understanding and predicting other people's affective and cognitive empathy and the nature of any emotional response to other people. Finally, among emotion-relevant performance tasks, which consist in evaluating emotional response to viewing photographs or videos, the Multifaceted Empathy Test (MET) [58] allows differentiating between mental state understanding (cognitive empathy) and subjective emotional response (affective empathy).

Deficits of social perception may be manifested as a deficit in identifying others' emotions, and this dysfunction may be assessed through the presentation of static photographs of high-intensity facial expressions. In this regard, the most commonly used task is the Ekman Faces, the one for assessing emotion labelling and discrimination [59]: participants are asked to identify which emotion is shown by a picture of a face and whether two faces show the same or different emotions. Moreover, to evaluate the intensity of a facial expression, the "Facial Expressions of Emotion: Stimuli and Tests" includes images that vary in their emotional intensity, enabling clinicians to create tasks that are graded in difficulty. The breadth and specificity of difficulties in recognizing emotions can be assessed with batteries of tests, such as the Comprehensive Affect Testing System [60] and the Florida Affect Battery [61], which use not only visual stimuli, but also auditory. Both of these batteries incorporate multiple subtasks that assess the ability to process visual (facial expressions), auditory (prosody), and visual-auditory (simultaneous facial expressions and prosody) emotional information.

The evaluation of the ability to integrate social perceptual cues with contextual information that forms part of normal social encounters can also be clinically useful. One measure that can be used for such an assessment is the Emotion Evaluation Test, which forms part of TASIT Part 1 [52], evaluating the ability to recognize emotions from dynamic, multimodal stimuli that are embedded into specific social scenarios. In particular, participants are shown videos in which an actor interprets one of seven basic emotions, sometimes with ambiguous dialogue, sometimes without any dialogue and they are asked to identify the emotional expression depicted.

In summary, when social cognitive dysfunction is suspected on the basis of clinical evidence, at least one measure of each of the four social cognitive domains should be evaluated [5] and, if specific social cognitive deficits are identified, a more comprehensive assessment that focuses on the domain(s) in question should be conducted. In this regard, Table 1 summarizes the abovementioned assessment tools, reporting the neurological disorders in which impairment of social cognition domains has been explored and the respective neuroanatomical correlates of these dysfunctions. The selection of the more appropriate protocol should be guided by the clinical validity of the tests to be administered (i.e., sensitivity and specificity for the neurological disorder of interest) and by the existence of population norms [5], and potential disadvantages may be linked to the lack of population norms in the case of some measures.

2. Social Cognition Abnormalities in Neurodegenerative Disorders

2.1. Amyotrophic Lateral Sclerosis-Frontotemporal Disease Spectrum Disorders (ALS-FTSD)

2.1.1. Frontotemporal Lobar Degeneration (FTLD). Social cognition has been reported as selectively vulnerable in FTLD, a term that grouped a clinically and pathologically complex spectrum of non-Alzheimer neurodegenerative disorders featured by selective and progressive atrophy of frontal, insular, and temporal brain lobes [62]. In the late 19th century, this complex group of disorders was denominated as Pick's disease in homage to Arnold Pick who helped in the study and description of these disorders. Although FTLD is considerably uncommon compared to Alzheimer's disease, this disease spectrum is one of the most important causes of young onset dementia and entails high clinical and socioeconomic costs [63].

Three major FTLD clinical syndromes, described considering the predominant clinical manifestations, are the bvFTD, mainly featured by disturbances in social behavior and in executive functioning [64, 65]; the primary progressive aphasias (PPAs) (semantic variant (svPPA), nonfluent agrammatic variant (nfvPPA), and logopenic variant), a group of disorders mainly characterized by linguistic and behavioral alterations [66]); and the syndromes characterized by the cooccurrence of FTLD with neurological disorders

Table 1: Social cognition domains with the related assessment tools for clinical and research investigation of social cognition deficits in neurodegenerative diseases.

Social cognition domains	Assessment tools	Neurodegenerative diseases with impairment of social cognition domains	Neuroanatomic correlates of social cognition dysfunctions in neurodegenerative diseases
Theory of mind	False-belief tasks, Faux-Pas Test, RMET, Strange Stories Test, TASIT	bvFTD	Ventromedial, dorsolateral, and ventrolateral prefrontal cortex, OFC, temporoparietal junction [42, 43, 115-119]
		nfvPPA	Temporal pole, insular cortex [113]
		svPPA	Left temporal lobe, medial frontal cortex [113]
		ALS	Dorsomedial and dorsolateral prefrontal cortex, supplementary motor areas [137]
		PD	Bilateral cingulate gyri, middle and inferior frontal gyri, fusiform and superior temporal gyri, bilateral parietal and bilateral occipital lobes [212, 213]
		PSP	Right inferior frontal gyrus, anterior medial frontal cortex [188]
		CBS	Right frontal-temporal-parietal cortices [214]
		AD	Superior temporal sulcus, posterior cingulate cortex, precuneus [42]
Empathy	EPT, EQ, IRI-EC, IRI-PT, MET	bvFTD, ALS, AD/MCI	Anterior cingulate, frontoinsular cortices [139, 115-119, 234]
Social perception	Ekman Faces test, TASIT, Comprehensive Affect Testing System, Florida Affect Battery	bvFTD	Anterior cingulate, orbitofrontal and medial prefrontal cortex, insula, striatum, and amygdala (SLN) [42, 43, 109, 115-119]
		nfvPPA	Posterior fusiform gyri, bilateral insular cortex, anterior temporal lobe [112]
		svPPA	Left temporal cortex, amygdala [112]
		ALS	Right inferior longitudinal fasciculus, inferior frontooccipital fasciculus [147, 148]
		PD	Orbitofrontal cortex, right and left superior frontal gyri, bilateral posterior cingulate gyri, somatosensory cortices, amigdala [206-209]
		PSP	Right inferior frontal gyrus [188]
		CBS	Paracentral gyrus, precuneus [163]
		AD	Temporoparietal regions [222-224]
Social behavior	AES, FBI, FrSBe scale, NPI, SDS, SIRS	bvFTD, ALS, PD, AD	Ventromedial and lateral prefrontal cortex, fronto-temporo-insular areas, anterior cingulate cortex [21, 22, 118, 129, 130, 222]

AD = Alzheimer's disease; AES = apathy evaluation scale; ALS = amyotrophic lateral sclerosis; bvFTD = behavioral variant frontotemporal dementia; CBS = corticobasal syndrome; EQ = Empathy Quotient; FrSBe = Frontal Systems Behavior; FBI = Frontal Behavioral Inventory; IRI-EC = Interpersonal Reactivity Inventory-Empathic Concern; IRI-PT = Interpersonal Reactivity Inventory-Perspective-Taking; MCI = mild cognitive impairment; MET = Multifaceted Empathy Test; NPI = Neuropsychiatric Inventory; OFC = orbitofrontal cortex; PD = Parkinson's disease; PSP = progressive supranuclear palsy; RMET = Reading the Mind in the Eyes Test; SDS = Socioemotional Dysfunction Scale; SIRS = Social Impairment Rating Scale; TASIT-S = The Awareness of Social Inference Test.

mainly affecting cortical and subcortical brain areas, including amyotrophic lateral sclerosis (ALS) [67], progressive supranuclear palsy (PSP), and the corticobasal syndrome (CBS) [63], which mainly affect motor functions, but also impact social behavior.

(1) Alterations in the Four Domains of Social Cognition. Social cognition deficits are pervasive in FTLD. However, among the aforementioned syndromes, dysfunctions in social interaction processes have been mostly described in patients with bvFTD [64, 65]. In particular, six core symptoms are recognized in the revised diagnostic criteria [64]: (i) early (i.e., within the first three years of symptom onset) behavioral disinhibition, for example, socially inappropriate behavior, loss of manners or decorum, or impulsive actions; (ii) early apathy or inertia; (iii) early loss of sympathy or empathy, for example, diminished response to other people's needs and feelings and diminished social interest; (iv) early perseverative, stereotyped, or compulsive/ritualistic behavior, for example, repetitive movements and stereotypy of speech; (v) hyperorality and dietary changes, for example, altered food preferences, binge eating, and oral exploration of inedible objects; and (vi) executive dysfunction; with at least 3 of these 6 features required for a diagnosis of bvFTD.

In bvFTD patients, impairments have been described in different social cognitive processes associated with previous behaviors ranging from basic affective to more high-order and reflexive processes [65, 68-71] and, interestingly, bvFTD has been proposed as a disease model for studying interactions between emotion processing, social cognition, and interoception [72]. In particular, with regard to basic social cognitive processes, bvFTD patients can exhibit emotion-processing alterations, including abnormalities of the perception of emotional and social cues [73-76], altered empathic concern [77], and alterations in affective expression that includes the presence of apathy or, by contrast, euphoric mood states, overfamiliarity, jocularity, and silliness [78, 79]. Furthermore, the bvFTD patients may present disturbances in the more reflexive social cognitive processes including reduced theory of mind abilities [43], mentalizing deficits [80], diminished prosocial sentiments [81], and reduced long-term cooperative behaviors [70, 82, 83]. Recently, impaired performances at RMET have been revealed to better discriminate bvFTD patients from healthy subjects or Alzheimer's disease patients than altered performances in executive tests, thereby underlining the relevance of social cognition abnormalities in bvFTD diagnosis [84-89]. In particular, executive function tests, such as Stroop task and Trail Making Test, have been shown to be less disease specific than social cognition tests, such as the RMET, for the differential diagnosis across different forms of dementia [85-89]. In support of this, recent meta-analyses confirmed the central role of ToM in bvFTD diagnosis by showing significantly higher and domain-specific impairments of ToM (and emotion recognition) in bvFTD in comparison to control subjects and Alzheimer's disease [90] or other clinical conditions including multiple psychiatric, neurological, and developmental disorders [91]. However, questionnaires that also account for behavioral disorders, such as apathy evaluation scale (AES) [92] and FrSBe scale, especially in the informant-report version, have been shown to significantly differentiate bvFTD patients from healthy controls [84]. Of note, some of the most frequent behavioral symptoms in bvFTD, including apathy, impulsivity, and disinhibition, have been associated to implicit difficulties in social interaction and alterations in the processing of social cues, suggesting a tight interplay between social cognition and neuropsychiatric symptoms in this condition [68, 93]. Thus, the apathetic presentation of bvFTD includes patients who have a lack of interest in their social surroundings as they present difficulty in initiating, planning, and motivating social behavior, related to atrophy in frontal areas and basal ganglia [93-95]. Along this vein, impulsive and disinhibited bvFTD patients exhibit inappropriate social behavior including undue familiarity, disorganized behaviors, and sexual acting out related to impaired mechanisms of cognitive control as a consequence to atrophy in the OFC, frontal ventromedial, and cingulate cortices and anterior temporal areas [96].

Alterations in the social cognitive process can also transfer to moral domains in bvFTD patients, who may show altered moral judgments, displaying more utilitarian judgments in the face of moral dilemmas [97, 98], a pattern also observed in extreme criminal terrorists [99]. Moreover, these patients can display increased antisocial and criminal behavior [100, 101], as well as a relatively high incidence of legal violations [102] and a heightened expression of counter-empathy emotions such as envy and gloating for others' misfortunes [103].

With regard to the ability to make judgements about others' behavior, attitudes, and emotions (i.e., social perception and empathy domains), patients with bvFTD may experience impaired emotion recognition, empathy, and sarcasm detection [73, 77, 104, 105]. In particular, performance on the newly developed TASIT-S, regarding emotion recognition and sarcasm detection, has been revealed impaired in bvFTD and relatively intact in AD [14]. However, although most studies have focused on the verbal categorization of facial expressions [106], deficits have also been reported under different task conditions and stimulus modalities including vocal [107], bodily [108], and musical [109] expressions of emotion. Moreover, the emotion recognition of film stimuli is also impaired [75, 110], although the psychological reactivity to negative film stimuli does not appear to differ from controls [75]. In addition to these deficits in recognizing emotions in others, bvFTD patients have also shown abnormal emotion suppression, emotion generation, and experience of self-conscious emotion, as revealed for bvFTD patients viewing disgust-invoking stimuli, who have been shown to display reduced facial expressions of disgust, reduced physiological reactivity, and reduced self-reported experience of disgust, compared to controls [111]. Furthermore, a deficit in social context processing was observed in the performance of FTLD patients in the empathy for pain task (EPT) [77], a suitable instrument that evaluates empathy in the context of intentional/accidental harm. Accidental pain situations are less clear and explicit; hence, they require greater demands to ascertain the action's intentionality and integration of contextual information. When performing the EPT, the FTLD patients do not easily discriminate between accidental and intentional situations revealing difficulties in integrating social context cues and agents' intentionality [73].

With regard to linguistic variants of FTLD, namely PPAs including svPPA and nfvPPA, some evidence also revealed alterations in several social cognitive processes. Several reports showed deficits in face and emotion recognition, and in ToM processes in both svPPA and nfvPPA [109, 112-114].

(2) Neuroanatomical Bases of Social Cognition Impairment in FTLD and Network-Based Approaches. Most of the aforementioned behavioral alterations might reflect a general disturbance in different neural networks. To date, it has been reported that the functioning of three neural networks can be altered in FTLD, including the salience network, the dorsal attention network, and the default mode network. Firstly, the salience network (SLN) [115] composed of the anterior cingulate, insula, striatum, and amygdala, which is activated in healthy subjects during tasks requiring attentional selection, task switching, and self-regulation of behavior, has been reported as impaired in FTLD as a consequence of atrophy over the main hubs of SLN [115]. In particular, the insula, a key region of SLN, is highly connected with the anterior

portion connecting with the lateral OFC, while the posterior portion connects with the superior temporal cortex; in bvFTD, both the ventral (frontoinsular) and dorsal areas of the anterior insular are affected [116]. Degeneration of these connected areas has been shown to be related to the impairment of emotion recognition and processing [109, 117], social cognition [118], and interoception [119] in bvFTD.

Secondly, it has been reported that in FTLD there is an abnormal increased connectivity in other networks including the dorsal attention network and default-mode network (DMN) [120]. Alterations in connectivity patterns of those networks seem to be at the core of the decline in executive functions and attention, as well as apathy in patients with FTLD [120, 121]. Thirdly, clinical alterations in FTLD have been associated to a disorder of functional frontolimbic disconnection leading to a compensatory hyperconnectivity in prefrontal areas in response to the absence of affective feedback during the planning and execution of behavior [121].

More recently, an integrative model suggested that the functioning of a network known as the social context network (SCN), composed by fronto-temporo-insular areas, might explain the social cognitive, executive, and behavioral alterations in FTLD [68, 122-124]. Arguably, in control subjects, the SCN favors (a) to update context cues to make predictions, (b) to consolidate context-target associative learning, and (c) to coordinate internal and external milieus [68, 122].

In linguistic variants, comparative analysis of regional gray matter related to social cognition deficits have revealed a differential pattern of fronto-insulo-temporal atrophy in bvFTD, in contrast to a set of dissociable insulo-temporal areas for svPPA and for nfvPPA [112]. Thus, face and emotion recognition impairments in nfvPPA were related to the atrophy of the bilateral posterior fusiform gyrus, bilateral insular cortex, and anterior temporal lobe [112]. Conversely, emotion recognition deficits in svPPA have been associated to atrophy in left temporal structures and also to amygdala atrophy [125]. Finally, deficits in ToM in nfvPPA have been associated with temporal pole and insular cortex degeneration. In contrast, theory of mind disturbances in svPPA are consistent with the patients' atrophy in the left temporal lobe and the medial frontal cortex [113].

Taken together, the integration of the study of social cognitive factors, such as emotion processing, empathy, ToM, moral cognition, and sociobehavioral regulation, are considered as the current target to assess complex behaviors in FTLD. In fact, a deep comprehension of the neurocognitive processes that subsume the interplay between the sociomoral cognition, the executive function, and the behavior seems to be the most robust way to create new perspectives for the diagnosis and new targets of intervention in FTLD.

2.1.2. Amyotrophic Lateral Sclerosis and Its Disease Spectrum. The presence of impaired social cognition in ALS, with or without dementia, provides additional evidence in favour of the existence of an ALS-FTLD continuum and appears to have crucial implications for patients' and caregivers' training from early disease stages. ALS, the most common motor neuron disease, has been traditionally classified as a disease of the motor system. However, cognitive and behavioral dysfunctions are now recognized as an integral part of ALS-related clinical syndrome [67, 126]. In particular, about 50–60% among ALS patients may develop frontotemporal dysfunctions [67, 127], mostly characterized by executive and language impairment, variable memory dysfunctions, and/or behavioral impairment [67, 128]. Apathy is the most pronounced ALS-related behavioral change [129], while disinhibition and disorganization have been less frequently reported [130]. In addition, approximately up to 15% of ALS patients will either present with or develop FTLD, exhibiting a strong clinical and pathological overlap between ALS and FTLD [131]. Thus, the abovementioned heterogeneity results in different categorization groups across a spectrum of disease, including cognitive impairment, behavioral impairment, and ALS-FTLD [67, 131].

Impaired social cognition is now recognized as a part of the cognitive phenotype of ALS, despite the fact that there is significant heterogeneity in tasks used to study social cognition. During the last decades, an increasing body of studies focus on patients' performance in tests related to social cognition [67] and also evaluated its neuroanatomical correlates [132]. On the other hand, social cognition is included in an ALS cognitive screening testing (i.e., Edinburg Cognitive and Behavioral ALS Screen (ECAS); [133]) and in the "Axis II: Defining the neuropsychological deficits" of the recently suggested diagnostic criteria for ALS-frontotemporal spectrum disorders (ALS-FTSD) [67]. Moreover, the evaluation of social cognition in ALS-FTSD may have an utmost importance in clinical settings, given the potential effects of its impairment on patients' quality of life and ability to engage in end-of-life decisions [134-136]. However, it is still debatable whether social cognition deficits are independent of other cognitive deficits in ALS or are part of the executive deficits or not [137-143] and to what degree they are associated with other cognitive deficits, including memory function [136]. Of note, a subgroup of ALS patients without dementia has been found to present impaired social cognition without executive dysfunction [140].

(1) Alterations in the Four Domains of Social Cognition. Changes in emotion-processing ability and reduced capacity in the emotional recognition of facial expressions (i.e., mostly related to negative emotions, including fear, anger, and disgust [144, 145]) is more likely in patients with ALS-FTLD [141, 146-148]. In particular, the latter, in association with the fact that the severity of social cognition deficits is much more pronounced and widespread in FTLD patients [149, 150], corroborates the existence of a considerable clinical overlapping between ALS and FTLD.

Social behavior dysfunction in ALS mainly includes apathy [141]. Moreover, loss of empathy [141], deficits in emotion processing [147, 151-153] and emotional empathy attribution [139], and compromised ability to make social inferences [142, 146] have also been described in nondemented ALS patients.

Patients with ALS show difficulty on tests tapping onto ToM components, exhibiting impaired abilities (i) to describe the intentions and feeling of characters [139, 142, 154], (ii) to identify and explain social faux pas [155], and (iii) to estimate preferences for objects based on the interpretation of eye gaze direction [141, 156].

Even though previous evidence revealed a more pronounced impairment in affective rather than cognitive component of ToM [157], Trojsi et al. [136] found that both cognitive and affective ToM may be impaired in the early disease stages by simultaneously comparing both ToM components [136]. Of note, cognitive ToM impairments have been mostly linked to a more general executive dysfunction [154].

Clinical variables have been directly or indirectly related to patients' ToM and other social abilities. For instance, the majority of studies with impairments include patients with an average duration of 30 months [141, 142, 155], bulbar onset [156], and/or cognitive impairment [142, 146]. With regard to the latter, it is still unclear whether social cognitive impairment is independent of other cognitive deficits (particularly executive dysfunction) or not. In particular, Watermeyer et al. [143] revealed that impaired social cognition in ALS has been mainly attributed to primary executive dysfunction, found to be the main predictor of social cognition performance above and beyond demographics, behavior, mood, and personality variables. Severe deficits in both cognitive and affective ToM have been proven to be related to apathy and impaired verbal fluency and naming [157], while early in the disease course impaired ToM has been associated to executive dysfunction [137]. On the other hand, there are several studies that failed to find an association between social cognition/ToM and executive impairment [137, 141, 155]. In this regard, Trojsi et al. [136] recently reported that both cognitive and affective ToM components are associated with nonexecutive impairment, including memory prose and visuospatial ability.

(2) Neuroanatomical Bases of Social Cognition Impairment in ALS. Some multimodal studies have directly addressed in vivo the degeneration of social brain networks in ALS, using neuroimaging techniques tailored to the study of structural changes (gray matter, white matter) [139, 148] and functional alternations (fMRI) [132]. Evidence was related to the emotion circuits, including amygdala and medial prefrontal, OFC and anterior cingulate cortices, and "mentalizing" and "empathy" networks. In particular, patterns of gray matter atrophy in anterior cingulate and right frontoinsular cortices were found significantly associated with emotional and empathy performances in nondemented ALS patients [139]. Moreover, a significant decline of emotion recognition skills (particularly affecting the identification of negative emotions) has been found related to microstructural changes (measured through fractional anisotropy) in right inferior longitudinal fasciculus and inferior frontooccipital fasciculus in nondemented ALS patients [148]. Interestingly, also in ALS patients the right hemisphere has been confirmed to play a key role in the identification of others' emotions, especially those negative, with specific damage of ventral associative tracts connecting frontal, temporal, limbic, and occipital areas [147].

Focusing on the cognitive ToM component, Carluer et al. [137] detected significant correlations between cognitive ToM deficit (i.e., false-belief task) and brain metabolic rate of glucose consumption in the bilateral dorsomedial and dorsolateral prefrontal cortex, as well as in supplementary motor areas. These findings are in line with the involvement of dorsomedial and dorsolateral prefrontal areas in cognitive ToM [158, 159], as well as the contribution of the supplementary motor area in the "mirror neuron system" [160].

2.2. Parkinson's Disease and Parkinsonisms. Parkinson's disease (PD), mainly characterized by motor symptoms (i.e., resting tremor, bradykinesia, rigidity, and postural instability), may exhibit early nonmotor symptoms, including neuropsychiatric symptoms, sleep problems, and cognitive deficits, hypothesized to be secondary to the loss of dopaminergic neurons in the substantia nigra and the consequent hypostimulation of the prefrontal cortex [161]. Among nonmotor domains, social cognition has been explored in PD, especially with regard to emotion recognition and ToM abilities. However, emerging evidence has underlined the severity of nonmotor symptoms of PSP and CBS, which may substantially impact on social interactions and contribute to alter emotion recognition [162, 163].

2.2.1. Alterations in the Four Domains of Social Cognition. As for emotion recognition in PD, several studies [164-169] revealed emotion recognition deficits in PD patients when compared to matched healthy controls. However, other studies failed to find these deficits [170-174]. A recent meta-analytic review [175], which investigated the emotion recognition from faces and voices in PD, revealed significant and modest deficits of this ability in nondemented PD patients, independently from the level of motor disability. Furthermore, several studies revealed that PD patients were more impaired in recognizing negative emotions (anger, disgust, fear, and sadness) than positive ones (happiness, surprise) [176], while other studies suggested that the recognition of negative emotions may be impaired mainly in the early stages of PD and, then, this impairment has been shown to mainly affect the positive ones [177]. In particular, Hipp et al. [178] showed that, at the early stages, PD patients might be still prone to compensate the deficient input of low contrast sensitivity that is crucial for the appreciation of negative facial emotions.

Impairments of facial emotion recognition in PD patients were found to be independent of depressive symptoms [167, 179-181], executive deficits [179, 180], and clinical aspects (i.e., disease duration and severity, [180]). Moreover, some studies revealed that emotion recognition abnormalities may occur after subthalamic nucleus stimulation [182-185], probably due to alterations of projections to cortical areas, particularly the OFC, which has been already implicated in emotion recognition [186]. However, a recent study of Albuquerque et al. [187] did not confirm these findings in advanced PD.

With regard to PSP and CBS, also belonging to the FTLD spectrum of neurodegeneration (i.e., abnormal function/levels of the microtubule associated protein tau), patients affected by PSP may exhibit impaired facial (i.e., sadness and sadness) and voice emotion recognition [188, 189] as well as CBS patients, who may exhibit difficulties in recognizing disgust, sadness, surprise, and happiness, but not anger and fear [163]. Moreover, half of the PSP patients reported that social impairments negatively impacted their quality of life [190] and, in this regard, this self-perceived social impairment may be the result of the loss of emotion knowledge or breakdown of higher-order social inferences, known as "theory of mind," as observed in FTLD [105]. In support of this overlap of social cognition impairment between FTLD and PSP, Shany-Ur et al. [191] assessed socioemotional comprehension, including visual perspective taking, belief representation, and emotion reading in a population of neurodegenerative patients, including patients with FTLD and PSP, using the Social Inference-Enriched (SI-E) and Social Inference-Minimal (SI-M) subtests of the TASIT [52]. They revealed that both patients with bvFTD and with PSP had significantly poorer scores than healthy controls on the TASIT SI-E "think" questions across verbal cue items, indicating an impaired ability to represent others' verbalized opinions/beliefs, and on the TASIT SI-E "do" questions across all items, indicating impaired ability to comprehend others' intentions. In particular, impairment of the comprehension of insincere communication and sarcasm was observed in PSP as well as in bvFTD patients, though to a major extent in patients with bvFTD [191]. Of note, failure to comprehend complex social interactions has been demonstrated to exacerbate patients' poor social self-monitoring and aberrant social behavior, thereby severely impacting interpersonal communication and patients' management [192]. Conversely, in CBS observation of facial apraxia, which results in the inability to express facial emotional expressions [193], and flat aprosodic speech [194] may reflect a compromised ability to express emotions.

Several studies explored the two different subcomponents of ToM (i.e., affective and cognitive subcomponents) in PD patients and revealed deficits of both across the entire disease course [169, 195-198]. Importantly, Peron et al. [199] found no different performance on ToM tasks between medicated and nonmedicated PD patients at early stages, suggesting that ToM deficits could be observed in PD patients when the degenerative process has spread beyond the dopaminergic pathways, but not in the early PD patients, in whom neuronal loss is limited to the nigrostriatal and mesolimbic dopaminergic systems. However, more recent studies did not confirm these findings, but revealed the occurrence of impairment of cognitive ToM in both medicated and unmedicated PD [196, 200], whereas other studies showed impairment of affective ToM [195] or deficits of both ToM subcomponents [198, 201].

Deficits of the cognitive ToM subcomponent have been found associated predominantly with executive dysfunction [198, 200, 202-204]. Conversely, Roca et al. [196] did not find any association between cognitive ToM, depression, executive dysfunctions, and medication usage. With regard to deficits of the affective ToM subcomponent, they have been associated with apathy [198] and reduced quality of life [201] and may be predicted by poor cognitive status and the dysfunction of visuospatial abilities [205].

2.2.2. Neuroanatomical Bases of Social Cognition Impairment in PD and Parkinsonisms. With regard to structural neural bases of the deficits in facial emotion recognition, Ibarretxe-Bilbao et al. [206] revealed an association between these deficits and reduced volume in OFC, associated to the degeneration of OFC and amygdala. More recently, Baggio et al. [207] confirmed the pivotal role of abnormalities within these areas in impaired facial emotion recognition and also found that poor sadness, disgust, and anger identification were also related to dysfunction in other cortical regions, such as postcentral and right occipital fusiform gyri, ventral striatum, subgenual cortex, and anterior cingulate cortex.

Previous neuroimaging studies, focusing on functional changes associated with the impaired recognition of emotions in PD patients, revealed that the impaired emotional facial recognition network was characterized by a decreased metabolism within the bilateral posterior cingulate gyrus (BA 31), right superior frontal gyrus (BAs 10, 9, and 6), and left superior frontal gyrus (BAs 10 and 11) [208]. Furthermore, Wabnegger et al. [209] found that, when compared to healthy subjects, PD patients showed a stronger activation in somatosensory cortices, which are involved in decoding emotional states by internally generating somatosensory representations that simulate how one feels when displaying a certain facial expression and, therefore, may be substantially involved in emotion recognition (Figure 1).

With regard to parkinsonisms, impaired emotion recognition in PSP patients have been associated with gray matter atrophy in the right inferior frontal gyrus [188], while in CBS neuroimaging analyses revealed that emotion-processing deficits were associated with the atrophy of the paracentral gyrus/precuneus region, as well as of the basal ganglia [163]. PSP patients have been proven to exhibit mild but significant focal deficits in social cognition [191], which is consistent with evidence showing that they may often manifest behavioral and personality changes, hypothesized to occur as a result of a disconnection between subcortical structures and the prefrontal cortex [210, 211].

With regard to neural correlates of ToM deficits in PD, Péron et al. [212] revealed a significant association between impaired ToM abilities and decreased cerebral glucose metabolism in brain areas belonging to the "ToM network" (i.e., bilateral cingulate gyri, middle and inferior frontal gyri, fusiform and superior temporal gyri, and bilateral parietal and bilateral occipital lobes). In addition, Diez-Ciranda et al. [213] observed that reduced gray matter volume in the precentral and postcentral gyrus and in the middle and inferior frontal gyri may be involved in ToM deficits in PD. Moreover, these authors reported an association between ToM impairment and alterations of white matter in the superior longitudinal fasciculus, adjacent to the parietal lobe, and of the white matter adjacent to the frontal lobe.

In atypical parkinsonisms, ToM abilities have been poorly explored. In detail, impaired ToM abilities have been described in PSP patients [188] and found to be related to grey matter atrophy in the right inferior frontal gyrus and in the anterior medial frontal cortex, both associated to the ToM domain. Finally, Poletti and Bonuccelli [214]

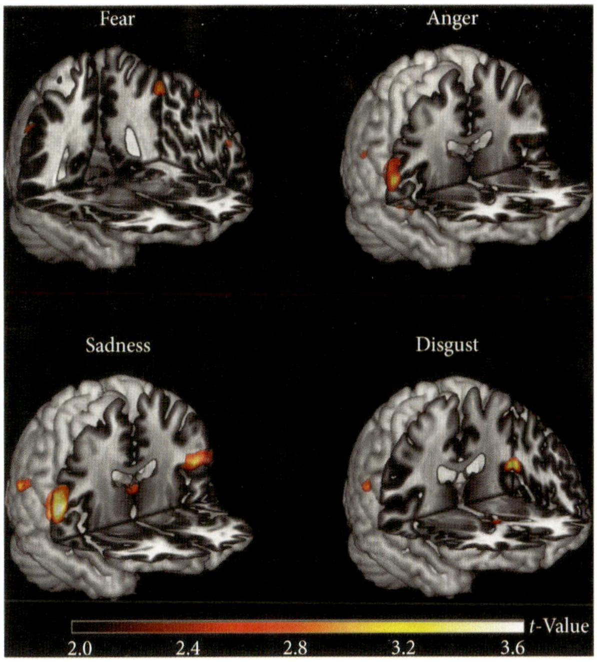

FIGURE 1: Regions showing increased fMRI activation in nonmedicated, nondemented PD patients ($n = 17$) compared to healthy controls ($n = 22$). PD patients may exhibit a general stronger recruitment of parietal regions when observing pictures of facial expressions depicting disgust, fear, sadness, and anger (image reproduced from Wabnegger et al. [209] under the Creative Commons license (CC-BY), no permission needed).

described a case of affective ToM impairment in a case of clinically diagnosed CBS with a bilateral 18-FDG positron emission tomography hypometabolism in the frontal-temporal-parietal cortices, more marked in the right hemisphere. However, no data have been reported about ToM abnormalities in patients affected by multisystem atrophy.

2.3. Alzheimer's Disease. Alzheimer's disease (AD), the most frequent neurodegenerative dementia and the first cause of neurocognitive disorder in the world, is typically characterized by an early and progressive episodic memory loss. From the neuropathological point of view, the progressive neurodegeneration initially affects the hippocampi, the entorhinal and posterior cingulate cortices, and, subsequently, the entire temporal, parietal, and frontal cortices [215]. Following this anatomical pathway, social cognition dysfunctions can occur during the course of the disease, particularly in the moderate-severe stages [216]. In contrast, earlier in the disease, social incongruities appear largely modulated by general cognitive decline in memory, language, and executive domains, rather than a genuine social dysfunction [217].

In particular, although considerably less common than in bvFTD, AD patients may present impaired social behavior, ToM, loss of empathy, facial emotion recognition, and inaccurate self-awareness, and, although uncommon as first symptoms, among alterations of social behavior, disinhibition, social awkwardness, and apathy have been reported, respectively, in 6.9%, 5%, and 2% of cases [218].

2.3.1. Alterations in the Four Domains of Social Cognition. With regard to apathy and disinhibition, associated with AD severity, one of the most common tools for social/behavior evaluation in dementia, the Neuropsychiatric Inventory (NPI) [219], has been used in combination with the Clinical Dementia Rating (CDR) scale [220], which is a disease severity scale, ranging from 0 (no impairment) to 2 (severe impairment). Several NPI dimensions, but in particular apathy and disinhibition, were correlated with the CDR score. Moreover, apathy was the most prevalent in all CDR groups and the only symptom with frequencies exceeding 50% in AD patients with CDR 0.5, 1, and 2 [221].

Other types of social disturbances are rarely described in AD, such as criminal behaviors, which are more recurrent in bvFTD [101]. In fact, rarely, AD patients may present an atypical, bvFTD-like clinical profile in very early stages of disease. However, this presentation is characterized by a milder and more restricted behavioral profile than in bvFTD, with high cooccurrence of memory dysfunction and dysexecutive abnormalities, and a pattern of atrophy centered on temporoparietal regions, as in typical AD [222].

Deficits in recognizing others' emotions are reported in AD [223] and in its prodromal stage, the so-called mild cognitive impairment (MCI) [224]. Most emotion recognition studies have required participants to identify emotional expressions in pictures producing mixed results, with evidence of both impaired [223, 225-227] and intact [228, 229] recognition overall. When considering specific emotions, the findings are also inconsistent. More recently, a large sample of neurodegenerative patients, including AD, was studied by using short films instead of photographs [229]. This study revealed that emotion recognition was indistinguishable by comparing the AD group to healthy controls. However, in this regard, it should be kept in mind that concomitant basic and high-level visual and visuospatial difficulties in AD may negatively impact facial recognition, which in turn translate in an impaired emotion recognition [230].

ToM deficits are reported in AD [231, 232], although ToM alterations in AD remains a controversial subject. Specifically, performances at ToM tests have been revealed to not reflect a genuine ToM deficit, rather a deficit mediated by general (and particularly executive) cognitive decline [233].

Loss of empathy has also been reported in AD, particularly as the so-called cognitive empathy (i.e., the ability to understand) in the context of a relative preservation of affective empathy (i.e., the ability to share) [234]. This pattern of spared/impaired types of empathy has been shown to be related to the vulnerability of a distributed network of regions, centered on the frontoinsular cortices, the integrity of which in AD is crucial for preserved social functioning [234].

Finally, AD patients may also present poor self-awareness of their functional limitations that may exacerbate their behavior abnormalities, as well as the reliability of the patient [235]. Self-awareness can be easily tested by asking the patient for a description of themselves, using a scale rating their competency across different domains (i.e., daily living activities and cognitive/emotional interpersonal control) (such as the Patient Competency Rating Scale) [235]. In particular, AD patients resulted in being more prone to overestimate cognitive and emotional functioning in comparison to bvFTD patients who may overestimate their functioning in all domains [235].

3. Conclusions and Future Perspectives

Abnormal interpersonal behavior is commonly observed in clinical practice, representing part of the core diagnostic criteria for many clinical disorders. Therefore, to overcome the potential consequences related to social isolation, known to be a risk factor for morbidity and mortality [2], social cognitive intervention may be prospected to reduce the negative impact of such disabilities on mental health, improving the ability to form and consolidate interpersonal networks. Among these strategies, targeted training programs may be implemented on the basis of the recent evidence of structural plasticity in well-known socioaffective and sociocognitive brain networks after training-induced behavioral improvements in healthy adults [236] and of potential advantages from targeted training programs on emotion recognition in neurodegenerative patients [104, 237].

Recently, increasing interest has been addressed to the potential benefits of pharmacotherapy on social cognition deficits, such as the potential effects of the peripheral administration of exogenous oxytocin, shown to exert prosocial effects [238-241], probably mediated by the modulation of the serotonergic system [239].

Another emerging approach is related to the use of brain stimulation techniques, such as theta burst and high-frequency repetitive transcranial magnetic stimulation (rTMS), to modulate empathy-related brain activity. In particular, rTMS sessions, by stimulating the bilateral medial prefrontal cortex, have been revealed to be useful in improving self-reported social functioning in the case of autism spectrum disorders [242] and major depressive disorders [243].

Finally, given the critical role of caregivers' wellbeing and collaboration in any therapeutic and rehabilitation plan, treatment efforts should also be directed towards ensuring the availability of appropriate education and support for them.

References

[1] R. Adolphs, "The social brain: neural basis of social knowledge," *Annual Review of Psychology*, vol. 60, no. 1, pp. 693–716, 2009.

[2] S. Cacioppo, J. P. Capitanio, and J. T. Cacioppo, "Toward a neurology of loneliness," *Psychological Bulletin*, vol. 140, no. 6, pp. 1464–1504, 2014.

[3] F. Adolfi, B. Couto, F. Richter et al., "Convergence of interoception, emotion, and social cognition: a two-fold fMRI meta-analysis and lesion approach," *Cortex*, vol. 88, pp. 124–142, 2017.

[4] R. Adolphs, S. Baron-Cohen, and D. Tranel, "Impaired recognition of social emotions following amygdala damage," *Journal of Cognitive Neuroscience*, vol. 14, no. 8, pp. 1264–1274, 2002.

[5] J. D. Henry, W. von Hippel, P. Molenberghs, T. Lee, and P. S. Sachdev, "Clinical assessment of social cognitive function in neurological disorders," *Nature Reviews Neurology*, vol. 12, no. 1, pp. 28–39, 2016.

[6] L. Brothers, "The social brain: a project for integrating primate behaviour and neurophysiology in a new domain," *Concepts Neuroscience*, vol. 1, pp. 27–51, 1990.

[7] J. V. Haxby, E. A. Hoffman, and M. I. Gobbini, "The distributed human neural system for face perception," *Trends in Cognitive Sciences*, vol. 4, no. 6, pp. 223–233, 2000.

[8] R. Adolphs, "What does the amygdala contribute to social cognition?," *Annals of the New York Academy of Sciences*, vol. 1191, no. 1, pp. 42–61, 2010.

[9] A. W. Young, J. P. Aggleton, D. J. Hellawell, M. Johnson, P. Broks, and J. R. Hanley, "Face processing impairments after amygdalotomy," *Brain*, vol. 118, no. 1, pp. 15–24, 1995.

[10] J. E. LeDoux, "Emotion circuits in the brain," *Annual Review of Neuroscience*, vol. 23, no. 1, pp. 155–184, 2000.

[11] L. Pessoa, "On the relationship between emotion and cognition," *Nature Reviews Neuroscience*, vol. 9, no. 2, pp. 148–158, 2008.

[12] K. H. Lee, T. F. D. Farrow, S. A. Spence, and P. W. R. Woodruff, "Social cognition, brain networks and schizophrenia," *Psychological Medicine*, vol. 34, no. 3, pp. 391–400, 2004.

[13] P. Mukherjee, H. C. Whalley, J. W. McKirdy et al., "Altered amygdala connectivity within the social brain in schizophrenia," *Schizophrenia Bulletin*, vol. 40, no. 1, pp. 152–160, 2014.

[14] F. Kumfor, C. Honan, S. McDonald, J. L. Hazelton, J. R. Hodges, and O. Piguet, "Assessing the "social brain" in dementia: applying TASIT-S," *Cortex*, vol. 93, pp. 166–177, 2017.

[15] A. Bejanin, G. Chételat, M. Laisney et al., "Distinct neural substrates of affective and cognitive theory of mind impairment in semantic dementia," *Social Neuroscience*, vol. 12, no. 3, pp. 287–302, 2017.

[16] E. A. H. von dem Hagen, R. S. Stoyanova, S. Baron-Cohen, and A. J. Calder, "Reduced functional connectivity within and between "social" resting state networks in autism spectrum conditions," *Social Cognitive and Affective Neuroscience*, vol. 8, no. 6, pp. 694–701, 2013.

[17] N. M. Kleinhans, T. Richards, L. Sterling et al., "Abnormal functional connectivity in autism spectrum disorders during face processing," *Brain*, vol. 131, no. 4, pp. 1000–1012, 2008.

[18] M. A. Patriquin, T. DeRamus, L. E. Libero, A. Laird, and R. K. Kana, "Neuroanatomical and neurofunctional markers of social cognition in autism spectrum disorder," *Human Brain Mapping*, vol. 37, no. 11, pp. 3957–3978, 2016.

[19] M. Roy, D. Shohamy, and T. D. Wager, "Ventromedial prefrontal-subcortical systems and the generation of affective meaning," *Trends in Cognitive Sciences*, vol. 16, no. 3, pp. 147–156, 2012.

[20] K. C. Berridge and M. L. Kringelbach, "Neuroscience of affect: brain mechanisms of pleasure and displeasure," *Current Opinion in Neurobiology*, vol. 23, no. 3, pp. 294–303, 2013.

[21] I. Cristofori, W. Zhong, V. Mandoske et al., "Brain regions influencing implicit violent attitudes: a lesion-mapping

study," *Journal of Neuroscience*, vol. 36, no. 9, pp. 2757–2768, 2016.

[22] J. S. Beer, O. P. John, D. Scabini, and R. T. Knight, "Orbitofrontal cortex and social behavior: integrating self-monitoring and emotion-cognition interactions," *Journal of Cognitive Neuroscience*, vol. 18, no. 6, pp. 871–879, 2006.

[23] C. A. Hill, S. Suzuki, R. Polania, M. Moisa, J. P. O'Doherty, and C. C. Ruff, "A causal account of the brain network computations underlying strategic social behavior," *Nature Neuroscience*, vol. 20, no. 8, pp. 1142–1149, 2017.

[24] D. Dodell-Feder, J. Koster-Hale, M. Bedny, and R. Saxe, "fMRI item analysis in a theory of mind task," *NeuroImage*, vol. 55, no. 2, pp. 705–712, 2011.

[25] R. Saxe, "Why and how to study Theory of Mind with fMRI," *Brain Research*, vol. 1079, no. 1, pp. 57–65, 2006.

[26] L. Young and R. Saxe, "An FMRI investigation of spontaneous mental state inference for moral judgment," *Journal of Cognitive Neuroscience*, vol. 21, no. 7, pp. 1396–1405, 2009.

[27] D. Schneider, V. P. Slaughter, S. I. Becker, and P. E. Dux, "Implicit false-belief processing in the human brain," *NeuroImage*, vol. 101, pp. 268–275, 2014.

[28] A. M. Kovacs, S. Kühn, G. Gergely, G. Csibra, and M. Brass, "Are all beliefs equal? Implicit belief attributions recruiting core brain regions of theory of mind," *PLoS One*, vol. 9, no. 9, article e106558, 2014.

[29] D. C. Hyde, M. Aparicio Betancourt, and C. E. Simon, "Human temporal-parietal junction spontaneously tracks others' beliefs: a functional near-infrared spectroscopy study," *Human Brain Mapping*, vol. 36, no. 12, pp. 4831–4846, 2015.

[30] G. Hein and T. Singer, "I feel how you feel but not always: the empathic brain and its modulation," *Current Opinion in Neurobiology*, vol. 18, no. 2, pp. 153–158, 2008.

[31] J. Decety and J. M. Cowell, "The complex relation between morality and empathy," *Trends in Cognitive Sciences*, vol. 18, no. 7, pp. 337–339, 2014.

[32] C. Lamm, J. Decety, and T. Singer, "Meta-analytic evidence for common and distinct neural networks associated with directly experienced pain and empathy for pain," *NeuroImage*, vol. 54, no. 3, pp. 2492–2502, 2011.

[33] C. Korponay, M. Pujara, P. Deming et al., "Impulsive antisocial psychopathic traits linked to increased volume and functional connectivity within prefrontal cortex," *Social Cognitive and Affective Neuroscience*, vol. 12, no. 7, pp. 1169–1178, 2017.

[34] S. V. Abram, K. M. Wisner, J. M. Fox et al., "Fronto-temporal connectivity predicts cognitive empathy deficits and experiential negative symptoms in schizophrenia," *Human Brain Mapping*, vol. 38, no. 3, pp. 1111–1124, 2017.

[35] M. Iacoboni, R. P. Woods, M. Brass, H. Bekkering, J. C. Mazziotta, and G. Rizzolatti, "Cortical mechanisms of human imitation," *Science*, vol. 286, no. 5449, pp. 2526–2528, 1999.

[36] J. Decety, T. Chaminade, J. Grèzes, and A. N. Meltzoff, "A PET exploration of the neural mechanisms involved in reciprocal imitation," *NeuroImage*, vol. 15, no. 1, pp. 265–272, 2002.

[37] M. C. Keuken, A. Hardie, B. T. Dorn et al., "The role of the left inferior frontal gyrus in social perception: an rTMS study," *Brain Research*, vol. 1383, pp. 196–205, 2011.

[38] P. G. Enticott, P. J. Johnston, S. E. Herring, K. E. Hoy, and P. B. Fitzgerald, "Mirror neuron activation is associated with facial emotion processing," *Neuropsychologia*, vol. 46, no. 11, pp. 2851–2854, 2008.

[39] N. Hadjikhani, R. M. Joseph, J. Snyder, and H. Tager-Flusberg, "Anatomical differences in the mirror neuron system and social cognition network in autism," *Cerebral Cortex*, vol. 16, no. 9, pp. 1276–1282, 2006.

[40] I. Fishman, C. L. Keown, A. J. Lincoln, J. A. Pineda, and R. A. Müller, "Atypical cross talk between mentalizing and mirror neuron networks in autism spectrum disorder," *Journal of the American Medical Association Psychiatry*, vol. 71, no. 7, pp. 751–760, 2014.

[41] M. Schulte-Rüther, E. Otte, K. Adigüzel et al., "Intact mirror mechanisms for automatic facial emotions in children and adolescents with autism spectrum disorder," *Autism Research*, vol. 10, no. 2, pp. 298–310, 2017.

[42] M. Poletti, I. Enrici, and M. Adenzato, "Cognitive and affective Theory of Mind in neurodegenerative diseases: neuropsychological, neuroanatomical and neurochemical levels," *Neuroscience & Biobehavioral Reviews*, vol. 36, no. 9, pp. 2147–2164, 2012.

[43] M. Adenzato, M. Cavallo, and I. Enrici, "Theory of mind ability in the behavioural variant of frontotemporal dementia: an analysis of the neural, cognitive, and social levels," *Neuropsychologia*, vol. 48, no. 1, pp. 2–12, 2010.

[44] M. L. Schroeter, "Considering the frontomedian cortex in revised criteria for behavioural variant frontotemporal dementia," *Brain*, vol. 135, no. 4, pp. e213–e212, 2012.

[45] M. L. Schroeter, B. Vogt, S. Frisch et al., "Executive deficits are related to the inferior frontal junction in early dementia," *Brain*, vol. 135, no. 1, pp. 201–215, 2012.

[46] J. Grace and P. F. Malloy, *Frontal Systems Behavior Scale Professional Manual*, Psychological Assessment Resources, Lutz, FL, USA, 2001.

[47] A. Kertesz, N. Nadkarni, W. Davidson, and A. W. Thomas, "The Frontal Behavioral Inventory in the differential diagnosis of frontotemporal dementia," *Journal of the International Neuropsychological Society*, vol. 6, no. 4, pp. 460–468, 2000.

[48] J. P. Barsuglia, N. C. Kaiser, S. S. Wilkins et al., "A scale of socioemotional dysfunction in frontotemporal dementia," *Archives of Clinical Neuropsychology*, vol. 29, no. 8, pp. 793–805, 2014.

[49] J. D. Henry, W. von Hippel, and K. Baynes, "Social inappropriateness, executive control, and aging," *Psychology and Aging*, vol. 24, no. 1, pp. 239–244, 2009.

[50] K. C. Bickart, M. Brickhouse, A. Negreira, D. Sapolsky, L. F. Barrett, and B. C. Dickerson, "Atrophy in distinct corticolimbic networks in frontotemporal dementia relates to social impairments measured using the Social Impairment Rating Scale," *Journal of Neurology, Neurosurgery & Psychiatry*, vol. 85, no. 4, pp. 438–448, 2014.

[51] H. Wimmer and J. Perner, "Beliefs about beliefs: representation and constraining function of wrong beliefs in young children's understanding of deception," *Cognition*, vol. 13, no. 1, pp. 103–128, 1983.

[52] S. McDonald, S. Flanagan, J. Rollins, and J. Kinch, "TASIT: a new clinical tool for assessing social perception after traumatic brain injury," *The Journal of Head Trauma Rehabilitation*, vol. 18, no. 3, pp. 219–238, 2003.

[53] F. G. E. Happé, "An advanced test of theory of mind: understanding of story characters' thoughts and feelings by able autistic, mentally handicapped, and normal children and adults," *Journal of Autism and Developmental Disorders*, vol. 24, no. 2, pp. 129–154, 1994.

[54] V. E. Stone, S. Baron-Cohen, and R. T. Knight, "Frontal lobe contributions to theory of mind," *Journal of Cognitive Neuroscience*, vol. 10, no. 5, pp. 640–656, 1998.

[55] S. Baron-Cohen, S. Wheelwright, J. Hill, Y. Raste, and I. Plumb, "The "Reading the Mind in the Eyes" test revised version: a study with normal adults, and adults with Asperger syndrome or high-functioning autism," *Journal of Child Psychology and Psychiatry*, vol. 42, no. 2, pp. 241–251, 2001.

[56] M. H. Davis, "Measuring individual-differences in empathy—evidence for a multidimensional approach," *Journal of Personality and Social Psychology*, vol. 44, no. 1, pp. 113–126, 1983.

[57] S. Baron-Cohen and S. Wheelwright, "The empathy quotient: an investigation of adults with Asperger syndrome or high functioning autism, and normal sex differences," *Journal of Autism and Developmental Disorders*, vol. 34, no. 2, pp. 163–175, 2004.

[58] I. Dziobek, K. Rogers, S. Fleck et al., "Dissociation of cognitive and emotional empathy in adults with Asperger syndrome using the Multifaceted Empathy Test (MET)," *Journal of Autism and Developmental Disorders*, vol. 38, no. 3, pp. 464–473, 2008.

[59] P. Ekman and W. V. Friesen, *Pictures of Facial Affect*, Consulting Psychologists Press, Palo Alto, CA, USA, 1976.

[60] K. B. Froming, M. Levy, S. G. Schaffer, and P. Ekman, *Comprehensive Affect Testing System (CATS)*, Psychology Software Inc, Gainesville, FL, USA, 2006.

[61] D. Bowers, L. X. Blonder, and K. M. Heilman, *Florida Affect Battery*, Center for Neuropsychological Studies, 1999.

[62] J. D. Warren, J. D. Rohrer, and M. N. Rossor, "Frontotemporal dementia," *BMJ*, vol. 347, article F4827, 2013.

[63] I. T. S. Coyle-Gilchrist, K. M. Dick, K. Patterson et al., "Prevalence, characteristics, and survival of frontotemporal lobar degeneration syndromes," *Neurology*, vol. 86, no. 18, pp. 1736–1743, 2016.

[64] K. Rascovsky, J. R. Hodges, D. Knopman et al., "Sensitivity of revised diagnostic criteria for the behavioural variant of frontotemporal dementia," *Brain*, vol. 134, no. 9, pp. 2456–2477, 2011.

[65] O. Piguet, M. Hornberger, E. Mioshi, and J. R. Hodges, "Behavioural-variant frontotemporal dementia: diagnosis, clinical staging, and management," *Lancet Neurology*, vol. 10, no. 2, pp. 162–172, 2011.

[66] M. L. Gorno-Tempini, A. E. Hillis, S. Weintraub et al., "Classification of primary progressive aphasia and its variants," *Neurology*, vol. 76, no. 11, pp. 1006–1014, 2011.

[67] M. J. Strong, S. Abrahams, L. H. Goldstein et al., "Amyotrophic lateral sclerosis-frontotemporal spectrum disorder (ALS-FTSD): revised diagnostic criteria," *Amyotrophic Lateral Sclerosis and Frontotemporal Degeneration*, vol. 18, no. 3–4, pp. 153–174, 2017.

[68] A. Ibáñez and F. Manes, "Contextual social cognition and the behavioral variant of frontotemporal dementia," *Neurology*, vol. 78, no. 17, pp. 1354–1362, 2012.

[69] A. Ibáñez, R. O. Kuljis, D. Matallana, and F. Manes, "Bridging psychiatry and neurology through social neuroscience," *World Psychiatry*, vol. 13, no. 2, pp. 148-149, 2014.

[70] A. Ibáñez, P. Billeke, L. de la Fuente, P. Salamone, A. M. Garcia, and M. Melloni, "Reply: towards a neurocomputational account of social dysfunction in neurodegenerative disease," *Brain*, vol. 140, no. 3, p. e15, 2017.

[71] W. W. Seeley, J. Zhou, and E. J. Kim, "Frontotemporal dementia: what can the behavioral variant teach us about human brain organization?," *Neuroscientist*, vol. 18, no. 4, pp. 373–385, 2012.

[72] J. Van den Stock and F. Kumfor, "Behavioural variant frontotemporal dementia: at the interface of interoception, emotion and social cognition?," *Cortex*, 2017.

[73] S. Baez, J. P. Morales, A. Slachevsky et al., "Orbitofrontal and limbic signatures of empathic concern and intentional harm in the behavioral variant frontotemporal dementia," *Cortex*, vol. 75, pp. 20–32, 2016.

[74] V. E. Sturm, J. S. Yokoyama, J. A. Eckart et al., "Damage to left frontal regulatory circuits produces greater positive emotional reactivity in frontotemporal dementia," *Cortex*, vol. 64, pp. 55–67, 2015.

[75] K. H. Werner, N. A. Roberts, H. J. Rosen et al., "Emotional reactivity and emotion recognition in frontotemporal lobar degeneration," *Neurology*, vol. 69, no. 2, pp. 148–155, 2007.

[76] M. H. Cohen, A. M. Carton, C. J. Hardy et al., "Processing emotion from abstract art in frontotemporal lobar degeneration," *Neuropsychologia*, vol. 81, pp. 245–254, 2016.

[77] S. Baez, F. Manes, D. Huepe et al., "Primary empathy deficits in frontotemporal dementia," *Frontiers in Aging Neuroscience*, vol. 6, p. 262, 2014.

[78] R. W. Levenson, V. E. Sturm, and C. M. Haase, "Emotional and behavioral symptoms in neurodegenerative disease: a model for studying the neural bases of psychopathology," *Annual Review of Clinical Psychology*, vol. 10, no. 1, pp. 581–606, 2014.

[79] S. C. Lanata and B. L. Miller, "The behavioural variant frontotemporal dementia (bvFTD) syndrome in psychiatry," *Journal of Neurology, Neurosurgery & Psychiatry*, vol. 87, no. 5, pp. 501–511, 2016.

[80] S. P. Caminiti, N. Canessa, C. Cerami et al., "Affective mentalizing and brain activity at rest in the behavioral variant of frontotemporal dementia," *Neuroimage: Clinical*, vol. 9, pp. 484–497, 2015.

[81] J. Moll, R. Zahn, R. de Oliveira-Souza et al., "Impairment of prosocial sentiments is associated with frontopolar and septal damage in frontotemporal dementia," *NeuroImage*, vol. 54, no. 2, pp. 1735–1742, 2011.

[82] C. O'Callaghan, M. Bertoux, M. Irish et al., "Fair play: social norm compliance failures in behavioural variant frontotemporal dementia," *Brain*, vol. 139, no. 1, pp. 204–216, 2016.

[83] M. Melloni, P. Billeke, S. Baez et al., "Your perspective and my benefit: multiple lesion models of self-other integration strategies during social bargaining," *Brain*, vol. 139, no. 11, pp. 3022–3040, 2016.

[84] M. L. Schroeter, S. Pawelke, S. Bisenius et al., "A modified Reading the Mind in the Eyes Test predicts behavioral variant frontotemporal dementia better than executive function tests," *Frontiers in Aging Neuroscience*, vol. 10, p. 11, 2018.

[85] C. Gregory, S. Lough, V. Stone et al., "Theory of mind in patients with frontal variant frontotemporal dementia and

Alzheimer's disease: theoretical and practical implications," *Brain*, vol. 125, no. 4, pp. 752–764, 2002.

[86] T. Torralva, C. M. Kipps, J. R. Hodges et al., "The relationship between affective decision-making and theory of mind in the frontal variant of fronto-temporal dementia," *Neuropsychologia*, vol. 45, no. 2, pp. 342–349, 2007.

[87] T. Torralva, M. Roca, E. Gleichgerrcht, T. Bekinschtein, and F. Manes, "A neuropsychological battery to detect specific executive and social cognitive impairments in early frontotemporal dementia," *Brain*, vol. 132, no. 5, pp. 1299–1309, 2009.

[88] E. Gleichgerrcht, T. Torralva, M. Roca, and F. Manes, "Utility of an abbreviated version of the executive and social cognition battery in the detection of executive deficits in early behavioral variant frontotemporal dementia patients," *Journal of the International Neuropsychological Society*, vol. 16, no. 4, pp. 687–694, 2010.

[89] C. Buhl, J. Stokholm, and A. Gade, "Clinical utility of short social cognitive tests in early differentiation of behavioral variant frontotemporal dementia from Alzheimer's disease," *Dementia and Geriatric Cognitive Disorders Extra*, vol. 3, no. 1, pp. 376–385, 2013.

[90] J. D. Henry, L. H. Phillips, and C. von Hippel, "A meta-analytic review of theory of mind difficulties in behavioural-variant frontotemporal dementia," *Neuropsychologia*, vol. 56, pp. 53–62, 2014.

[91] J. Cotter, K. Granger, R. Backx, M. Hobbs, C. Y. Looi, and J. H. Barnett, "Social cognitive dysfunction as a clinical marker: a systematic review of meta-analyses across 30 clinical conditions," *Neuroscience & Biobehavioral Reviews*, vol. 84, pp. 92–99, 2018.

[92] R. S. Marin, R. C. Biedrzycki, and S. Firinciogullari, "Reliability and validity of the apathy evaluation scale," *Psychiatry Research*, vol. 38, no. 2, pp. 143–162, 1991.

[93] H. Santamaria-Garcia, P. Reyes, A. Garcia et al., "First symptoms and neurocognitive correlates of behavioral variant frontotemporal dementia," *Journal of Alzheimer's Disease*, vol. 54, no. 3, pp. 957–970, 2016.

[94] G. Zamboni, E. D. Huey, F. Krueger, P. F. Nichelli, and J. Grafman, "Apathy and disinhibition in frontotemporal dementia: insights into their neural correlates," *Neurology*, vol. 71, no. 10, pp. 736–742, 2008.

[95] P. J. Eslinger, P. Moore, S. Antani, C. Anderson, and M. Grossman, "Apathy in frontotemporal dementia: behavioral and neuroimaging correlates," *Behavioural Neurology*, vol. 25, no. 2, 136 pages, 2012.

[96] M. Hornberger, J. Geng, and J. R. Hodges, "Convergent grey and white matter evidence of orbitofrontal cortex changes related to disinhibition in behavioural variant frontotemporal dementia," *Brain*, vol. 134, no. 9, pp. 2502–2512, 2011.

[97] S. Baez, P. Kanske, D. Matallana et al., "Integration of intention and outcome for moral judgment in frontotemporal dementia: brain structural signatures," *Neurodegenerative Diseases*, vol. 16, no. 3–4, pp. 206–217, 2016.

[98] S. Baez, B. Couto, T. Torralva et al., "Comparing moral judgments of patients with frontotemporal dementia and frontal stroke," *Journal of the American Medical Association Neurology*, vol. 71, no. 9, pp. 1172–1176, 2014.

[99] S. Baez, E. Herrera, A. M. Garcia, F. Manes, L. Young, and A. Ibáñez, "Outcome-oriented moral evaluation in terrorists," *Nature Human Behaviour*, vol. 1, no. 6, article 0118, pp. 1–8, 2017.

[100] R. de Oliveira-Souza, R. D. Hare, I. E. Bramati et al., "Psychopathy as a disorder of the moral brain: fronto-temporo-limbic grey matter reductions demonstrated by voxel-based morphometry," *NeuroImage*, vol. 40, no. 3, pp. 1202–1213, 2008.

[101] M. Liljegren, G. Naasan, J. Temlett et al., "Criminal behavior in frontotemporal dementia and Alzheimer disease," *Journal of the American Medical Association Neurology*, vol. 72, no. 3, pp. 295–300, 2015.

[102] M. F. Mendez, "The unique predisposition to criminal violations in frontotemporal dementia," *The Journal of the American Academy of Psychiatry and the Law*, vol. 38, no. 3, pp. 318–323, 2010.

[103] H. Santamaria-Garcia, S. Baez, P. Reyes et al., "A lesion model of envy and Schadenfreude: legal, deservingness and moral dimensions as revealed by neurodegeneration," *Brain*, vol. 140, no. 12, pp. 3357–3377, 2017.

[104] F. Kumfor, L. Miller, S. Lah et al., "Are you really angry? The effect of intensity on facial emotion recognition in frontotemporal dementia," *Social Neuroscience*, vol. 6, no. 5–6, pp. 502–514, 2011.

[105] C. M. Kipps, P. J. Nestor, J. Acosta-Cabronero, R. Arnold, and J. R. Hodges, "Understanding social dysfunction in the behavioural variant of frontotemporal dementia. The role of emotion and sarcasm processing," *Brain*, vol. 132, no. 3, pp. 592–603, 2009.

[106] F. Kumfor and O. Piguet, "Disturbance of emotion processing in frontotemporal dementia: a synthesis of cognitive and neuroimaging findings," *Neuropsychology Review*, vol. 22, no. 3, pp. 280–297, 2012.

[107] J. S. Snowden, N. A. Austin, S. Sembi, J. C. Thompson, D. Craufurd, and D. Neary, "Emotion recognition in Huntington's disease and frontotemporal dementia," *Neuropsychologia*, vol. 46, no. 11, pp. 2638–2649, 2008.

[108] J. Van den Stock, F. L. De Winter, B. de Gelder et al., "Impaired recognition of body expressions in the behavioral variant of frontotemporal dementia," *Neuropsychologia*, vol. 75, pp. 496–504, 2015.

[109] R. Omar, S. M. D. Henley, J. W. Bartlett et al., "The structural neuroanatomy of music emotion recognition: evidence from frontotemporal lobar degeneration," *NeuroImage*, vol. 56, no. 3, pp. 1814–1821, 2011.

[110] M. S. Goodkind, V. E. Sturm, E. A. Ascher et al., "Emotion recognition in frontotemporal dementia and Alzheimer's disease: a new film-based assessment," *Emotion*, vol. 15, no. 4, pp. 416–427, 2015.

[111] J. A. Eckart, V. E. Sturm, B. L. Miller, and R. W. Levenson, "Diminished disgust reactivity in behavioral variant frontotemporal dementia," *Neuropsychologia*, vol. 50, no. 5, pp. 786–790, 2012.

[112] B. Couto, F. Manes, P. Montañés et al., "Structural neuroimaging of social cognition in progressive non-fluent aphasia and behavioral variant of frontotemporal dementia," *Frontiers in Human Neuroscience*, vol. 7, p. 467, 2013.

[113] C. Duval, A. Bejanin, P. Piolino et al., "Theory of mind impairments in patients with semantic dementia," *Brain*, vol. 135, no. 1, pp. 228–241, 2012.

[114] H. J. Rosen, R. J. Perry, J. Murphy et al., "Emotion comprehension in the temporal variant of frontotemporal dementia," *Brain*, vol. 125, no. 10, pp. 2286–2295, 2002.

[115] G. S. Day, N. A. Farb, D. F. Tang-Wai et al., "Salience network resting-state activity: prediction of frontotemporal dementia progression," *Journal of the American Medical Association Neurology*, vol. 70, no. 10, pp. 1249–1253, 2013.

[116] W. W. Seeley, "Anterior insula degeneration in frontotemporal dementia," *Brain Structure and Function*, vol. 214, no. 5–6, pp. 465–475, 2010.

[117] F. Kumfor, M. Irish, J. R. Hodges, and O. Piguet, "Discrete neural correlates for the recognition of negative emotions: insights from frontotemporal dementia," *PLoS One*, vol. 8, no. 6, article e67457, 2013.

[118] S. Baez, C. Pinasco, M. Roca et al., "Brain structural correlates of executive and social cognition profiles in behavioral variant frontotemporal dementia and elderly bipolar disorder," *Neuropsychologia*, 2017.

[119] I. Garcia-Cordero, L. Sedeño, L. de la Fuente et al., "Feeling, learning from and being aware of inner states: interoceptive dimensions in neurodegeneration and stroke," *Philosophical Transactions of the Royal Society B: Biological Sciences*, vol. 371, no. 1708, article 20160006, 2016.

[120] R. Rytty, J. Nikkinen, L. Paavola et al., "GroupICA dual regression analysis of resting state networks in a behavioral variant of frontotemporal dementia," *Frontiers in Human Neuroscience*, vol. 7, p. 461, 2013.

[121] N. A. S. Farb, C. L. Grady, S. Strother et al., "Abnormal network connectivity in frontotemporal dementia: evidence for prefrontal isolation," *Cortex*, vol. 49, no. 7, pp. 1856–1873, 2013.

[122] S. Baez, A. M. Garcia, and A. Ibáñez, "The social context network model in psychiatric and neurological diseases," *Current Topics in Behavioral Neurosciences*, vol. 30, pp. 379–396, 2017.

[123] L. Sedeño, B. Couto, I. García-Cordero et al., "Brain network organization and social executive performance in frontotemporal dementia," *Journal of the International Neuropsychological Society*, vol. 22, no. 2, pp. 250–262, 2016.

[124] W. W. Seeley, R. Crawford, K. Rascovsky et al., "Frontal paralimbic network atrophy in very mild behavioral variant frontotemporal dementia," *Archives of Neurology*, vol. 65, no. 2, pp. 249–255, 2008.

[125] J. L. Whitwell, E. L. Sampson, H. C. Watt, R. J. Harvey, M. N. Rossor, and N. C. Fox, "A volumetric magnetic resonance imaging study of the amygdala in frontotemporal lobar degeneration and Alzheimer's disease," *Dementia and Geriatric Cognitive Disorders*, vol. 20, no. 4, pp. 238–244, 2005.

[126] S. Tsermentseli, P. N. Leigh, and L. H. Goldstein, "The anatomy of cognitive impairment in amyotrophic lateral sclerosis: more than frontal lobe dysfunction," *Cortex*, vol. 48, no. 2, pp. 166–182, 2012.

[127] A. Montuschi, B. Iazzolino, A. Calvo et al., "Cognitive correlates in amyotrophic lateral sclerosis: a population-based study in Italy," *Journal of Neurology, Neurosurgery & Psychiatry*, vol. 86, no. 2, pp. 168–173, 2015.

[128] E. Beeldman, J. Raaphorst, M. Klein Twennaar, M. de Visser, B. A. Schmand, and R. J. de Haan, "The cognitive profile of ALS: a systematic review and meta-analysis update," *Journal of Neurology, Neurosurgery & Psychiatry*, vol. 87, no. 6, pp. 611–619, 2016.

[129] A. B. Grossman, S. Woolley-Levine, W. G. Bradley, and R. G. Miller, "Detecting neurobehavioral changes in amyotrophic lateral sclerosis," *Amyotrophic Lateral Sclerosis*, vol. 8, no. 1, pp. 56–61, 2007.

[130] M. Witgert, A. R. Salamone, A. M. Strutt et al., "Frontal-lobe mediated behavioral dysfunction in amyotrophic lateral sclerosis," *European Journal of Neurology*, vol. 17, no. 1, pp. 103–110, 2010.

[131] J. R. Burrell, G. M. Halliday, J. J. Kril et al., "The frontotemporal dementia motor neuron disease continuum," *The Lancet*, vol. 388, no. 10047, pp. 919–931, 2016.

[132] J. Keller, S. Bohm, H. E. A. Aho-Ozhan et al., "Functional reorganization during cognitive function tasks in patients with amyotrophic lateral sclerosis," *Brain Imaging and Behavior*, 2017.

[133] S. Abrahams, J. Newton, E. Niven, J. Foley, and T. H. Bak, "Screening for cognition and behaviour changes in ALS," *Amyotrophic Lateral Sclerosis and Frontotemporal Degeneration*, vol. 15, no. 1–2, pp. 9–14, 2014.

[134] S. Körner, K. Kollewe, S. Abdulla, A. Zapf, R. Dengler, and S. Petri, "Interaction of physical function, quality of life and depression in amyotrophic lateral sclerosis: characterization of a large patient cohort," *BMC Neurology*, vol. 15, no. 1, p. 84, 2015.

[135] D. Lulé, B. Ehlich, D. Lang et al., "Quality of life in fatal disease: the flawed judgement of the social environment," *Journal of Neurology*, vol. 260, no. 11, pp. 2836–2843, 2013.

[136] F. Trojsi, M. Siciliano, A. Russo et al., "Theory of mind and its neuropsychological and quality of life correlates in the early stages of amyotrophic lateral sclerosis," *Frontiers in Psychology*, vol. 7, p. 1934, 2016.

[137] L. Carluer, A. Mondou, M. S. Buhour et al., "Neural substrate of cognitive theory of mind impairment in amyotrophic lateral sclerosis," *Cortex*, vol. 65, pp. 19–30, 2015.

[138] M. Cavallo, M. Adenzato, S. E. Macpherson, G. Karwig, I. Enrici, and S. Abrahams, "Evidence of social understanding impairment in patients with amyotrophic lateral sclerosis," *PLoS One*, vol. 6, no. 10, article e25948, 2011.

[139] C. Cerami, A. Dodich, N. Canessa et al., "Emotional empathy in amyotrophic lateral sclerosis: a behavioural and voxel-based morphometry study," *Amyotrophic Lateral Sclerosis and Frontotemporal Degeneration*, vol. 15, no. 1–2, pp. 21–29, 2014.

[140] M. Consonni, E. Catricala, E. Dalla Bella, V. C. Gessa, G. Lauria, and S. F. Cappa, "Beyond the consensus criteria: multiple cognitive profiles in amyotrophic lateral sclerosis?," *Cortex*, vol. 81, pp. 162–167, 2016.

[141] A. Girardi, S. E. Macpherson, and S. Abrahams, "Deficits in emotional and social cognition in amyotrophic lateral sclerosis," *Neuropsychology*, vol. 25, no. 1, pp. 53–65, 2011.

[142] M. Staios, F. Fisher, A. K. Lindell, B. Ong, J. Howe, and K. Reardon, "Exploring sarcasm detection in amyotrophic lateral sclerosis using ecologically valid measures," *Frontiers in Human Neuroscience*, vol. 7, p. 178, 2013.

[143] T. J. Watermeyer, R. G. Brown, K. C. L. Sidle et al., "Executive dysfunction predicts social cognition impairment in amyotrophic lateral sclerosis," *Journal of Neurology*, vol. 262, no. 7, pp. 1681–1690, 2015.

[144] H. E. A. Aho-Özhan, J. Keller, J. Heimrath et al., "Perception of emotional facial expressions in amyotrophic lateral sclerosis (ALS) at behavioural and brain metabolic level," *PLoS One*, vol. 11, no. 10, article e0164655, 2016.

[145] A. Sedda, "Disorders of emotional processing in amyotrophic lateral sclerosis," *Current Opinion in Neurology*, vol. 27, no. 6, pp. 659–665, 2014.

[146] S. A. Savage, P. Lillo, F. Kumfor, M. C. Kiernan, O. Piguet, and J. R. Hodges, "Emotion processing deficits distinguish pure amyotrophic lateral sclerosis from frontotemporal dementia," *Amyotrophic Lateral Sclerosis and Frontotemporal Degeneration*, vol. 15, no. 1–2, pp. 39–46, 2014.

[147] A. Palmieri, M. Naccarato, S. Abrahams et al., "Right hemisphere dysfunction and emotional processing in ALS: an fMRI study," *Journal of Neurology*, vol. 257, no. 12, pp. 1970–1978, 2010.

[148] C. Crespi, C. Cerami, A. Dodich et al., "Microstructural white matter correlates of emotion recognition impairment in amyotrophic lateral sclerosis," *Cortex*, vol. 53, pp. 1–8, 2014.

[149] E. Bora, M. Walterfang, and D. Velakoulis, "Theory of mind in behavioural-variant frontotemporal dementia and Alzheimer's disease: a meta-analysis," *Journal of Neurology, Neurosurgery & Psychiatry*, vol. 86, no. 7, pp. 714–719, 2015.

[150] E. Bora, D. Velakoulis, and M. Walterfang, "Meta-analysis of facial emotion recognition in behavioral variant frontotemporal dementia: comparison with Alzheimer disease and healthy controls," *Journal of Geriatric Psychiatry and Neurology*, vol. 29, no. 4, pp. 205–211, 2016.

[151] E. K. Zimmerman, P. J. Eslinger, Z. Simmons, and A. M. Barrett, "Emotional perception deficits in amyotrophic lateral sclerosis," *Cognitive and Behavioral Neurology*, vol. 20, no. 2, pp. 79–82, 2007.

[152] B. Papps, S. Abrahams, P. Wicks, P. N. Leigh, and L. H. Goldstein, "Changes in memory for emotional material in amyotrophic lateral sclerosis (ALS)," *Neuropsychologia*, vol. 43, no. 8, pp. 1107–1114, 2005.

[153] H. Schmolck, D. Mosnik, and P. Schulz, "Rating the approachability of faces in ALS," *Neurology*, vol. 69, no. 24, pp. 2232–2235, 2007.

[154] Z. C. Gibbons, J. S. Snowden, J. C. Thompson, F. Happé, A. Richardson, and D. Neary, "Inferring thought and action in motor neurone disease," *Neuropsychologia*, vol. 45, no. 6, pp. 1196–1207, 2007.

[155] S. L. Meier, A. J. Charleston, and L. J. Tippett, "Cognitive and behavioural deficits associated with the orbitomedial prefrontal cortex in amyotrophic lateral sclerosis," *Brain*, vol. 133, no. 11, pp. 3444–3457, 2010.

[156] T. Burke, M. Elamin, P. Bede et al., "Discordant performance on the "Reading the Mind in the Eyes" test based on disease onset in amyotrophic lateral sclerosis," *Amyotrophic Lateral Sclerosis and Frontotemporal Degeneration*, vol. 17, no. 7–8, pp. 467–472, 2016.

[157] E. J. van der Hulst, T. H. Bak, and S. Abrahams, "Impaired affective and cognitive theory of mind and behavioural change in amyotrophic lateral sclerosis," *Journal of Neurology, Neurosurgery & psychiatry*, vol. 86, no. 11, pp. 1208–1215, 2015.

[158] H. L. Gallagher and C. D. Frith, "Functional imaging of "theory of mind"," *Trends in Cognitive Sciences*, vol. 7, no. 2, pp. 77–83, 2003.

[159] A. Abu-Akel and S. Shamay-Tsoory, "Neuroanatomical and neurochemical bases of theory of mind," *Neuropsychologia*, vol. 49, no. 11, pp. 2971–2984, 2011.

[160] F. Filimon, J. D. Nelson, D. J. Hagler, and M. I. Sereno, "Human cortical representations for reaching: mirror neurons for execution, observation, and imagery," *NeuroImage*, vol. 37, no. 4, pp. 1315–1328, 2007.

[161] E. C. Wolters, "Non-motor extranigral signs and symptoms in Parkinson's disease," *Parkinsonism & Related Disorders*, vol. 15, Supplement 3, pp. S6–12, 2009.

[162] F. E. Pontieri, F. Assogna, A. Stefani et al., "Sad and happy facial emotion recognition impairment in progressive supranuclear palsy in comparison with Parkinson's disease," *Parkinsonism & Related Disorders*, vol. 18, no. 7, pp. 871–875, 2012.

[163] F. Kumfor, L. A. Sapey-Triomphe, C. E. Leyton, J. R. Burrell, J. R. Hodges, and O. Piguet, "Degradation of emotion processing ability in corticobasal syndrome and Alzheimer's disease," *Brain*, vol. 137, no. 11, pp. 3061–3072, 2014.

[164] W. W. Beatty, D. E. Goodkin, W. S. Weir, R. D. Staton, N. Monson, and P. A. Beatty, "Affective judgments by patients with Parkinson's disease or chronic progressive multiple sclerosis," *Bulletin of the Psychonomic Society*, vol. 27, no. 4, pp. 361–364, 1989.

[165] A. Ariatti, F. Benuzzi, and P. Nichelli, "Recognition of emotions from visual and prosodic cues in Parkinson's disease," *Neurological Sciences*, vol. 29, no. 4, pp. 219–227, 2008.

[166] L. X. Blonder, R. E. Gur, and R. C. Gur, "The effects of right and left hemiparkinsonism on prosody," *Brain and Language*, vol. 36, no. 2, pp. 193–207, 1989.

[167] M. De Risi, G. Di Gennaro, A. Picardi et al., "Facial emotion decoding in patients with Parkinson's disease," *The International Journal of Neuroscience*, vol. 128, no. 1, pp. 71–78, 2017.

[168] E. Herrera, F. Cuetos, and J. Rodríguez-Ferreiro, "Emotion recognition impairment in Parkinson's disease patients without dementia," *Journal of the Neurological Sciences*, vol. 310, no. 1–2, pp. 237–240, 2011.

[169] C. Xi, Y. Zhu, Y. Mu et al., "Theory of mind and decision-making processes are impaired in Parkinson's disease," *Behavioural Brain Research*, vol. 279, pp. 226–233, 2015.

[170] R. Adolphs, R. Schul, and D. Tranel, "Intact recognition of facial emotion in Parkinson's disease," *Neuropsychology*, vol. 12, no. 2, pp. 253–258, 1998.

[171] J. F. Caekebeke, A. Jennekens-Schinkel, M. E. Van der Linden, O. J. Buruma, and R. A. Roos, "The interpretation of dysprosody in patients with Parkinson's disease," *Journal of Neurology, Neurosurgery & Psychiatry*, vol. 54, no. 2, pp. 145–148, 1991.

[172] P. Madeley, A. W. Ellis, and R. H. S. Mindham, "Facial expressions and Parkinson's disease," *Behavioural Neurology*, vol. 8, no. 2, 119 pages, 1995.

[173] M. D. Pell and C. L. Leonard, "Facial expression decoding in early Parkinson's disease," *Cognitive Brain Research*, vol. 23, no. 2–3, pp. 327–340, 2005.

[174] R. Ille, A. Wabnegger, P. Schwingenschuh et al., "Intact emotion recognition and experience but dysfunctional emotion regulation in idiopathic Parkinson's disease," *Journal of the Neurological Sciences*, vol. 361, pp. 72–78, 2016.

[175] H. M. Gray and L. Tickle-Degnen, "A meta-analysis of performance on emotion recognition tasks in Parkinson's disease," *Neuropsychology*, vol. 24, no. 2, pp. 176–191, 2010.

[176] A. Sedda, S. Petito, M. Guarino, and A. Stracciari, "Identification and intensity of disgust: distinguishing visual, linguistic and facial expressions processing in Parkinson disease," *Behavioural Brain Research*, vol. 330, pp. 30–36, 2017.

[177] C. Y. Lin, Y. M. Tien, J. T. Huang, C. H. Tsai, and L. C. Hsu, "Degraded impairment of emotion recognition in Parkinson's disease extends from negative to positive emotions," *Behavioural Neurology*, vol. 2016, Article ID 9287092, 8 pages, 2016.

[178] G. Hipp, N. J. Diederich, V. Pieria, and M. Vaillant, "Primary vision and facial emotion recognition in early Parkinson's disease," *Journal of the Neurological Sciences*, vol. 338, no. 1–2, pp. 178–182, 2014.

[179] A. Saenz, A. Doé de Maindreville, A. Henry, S. de Labbey, S. Bakchine, and N. Ehrlé, "Recognition of facial and musical emotions in Parkinson's disease," *European Journal of Neurology*, vol. 20, no. 3, pp. 571–577, 2013.

[180] I. Enrici, M. Adenzato, R. B. Ardito et al., "Emotion processing in Parkinson's disease: a three-level study on recognition, representation, and regulation," *PLoS One*, vol. 10, no. 6, article e0131470, 2015.

[181] J. Pietschnig, L. Schröder, I. Ratheiser et al., "Facial emotion recognition and its relationship to cognition and depressive symptoms in patients with Parkinson's disease," *International Psychogeriatrics*, vol. 28, no. 7, pp. 1165–1179, 2016.

[182] I. Biseul, P. Sauleau, C. Haegelen et al., "Fear recognition is impaired by subthalamic nucleus stimulation in Parkinson's disease," *Neuropsychologia*, vol. 43, no. 7, pp. 1054–1059, 2005.

[183] D. Drapier, J. Péron, E. Leray et al., "Emotion recognition impairment and apathy after subthalamic nucleus stimulation in Parkinson's disease have separate neural substrates," *Neuropsychologia*, vol. 46, no. 11, pp. 2796–2801, 2008.

[184] J. Péron, I. Biseul, E. Leray et al., "Subthalamic nucleus stimulation affects fear and sadness recognition in Parkinson's disease," *Neuropsychology*, vol. 24, no. 1, pp. 1–8, 2010.

[185] F. Le Jeune, J. Péron, I. Biseul et al., "Subthalamic nucleus stimulation affects orbitofrontal cortex in facial emotion recognition: a PET study," *Brain*, vol. 131, no. 6, pp. 1599–1608, 2008.

[186] R. Adolphs, "Recognizing emotion from facial expressions: psychological and neurological mechanisms," *Behavioral and Cognitive Neuroscience Reviews*, vol. 1, no. 1, pp. 21–62, 2002.

[187] L. Albuquerque, M. Coelho, M. Martins et al., "STN-DBS does not change emotion recognition in advanced Parkinson's disease," *Parkinsonism & Related Disorders*, vol. 20, no. 2, pp. 166–169, 2014.

[188] B. C. P. Ghosh, A. J. Calder, P. V. Peers et al., "Social cognitive deficits and their neural correlates in progressive supranuclear palsy," *Brain*, vol. 135, no. 7, pp. 2089–2102, 2012.

[189] B. C. P. Ghosh, J. B. Rowe, A. J. Calder, J. R. Hodges, and T. H. Bak, "Emotion recognition in progressive supranuclear palsy," *Journal of Neurology, Neurosurgery & Psychiatry*, vol. 80, no. 10, pp. 1143–1145, 2009.

[190] A. Schrag, C. Selai, J. Davis, A. J. Lees, M. Jahanshahi, and N. Quinn, "Health-related quality of life in patients with progressive supranuclear palsy," *Movement Disorders*, vol. 18, no. 12, pp. 1464–1469, 2003.

[191] T. Shany-Ur, P. Poorzand, S. N. Grossman et al., "Comprehension of insincere communication in neurodegenerative disease: lies, sarcasm, and theory of mind," *Cortex*, vol. 48, no. 10, pp. 1329–1341, 2012.

[192] E. Winner, H. Brownell, F. Happe, A. Blum, and D. Pincus, "Distinguishing lies from jokes: theory of mind deficits and discourse interpretation in right hemisphere brain-damaged patients," *Brain and Language*, vol. 62, no. 1, pp. 89–106, 1998.

[193] B. M. Kluger and K. M. Heilman, "Dysfunctional facial emotional expression and comprehension in a patient with corticobasal degeneration," *Neurocase*, vol. 13, no. 3, pp. 165–168, 2007.

[194] A. Kertesz and P. McMonagle, "Behavior and cognition in corticobasal degeneration and progressive supranuclear palsy," *Journal of the Neurological Sciences*, vol. 289, no. 1–2, pp. 138–143, 2010.

[195] M. Poletti, A. Vergallo, M. Ulivi, A. Sonnoli, and U. Bonuccelli, "Affective theory of mind in patients with Parkinson's disease," *Psychiatry and Clinical Neurosciences*, vol. 67, no. 4, pp. 273–276, 2013.

[196] M. Roca, T. Torralva, E. Gleichgerrcht et al., "Impairments in social cognition in early medicated and unmedicated Parkinson disease," *Cognitive and Behavioral Neurology*, vol. 23, no. 3, pp. 152–158, 2010.

[197] G. Santangelo, C. Vitale, D. Errico, D. Grossi, L. Trojano, and P. Barone, "Affective theory of mind in patients with Parkinson's disease: comment," *Psychiatry and Clinical Neurosciences*, vol. 68, no. 3, p. 242, 2014.

[198] G. Santangelo, C. Vitale, L. Trojano et al., "Neuropsychological correlates of theory of mind in patients with early Parkinson's disease," *Movement Disorders*, vol. 27, no. 1, pp. 98–105, 2012.

[199] J. Péron, S. Vicente, E. Leray et al., "Are dopaminergic pathways involved in theory of mind? A study in Parkinson's disease," *Neuropsychologia*, vol. 47, no. 2, pp. 406–414, 2009.

[200] R. L. Yu, R. M. Wu, M. J. Chiu, C. H. Tai, C. H. Lin, and M. S. Hua, "Advanced Theory of Mind in patients at early stage of Parkinson's disease," *Parkinsonism & Related Disorders*, vol. 18, no. 1, pp. 21–24, 2012.

[201] M. E. Bodden, B. Mollenhauer, C. Trenkwalder et al., "Affective and cognitive Theory of Mind in patients with Parkinson's disease," *Parkinsonism & Related Disorders*, vol. 16, no. 7, pp. 466–470, 2010.

[202] E. Bora, M. Walterfang, and D. Velakoulis, "Theory of mind in Parkinson's disease: a meta-analysis," *Behavioural Brain Research*, vol. 292, no. 1, pp. 515–520, 2015.

[203] L. Nobis, K. Schindlbeck, F. Ehlen et al., "Theory of mind performance in Parkinson's disease is associated with motor and cognitive functions, but not with symptom lateralization," *Journal of Neural Transmission*, vol. 124, no. 9, pp. 1067–1072, 2017.

[204] A. Costa, A. Peppe, M. Martini et al., "Parkinsonian patients with deficits in the dysexecutive spectrum are impaired on theory of mind tasks," *Behavioural Neurology*, vol. 27, no. 4, 533 pages, 2013.

[205] A. McKinlay, M. Albicini, and P. S. Kavanagh, "The effect of cognitive status and visuospatial performance on affective theory of mind in Parkinson's disease," *Neuropsychiatric Disease and Treatment*, vol. 9, pp. 1071–1076, 2013.

[206] N. Ibarretxe-Bilbao, C. Junque, E. Tolosa et al., "Neuroanatomical correlates of impaired decision-making and facial emotion recognition in early Parkinson's disease," *European Journal of Neuroscience*, vol. 30, no. 6, pp. 1162–1171, 2009.

[207] H. C. Baggio, B. Segura, N. Ibarretxe-Bilbao et al., "Structural correlates of facial emotion recognition deficits in

Parkinson's disease patients," *Neuropsychologia*, vol. 50, no. 8, pp. 2121–2128, 2012.

[208] G. Robert, F. Le Jeune, T. Dondaine et al., "Apathy and impaired emotional facial recognition networks overlap in Parkinson's disease: a PET study with conjunction analyses," *Journal of Neurology, Neurosurgery & Psychiatry*, vol. 85, no. 10, pp. 1153–1158, 2014.

[209] A. Wabnegger, R. Ille, P. Schwingenschuh et al., "Facial emotion recognition in Parkinson's disease: an fMRI investigation," *PLoS One*, vol. 10, no. 8, article e0136110, 2015.

[210] J. Grafman, I. Litvan, C. Gomez, and T. N. Chase, "Frontal lobe function in progressive supranuclear palsy," *Archives of Neurology*, vol. 47, no. 5, pp. 553–558, 1990.

[211] L. D. Kaat, A. J. W. Boon, W. Kamphorst, R. Ravid, H. J. Duivenvoorden, and J. C. van Swieten, "Frontal presentation in progressive supranuclear palsy," *Neurology*, vol. 69, no. 8, pp. 723–729, 2007.

[212] J. Péron, F. Le Jeune, C. Haegelen et al., "Subthalamic nucleus stimulation affects theory of mind network: a PET study in Parkinson's disease," *PLoS One*, vol. 5, no. 3, article e9919, 2010.

[213] M. Díez-Cirarda, N. Ojeda, J. Peña et al., "Neuroanatomical correlates of Theory of Mind deficit in Parkinson's disease: a multimodal imaging study," *PLoS One*, vol. 10, no. 11, article e0142234, 2015.

[214] M. Poletti and U. Bonuccelli, "Impairment of affective theory of mind in corticobasal degeneration," *The Journal of Neuropsychiatry and Clinical Neurosciences*, vol. 24, no. 1, p. E7, 2012.

[215] G. B. Frisoni, N. C. Fox, C. R. Jack, P. Scheltens, and P. M. Thompson, "The clinical use of structural MRI in Alzheimer disease," *Nature Reviews Neurology*, vol. 6, no. 2, pp. 67–77, 2010.

[216] F. Kumfor, M. Irish, C. Leyton et al., "Tracking the progression of social cognition in neurodegenerative disorders," *Journal of Neurology, Neurosurgery & Psychiatry*, vol. 85, no. 10, pp. 1076–1083, 2014.

[217] A. Dodich, C. Cerami, C. Crespi et al., "Differential impairment of cognitive and affective mentalizing abilities in neurodegenerative dementias: evidence from behavioral variant of frontotemporal dementia, Alzheimer's disease, and mild cognitive impairment," *Journal of Alzheimer's Disease*, vol. 50, no. 4, pp. 1011–1022, 2016.

[218] M. Lindau, O. Almkvist, J. Kushi et al., "First symptoms—frontotemporal dementia versus Alzheimer's disease," *Dementia and Geriatric Cognitive Disorders*, vol. 11, no. 5, pp. 286–293, 2000.

[219] J. L. Cummings, M. Mega, K. Gray, S. Rosenberg-Thompson, D. A. Carusi, and J. Gornbein, "The Neuropsychiatric Inventory: comprehensive assessment of psychopathology in dementia," *Neurology*, vol. 44, no. 12, pp. 2308–2314, 1994.

[220] J. C. Morris, "The Clinical Dementia Rating (CDR): current version and scoring rules," *Neurology*, vol. 43, no. 11, pp. 2412–2414, 1993.

[221] H. Kazui, K. Yoshiyama, H. Kanemoto et al., "Differences of behavioral and psychological symptoms of dementia in disease severity in four major dementias," *PLoS One*, vol. 11, no. 8, article e0161092, 2016.

[222] R. Ossenkoppele, Y. A. L. Pijnenburg, D. C. Perry et al., "The behavioural/dysexecutive variant of Alzheimer's disease: clinical, neuroimaging and pathological features," *Brain*, vol. 138, no. 9, pp. 2732–2749, 2015.

[223] N. L. Cadieux and K. W. Greve, "Emotion processing in Alzheimer's disease," *Journal of the International Neuropsychological Society*, vol. 3, no. 5, pp. 411–419, 1997.

[224] E. Teng, P. H. Lu, and J. L. Cummings, "Deficits in facial emotion processing in mild cognitive impairment," *Dementia and Geriatric Cognitive Disorders*, vol. 23, no. 4, pp. 271–279, 2007.

[225] M. S. Albert, C. Cohen, and E. Koff, "Perception of affect in patients with dementia of the Alzheimer type," *Archives of Neurology*, vol. 48, no. 8, pp. 791–795, 1991.

[226] J. Allender and A. W. Kaszniak, "Processing of emotional cues in patients with dementia of the Alzheimer's type," *The International Journal of Neuroscience*, vol. 46, no. 3-4, pp. 147–155, 1989.

[227] A. Shimokawa, N. Yatomi, S. Anamizu, S. Torii, H. Isono, and Y. Sugai, "Recognition of facial expressions and emotional situations in patients with dementia of the Alzheimer and vascular types," *Dementia and Geriatric Cognitive Disorders*, vol. 15, no. 3, pp. 163–168, 2003.

[228] H. Burnham and E. Hogervorst, "Recognition of facial expressions of emotion by patients with dementia of the Alzheimer type," *Dementia and Geriatric Cognitive Disorders*, vol. 18, no. 1, pp. 75–79, 2004.

[229] I. Lavenu, F. Pasquier, F. Lebert, H. Petit, and M. v. der Linden, "Perception of emotion in frontotemporal dementia and Alzheimer disease," *Alzheimer Disease & Associated Disorders*, vol. 13, no. 2, pp. 96–101, 1999.

[230] I. Spoletini, C. Marra, F. D. Iulio et al., "Facial emotion recognition deficit in amnestic mild cognitive impairment and Alzheimer disease," *The American Journal of Geriatric Psychiatry*, vol. 16, no. 5, pp. 389–398, 2008.

[231] M. Freedman, M. A. Binns, S. E. Black, C. Murphy, and D. T. Stuss, "Theory of mind and recognition of facial emotion in dementia: challenge to current concepts," *Alzheimer Disease & Associated Disorders*, vol. 27, no. 1, pp. 56–61, 2013.

[232] N. Moreau, S. Rauzy, F. Viallet, and M. Champagne-Lavau, "Theory of mind in Alzheimer disease: evidence of authentic impairment during social interaction," *Neuropsychology*, vol. 30, no. 3, pp. 312–321, 2016.

[233] S. Ramanan, L. C. de Souza, N. Moreau et al., "Determinants of theory of mind performance in Alzheimer's disease: a data-mining study," *Cortex*, vol. 88, pp. 8–18, 2017.

[234] N. Dermody, S. Wong, R. Ahmed, O. Piguet, J. R. Hodges, and M. Irish, "Uncovering the neural bases of cognitive and affective empathy deficits in Alzheimer's disease and the behavioral-variant of frontotemporal dementia," *Journal of Alzheimer's Disease*, vol. 53, no. 3, pp. 801–816, 2016.

[235] T. Shany-Ur, N. Lin, H. J. Rosen, M. Sollberger, B. L. Miller, and K. P. Rankin, "Self-awareness in neurodegenerative disease relies on neural structures mediating reward-driven attention," *Brain*, vol. 137, no. 8, pp. 2368–2381, 2014.

[236] S. L. Valk, B. C. Bernhardt, F. M. Trautwein et al., "Structural plasticity of the social brain: differential change after socio-affective and cognitive mental training," *Science Advances*, vol. 3, no. 10, article e1700489, 2017.

[237] C. L. Kempnich, D. Wong, N. Georgiou-Karistianis, and J. C. Stout, "Feasibility and efficacy of brief computerized training to improve emotion recognition in premanifest and early-symptomatic Huntington's disease," *Journal of*

the International Neuropsychological Society, vol. 23, no. 4, pp. 314–321, 2017.

[238] S. Yao, B. Becker, W. Zhao et al., "Oxytocin modulates attention switching between interoceptive signals and external social cues," *Neuropsychopharmacology*, vol. 43, no. 2, pp. 294–301, 2017.

[239] M. Fukai, T. Hirosawa, M. Kikuchi et al., "Oxytocin effects on emotional response to others' faces via serotonin system in autism: a pilot study," *Psychiatry Research*, vol. 267, pp. 45–50, 2017.

[240] M. Timmermann, H. Jeung, R. Schmitt et al., "Oxytocin improves facial emotion recognition in young adults with antisocial personality disorder," *Psychoneuroendocrinology*, vol. 85, pp. 158–164, 2017.

[241] K. J. Parker, O. Oztan, R. A. Libove et al., "Intranasal oxytocin treatment for social deficits and biomarkers of response in children with autism," *Proceedings of the National Academy of Sciences of the United States of America*, vol. 114, no. 30, pp. 8119–8124, 2017.

[242] P. G. Enticott, H. A. Kennedy, A. Zangen, and P. B. Fitzgerald, "Deep repetitive transcranial magnetic stimulation associated with improved social functioning in a young woman with an autism spectrum disorder," *Journal of Electroconvulsive Therapy*, vol. 27, no. 1, pp. 41–43, 2011.

[243] M. T. Berlim, A. McGirr, M. M. Beaulieu, and G. Turecki, "Theory of mind in subjects with major depressive disorder: is it influenced by repetitive transcranial magnetic stimulation?," *World Journal of Biological Psychiatry*, vol. 13, no. 6, pp. 474–479, 2012.

12

Determination of Care Burden of Caregivers of Patients with Multiple Sclerosis in Turkey

Serpil Özmen[1] and Afife Yurttaş[2]

[1]*Narman Technical College, Atatürk University, Erzurum, Turkey*
[2]*Faculty of Nursing, Atatürk University, Erzurum, Turkey*

Correspondence should be addressed to Afife Yurttaş; afife-72@hotmail.com

Academic Editor: Luigi Trojano

The aim of this study was to determine the care burden of caregivers of patients with multiple sclerosis in Turkey. This descriptive study was conducted with 92 caregivers. To collect data, information form and Zarit Caregiver Burden Interview (ZCBI) were used. Most of the caregivers (65.2%) were females and 71.7% of them were married. The average age of caregivers was 38 and above. The mean ZCBI score of caregivers was 25.44 ± 9.50. The ZCBI score was significantly higher in caregivers providing care for more than six years (28.09 ± 10.16). Additionally, the ZCBI score was significantly higher in caregivers providing care 3-4 hours per day (32.23 ± 8.37) and providing physical care (29.28 ± 5.18).

1. Introduction

Multiple sclerosis (MS) is a chronic demyelinating disease of the central nervous system, which affects the brain, the spinal cord, and the optic nerves. MS does not directly affect the peripheral nerves [1]. Diagnostic criteria for MS have evolved over the past 50 years [2–5]. In the early 1900s, a few of MS have been reported, which is an admission to neurological clinics [6]. In 1996, the US National Multiple Sclerosis Society Advisory Committee on Clinical Trials in MS defined the clinical subtypes of MS. The committee standardized four subtypes of MS: relapsing-remitting, primary-progressive, secondary-progressive, and progressive-relapsing [7]. This disease affects 2.5 million people around the world and approximately 35,000 people in Turkey [8].

At the time of diagnosis, many patients with MS are in stable relationships, which are inevitably affected by the advancing disease. The caregivers have to cope with not only the presence of the disease but also the added fact of an unpredictable prognosis, including the possibility that their caregivers may become severely physically and cognitively impaired [9–11]. Also, there are a lot of reasons increasing burden of caregivers of patients with MS in our country. In Turkey, patients and caregivers cannot benefit adequately from the primary healthcare system due to a lack of trained personnel with expertise in MS. It gives care for patients with MS in hospitals and rehabilitation centers. However, caregivers cannot benefit from these centers due to various reasons. These reasons include the limited financial of patients and their families, difficulty of reaching hospitals in these provinces and a high patient population. Both patients with MS and their caregivers may experience financial difficulties due to having a chronic disease and living in the same home [10–12]. Therefore, emotional, physical, and financial support should be given to caregivers [13–15].

Besides these, due to the cultural structure of Turkish society, usually the family members are responsible for providing care to patients. On the other hand, although care was provided by the spouses of male patients with MS, unfortunately husbands of female patients do not take responsibility for the care of their wives. Moreover, male caregivers sometimes get divorced from their wives, fearing that they cannot have children and fulfill family responsibilities. This especially increases the burden of care of the female patients with MS and their families [16].

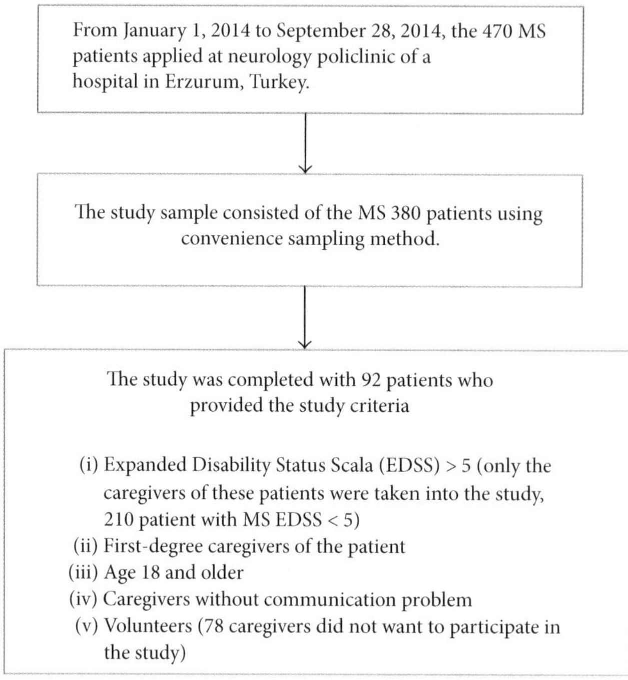

Figure 1: The flowchart of the study.

As professionals, nurses have an important role in the implementation of care in healthcare services. It is necessary for nurses to establish healthy or nurse-patient relationship on well-established bases so that nurses can give meaningful care to healthy individuals or their patients and their families in frequently changing health practices [17].

It is thought that the level of burnout will decrease and living standards will improve as a result of the social support provided to relatives of patients with MS. Nurses have very important responsibilities in order to develop a network of social support between relatives of patients. Informing caregivers of patients with MS about their care, training them to provide care, and teaching coping strategies may reduce the burnout of caregivers [16].

Many of the previous studies have focused on the care and quality life of patients with MS, but there are a limited number of studies investigating the care burden of caregivers of patients with MS in Turkey. Therefore, this study was conducted to determine the care burden of caregivers of patients with MS in Turkey. We think that this research will contribute to the literature.

2. Materials and Methods

2.1. Participants and Recruitment Procedure. This study was conducted at neurology policlinic of a hospital in Erzurum, Turkey, between January 1, 2014, and September 28, 2014. Between these dates, the 470 MS patients applied to the neurology policlinic. The study sample consisted of 380 patients using sampling method [18]. The caregivers were selected through convenience sampling. Inclusion criteria were as follows: Expanded Disability Status Scale (EDSS) > 5 (only the caregivers of these patients were taken into the study), first-degree caregivers of the patient, age of 18 and older, caregivers without communication problem, and volunteers. Eventually, the study was completed with 92 patients with MS. Figure 1 shows the flowchart of the study.

2.2. Ethical Consideration. Caregivers were informed about the purpose of this study upon inclusion in the database and consent was obtained after oral and written information.

The local ethical committee of the University of Atatürk, Erzurum, Turkey, approved the study (IRB; AU 2014.12.2/b). The study was conducted according to the Declaration of Helsinki.

2.3. Measurements

2.3.1. The Information Form. The information form was prepared by the researchers using the literature [19–29]. In the information, there were questions including age, gender, marital status, educational status, and problems experienced during care.

2.3.2. Zarit Caregiver Burden Interview (ZCBI). The ZCBI was developed by Zarit and colleagues in 1980. It consists of 22 items. In its 22-item version, the highest score is 88 and lowest score is 0. Higher scores indicate greater burden. The ZCBI measures subjective burden in terms of the degree to which the caregiver experiences physical, psychological, emotional, social, and financial problems as a result of their caregiving role. The Cronbach's alpha of ZCBI ranges from 0.85 to 0.94 [30].

The Turkish validity and reliability of the scale was performed by Ozer et al. in 2012 and the Cronbach's alpha value is in the range of 0.82 [31]. Our research Cronbach's alpha value is 0.85.

Many studies have been carried evaluating the care burden of caregivers of patients in the world and Turkey. The majority of these studies have used ZCBI [19–29].

2.4. Data Collection/Procedure. An information form and ZCBI were administered to the caregivers in a patient education class of neurology service. The instructions were made using face-to-face interviews by researchers. The caregivers were asked to mark the most suitable statement for each item of the scale and the information form. It took approximately 30–35 minutes responding the information form and ZCBI.

2.5. Data Analysis. Data analysis was performed by using the Statistical Package for the Social Sciences (SPSS) 16 packet program. We used Kruskal-Wallis test and Mann-Whitney *U* test to compare continuous variables in independent groups. $P < 0.05$ for the results was considered statistically significant.

3. Results

A large part of caregivers enrolled in the present study were women, married, and unemployed; most of them had children and some of them a relatively high number of children. Half of the caregivers had a social insurance. In addition, one in four of them was the spouse of the patient. A large of caregivers lived with the patient (Table 1).

The vast majority of caregivers had information about MS. In addition, more than half of them had information about MS treatment and care. Approximately one-third of them gave care more than six years to patient with MS patient and one-third of the caregivers gave this care at the patient's home. A large part of caregivers did not find enough this care. Most of the caregivers gave physical, social, and economic care to patient with MS (Table 2).

The mean scores of caregivers who had social insurance from the pension fund were higher than the other groups (27.61 ± 10.71). The mean scores of the caregivers who were spouses of the patients were higher than the other groups (27.16 ± 10.62). The mean scores of the caregivers who did not live with the patient (26.56 ± 8.85) were higher (Table 3).

The mean scores of the caregivers who received MS-related information (25.83 ± 8.82), who received this information from healthcare worker (26.13 ± 9.00), and who found the received information sufficient (25.87 ± 8.18) were higher and no statistically significant difference was found between the mean scores. The mean scores of the caregivers, who were care providing their patients for more than 6 years, (28.09 ± 10.16) were higher. The mean scores of the caregivers who provided care at the patient's house (26.00 ± 11.33) were higher (Table 4).

The mean scores of caregivers who provided care for 3-4 hours per day (32.23 ± 8.37) and provided physical care (29.28 ± 5.18) were higher. The mean scores of the caregivers, who did not consider the time spent for care sufficient (36.25 ± 12.14) and who expressed that more than one person provided support for the care (26.95 ± 10.86), were higher than the other groups (Table 4).

Table 1: Demographic characteristics of caregivers.

Demographic characteristics	*n*	%
Age		
18–27	27	29.4
28–37	22	23.9
38 or above	43	46.7
Gender		
Female	60	65.2
Male	32	34.8
Education level		
Literate	12	13.0
Primary school	45	48.9
High school	11	12.0
University	24	26.1
Occupation		
Working	32	34.8
Non-working	60	65.2
Working status		
Worker	19	59.3
Officer	13	40.7
Marital status		
Married	66	71.7
Single	26	28.3
Having children		
Yes	61	66.3
No	31	33.7
Number of children ($n = 61$)		
1-2	22	36.1
3-4	23	37.7
5 and above	16	26.2
Social insurance		
Green card	18	19.6
Social insurance	50	54.3
Pension fund	18	19.6
Self-employed	6	6.5
The degree of proximity to patient		
Parents	29	31.5
Spouse	25	27.2
Son/daughter	22	23.9
Sibling	16	17.4
Living situations with patients		
Yes	69	75.0
No	23	25.0
The number of family members living together		
2-3	30	32.6
4-5	37	40.2
6 and above	25	27.2
Having any disease		
Yes	17	18.5
No	75	81.5

TABLE 2: Level of information about MS of the caregiver sample.

Features	n	%
Having information about MS		
Yes	60	65.2
No	32	34.8
Having information about MS treatment		
Yes	56	60.9
No	36	39.1
Need information about MS care		
Yes	51	55.4
No	41	44.6
Getting information about MS		
Yes	55	59.8
No	37	40.2
Who did give your information about MS? ($n = 55$)		
Healthcare worker	51	92.7
Internet	4	7.3
Is your information enough? ($n = 55$)		
Yes	40	72.7
No	15	27.3
Duration of care given for MS		
Less than 1 year	17	18.5
1–5 years	42	45.7
More than 6 years	33	35.8
Where did you give MS care?		
At hospital	3	3.3
At home of patients with MS	36	39.1
At home of caregivers	32	34.8
Both at hospital and at home	21	22.8
Duration of care given to the patient		
1-2 hours	38	41.3
2-3 hours	25	27.2
3-4 hours	17	18.5
4-5 hours	8	8.7
All day	4	4.3
Do you find enough time spending for care?		
Yes	88	95.7
No	4	4.3
Which areas do you care?		
Psychological	8	8.7
Physical	7	7.6
Psychological, social, and economic	77	83.7

4. Discussion

In the study, it was found that the majority of caregivers were females. This result can be interpreted to say that caregiving is traditionally known a responsibility of the woman and also women consider caregiving the continuation of their older responsibilities, whereas men are strangers to the caregiving responsibility. Studies have revealed that the majority of caregivers were women and patient's spouses [32, 33].

The majority of caregivers lived in the same house with the patient. In addition, majority of caregivers had children and majority of them had 4-5 family members living with them. This may be associated with the fact that the caregivers were mostly patients' parents or spouses. In a similar study, it was found that the majority of caregivers and patients lived in the same house [34].

When ZCBI scores were compared to each other according to the caregivers' status of living with patients in the same house, the mean scores of the caregivers living in separate environments and who had 4-5 family members living with them were higher. This may make us think that the caregivers who lived in the same house environment with their patients may be more useful in terms of the continuity of the care. This result of our study shows similarity with the results of other studies in the literature [24, 35].

The minority of the caregivers included in the study provided care also for other individuals in need of care and these persons were the caregivers' parents or spouses. In a similar study reported that the caregivers also provided other people with care and the individuals they provided care for were their parents, spouses, and children [36].

It was determined that 45.0% of caregivers provided the patients with care for 1–5 years and 1-2 hours per day and they found the time spent for the care sufficient. Acccording to the study conducted by National MS Society in 2012, it was found that while 35.0% of caregivers provided their patients with care for 1–10 hours, 3% provided the care for 81 hours and above [37]. In another study, 50% of caregivers provided their patients with care for 1–5 hours [38].

It was determined that majority of the caregivers supported their patients from psychological, social, economic, and physical aspects, whereas minority of them supported only the physical needs of their patients. Carod-Artal et al. found that those who provided primary care within the care process gave support to their patients mostly in terms of coping with the disease and in psychological aspects [28]. It was also reported in another study that patients not only felt physically incompetent but also were affected in psychosocial aspect and supporting the patients in psychosocial aspect may be important in order to increase their life qualities [29].

The mean scores received by the employed patient relatives, included in the study, from the ZCBI were found to be higher compared to patient relatives who were unemployed. This situation may be associated with the fact that the caregiver had difficulties in the caregiving procedure due to the additional roles added to the roles of the caregiver. Zarit et al. emphasized that employment caused stress on caregivers, and accordingly, risk of depression may increase among caregivers; in addition, caregivers may feel exhausted and tired, and serious increase in health problems such as insomnia, diabetes, and arthritis and decrease in social bonds may be present [30].

The mean scores received by the participating caregivers aged 38 and over from the ZCBI were found to be higher compared to the other age groups. In contrast to this

TABLE 3: ZCBI mean scores ± SD as a function of demographic characteristics of caregivers and summary of statistical comparisons.

Features	$X \pm SD$	Test and P value
Age		
18–27	22.70 ± 8.26	
28–37	24.36 ± 9.78	KW = 4.97
38 or above	27.72 ± 9.73	$P > 0.05^*$
Gender		
Female	24.88 ± 9.50	$t = 0.77$
Male	26.50 ± 9.56	$P > 0.05$
Education level		
Literate	28.58 ± 6.69	
Primary school	26.73 ± 10.37	KW = 6.01
High school	24.45 ± 9.22	$P > 0.05$
University	21.91 ± 8.43	
Occupation		
Working	23.68 ± 7.21	$t = 1.30$
Non-working	26.38 ± 10.45	$P > 0.05$
Working status		
Worker	23.89 ± 7.57	$t = 0.19$
Officer	23.38 ± 6.93	$P > 0.05$
Marital status		
Married	26.39 ± 9.30	MW-U = 672.00
Single	23.03 ± 9.75	$P > 0.05$
Having children		
Yes	27.29 ± 9.41	$t = 2.70$
No	21.80 ± 8.71	$P < 0.05$
Number of children ($n = 61$)		
1-2	28.22 ± 10.95	
3-4	26.13 ± 9.96	KW = 0.78
5 and above	27.68 ± 6.11	$P > 0.05$
Social insurance		
Green card	27.55 ± 11.45	
Social insurance	23.92 ± 7.77	KW = 2.05
Pension fund	27.61 ± 10.71	$P > 0.05$
Self-employed	25.33 ± 12.59	
The degree of proximity to patient		
Parents	24.82 ± 8.03	
Spouse	27.16 ± 10.62	KW = 0.60
Son/daughter	26.68 ± 9.89	$P > 0.05$
Sibling	22.18 ± 9.50	
Living situations with patients		
Yes	25.07 ± 9.74	MW-U = 724.00
No	26.56 ± 8.85	$P > 0.05$
The number of family members living together		
2-3	25.40 ± 8.77	KW = 0.19
4-5	26.37 ± 11.02	$P > 0.05$
6 and above	24.12 ± 7.99	
Ownership of any disease		
Yes	29.23 ± 8.28	MW-U = 419.50
No	24.58 ± 9.60	$\mathbf{P < 0.05}$

*NS = not significant.

information, the studies have reported that age affects the care burden and younger caregivers experience heavier burdens [31].

When the mean score received from ZCBI was examined in terms of gender and marital status, it was observed that patient relatives who were males and married had higher mean scores. In the study entitled "Caregiver burden among informal caregivers assisting people with multiple sclerosis" conducted by Buchanan et al., it was found that the burden of male caregivers was higher than women [32]. Contrary to this, another study reported that the risk of experiencing emotional burden was higher among women compared to men and their life qualities were lower than men [33].

Among the caregivers included in the study, the care burden mean scores of spouses were found to be higher than other relatives. Previous studies reported that care was mostly provided by spouses and this process was considered as limiting the social life for both men and women. Also, disorders such as depression and anxiety were observed to be increasing in spouses during the process of caregiving [34, 35]. Figved et al. found that the spouses providing the care to MS patients experienced more distress compared to other groups and their life qualities were lower [36].

It was found that the mean scores of the caregivers, providing their patients with care for six years and longer during the care process, were higher than other groups, which caused a significant difference. Özyeşil et al. [37] indicated that there was a positive correlation between continuous and long care process and the developmental burden, physical burden, social burden, and emotional burden of caregivers.

Among caregivers included in this study, the mean scores of those who had any disease were higher than healthy caregivers, which caused a significant difference. In the study of Taşdelen and Ateş [38], it was found that half of the caregivers had a chronic disease. The study by Özmen and Yurttaş showed that the majority of caregivers had a disease [39]. Since caregivers devote themselves to the care procedure, it can be said that they may neglect their own diseases and treatments. Consequently, providing someone else with care in addition to their own health problems may create burden on caregivers.

The results of the study are limited to caregivers of patients with MS at the university hospital where the study was conducted. Furthermore, other limitations of the study include a small sample and a single center.

5. Conclusions

In conclusion, our study showed that the ZCBI score increased as the age of caregivers increased. The caregivers

TABLE 4: ZCBI mean scores ± SD as a function of level of information about MS and summary of statistical comparisons.

Features	$X \pm SD$	Test and P value
Having information about MS		
Yes	25.31 ± 9.15	$t = 1.17$
No	25.68 ± 10.26	$P > 0.05^*$
Having information about MS treatment		
Yes	25.21 ± 9.04	$t = 0.29$
No	25.80 ± 10.30	$P > 0.05$
Need information about MS care		
Yes	26.03 ± 10.6	$t = 0.66$
No	24.70 ± 7.85	$P > 0.05$
Getting information about MS		
Yes	25.83 ± 8.82	$t = 0.47$
No	24.86 ± 10.52	$P > 0.05$
Who did give your information about MS? ($n = 55$)		
Healthcare worker	26.13 ± 9.00	MW-U = 65.00
Internet	22.00 ± 5.35	$P > 0.05$
Is your information enough? ($n = 55$)		
Yes	25.87 ± 8.18	MW-U = 283.50
No	25.73 ± 10.67	$P > 0.05$
Duration of care given for MS		
Less than 1 year	20.64 ± 7.76	KW = 6.79
1–5 years	25.30 ± 8.99	$\mathbf{P < 0.05}$
More than 6 years	28.09 ± 10.16	
Where did you give MS care?		
At hospital	24.00 ± 7.00	KW = 0.21
At home of patients with MS	26.00 ± 11.33	$P > 0.05$
At home of caregivers	24.75 ± 8.87	
Both at hospital and at home	25.76 ± 7.56	
Duration of care given to the patient		
1-2 hours	22.78 ± 7.59	
2-3 hours	25.16 ± 10.77	KW = 12.95
3-4 hours	32.23 ± 8.37	$\mathbf{P < 0.05}$
4-5 hours	22.50 ± 8.65	
All day	29.50 ± 12.39	
Do you find enough time spending for care?		
Yes	24.95 ± 9.15	MW-U = 77.50
No	36.25 ± 12.14	$P > 0.05$
Which areas do you care?		
Psychological	17.25 ± 6.34	
Physical	29.28 ± 5.18	KW = 7.72
Psychological, social, and economic	25.94 ± 9.67	$\mathbf{P < 0.05}$

*NS = not significant.

who care for longer than six years had a higher ZCBI mean scores. In line with these results, caregivers' burden and affecting factors should be identified in future research with a large sample. The nursing care should include not only patients but also their caregivers. Additionally, information and education about MS should also be given to caregivers.

Additional Points

This research was accepted as a master thesis (January 22, 2015).

Ethical Approval

The study was approved by the Ethics Committee of the Faculty of Health Sciences with reference number (11.12. 2013/169).

Authors' Contributions

Afife Yurttaş and Serpil Özmen performed the study design, analyzed the data, and drafted the manuscript. Serpil Özmen performed the data collection.

References

[1] R. Bakshi, "Fatigue associated with multiple sclerosis: diagnosis, impact and management," *Multiple Sclerosis*, vol. 9, no. 3, pp. 219–227, 2003.

[2] G. A. Schumacher, G. Beeve, R. F. Kibler et al., "Problems of experimental trials of therapy in multiple sclerosis: report by the panel on the evaluation of experimental trials of therapy in multiple sclerosis," *Annals of the New York Academy of Sciences*, vol. 122, no. 1, pp. 552–568, 1965.

[3] C. M. Poser, D. W. Paty, L. C. Scheinberg et al., "New diagnostic criteria for multiple sclerosis: guidelines for research protocols," *Annals of Neurology*, vol. 13, no. 3, pp. 227–231, 1983.

[4] W. I. McDonald, A. Compston, G. Edan et al., "Recommended diagnostic criteria for multiple sclerosis: guidelines from the international panel on the diagnosis of multiple sclerosis," *Annals of Neurology*, vol. 50, no. 1, pp. 121–127, 2001.

[5] C. H. Polman, S. C. Reingold, G. Edan et al., "Diagnostic criteria for multiple sclerosis: 2005 revisions to the "McDonald Criteria"," *Annals of Neurology*, vol. 58, no. 6, pp. 840–846, 2005.

[6] A. Compston and A. Coles, "Multiple sclerosis," *Lancet*, vol. 359, no. 9313, pp. 1221–1231, 2002.

[7] F. D. Lublin, S. C. Reingold, and National Multiple Sclerosis Society (USA) Advisory Committee on Clinical Trials of New Agents in Multiple Sclerosis, "Defining the clinical course of multiple sclerosis: results of an international survey," *Neurology*, vol. 46, no. 4, pp. 907–911, 1996.

[8] M. Mollaoglu, "Multiple sclerosis and care," in *Chronic Diseases and Care*, Z. Durna, Ed., pp. 261–276, Nobel Medical Publishing, Istanbul, 2012.

[9] L. P. McKeown, A. P. Porter-Armstrong, and G. D. Baxter, "The needs and experiences of caregivers of individuals with

multiple sclerosis: a systematic review," *Clinical Rehabilitation*, vol. 17, no. 3, pp. 234–248, 2003.

[10] A. F. Alshubaili, J. U. Ohaeri, A. W. Awadalla, and A. A. Mabrouk, "Family caregiver quality of life in multiple sclerosis among Kuwaitis: a controlled study," *BMC Health Services Research*, vol. 8, no. 1, p. 206, 2008.

[11] M. Aymerich, I. Guillamón, and A. J. Jovell, "Health-related quality of life assessment in people with multiple sclerosis and their family caregivers. A multicenter study in Catalonia (Southern Europe)," *Patient Preference and Adherence*, vol. 3, pp. 311–321, 2009.

[12] M. Buhse, "Assessment of caregiver burden in families of persons with multiple sclerosis," *The Journal of Neuroscience Nursing*, vol. 40, no. 1, pp. 25–31, 2008.

[13] R. W. Toseland, G. Smith, and P. Mccalion, "Family caregivers of the frail elderly," in *Handbook of Social Work Practice with Vulnerable and Resilient Population*, A. Gıtterman, Ed., pp. 99–109, Columbia University Press, New York, NY, USA, 2nd edition, 2001.

[14] Z. Tülek, "Nursing care of patients with multiple sclerosis," *Cumhuriyet University Nursing Journal*, vol. 11, no. 2, pp. 25–32, 2007.

[15] C. S. Rehinhard, B. Given, N. Huhtala Petlick, and A. Bemis, "Supporting family caregivers in providing care, family caregiving-caregiver assessment," in *Patient Safety and Quality: An Evidence-Based Handbook for Nurses*, R. G. Hughes, Ed., vol. 14, pp. 1–64, Rockville, MD, USA, 3rd edition, 2008.

[16] N. Dayapoğlu and M. Tan, "The care burden and social support levels of caregivers of patients with multiple sclerosis," *Kontakt*, vol. 19, no. 1, pp. e17–e23, 2017.

[17] P. A. Potter and A. G. Perry, *Caring in Nursing Practice, Fundamentals of Nursing*, Mosby Inc, St. Louis, GA, USA, 6th edition, 2005.

[18] *The Research Advisor*, (January, 2018 http://research-advisors.com).

[19] Ö. Küçükgüçlü, A. Esen, and G. Yener, "The reliability and validity of the caregiver burden inventory in Turkey," *Journal of Neurological Sciences*, vol. 26, no. 1, pp. 60–73, 2009.

[20] F. Çetinkaya and A. Karadakovan, "Investigation of care burden in dementia patient caregivers," *Turkish Journal of Geriatrics*, vol. 15, no. 2, pp. 171–178, 2012.

[21] A. Zaybak, Ü. Güneş, E. Günay İsmailoğlu, and E. Ülker, "The determination of burden care of caregivers for bedridden patients," *Anatolian Journal of Nursing and Health Sciences*, vol. 15, no. 1, pp. 48–54, 2012.

[22] M. Atagün, Ö. D. Balaban, Z. Atagün, M. Elagöz, and A. Y. Özpolat, "Caregiver burden in chronic diseases," *Current Approaches in Psychiatry*, vol. 3, no. 3, pp. 513–552, 2011.

[23] M. Mollaoğlu, F. Tuncay O, and T. K. Fertelli, "Care burden of care givers of stroke patients and related factors," *Dokuz Eylul University School of Nursing Electronic Journal*, vol. 4, no. 3, pp. 125–130, 2011.

[24] H. Tel, D. Demirkol, S. Kara, and D. Aydın, "Care burden and quality of life among the caregivers of patients with COPD," *Turkish Thoracic Journal*, vol. 13, no. 3, pp. 87–92, 2012.

[25] E. Yildiz, S. A. Karakaş, Z. Güngörmüş, and M. Cengiz, "Levels of care burden and self-efficacy for informal caregiver of patients with cancer," *Holistic Nursing Practice*, vol. 31, no. 1, pp. 7–15, 2017.

[26] J. Hileman, N. Lackey, and R. Hassanien, "Identifying the needs of home caregivers of patients with cancer," *Oncology Nursing Form*, vol. 19, no. 5, pp. 771–777, 1992.

[27] H. P. Ma, H. J. Lu, X. Y. Xiong, J. Y. Yao, and Z. Yang, "The investigation of care burden and coping style in caregivers of spinal cord injury patients," *International Journal of Nursing Sciences*, vol. 1, no. 2, pp. 185–190, 2014.

[28] F. J. Carod-Artal, L. Ferreira Coral, D. S. Trizotto, and C. Menezes Moreira, "Burden and perceived health status among caregivers of stroke patients," *Cerebrovascular Diseases*, vol. 28, no. 5, pp. 472–480, 2009.

[29] A. Iavarone, A. R. Ziello, F. Pastore, A. M. Fasanaro, and C. Poderico, "Caregiver burden and coping strategies in caregivers of patients with Alzheimer's disease," *Neuropsychiatric Disease and Treatment*, vol. 10, pp. 1407–1413, 2014.

[30] S. H. Zarit, K. E. Reever, and J. Bach-Peterson, "Relatives of the impaired elderly: correlates of feelings of burden," *The Gerontologist*, vol. 20, no. 6, pp. 649–655, 1980.

[31] N. Ozer, A. Yurttaş, and R. Ç. Akyil, "Psychometric evaluation of the Turkish version of the Zarit Burden Interview in family caregivers of inpatients in medical and surgical clinics," *Journal of Transcultural Nursing*, vol. 23, no. 1, pp. 65–71, 2012.

[32] R. J. Buchanan, R. Dagmar, and C. Huangh, "Caregiver burden among informal caregivers assisting people with multiple sclerosis," *International Journal of MS Care*, vol. 13, no. 2, pp. 76–83, 2011.

[33] İ. Altun, *Strain State in the Event of Caring for Sick Relatives*, First National Home Health Care Congress Abstract Book, İstanbul, 1998.

[34] S. Yıldırım, E. Engin, and V. A. Başkaya, "The burden of caregivers of stroke patients and the factors affecting the burden," *Archives of Neuropsychiatry*, vol. 50, no. 2, pp. 169–174, 2013.

[35] F. Yaşar, *Requirements of the Individuals with Chronic Obstructive Pulmonary Disease in Primary Care Transmitter Identification of Factors Affecting Care Charges. Institute of Health Sciences, Nursing Department*, Baskent University, M.Sc., Ankara, 2008.

[36] N. Figved, K. M. Myhr, J. P. Larsen, and D. Aarsland, "Caregiver burden in multiple sclerosis: the impact of neuropsychiatric symptoms," *Journal of Neurology, Neurosurgery, & Psychiatry*, vol. 78, no. 10, pp. 1097–1102, 2007.

[37] Z. Özyeşil, A. Oluk, and D. Çakmak, "State and trait anxiety levels of load procedure giving care to elderly patients," *Anatolian Journal of Psychiatric Nursing*, vol. 15, pp. 39–44, 2014.

[38] P. Taşdelen and M. Ateş, "Evaluation of the burden of caregivers and home care needs of patients requiring care," *Journal of Nursing Research and Development*, vol. 12, no. 9, pp. 22–29, 2012.

[39] S. Özmen and A. Yurttaş, *Assessment of Caregiver Burden of Patients with Multiple Sclerosis, {M.S.thesis}*, Atatürk University Health Sciences Institute, Erzurum, Turkey, 2015.

Neural Basis of Depression Related to a Dominant Right Hemisphere: A Resting-State fMRI Study

Mi Li,[1,2] Hongpei Xu,[1,2] and Shengfu Lu[1,2,3]

[1]*Laboratory of Intelligent Science & Technology, Department of Automation, Faculty of Information Technology, Beijing University of Technology, Beijing 100024, China*
[2]*Beijing International Collaboration Base on Brain Informatics and Wisdom Services, Beijing 100024, China*
[3]*Beijing Advanced Innovation Centre for Future Internet Technology, Beijing University of Technology, Beijing 100024, China*

Correspondence should be addressed to Shengfu Lu; lusf@bjut.edu.cn

Academic Editor: Laura Piccardi

Background. In the past, studies on the lateralization of the left and right hemispheres of the brain suggested that depression is dominated by the right hemisphere of the brain, but the neural basis of this theory remains unclear. *Method.* Functional magnetic resonance imaging of the brain was performed in 22 depressive patients and 15 healthy controls. The differences in the mean values of the regional homogeneity (ReHo) of two groups were compared, and the low-frequency amplitudes of these differential brain regions were compared. *Results.* The results show that compared with healthy subjects, depressive patients had increased ReHo values in the right superior temporal gyrus, right middle temporal gyrus, left inferior temporal gyrus, left middle temporal gyrus, right middle frontal gyrus, triangular part of the right inferior frontal gyrus, orbital part of the right inferior frontal gyrus, right superior occipital gyrus, right middle occipital gyrus, bilateral anterior cingulate, and paracingulate gyri; reduced ReHo values were seen in the right fusiform gyrus, left middle occipital gyrus, left lingual gyrus, and left inferior parietal except in the supramarginal and angular gyri. *Conclusions.* The results show that regional homogeneity mainly occurs in the right brain, and the overall performance of the brain is such that right hemisphere synchronization is enhanced while left hemisphere synchronization is weakened. ReHo abnormalities in the resting state can predict abnormalities in individual neurological activities that reflect changes in the structure and function of the brain; abnormalities shown with this indicator are the neuronal basis for the phenomenon that the right hemisphere of the brain has a dominant effect on depression.

1. Introduction

Previous studies revealed a link between the left and right cerebral hemispheres and depression, providing a better understanding of the neuropathology of depression. Liotti and Tucker's results of a side-by-side simple response task showed that the left visual field response is impaired in healthy people with a depressive mood and in mild unipolar depressive patients, while the right visual field of healthy people with a depressive mood and in mild unipolar depressive patients did not show a slow response time for the viewing material [1]. A related EEG study in emotion recognition tasks also found that higher right frontal activity was associated with negative emotions and higher left frontal activity was associated with positive emotions [2]. When the healthy subjects were induced to experience negative emotions, the alpha power of the right frontal lobe was more inhibited than the left frontal lobe was, whereas in cases of positive emotions, the asymmetry of alpha power in the relevant region showed opposite results. These findings indicate that individuals with higher right frontal lobe activity have stronger negative emotions than individuals with higher left frontal lobe activity have [3–5]. The above findings discuss the relationship between the left and right hemispheres and emotions. The right frontal activity is enhanced in depressive patients or healthy subjects who were induced to experience depressive emotions.

There are also differences in information processing between the left hemisphere and the right hemisphere. The information processing of the left hemisphere is characterized by sequence, analysis, and logic; the information processed by the right hemisphere is parallel, holistic, and intuitive [6]. Based on the differences between left and right brain information processing, many experiments were designed to determine the characteristics of different hemispheric cognitive functions. The tachistoscopic visual half-field technique [7] and the dichotic listening technique [8] have been used to examine the effects of each hemisphere in visual and auditory processing. Bruder et al. used dichotic listening and visual half-field tasks to detect the perceptual asymmetry of depressive patients. The results showed that the perceived asymmetry of depressive patients was consistent with the hypothesis of right hemisphere dysfunction [9]. Similarly, in a study by Kaprinis et al., 26 patients with bipolar disorder were subjected to a dichotic test during a manic phase and after recovery; the manic phase showed a significant left ear (right hemisphere) advantage, and after recovery, patients shifted to a right ear advantage. These results show that a characteristic of manic disorder is the overactivation of right hemisphere function [10]. EEG and neuroimaging studies have also been extensively used in the study of hemispheric lateralization in depression. Flor-Henry et al. used EEG to analyze the differences between the left and right hemispheres of subjects in a resting state and during language and spatial cognitive tasks, and the results showed that negative emotions and depression were associated with relatively high activity in the frontal cortex of the right hemisphere [11]. Relevant neuroimaging studies reported that patients with unipolar depression are characterized by metabolic decline in the left brain and metabolic enhancement in the right brain [12]. The severity of depression is positively correlated with the metabolic enhancement of the right hemisphere [13]. The high activity in the right frontal lobe and the relatively low activity in the left frontal lobe in depressed patients have been confirmed in most surveys, with only a few exceptions [14]. A functional right hemisphere can make individuals overcome negative emotions and prevent the development of depression [15].

Bruder et al. systematically reviewed evidence of left and right brain asymmetry in electrophysiological (EEG and event-related potential), behavioral (dichotic and visual perceptual asymmetry), and neuroimaging (PET, MRI, and NIRS) and discussed that individual differences in left and right brain function measurements in patients with depression are related to the clinical diagnosis of subtypes of depression, anxiety disorders, and clinical response to antidepressant drugs or cognitive behavioral therapy [16]. Bruder et al. found that depressed patients with an anxiety disorder exhibited a frontal alpha asymmetry, whereas nonanxious depressed patients did not show this asymmetry [17]. Gold et al. found that frontal asymmetry was significantly associated with the degree of anxiety rather than the severity of depression [18]. Some studies have also found that the parietal region of depressed or previously depressed individuals has an opposite asymmetry compared to the frontal lobe (i.e., the right hemisphere has less activity than the left hemisphere) relative to the subjects of no depression [19, 20]. However, right parietal lobe activity of depressed patients with an anxiety disorder increases or offsets relatively less right parietal lobe activity in adolescents and adults [21]. Alpha asymmetry in patients with major depression and comorbid anxiety indicates that the right side has more activity than the left parietal lobe has, whereas patients with "pure" depression show less activity on the right parietal lobe [16]. It shows that the activity of the parietal lobe is related to depression and whether there is comorbid anxiety.

Previous studies have found abnormal lateralization of right and left hemisphere activity or function in depressive disorders, but the literature does not provide a detailed description of the neurological basis of depression associated with the high activity in the right hemisphere. Zang et al. proposed a regional homogeneity method to understand brain function in the resting state. Abnormalities are associated with temporal changes in neural activity of local areas and can be used to detect abnormal activity throughout the brain [22]. High ReHo values indicate that high synchronous oscillations of neurons in ALFF are directly related to the intensity of spontaneous neural activity in energy metabolism at resting state [23]. Kong et al. compared the differences in ReHo and low-frequency amplitude (ALFF) in brain regions before and after treatment with electroconvulsive therapy (ECT) in elderly patients with major depressive disorder (MDD); results show that ECT may affect brain function in elderly patients with MDD at resting state [24]. Yao et al. compared the ReHo of bipolar depression (BD), unipolar depression (UD), and healthy controls (HC) in the whole brain. The results show that the left frontal cluster (LFC) had significant differences among the three groups of subjects and the left temporal cluster (LTC) has a significant difference between BD and UD; the cuneus may provide neurological signs of depression in patients with BD and UD [25]. Peng et al. studied the ReHo of whole brain fMRI in patients with major depression and healthy controls at rest, and the results show that the ReHo values of the left thalamus, left temporal lobe, left cerebellar posterior lobe, and bilateral occipital lobe in patients with depression were significantly lower than in healthy subjects, suggesting abnormal activity in these brain regions [26]. Liu et al. found that the ReHo values of the right insula and left cerebellum of patients with MDD and high-risk MDD were significantly lower than those of healthy controls [27]. Guo et al. studied ReHo values in the brain regions of the first-time, initial, short-term, and treatment-responsive depression patients at resting state to detect abnormal marginal cortical networks in the MDD; the results show that the marginal cortical networks in first-time, initial, short-term, and treatment-responsive MDD patients are abnormal [28]. Wu et al. compared ReHo values of resting-state fMRI in treatment-refractory depression (TRD), depressed but not treatment-refractory (NDD), and healthy controls; the results show that compared with the healthy control group, the ReHo values within temporolimbic structures in the two depression groups were large and the ReHo values in the frontal, parietal, and posterior fusiform cortices and caudate were small; patients with TRD have more ReHo-modified brain regions than those with NDD have, demonstrating the feasibility of using ReHo as a research and clinical tool to monitor persistent cerebral dysfunction in depression [29]. Yao et al. used the ReHo method to explore the brain activity characteristics of MDD patients in resting state; the results showed that the severity of anxiety was positively related to ReHo in the right insula; the degree of cognitive impairment is positively correlated with ReHo in the right frontal cortex and left anterior cingulate gyrus; late severity was positively associated with ReHo in the right posterior cingulate gyrus and the right insula; the severity of sleep disorders was positively correlated with ReHo in the dorsomedial anterior cingulate gyrus; and desperate severity is positively correlated with right ventral anterior cingulate gyrus and right inguinal reanimation [30]. Liang et al. studied changes in brain activation patterns in bipolar disorder (BD) and unipolar depression (UD) patients. The results show some overlap in ReHo between UD and BD groups; however, significant differences in the thalamus of BD can assist in detecting functional defects and distinguish clinical and pathophysiological signs of BD and UD [31].

To explore the highly activated neural basis of the right hemisphere of depression, this paper analyzed and compared ReHo values across the entire brain area between patients with depression and healthy controls and extracted the amplitude of low-frequency fluctuation (ALFF) of the brain areas that showed significant differences in ReHo measures between depressed patients and the control group to verify our guess.

2. Materials and Methods

2.1. Subjects. A total of 22 depressed patients and 15 healthy controls were recruited from the Anding Hospital in Beijing, China. All participants' diagnostic evaluations were conducted using DSM-IV-based Mini International Neuropsychiatric Interview 6.0 (MINI 6.0) by clinically trained and experienced evaluators [32]. Physiological reports were performed on MDD and HC groups using a nine-item patient health questionnaire (PHQ-9). The demographic and clinical characteristics of the subjects are given in Table 1. Depressive patients suffer from severe anxiety (generalized anxiety diso rder > 10) in this paper. Exclusion criteria were the following: (1) depressive patients with a history of any manic episode or any major mental illness on axis I or axis II, (2) simultaneously suffering from a severe disease or primary nervous system disorder, (3) a history of loss of consciousness due to head injury, (4) abuse or dependence on alcohol or other substances, and (5) MRI contraindications.

2.2. MRI Data Acquisition. The fMRI data were collected by a Siemens Trio Tim 3T scanner. Functional data were scanned by a gradient plane echo pulse sequence. The head of the subject was fixed with a sponge pad to reduce the effects of head movement on the experimental results. During the resting-state scan, subjects kept their eyes closed, were sober, and relaxed their bodies. The scanning parameters were as follows: TR (scanning repetition time)= 2000 ms, TE (echo time)= 30 ms, FOV (field of view)= 224 mm × 224 mm, FA (rotation angle)= 90°, matrix = 64 × 64, gap (spacing of layers)= 0 mm, a total of 33 layers of axial images covering the whole brain, and a voxel size = 3.5 mm × 3.5 mm × 3.5 mm. The scan time of each subject was 860 seconds, 860 functional images frames were collected, and the corresponding BOLD signal contained 430 time points.

2.3. Image Preprocessing. Image preprocessing was completed on a MATLAB platform using SPM12 Software (Wellcome Trust Center for Neuroimaging, London, UK; http://www.fil.ion.ucl.ac.uk/spm/ext/) and REST toolkit. To eliminate the instability of the magnetic field at the beginning of the scan, the data from the first ten time points were removed, and only the remaining 420 time points were processed and analyzed. The main steps of image preprocessing are described below. (1) Slice-timing correction was performed to correct the layer time to eliminate the error caused by the removal of sequences at the beginning of the scan. (2) Realignment was performed to correct the differences in head translation or rotation during data collection. If the degree of translation or rotation of the subjects was within a certain range, the artifacts and errors produced by the head movement could be eliminated by realignment. If the degree of translation or rotation was too large and could not be eliminated by software corrections, the subjects were removed. In this study, the standard translation was less than 2.0 mm and the rotation angle was less than 2.0°; ultimately, four subjects were excluded. (3) Coregistration was performed, where the images obtained at different times were aligned in space and time. (4) Data were normalized, where different subjects' fMRI images were registered to the MNI standard brain anatomical template to correct for individual differences in brain structure. The specific steps were as follows: first, the 3D structural image of each subject was matched with the functional image of the resting state, and then the 3D structural image was divided into gray matter, white matter, and cerebrospinal fluid. The parameters of the structural image for the standard template were written into the aligned functional image; at the same time, if the functional image needed to be resliced, the voxel size of the reslice was $3 \times 3 \times 3\ \mathrm{mm}^3$. (5) Detrending was performed to remove the linear trend produced by a rise in temperature due to the machine working or adaptation of the subject over time. (6) The resting-state BOLD signal was filtered using a filter with a frequency band of 0.01 to 0.1. This frequency range mainly reflects the spontaneous activity of nerve cells. (7) Smoothing was performed to reduce the spatial structural differences between subjects, improving the signal-to-noise ratio. The spatial normalization of the image was carried out with 4 mm full width at half-maximum Gaussian space smoothing, which improves the validity of the statistical tests. (8) ReHo and ALFF were calculated, where the brain data of the subjects were calculated after the abovementioned processing steps. It should be noted that the smoothing was done after the calculation of ReHo. Because the consistency of a voxel and its surrounding voxels will increase after smoothing, the ReHo analysis must first calculate the Kendall harmony coefficient of each voxel and then the ReHo diagram should be smoothed to eliminate the standardization of small errors and improve the signal-to-noise ratio (using 4 × 4 × 4 mm Gaussian kernel). The calculation of ALFF needs to follow the smoothing step, and then the time series of each voxel in the image should be converted into a frequency range

TABLE 1: Demographic and clinical characteristics of depression patients and healthy controls.

Variables (mean ± SD)	Depression ($n = 16$)	Healthy controls ($n = 14$)	t/χ^2	P value	Cohen's d
Gender (M : F)	9 : 7	7 : 7	0.12	0.73	
Age (years)	27.38 ± 7.62	30.43 ± 8.50	1.04	0.31	−0.38
Age range	16–43	23–47			
Education level (years)	13.06 ± 3.62	15.00 ± 4.30	1.34	0.19	−0.49
PHQ-9	16.63 ± 5.33	3.29 ± 2.79	8.41	0.00	3.14

PHQ-9: 9-item patient health questionnaire.

using a Fourier transform to obtain a frequency power spectrum, where the peak area can be regarded as the amount of energy. The power spectrum of the signal with a frequency range of 0.01–0.1 Hz was squared to obtain ALFF.

2.4. Regional Homogeneity (ReHo) Analysis. Regional homogeneity is a brain imaging method based on functional magnetic resonance imaging data. Assuming that the temporal sequence of the selected voxel is similar in time to the adjacent 26 voxels, an increase in the indicator implies that the local neuronal activity tends to be synchronized. Conversely, this metric can show disorders over time. ReHo is calculated by Kendall's concordance coefficient (KCC). The formula for calculation is as follows:

$$W = \frac{\sum_{i=1}^{n} (R_i)^2 - n(\bar{R})^2}{(1/2)K^2(n^3 - n)}, \qquad (1)$$

where W represents Kendall's concordance coefficient of a specific point, which ranges from 0 to 1, indicating the regional homogeneity of the BOLD signal from weak to strong, respectively; n represents the number of time points, which in this paper was 420; K represents the total number of specific voxels and the surrounding voxels (which is 7,19,27), and in this paper K was 27; R_i is the total number of levels of voxels of each voxel at the ith time point; and $\bar{R}$ is the average of R. The closer the KCC value is to 1, the higher the synchronization of local neural activity in the brain and the more orderly the neural activity is.

2.5. Amplitude of Low-Frequency Fluctuation (ALFF). Electrophysiological studies show that the generation of low-frequency oscillations may be due to spontaneous neuronal activity. This spontaneous neuronal activity is physiologically significant, reflecting the rhythmic activity patterns a brain region produces by interacting with its connected brain regions. Thus, there is reason to believe that ALFF can serve as an indicator of brain characteristics. Low-frequency oscillations (LFO) are mainly observed with low-frequency amplitudes, and the low-frequency amplitude range selected for this study was between 0.01 and 0.1 Hz. The low-frequency amplitude was calculated as follows:

$$\text{ALFF} = \sum_{K:f_k \in [0.01,\ 0.1]} \sqrt{\frac{a_k(f)^2 + b_k(f)^2}{N}}. \qquad (2)$$

This formula calculation is the sum of the amplitude at a given frequency, where a_k and b_k are coefficients corresponding to different frequencies and N is the total number of voxels. In this paper, we did not directly analyze the whole brain ALFF but extracted the low-frequency amplitude (ALFF) of the brain areas that showed significant differences in ReHo measures between depressed patients and the control group. Differences between groups were tested using two-sample t-tests.

3. Results

3.1. Subjects. Twenty-two depressive patients and 15 healthy subjects completed the fMRI scan. One patient and 1 healthy subject were excluded due to incomplete data at the functional imaging time point. Four patients were excluded due to excessive head movements, and 1 patient was excluded due to a lack of spatially standardized results, leaving 16 patients and 14 healthy subjects.

3.2. ReHo: Depression versus Healthy Subjects. The ReHo brain data of the depression group and the healthy control group were analyzed by two-sample t-tests [26, 29]. The results showed that compared with the healthy control group, the brain BOLD signal of the depression group in the resting state was significantly different. As shown in Figure 1 and Table 2, the ReHo values were higher in depressed patients in the right superior temporal gyrus, right middle temporal gyrus, left inferior temporal gyrus, left middle temporal gyrus, right middle frontal gyrus, triangular part of the right inferior frontal gyrus, orbital part of the right inferior frontal gyrus, right superior occipital gyrus, right middle occipital gyrus, bilateral anterior cingulate, and paracingulate gyri, and values were reduced in the right fusiform gyrus, left middle occipital gyrus, left lingual gyrus, and left inferior parietal except for the supramarginal and angular gyri. In Figure 1, the colored area represents the brain regions with differences in ReHo between patients with depression and healthy subjects; the differences include both the increased ReHo brain area and the reduced ReHo brain area of depression.

In the multibaseline 3D graph (the multifiducial map gives a smoother map and the best estimate of spatial localization), Figure 2 shows regions where the ReHo value in the depressed patients was greater than in the healthy control group, and Figure 3 shows regions where ReHo values were

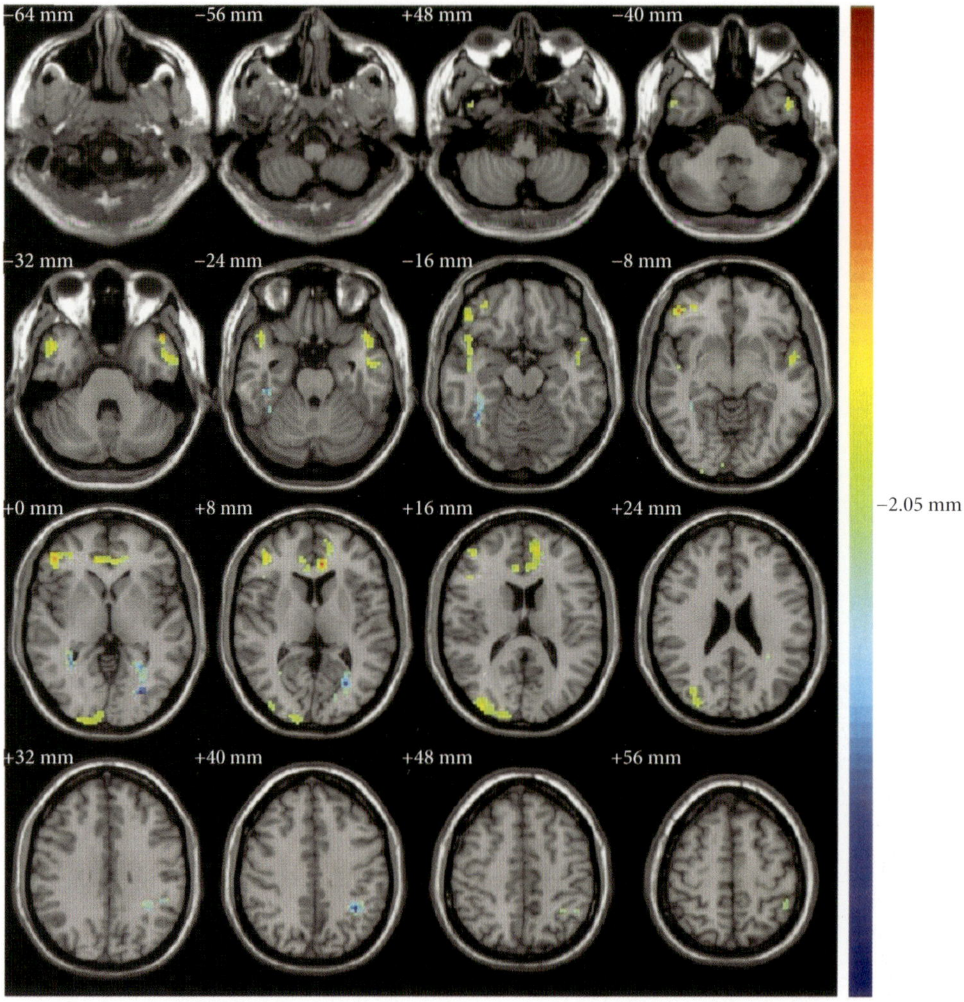

FIGURE 1: Brain regions with increased/decreased regional homogeneity (ReHo) (patients versus controls, independent t-test, $P < 0.05$, cluster size > 8 voxels; the left side of each brain image in the figure shows the right brain and the right side shows the left brain, and the color from blue to red indicates that the significant difference is from small to large).

greater in healthy controls than in the depressed patients. Finally, the low-frequency amplitude (ALFF) of the brain regions with significant differences in ReHo measures between the depression group and the healthy control group was extracted for two-sample t-tests. The results are shown in Table 3. The ALFF for the depression group was higher in the left middle temporal gyrus, while the other brain regions were not significantly different from the controls.

4. Discussion

In this study of resting-state fMRI, we used the regional homogeneity (ReHo) method to analyze fMRI data. This indicator can measure the time consistency of local blood oxygen level-dependent signals and reflect the time consistency of neural activity. The results show that there are synchronal abnormalities in some brain areas of depressive patients in the resting state.

Compared with the healthy subjects, we found that the ReHo value in the depression group was higher in the right middle frontal gyrus, triangular part of the right inferior frontal gyrus, and orbital part of the right inferior frontal gyrus; the frontal lobe region showed the most intense activation (the highest peak area was located in the orbital part of the inferior frontal gyrus, $t = 6.45$). Frontal lobe activity is related to the characteristics of depressive patients, including functional abnormalities, emotional adjustments, and cognitive controls [19]. To date, frontal lobes have been identified as one of the most consistent areas associated with MDD [33]. Yao et al. found that the ReHo value of major depressive patients with anxiety disorder was reduced in the left middle frontal gyrus, but no abnormalities were found in the right middle frontal gyrus [30, 34]; however, this paper has not completely ruled out the effect of antidepressants on brain activity in depressed patients which is likely to cause different findings with our paper.

The ReHo values in the depression group of the current study were increased in the right superior temporal gyrus, right middle temporal gyrus, left inferior temporal gyrus, and left middle temporal gyrus, as well as in the superior temporal gyrus. The right superior temporal gyrus is involved in the perception of facial expressions of emotion [35, 36] and

TABLE 2: Brain areas with significant ReHo differences between depression patients and controls.

Brain regions	Side	Brodmann areas	Coordinates (MNI) x	y	z	k	t statistic
Patients > control							
Middle frontal gyrus	Right	45/46	45	45	12	46	3.51
Inferior frontal gyrus, triangular part	Right	10/45	45	42	3	40	4.24
Middle frontal gyrus, orbital part	Right	47	48	42	−6	52	6.45
Temporal pole: superior temporal gyrus	Right	38	48	18	−18	45	3.44
Temporal pole: middle temporal gyrus	Right	20	45	12	−27	17	3.37
Temporal pole: middle temporal gyrus	Left	38	−48	18	−33	23	3.96
Inferior temporal gyrus	Left	20	−51	−6	−27	44	3.66
Superior occipital gyrus	Right	17	15	−102	6	33	2.84
Middle occipital gyrus	Right	19	36	−90	12	56	3.31
Anterior cingulate and paracingulate gyri	Left	24	−6	36	9	61	5.36
Anterior cingulate and paracingulate gyri	Right	32	12	39	3	44	3.52
Patients < control							
Fusiform gyrus	Right	37	33	−54	3	48	−3.67
Middle occipital gyrus	Left	19	−27	−78	0	8	−3.81
Lingual gyrus	Left	18	−18	−78	3	8	−2.05
Inferior parietal, except supramarginal and angular gyri	Left	40	−36	−52	42	57	−4.43

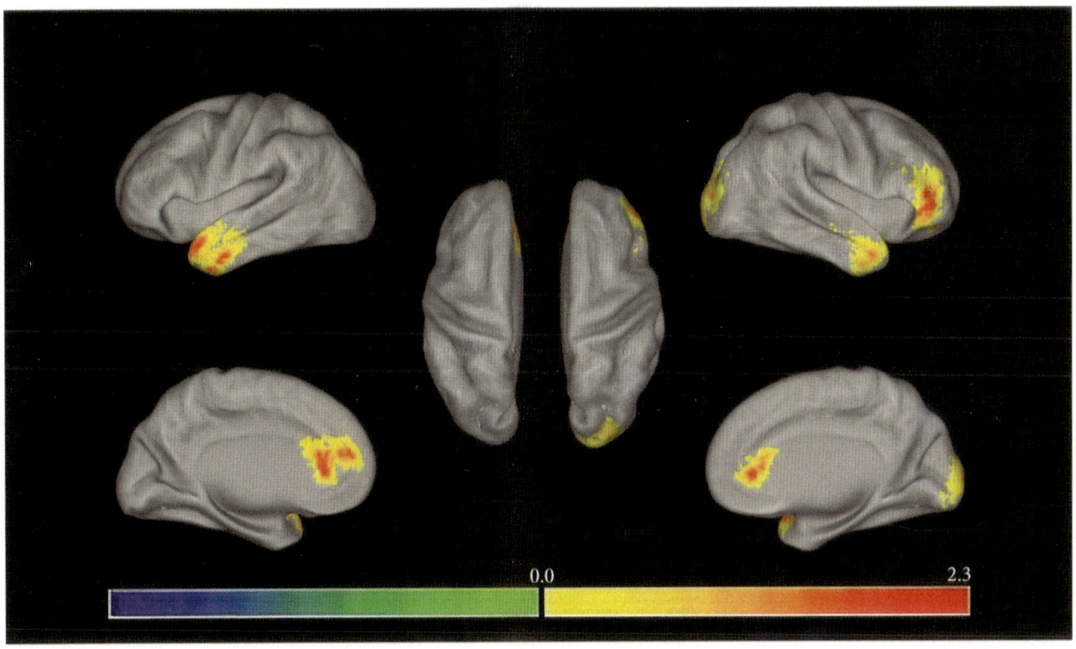

FIGURE 2: Regional homogeneity (ReHo) where depression group > control group (independent t-test, $P < 0.05$, cluster size > 8 voxels; the left half of the figure represents the left brain and the right half of the figure represents the right brain, and the color from blue to red represents that the significant difference is from small to large).

the left middle temporal gyrus, which is associated with text and language processing. Wu et al. have found results consistent with this study. Additional correlation analysis showed that anxiety symptoms were associated with dysfunction of the temporal lobe brain area [30, 37]. For example, other studies have reported that the ReHo value in depressive patients is reduced in the left superior temporal gyrus and the left temporal lobe [26], which is inconsistent with the results of this study. The paper's Hamilton Anxiety Scale (HAMA) < 14 indicates that patients with major depression may have anxiety but no obvious or no symptoms of anxiety; the statistical test results show that there is no significant difference in anxiety symptoms between patients with depression and healthy subjects, and our depressive patients have severe anxiety, indicating that differences of results may be related to anxiety.

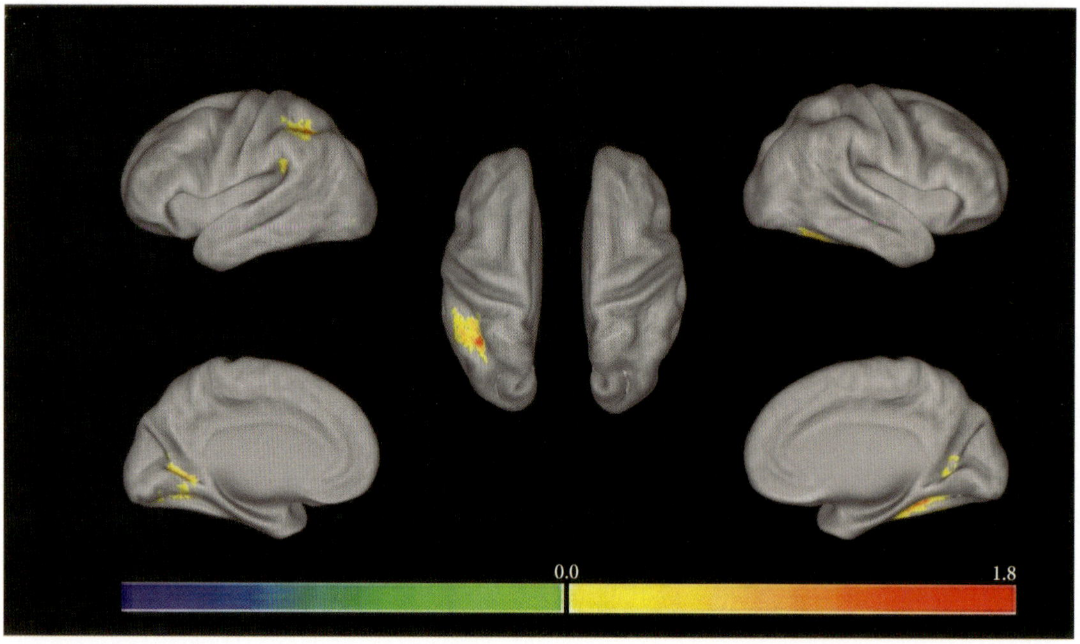

Figure 3: Regional homogeneity (ReHo) where depression group < control group (independent t-test, $P < 0.05$, cluster size > 8 voxels; the left half of the figure represents the left brain and the right half of the figure represents the right brain, and the color from blue to red represents that the significant difference is from small to large).

Table 3: ALFF differences in brain areas with significant ReHo differences between depression patients and controls.

Brain regions	Side	ALFF Depression	ALFF Control	t	P
Patients > control					
Middle frontal gyrus	Right	0.83 ± 0.08	0.85 ± 0.07	−0.64	0.53
Inferior frontal gyrus, triangular part	Right	0.72 ± 0.05	0.75 ± 0.09	−1.11	0.28
Middle frontal gyrus, orbital part	Right	0.82 ± 0.09	0.88 ± 0.12	−1.42	0.17
Temporal pole: superior temporal gyrus	Right	0.95 ± 0.14	0.99 ± 0.13	−0.88	0.38
Temporal pole: middle temporal gyrus	Right	0.57 ± 0.09	0.55 ± 0.07	0.45	0.66
Temporal pole: middle temporal gyrus	Left	0.69 ± 0.11	0.62 ± 0.08	2.19	0.04
Inferior temporal gyrus	Left	0.79 ± 0.27	0.77 ± 0.05	0.83	0.42
Superior occipital gyrus	Right	1.04 ± 0.12	1.05 ± 0.13	−0.24	0.81
Middle occipital gyrus	Right	1.04 ± 0.13	1.07 ± 0.15	−0.49	0.63
Anterior cingulate and paracingulate gyri	Left	0.78 ± 0.06	0.82 ± 0.05	−2.02	0.54
Anterior cingulate and paracingulate gyri	Right	0.92 ± 0.11	0.94 ± 0.07	−0.61	0.55
Patients < control					
Fusiform gyrus	Right	1.10 ± 0.08	1.09 ± 0.08	0.54	0.60
Middle occipital gyrus	Left	1.09 ± 0.12	1.09 ± 0.13	−0.13	0.90
Lingual gyrus	Left	1.15 ± 0.17	1.10 ± 012	0.86	0.40
Inferior parietal, except supramarginal and angular gyri	Left	0.98 ± 0.13	1.05 ± 0.09	−1.73	0.10

The ReHo value of the depression group was higher in the right superior occipital gyrus and right middle occipital gyrus and lower in the left lingual gyrus, bilateral anterior cingulate gyrus, and paracingulate gyri. These areas belong to the occipital lobe, and most of the functional areas of the occipital lobe are related to visual signal coding. The middle occipital gyrus participates in visual processing; the right anterior cingulate and paracingulate gyri, as well as the fusiform gyrus, as part of the marginal system are connected to the amygdala, orbital frontal cortex, and hippocampus and participate in the emotional system, and the left anterior cingulate and paracingulate gyri are responsible for the decision-making process. In a study by Peng et al. [26], the ReHo values of major depressive patients without anxiety were reduced in bilateral occipital lobes, and there were both increased and reduced areas in the current study; the reason for this difference, as described above, may be related to whether or not the depression suffers from anxiety.

The ReHo value of the depression group was reduced in the left inferior parietal, except the supramarginal and angular gyri; this area belongs to the parietal lobe. An EEG study found that patients with major depression and comorbid anxiety showed alpha asymmetry which indicates that the right side has more activity than the left parietal lobe has, whereas patients with "pure" depression show less activity on the right parietal lobe [16]. Bruder et al. reviewed the use of behavioral, EEG, and ERP measurement methods to indicate that there may be defects in right parietal lobe function in depressed patients, especially when dealing with emotional information [16].

The amplitude of low-frequency fluctuation (ALFF) is also commonly used as an indicator of abnormal brain activity. In this study, the amplitude of low-frequency fluctuation of the brain regions with significant differences in ReHo values between the depression group and the healthy subject group was extracted for two-sample t-tests. The results showed that the depression group ALFF was higher in the left middle temporal lobe, while the other brain regions were not significantly different between groups. The value of ALFF can directly reflect the strength of the brain's neural activity, and ReHo is an indirect measurement. Whether ReHo is enhanced or weakened indicates that the neural activity in a local area is synchronization abnormalities and the region's collaboration capacity is abnormal. Although the efficiency of the brain can decline, it is still able to complete its corresponding physiological functions. The synchronization abnormalities of local nerve activity above a certain limit will be expressed as neural activity abnormalities, and, at this point, the brain cannot complete its corresponding physiological functions. Although abnormalities in regional homogeneity cannot directly represent neural activity abnormalities, the regional homogeneity of a region with abnormal neural activity must be abnormal, which means that regional homogeneity can predict individual neural activity. From the regional homogeneity results, we found that abnormal areas occurred mainly in the right brain in depressed patients, and the overall brain synchronization performance was enhanced in the right hemisphere and attenuated in the left hemisphere. Based on these results, we can predict neurological activity trends in these patients' brains; that is, the spontaneous nerve activity in ReHo-enhanced brain regions in resting states may be enhanced. In contrast, spontaneous nerve activity in the brain area with ReHo attenuation may be diminished. The amplitude of low-frequency fluctuation (ALFF) of the brain regions with significant differences in ReHo values between the depression group and the healthy control group increased in the left temporal gyrus, indicating that the spontaneous nerve activity in this region was enhanced, thus validating our hypothesis. Furthermore, according to this trend of right hemisphere enhancement and left hemisphere attenuation of ReHo values, we can predict that the spontaneous nerve activity in the resting state of the brain as a whole shows right hemisphere enhancement and left hemisphere attenuation.

Related studies suggest that the physiological activation of the right hemisphere of the brain in depressive patients is accompanied by functional decline and deficiencies. The additional physiological activity in the right hemisphere is to overcome functional barriers. To be able to properly complete corresponding functions, the right brain of depressive patients must increase its activity level (but the result is futile). The increase and decrease of ReHo suggest that neuronal activity is disturbed, indicating that the structure and function of the corresponding brain area are changed. Abnormalities mainly occur in the right hemisphere, which is consistent with the previous studies showing the dominant role of the right hemisphere in depression. Regional homogeneity can predict abnormalities in neurological activity and reflect changes in the structure and function of the brain in the resting state. Abnormalities in this indicator are the neural basis of the phenomenon that the right hemisphere of the brain has a dominant effect on depression.

Acknowledgments

This work is supported by the National Natural Science Foundation of China (61602017 and 61420106005), the National Basic Research Program of China (2014CB744600), the Beijing Natural Science Foundation (4164080), the "Rixin Scientist" Foundation of Beijing University of Technology (2017-RX(1)-03), the Beijing Outstanding Talent Training Foundation (2014000020124G039), the International Science and Technology Cooperation Program of China (2013DFA32180), the special fund of Beijing Municipal Science and Technology Commission (Z171100000117004 and Z151100003915117), the Beijing Municipal Administration of Hospitals Clinical Medicine Development of Special Funding Support (ZYLX201607), and the Beijing Municipal Administration of Hospitals Ascent Plan (DFL20151801).

References

[1] M. Liotti and D. M. Tucker, "Right hemisphere sensitivity to arousal and depression," *Brain and Cognition*, vol. 18, no. 2, pp. 138–151, 1992.

[2] R. J. Davidson, "Affective style and affective disorders: perspectives from affective neuroscience," *Cognition and Emotion*, vol. 12, no. 3, pp. 307–330, 1998.

[3] A. J. Tomarken, R. J. Davidson, and J. B. Henriques, "Resting frontal brain asymmetry predicts affective responses to films," *Journal of Personality and Social Psychology*, vol. 59, no. 4, pp. 791–801, 1990.

[4] S. S. Sobotka, R. J. Davidson, and J. A. Senulis, "Anterior brain electrical asymmetries in response to reward and punishment," *Electroencephalography and Clinical Neurophysiology*, vol. 83, no. 4, pp. 236–247, 1992.

[5] A. J. Tomarken, R. J. Davidson, R. E. Wheeler, and R. C. Doss, "Individual differences in anterior brain asymmetry and fundamental dimensions of emotion," *Journal of Personality and Social Psychology*, vol. 62, no. 4, pp. 676–687, 1992.

[6] J. B. Hellige, "Hemispheric asymmetry: what's right and what's left," *Science*, vol. 261, pp. 1755–1757, 1993.

[7] M. Mishkin and D. G. Forgays, "Word recognition as a function of retinal locus," *Journal of Experimental Psychology*, vol. 43, no. 1, pp. 43–48, 1952.

[8] D. E. Broadbent, "The role of auditory localization in attention and memory span," *Journal of Experimental Psychology*, vol. 47, no. 3, pp. 191–196, 1954.

[9] G. E. Bruder, F. M. Quitkin, J. W. Stewart, C. Martin, M. M. Voglmaier, and W. M. Harrison, "Cerebral laterality and depression: differences in perceptual asymmetry among diagnostic subtypes," *Journal of Abnormal Psychology*, vol. 98, no. 2, pp. 177–186, 1989.

[10] G. Kaprinis, J. Nimatoudis, A. Karavatos, D. Kandylis, and S. Kaprinis, "Functional brain organization in bipolar affective patients during manic phase and after recovery: a digit dichotic listening study," *Perceptual and Motor Skills*, vol. 80, Supplement 3, pp. 1275–1282, 1995.

[11] P. Flor-Henry, J. C. Lind, and Z. J. Koles, "A source-imaging (low-resolution electromagnetic tomography) study of the EEGs from unmedicated males with depression," *Psychiatry Research: Neuroimaging*, vol. 130, no. 2, pp. 191–207, 2004.

[12] A. Janocha, W. Pilecki, M. Bolanowski et al., "Interhemispheric cerebral asymmetry detected by VEPS in diabetic patients with recognized depression," *Neuro Endocrinology Letters*, vol. 30, no. 1, pp. 119–124, 2009.

[13] S. Grimm, J. Beck, D. Schuepbach et al., "Imbalance between left and right dorsolateral prefrontal cortex in major depression is linked to negative emotional judgment: an fMRI study in severe major depressive disorder," *Biological Psychiatry*, vol. 63, no. 4, pp. 369–376, 2008.

[14] S. Debener, A. Beauducel, D. N. eacute et al., "Is resting anterior EEG alpha asymmetry a trait marker for depression?," *Neuropsychobiology*, vol. 41, no. 1, pp. 31–37, 2000.

[15] A. N. Schore, *Affect Regulation and the Origin of the Self: The Neurobiology of Emotional Development*, Routledge, 2015.

[16] G. E. Bruder, J. W. Stewart, and P. J. Mcgrath, "Right brain, left brain in depressive disorders: clinical and theoretical implications of behavioral, electrophysiological and neuroimaging findings," *Neuroscience & Biobehavioral Reviews*, vol. 78, pp. 178–191, 2017.

[17] G. E. Bruder, R. Fong, C. E. Tenke et al., "Regional brain asymmetries in major depression with or without an anxiety disorder: a quantitative electroencephalographic study," *Biological Psychiatry*, vol. 41, no. 9, pp. 939–948, 1997.

[18] C. Gold, J. Fachner, and J. Erkkilä, "Validity and reliability of electroencephalographic frontal alpha asymmetry and frontal midline theta as biomarkers for depression," *Scandinavian Journal of Psychology*, vol. 54, no. 2, pp. 118–126, 2013.

[19] J. B. Henriques and R. J. Davidson, "Regional brain electrical asymmetries discriminate between previously depressed and healthy control subjects," *Journal of Abnormal Psychology*, vol. 99, no. 1, pp. 22–31, 1990.

[20] A. S. REID, M. L. DUKE, and J. B. J. ALLEN, "Resting frontal electroencephalographic asymmetry in depression: inconsistencies suggest the need to identify mediating factors," *Psychophysiology*, vol. 35, no. 4, pp. 389–404, 1998.

[21] G. E. Bruder, J. W. Stewart, M. A. Mercier et al., "Outcome of cognitive–behavioral therapy for depression: relation to hemispheric dominance for verbal processing," *Journal of Abnormal Psychology*, vol. 106, no. 1, pp. 138–144, 1997.

[22] Y. Zang, T. Jiang, Y. Lu, Y. He, and L. Tian, "Regional homogeneity approach to fMRI data analysis," *NeuroImage*, vol. 22, no. 1, pp. 394–400, 2004.

[23] R. Qi, L. Zhang, S. Wu et al., "Altered resting-state brain activity at functional MR imaging during the progression of hepatic encephalopathy," *Radiology*, vol. 264, no. 1, pp. 187–195, 2012.

[24] X. M. Kong, S. X. Xu, Y. Sun et al., "Electroconvulsive therapy changes the regional resting state function measured by regional homogeneity (ReHo) and amplitude of low frequency fluctuations (ALFF) in elderly major depressive disorder patients: an exploratory study," *Psychiatry Research: Neuroimaging*, vol. 264, pp. 13–21, 2017.

[25] X. Yao, Z. Yin, F. Liu et al., "Shared and distinct regional homogeneity changes in bipolar and unipolar depression," *Neuroscience Letters*, vol. 673, pp. 28–32, 2018.

[26] D. H. Peng, K. D. Jiang, Y. R. Fang et al., "Decreased regional homogeneity in major depression as revealed by resting-state functional magnetic resonance imaging," *Chinese Medical Journal-Beijing*, vol. 124, no. 3, pp. 369–373, 2011.

[27] Z. Liu, C. Xu, Y. Xu et al., "Decreased regional homogeneity in insula and cerebellum: a resting-state fMRI study in patients with major depression and subjects at high risk for major depression," *Psychiatry Research: Neuroimaging*, vol. 182, no. 3, pp. 211–215, 2010.

[28] W. B. Guo, F. Liu, Z. M. Xue et al., "Abnormal neural activities in first-episode, treatment-naïve, short-illness-duration, and treatment-response patients with major depressive disorder: a resting-state fMRI study," *Journal of Affective Disorders*, vol. 135, no. 1-3, pp. 326–331, 2011.

[29] Q. Z. Wu, D. M. Li, W. H. Kuang et al., "Abnormal regional spontaneous neural activity in treatment-refractory depression revealed by resting-state fMRI," *Human Brain Mapping*, vol. 32, no. 8, pp. 1290–1299, 2011.

[30] Z. Yao, L. Wang, Q. Lu, H. Liu, and G. Teng, "Regional homogeneity in depression and its relationship with separate depressive symptom clusters: a resting-state fMRI study," *Journal of Affective Disorders*, vol. 115, no. 3, pp. 430–438, 2009.

[31] M. J. Liang, Q. Zhou, K. R. Yang et al., "Identify changes of brain regional homogeneity in bipolar disorder and unipolar depression using resting-state fMRI," *PLoS One*, vol. 8, no. 12, article e79999, 2013.

[32] D. V. Sheehan, K. H. Sheehan, R. D. Shytle et al., "Reliability and validity of the mini international neuropsychiatric interview for children and adolescents (MINI-KID)," *The Journal of Clinical Psychiatry*, vol. 71, no. 3, pp. 313–326, 2010.

[33] H. S. Mayberg, "Positron emission tomography imaging in depression: a neural systems perspective," *Neuroimaging Clinics of North America*, vol. 13, no. 4, pp. 805–815, 2003.

[34] Y. Yuan, Z. Zhang, F. Bai et al., "Abnormal neural activity in the patients with remitted geriatric depression: a resting-state functional magnetic resonance imaging study," *Journal of Affective Disorders*, vol. 111, no. 2-3, pp. 145–152, 2008.

[35] J. Radua, M. L. Phillips, T. Russell et al., "Neural response to specific components of fearful faces in healthy and schizophrenic adults," *NeuroImage*, vol. 49, no. 1, pp. 939–946, 2010.

[36] M. Sugiura, Y. Sassa, H. Jeong, K. Horie, S. Sato, and R. Kawashima, "Face-specific and domain-general characteristics of cortical responses during self-recognition," *NeuroImage*, vol. 42, no. 1, pp. 414–422, 2008.

A Comparative Study of Conventional Physiotherapy versus Robot-Assisted Gait Training Associated to Physiotherapy in Individuals with Ataxia after Stroke

Marcia Belas dos Santos,[1] **Clarissa Barros de Oliveira**,[2] **Arly dos Santos**,[1] **Cristhiane Garabello Pires**,[3] **Viviana Dylewski**,[2] **and Ricardo Mario Arida**[1]

[1]*Physiology Department, Universidade Federal de São Paulo (UNIFESP), São Paulo, SP, Brazil*
[2]*Physiotherapy Department, Associação de Assistência a Criança Deficiente (AACD), São Paulo, SP, Brazil*
[3]*Faculty of Medicine, University of Sao Paulo (USP), São Paulo, SP, Brazil*

Correspondence should be addressed to Marcia Belas dos Santos; mbelassantos@gmail.com

Academic Editor: Tauheed Ishrat

Objectives. To assess the influence of RAGT on balance, coordination, and functional independence in activities of daily living of chronic stroke survivors with ataxia at least one year of injury. *Methods.* It was a randomized controlled trial. The patients were allocated to either therapist-assisted gait training (TAGT) or robotic-assisted gait training (RAGT). Both groups received 3 weekly sessions of physiotherapy with an estimated duration of 60 minutes each and prescribed home exercises. The following outcome measures were evaluated prior to and after the completion of the 5-month protocol treatment: BBS, TUG test, FIM, and SARA. For intragroup comparisons, the Wilcoxon test was used, and the Mann–Whitney test was used for between-group comparison. *Results.* Nineteen stroke survivors with ataxia sequel after one year of injury were recruited. Both groups showed statistically significant improvement ($P < 0.05$) in balance, functional independencein, and general ataxia symptoms. There were no statistically significant differences ($P < 0.05$) for between-group comparisons both at baseline and after completion of the protocol. *Conclusions.* Chronic stroke patients with ataxia had significant improvements in balance and independence in activities of daily living after RAGT along with conventional therapy and home exercises. This trial was registered with trial registration number 39862414.6.0000.5505.

1. Introduction

Stroke is the third most common cause of death and the biggest factor for disability in adults of developing nations, just behind cancer and heart diseases [1]. Approximately 795,000 stroke cases occur every year in the USA [2] with 2-3% in the cerebellum area [3]. The loss of motor skills is one of the most common complaints of stroke survivors as approximately 75% of these patients have some walking disability that could result in high risk of falls [4, 5]. In a prospective study, 256 stroke patients were evaluated in the acute phase, with approximately 27% reporting at least one fall in a three-month period [6].

Impairment in the posterior circulation that involves the cerebellum or brainstem region may lead to damages in several important functions, such as balance, movement coordination, speech, hearing, ocular movement, and swallowing [7, 8]. Ataxia is an important sequela observed and recognized for its presentation as a loss of coordination, dysmetria, dysarthria, hypotonia, rebound phenomenon, and nystagmus [9]. Gait ataxia is described by a stumbling walking pattern, an irregular foot placement, an increased step, an enlarged stance, and an abnormal joint torque [10, 11].

When the depletion of balance ability is associated with decreased joint mobility, muscle tone problems, and loss of proprioception, there is an increase in the difficulty to perform activities of daily living for individuals with stroke injury [12]. Consequently, balance training is crucial for rehabilitation treatment. Conventional gait therapy (CGT), such as the Bobath concept, proprioceptive neuromuscular facilitation, therapist-assisted walking, and the use of braces or other devices are common treatment approaches [13]. Furthermore, high severity stroke patients with poor coordination in walking may benefit from treatment with a robotic device that allows task-focused training [14].

Robot-assisted gait training (RAGT) has been used since 1980 to assist patients with dysfunction in movement caused by neurological disorders [15]. This treatment is based on the body weight-supported treadmill (BWSTT) principle and achieves functional motor relearning through the repetitive practice of all different phases of gait [16]. Training the same movement repetitively enables the nervous system to develop circuits for better communication between the motor center and sensory pathways [17].

Treatment by RAGT compared with conventional treatment on the treadmill presents advantages, including training duration, more reproducible symmetrical gait patterns, operation by a single therapist, and a reduction in the energy expenditure imposed upon the therapists [18]. In addition, recent research revealed that robot-assisted treadmill training resulted in a more symmetrical muscle activity pattern in paretic patients compared with conventional treatment [5]. It is important to highlight that there have been very few investigations on RAGT in individuals with ataxia poststroke.

A systematic review on the efficacy of rehabilitation robotics for walking training in neurological disorders showed that patients injured by stroke had statistically significant amelioration in walking speed, functional abilities, and motor functions after treatment [19]. However, a study that compared treadmill training with both partial body weight support and robotic training revealed that therapy with partial body weight support was superior to robotic training for subjects with chronic stroke [20].

One of the possible drawbacks of treatment with RAGT may be the excessive passive guidance of device, which could potentially reduce patient effort and treatment effectiveness [21]. Additionally, another important factor is the patients' limited degree of freedom with the equipment, which could result in abnormal torque [18].

Considering the critical importance of the subject as well as the shortage and inconclusive information about it, this study aimed to assess the influence of robot-assisted gait training on balance and coordination and to verify the functional independence in activities of daily living of chronic stroke survivors with ataxia after at least one year of injury.

2. Methods

2.1. Subjects. This was a randomized controlled trial approved by the Universidade Federal do Estado de São Paulo (UNIFESP) ethics committee (number 933.112). All the patients who participated or their legal representatives gave written informed consent voluntarily without financial gains.

The inclusion criteria were stroke survivors with ataxia, minimum time of injury over 1 year (in the chronic phase of rehabilitation), cerebellar stroke verified by an initial MRI, clinical stability, presence of hemiplegia or quadriplegia motor impairment, and admission to the Associação de Assistência a Criança Deficiente (AACD) Rehabilitation Center from September 23, 2014, to December 20, 2015. Patients from both genders who were at least 18 years of age were accepted. A physician examined all the patients and described their diagnosis in medical records.

The exclusion criteria were physical disability that made training with the robotic device unsafe such as cognitive impairment, dementia, aphasia, presence of other orthopedic or neurosurgical problems in the lower extremities, pressure ulcers on the hips or lower extremities, weight higher than 120 kg, ataxia originated by progressive disease, and not accomplishing the proposed treatment.

The participants were allocated to each arm of this study using a weekly timetable, which illustrated a list of sessions available for the proposed treatment. This specific schedule was formulated given ten different schedule options per week. Depending on their preferable time session chosen, they were allocated to one of the two arms of this study: therapist-assisted gait training (TAGT) or RAGT. Each participant completed three sessions per week. Furthermore, their timeline was organized with the availability and capacity of the institution for both proposed interventions.

2.2. Evaluation Protocol. All participants were examined by a blinded evaluator at two-time points: before and after the protocol treatment was completed. The Berg Balance Scale (BBS), the Functional Independence Measure (FIM), the Timed Up and Go Test (TUG), and the Scale for the Assessment and Rating of Ataxia (SARA) were the tools used for baseline and outcome evaluation.

The BBS test is used to evaluate balance and risk of fall. The BBS focuses on static and dynamic balance, which includes 14 tasks with a maximum score of 56 [22, 23].

The TUG test evaluates sitting balance, transfers from sitting to standing, stability in ambulation, and gait course changes [24].

The FIM is used to assess neuropsychological and motor disability. This functional scale includes 18 items allocated into 6 domains: 2 cognitive and 4 motors. Each item has an increasing score from 1 to 7 (1 = maximum of functional dependence and 7 = maximum of functional independence). The minimum value of the entire range is 18, and the total score is 126 [22].

The SARA is used to assess the severity and treatment effectiveness of cerebellar ataxia. Some studies have shown its usefulness in stroke individuals [25, 26]. The total score ranges from 0 (no ataxia) to 40 (severe ataxia), and it is composed of the following 8 items [27]: 1 gait (0–8); 2 stance (0–6); 3 sitting (0–4); 4 speech disturbance (0–6); 5 finger chase (0–4); 6 nose finger test (0–4); 7 fast alternating hand movement (0–4); and 8 heel-shin slide (0–4); the four extremities are evaluated bilaterally, and the mean values are used to calculate the total score [26].

TABLE 1: Summary of demographic and baseline characteristics by intervention therapy.

Demographic and baseline characteristics	Therapist-assisted ($n = 8$) X (SD)	Robot-assisted ($n = 7$) X (SD)	P value
Mean age (year)	56.4 (11.8)	44.4 (12.7)	0.064
Gender, number (M/F)	6/2	5/2	0.876
Diagnosis, number (I/H)	2/6	2/5	0.876
Right side motor impairment, number	2	2	0.876
Left side motor impairment, number	2	2	0.876
Both side motor impairment, number	4	3	0.782
Onset (year)	10.5 (5.4)	4.8 (0.92)	0.021*

P value represents between-group differences. *Requirement for a statistically significant difference: $P < 0.05$. SD: standard deviation; M: male; F: female; I: ischemic; H: hemorrhagic.

2.3. Training Protocol. The patients were allocated into two groups according to the treatment received for gait training: therapist-assisted gait training (TAGT) and robot-assisted gait training (RAGT). Both groups were submitted to 3 intensive sessions of physiotherapy per week and were prescribed home exercises. Each group had 2 sessions of conventional physiotherapy and 1 session of gait training with an estimated duration of 60 minutes each. The TAGT was delivered over ground with the use of a walker device, if necessary. The RAGT was performed with a robot-driven exoskeleton orthosis equipment Lokomat® 5.0. In an automated electromechanical gait rehabilitation, the Lokomat device consists of a robotic gait orthosis combined with a harness-supported body weight system used in combination with a treadmill. The estimated protocol time was 5 months.

For both groups, the rehabilitation program consisted of muscle stretching and strengthening, balance training, postural stability control, sensory techniques, and functional daily activities. Furthermore, the patients were encouraged to continue practicing exercises at home. The professional in charge of the physiotherapy treatment was very knowledgeable and experienced in treating neurological disorders.

The main aim of RAGT was to improve the quality of movement and the coordination of both legs. The parameters were performed at a low speed (between 0.8 kph and 1.5 kph) and were adjusted gradually according to the patients' evolution. The body weight support was 50% of the patient weight at the beginning of the protocol treatment, which was gradually reduced until a minimum of 10% at the end the protocol training.

2.4. Statistical Analysis. All parametric results are illustrated as the mean ± standard deviation for each group in the tables and text. A level of significance of $P < 0.05$ was accepted for this study. The data were analyzed using change scores from pre- to posttraining with intragroup and between-group comparisons. Only data from subjects who completed the protocol training were used. The demographic characteristics (age and median onset time) were analyzed using the Mann–Whitney U test. Gender, the distribution of diagnosis, and side motor impairment were analyzed using the two-ratio test. The Wilcoxon test was used for intragroup comparisons, and the Mann–Whitney U test for between-group comparison. The data were analyzed using SPSS software V17, Minitab 16, and Excel Office 2010.

3. Results

A total of 19 patients were enrolled in this study from September 23, 2014, to December 20, 2015. The TAGT group contained 8 subjects. The RAGT group contained 11 subjects, of whom 4 were excluded for not complying with the protocol treatment criteria, leaving 7 subjects. The median age of all patients was 50.8 ± 13.3 years. The median onset time of all patients was 7.8 ± 4.8 years. The population studied was predominantly composed of hemorrhagic stroke patients ($P = 0.017$) (two-ratio test). The distribution of motor impairment side was homogeneous for both groups. The demographic distribution and baseline characteristics for each group are reported separately in Table 1.

After protocol treatment, both groups showed statistically significant improvement ($P < 0.05$) in balance, functional independence in daily living activities, and general ataxia sequela symptoms. Such betterment was evidenced by the intragroup comparison of all functional scales scores from pre- and posttreatment, which are described in Table 2.

Figure 1 shows the difference in the means of the SARA score for both TAGT and RAGT at baseline and after the conclusion of the protocol treatment. There was a significant improvement in the SARA score at the completion of the protocol training for both groups.

Although the two groups had different mean values for the functional scale scores (Table 2), there was no statistically significant difference for the between-group comparison at both baseline and after completion of the protocol treatment (BBS pre $P = 0.816$, post $P = 0.862$; TUG pre $P = 0.807$, post $P = 0.684$; FIM pre $P = 0.318$, post $P = 0.343$; and SARA pre $P = 0.817$, post: $P = 0.643$).

4. Discussion

In general, the major goal of a rehabilitation program is to improve gait capacity, which has been directly connected to the quality of life in poststroke patients [28]. Moreover, other frequently addressed complaints are postural instability and balance impairments, which are related to a loss in independence to perform activities of daily living [29].

Balance involves a range of motor skills that are directly connected to sensory-motor processes, functional contexts, and the environment [30]. Stroke is frequently associated with the impairment of these abilities. However, there are

TABLE 2: Outcome measures at baseline and after protocol treatment by intervention therapy.

Functional scale	Therapist-assisted		P value	Robot-assisted		P value
	Pre	Post		Pre	Post	
BBS	27.3 ± 10.8	35.5 ± 14.1	0.012*	26.6 ± 18.0	32.4 ± 18.8	0.018*
TUG	$0:28 \pm 0:11$	$0:22 \pm 0:10$	0.017*	$0:46 \pm 0.40$	$0:27 \pm 0:17$	0.011*
FIM	80.9 ± 9.6	85.4 ± 8.2	0.016*	73.9 ± 14.6	78.5 ± 12.9	0.042*
SARA	18.9 ± 6.8	15.4 ± 5.6	0.012*	18.7 ± 7.6	15.2 ± 6.8	0.018*

All values are shown as the mean ± SD. P value represents intragroup differences. *Requirement for a statistically significant difference: $P < 0.05$. The nonparametric Wilcoxon test was used to compare pre- and posttreatment measurements. BBS: Berg Balance Scale; TUG: Timed Up and Go Test reported in seconds; FIM: Functional Independence Measure; SARA: Scale Assessment and Rating of Ataxia.

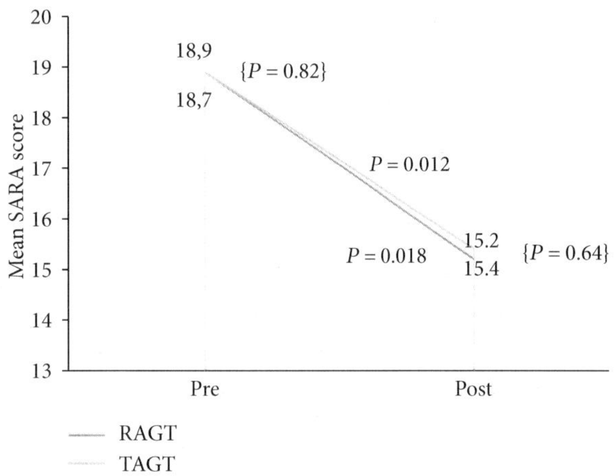

FIGURE 1: Changes in assessment and rating of ataxia. P value represents intragroup differences. Requirement for a statistically significant difference: $P < 0.05$. P value for between-group comparison: $\{P = 0.82; P = 0.64\}$. Requirement for a statistically significant difference: $P < 0.05$.

few studies that have reported the effect of RAGT on balance [18]. This research aimed to assess the influence of robot-assisted gait training on balance and to verify the functional independence in daily living activities of chronic stroke survivors with ataxia after at least one year of injury.

In the present study, we used the BBS and TUG tests to assess balance control. The results indicated a significant improvement in balance for both RAGT and TAGT groups. These findings agree with previous reports [18, 31, 32]. Furthermore, when the balance outcomes were compared between groups, that is, RAGT versus TAGT, no significant difference was demonstrated, which is also supported by several studies [18, 32–35]. In contrast, Dundar et al. showed greater improvement in balance for the group that received RAGT; their treatment protocol included patients with a stroke onset ranging from 28 days to 365 days, which differs from the current study that included only subjects with chronic stroke [22].

After the protocol treatment was completed, both RAGT and TAGT groups revealed a significant improvement in mean FIM scale results, which indicates that both strategies could be effective in improving independence in activities of daily living. Moreover, no significant difference was encountered when these outcomes were compared between groups. Tong et al. also compared the therapeutic effects of TAGT and RAGT interventions [32]. Our findings agree with regard to the improvement in general independence and the absence of significant differences for the intergroup comparison. On the contrary, other studies presented statistically superior improvement in general activities for the group that received RAGT [22, 28]. This discrepancy in the findings is still relatively unexplained and should be investigated further.

In the present study, an improvement in the SARA outcome measure after protocol treatment was observed in stroke patients with ataxia sequela, showing a better control in postural disorders. When the total SARA scores were compared between groups, there was no statistically significant difference. Only a few studies have focused on the assessment and rehabilitation treatment of ataxia disorders and have demonstrated the beneficial effects of rehabilitation programs [36, 37]. Although there are published investigations of different techniques, such as virtual reality, biofeedback, and treadmill exercise with or without body weight support [36–39], none have evaluated the effect of RAGT on chronic stroke patients with ataxia.

Gait ability is closely associated with balance control [40]. A systematic review concluded that RAGT may increase the chance of recovering independent walking ability in poststroke patients [22]. The greatest improvement in independent walking and walking speed was observed during the early months after stroke [22, 41].

A multicenter randomized clinical trial that compared RAGT with TAGT interventions in subjects affected by subacute stroke showed that TAGT rendered better outcomes for gait improvement [33]. Similarly, another comparative study showed greater improvements in overground walking speed in chronic stroke survivors who received TAGT [20].

In the last two decades, several studies have demonstrated different results regarding the effects of RAGT treatment for gait rehabilitation on poststroke individuals [14, 31, 33, 42, 43]. Robotic assistance is a valuable resource for recovering gait ability. Notwithstanding, only a few studies have investigated its effectiveness for balance recovery in chronic stroke survivors. Additionally, there is no published study that has specifically focused on treating ataxia with RAGT. This study has addressed this gap in knowledge and has contributed to the evidence that robotic therapy may also be an additional asset for the balance treatment of ataxic patients.

This study has some limitations. In particular, some limitations are related to the small sample size. Moreover, future studies should evaluate a longer follow-up time and patients in acute and subacute stroke phases. Additionally, we recommend that future studies should address the analysis of RAGT in larger samples with a comparative measurement and include patients in all stages of stroke. Furthermore, we also suggest the investigation of supplementary interventional methods to gain a comprehensive understanding of the balance control mechanism in ataxic patients.

5. Conclusions

This study concluded that chronic stroke patients with ataxia sequela had a significant improvement in balance and independence in activities of daily living after treatment with RAGT along with conventional therapy and home exercises. For this sample size, the outcomes were similar regardless of the applied treatment strategy, that is, RAGT or TAGT. Both treatment approaches should be included as options in balance rehabilitation programs for ataxic patients.

References

[1] A. Pennycott, D. Wyss, H. Vallery, V. Klamroth-Marganska, and R. Riener, "Towards more effective robotic gait training for stroke rehabilitation: a review," *Journal of NeuroEngineering and Rehabilitation*, vol. 9, no. 1, pp. 65–13, 2012.

[2] D. Lloyd-Jones, R. J. Adams, T. M. Brown et al., "Executive summary: heart disease and stroke statistics-2010 update: a report from the American heart association," *Circulation*, vol. 121, no. 7, pp. 948–954, 2010.

[3] U. Bultmann, D. Pierscianek, E. R. Gizewski et al., "Functional recovery and rehabilitation of postural impairment and gait ataxia in patients with acute cerebellar stroke," *Gait & Posture*, vol. 39, no. 1, pp. 563–569, 2014.

[4] B. Husemann, F. Müller, C. Krewer, S. Heller, and E. Koenig, "Effects of locomotion training with assistance of a robot-driven gait orthosis in hemiparetic patients after stroke: a randomized controlled pilot study," *Stroke*, vol. 38, no. 2, pp. 349–354, 2007.

[5] C. Krishnan, D. Kotsapouikis, Y. Y. Dhaher, and W. Z. Rymer, "Reducing robotic guidance during robot-assisted gait training improves gait function: a case report on a stroke survivor," *Archives of Physical Medicine and Rehabilitation*, vol. 94, no. 6, pp. 1202–1206, 2013.

[6] B. Indredavik, G. Rohweder, E. Naalsund, and S. Lydersen, "Medical complications in a comprehensive stroke unit and an early supported discharge service," *Stroke*, vol. 39, no. 2, pp. 414–420, 2008.

[7] S. Bonnì, V. Ponzo, C. Caltagirone, and G. Koch, "Cerebellar theta burst stimulation in stroke patients with ataxia," *Functional Neurology*, vol. 29, no. 1, pp. 41–45, 2014.

[8] S. Maeshima, A. Osawa, Y. Miyazaki, H. Takeda, and N. Tanahashi, "Functional outcome in patients with pontine infarction after acute rehabilitation," *Neurological Sciences*, vol. 33, no. 4, pp. 759–764, 2012.

[9] S. Datar and A. A. Rabinstein, "Cerebellar hemorrhage," *Neurologic Clinics*, vol. 32, no. 4, pp. 993–1007, 2014.

[10] W. Ilg, H. Golla, P. Thier, and M. A. Giese, "Specific influences of cerebellar dysfunctions on gait," *Brain*, vol. 130, no. 3, pp. 786–798, 2007.

[11] S. M. Morton, Y.-W. Tseng, K. M. Zackowski, J. R. Daline, and A. J. Bastian, "Longitudinal tracking of gait and balance impairments in cerebellar disease," *Movement Disorders*, vol. 25, no. 12, pp. 1944–1952, 2010.

[12] Z. Sawacha, E. Carraro, P. Contessa, A. Guiotto, S. Masiero, and C. Cobelli, "Relationship between clinical and instrumental balance assessments in chronic post-stroke hemiparesis subjects," *Journal of NeuroEngineering and Rehabilitation*, vol. 10, no. 1, p. 95, 2013.

[13] S. Hesse, "Treadmill training with partial body weight support after stroke: a review," *NeuroRehabilitation*, vol. 23, no. 1, pp. 55–65, 2008.

[14] D. Y. Cho, S.-W. Park, M. J. Lee, D. S. Park, and E. J. Kim, "Effects of robot-assisted gait training on the balance and gait of chronic stroke patients: focus on dependent ambulators," *Journal of Physical Therapy Science*, vol. 27, no. 10, pp. 3053–3057, 2015.

[15] S. Kubota, Y. Nakata, K. Eguchi et al., "Feasibility of rehabilitation training with a newly developed wearable robot for patients with limited mobility," *Archives of Physical Medicine and Rehabilitation*, vol. 94, no. 6, pp. 1080–1087, 2013.

[16] S. Jezernik, G. Colombo, T. Keller, H. Frueh, and M. Morari, "Robotic orthosis lokomat: a rehabilitation and research tool," *Neuromodulation: Technology at the Neural Interface*, vol. 6, no. 2, pp. 108–115, 2003.

[17] L. Wallard, G. Dietrich, Y. Kerlirzin, and J. Bredin, "Effects of robotic gait rehabilitation on biomechanical parameters in the chronic hemiplegic patients," *Neurophysiologie Clinique/Clinical Neurophysiology*, vol. 45, no. 3, pp. 215–219, 2015.

[18] E. Swinnen, D. Beckwée, R. Meeusen, J.-P. Baeyens, and E. Kerckhofs, "Does robot-assisted gait rehabilitation improve balance in stroke patients? A systematic review," *Topics in Stroke Rehabilitation*, vol. 21, no. 2, pp. 87–100, 2014.

[19] C. Tefertiller, B. Pharo, N. Evans, and P. Winchester, "Efficacy of rehabilitation robotics for walking training in neurological disorders: a review," *Journal of Rehabilitation Research & Development*, vol. 48, no. 4, pp. 387–416, 2011.

[20] T. G. Hornby, D. D. Campbell, J. H. Kahn, T. Demott, J. L. Moore, and H. R. Roth, "Enhanced gait-related improvements after therapist-versus robotic-assisted locomotor training in subjects with chronic stroke: a randomized controlled study," *Stroke*, vol. 39, no. 6, pp. 1786–1792, 2008.

[21] J. F. Israel, D. D. Campbell, J. H. Kahn, and T. G. Hornby, "Metabolic costs and muscle activity patterns during robotic- and therapist-assisted treadmill walking in individuals with incomplete spinal cord injury," *Physical Therapy*, vol. 86, no. 11, pp. 1466–1478, 2006.

[22] U. Dundar, H. Toktas, O. Solak, A. M. Ulasli, and S. Eroglu, "A comparative study of conventional physiotherapy versus robotic training combined with physiotherapy in patients with stroke," *Topics in Stoke Rehabilitation*, vol. 21, no. 6, pp. 453–461, 2014.

[23] S. T. Miyamoto, I. Lombardi Junior, K. O. Berg, L. R. Ramos, and J. Natour, "Brazilian version of the Berg balance scale," *Brazilian Journal of Medical and Biological Research*, vol. 37, no. 9, pp. 1411–1421, 2004.

[24] T. B. Hafsteinsdóttir, M. Rensink, and M. Schuurmans, "Clinimetric properties of the timed up and go test for patients with stroke: a systematic review," *Topics in Stroke Rehabilitation*, vol. 21, no. 3, pp. 197–210, 2014.

[25] B.-R. Kim, J.-Y. Lee, M. J. Kim, H. Jung, and J. Lee, "Korean version of the scale for the assessment and rating of ataxia in ataxic stroke patients," *Annals of Rehabilitation Medicine*, vol. 38, no. 6, pp. 742–751, 2014.

[26] B.-R. Kim, J.-H. Lim, S. A. Lee et al., "Usefulness of the scale for the assessment and rating of ataxia (SARA) in ataxic stroke patients," *Annals of Rehabilitation Medicine*, vol. 35, no. 6, pp. 772–780, 2011.

[27] P. Braga-Neto, C. Godeiro-Junior, L. A. Dutra, J. L. Pedroso, and O. G. P. Barsottini, "Translation and validation into Brazilian version of the scale of the assessment and rating of ataxia (SARA)," *Arquivos de Neuro-Psiquiatria*, vol. 68, no. 2, pp. 228–230, 2010.

[28] G. Taveggia, A. Borboni, C. Mulé, J. H. Villafañe, and S. Negrini, "Conflicting results of robot-assisted versus usual gait training during postacute rehabilitation of stroke patients: a randomized clinical trial," *International Journal of Rehabilitation Research*, vol. 39, no. 1, pp. 29–35, 2016.

[29] P. G. Lopes, J. A. F. Lopes, C. M. Brito, F. M. Alfieri, and L. Rizzo Battistella, "Relationships of balance, gait performance, and functional outcome in chronic stroke patients: a comparison of left and right lesions," *BioMed Research International*, vol. 2015, Article ID 716042, 8 pages, 2015.

[30] C. B. de Oliveira, I. R. de Medeiros, N. A. Frota, M. E. Greters, and A. B. Conforto, "Balance control in hemiparetic stroke patients: main tools for evaluation," *Journal of Rehabilitation Research & Development*, vol. 45, no. 8, pp. 1215–1226, 2008.

[31] L. Conesa, Ú. Costa, E. Morales et al., "An observational report of intensive robotic and manual gait training in sub-acute stroke," *Journal of NeuroEngineering and Rehabilitation*, vol. 9, no. 1, p. 13, 2012.

[32] R. K. Tong, M. F. Ng, and L. S. Li, "Effectiveness of gait training using an electromechanical gait trainer, with and without functional electric stimulation, in subacute stroke: a randomized controlled trial," *Archives of Physical Medicine and Rehabilitation*, vol. 87, no. 10, pp. 1298–1304, 2006.

[33] J. Hidler, D. Nichols, M. Pelliccio et al., "Multicenter randomized clinical trial evaluating the effectiveness of the lokomat in subacute stroke," *Neurorehabilitation and Neural Repair*, vol. 23, no. 1, pp. 5–13, 2009.

[34] D. Dias, J. Laíns, A. Pereira et al., "Can we improve gait skills in chronic hemiplegics? A randomised control trial with gait trainer," *Europa Medicophysica*, vol. 43, no. 4, pp. 499–504, 2007.

[35] M. F. W. Ng, R. K. Y. Tong, and L. S. W. Li, "A pilot study of randomized clinical controlled trial of gait training in subacute stroke patients with partial body-weight support electromechanical gait trainer and functional electrical stimulation: six-month follow-up," *Stroke*, vol. 39, no. 1, pp. 154–160, 2008.

[36] A. Marquer, G. Barbieri, and D. Pérennou, "The assessment and treatment of postural disorders in cerebellar ataxia: a systematic review," *Annals of Physical and Rehabilitation Medicine*, vol. 57, no. 2, pp. 67–78, 2014.

[37] K. Cernak, V. Stevens, R. Price, and A. Shumway-Cook, "Locomotor training using body-weight support on a treadmill in conjunction with ongoing physical therapy in a child with severe cerebellar ataxia," *Physical Therapy*, vol. 88, no. 1, pp. 88–97, 2007.

[38] J. E. Freund and D. M. Stetts, "Use of trunk stabilization and locomotor training in an adult with cerebellar ataxia: a single system design," *Physiotherapy Theory and Practice*, vol. 26, no. 7, pp. 447–458, 2010.

[39] D. V. Vaz, C. Schettino R de, T. R. Rolla de Castro, V. R. Teixeira, S. R. Cavalcanti Furtado, and E. de Mello Figueiredo, "Treadmill training for ataxic patients: a single-subject experimental design," *Clinical Rehabilitation*, vol. 22, no. 3, pp. 234–241, 2008.

[40] T. J. Kim, K. M. Seo, D.-K. Kim, and S. H. Kang, "The relationship between initial trunk performances and functional prognosis in patients with stroke," *Annals of Rehabilitation Medicine*, vol. 39, no. 1, pp. 66–73, 2015.

[41] J. Mehrholz, C. Werner, J. Kugler, and M. Pohl, "Electromechanical-assisted training for walking after stroke-review," *The Cochrane Collaboration*, no. 9, 2010.

[42] D. E. Uçar, N. Paker, and D. Buğdaycı, "Lokomat: a therapeutic chance for patients with chronic hemiplegia," *NeuroRehabilitation*, vol. 34, no. 3, pp. 447–453, 2014.

[43] B. H. Dobkin, "Progressive staging of pilot studies to improve phase III trials for motor interventions," *Neurorehabilitation and Neural Repair*, vol. 23, no. 3, pp. 197–206, 2009.

Effect of Voluntary Wheel Running on Striatal Dopamine Level and Neurocognitive Behaviors after Molar Loss in Rats

Linlin Zhang,[1] Yi Feng,[2] Wenliang Ji,[1] Jianzhang Liu,[3] and Kun Liu[1,4]

[1]*Capital University of Physical Education and Sports, Beijing 100191, China*
[2]*Beijing Xicheng District Desheng Community Health Service Center, Beijing 100120, China*
[3]*Peking University School and Hospital of Stomatology, Beijing 100081, China*
[4]*Department of Psychiatry, Yale University School of Medicine, New Haven, CT 06511, USA*

Correspondence should be addressed to Jianzhang Liu; liujianzhang@bjmu.edu.cn and Kun Liu; kun.liu@yale.edu

Linlin Zhang and Yi Feng contributed equally to this work.

Academic Editor: Francesca Trojsi

The aim of the present study is to evaluate the effect of voluntary wheel running on striatal dopamine level and behavior of cognition and emotion in molar loss rats. Twenty-four Sprague-Dawley rats were enrolled in this study and randomly divided into following 4 groups: control group (C group), molar loss group (ML group), 1-week physical exercise before molar loss group (1W-ML group), and 4-week physical exercise before molar loss group (4W-ML group). The rats both in 4W-ML and 1W-ML groups were placed in the voluntary running wheel in order to exercise for 4 weeks and 1 week, respectively. Then, the rats in 4W-ML, 1W-M, and ML groups received bilateral molar loss operation. After 10 days, striatal dopamine level was detected by in vivo microdialysis coupled with high-performance liquid chromatography (HPLC) and electrochemical detection. All the rats received behavior test after microdialysis detection. The behavior tests including passive avoidance test were used to assess cognition and elevated plus maze test for emotion. The results indicated that voluntary wheel running promoted striatal dopamine level in rats of molar loss. Behavioral data indicated that voluntary wheel running promoted cognition and emotion recovery after molar loss. Therefore, we concluded physical exercise significantly improved the neurocognitive behaviors and increased the striatal dopamine level after molar loss in rats.

1. Introduction

It is well established that tooth loss is a known risk factor of Alzheimer's disease (AD) [1]. As a common disorder in senior population, loss of teeth could adversely affect human cognition and emotion [2, 3]. Clinical medicine has established that tooth loss in patients can induce neuronal cell loss and memory impairment [4, 5]. Animal research also demonstrated that molar loss can cause the functional deterioration of cognition [6]. Previous studies have demonstrated that the rat with molar loss broke the balance of the cholinergic neuronal system and caused the impairment of cognition [7]. In addition, a preliminary quantitative study revealed that wide range of emotional effects was caused by tooth loss, such as loss of self-confidence and anxiety [8]. Further studies have shown that physical exercise, aerobic fitness exercise in particularly, had a positive effect on multiple aspects of brain function [9–11]. Neurochemistry studies indicated that physical exercise increased the antioxidant ability and glucose level to enhance cognition and emotion [12–14]. Neurobiology research also confirmed that aerobic exercise predominately employed the action of BDNF and the new growth of synaptic plasticity [15–17]. In addition, dopamine acts as a classic neurotransmitter in the brain, which plays an important role in cognitive and emotive aspects [18–20]. Numerous studies have shown that dopamine degeneration caused significant alteration in cognitive and emotive function by medicating striatal dopamine pathways [21-22]. Striatum is one of the four major dopamine pathways in the brain, partially involved in reward and in the reinforcement of memory consolidation. Degeneration of dopamine-producing neurons in striatum complex leads to diminished concentrations of dopamine in the nigrostriatal pathway, leading to reduce function and the characteristic symptoms, such as motor ability and cognitive impairment [23–25]. Therefore, this study was designed to explore the effect of voluntary wheel running on striatal dopamine level and neurocognitive behaviors after molar loss in rats. These findings may provide a theoretical basis for the clinical prevention of Alzheimer's disease.

2. Materials and Methods

2.1. Animals. Adult male Sprague-Dawley rats (3 months of age, weighting 300 ± 50 g at the time of surgery) were obtained from Experimental Animal Center of Peking University. Rats ($n = 24$) were enrolled in this study and randomly divided into following 4 groups: control group (C group, $n = 6$), molar loss group (ML group, $n = 6$), 1-week physical exercise before molar loss group (1W-ML group, $n = 6$), and 4-week physical exercise before molar loss group (4W-ML group, $n = 6$). The rats in both 4W-ML and 1W-ML groups were placed in the voluntary running wheel in order to exercise for 4 weeks or 1 week. Then, the rats in 4W-ML, 1W-ML, and ML groups received bilateral molar loss operation. In the C group, bilateral maxillary molar teeth remained intact. All rats were housed under 12 h light/dark cycle and had a sufficient amount of food and water.

2.2. Voluntary Wheel Running. The rats in both 4W-ML and 1W-ML groups received voluntary wheel running. Two rat groups were given free access to running wheels (wheel circumference, 100 cm; Harvard Apparatus) in their cages for 4 weeks or 1 week. A magnetic counter was installed to the running wheel in order to record wheel revolutions [26]. The distance was obtained by wheel revolutions multiplied by the circumference of the wheel. Those rats that cannot adapt new circumstances will be removed.

2.3. Molar Loss Surgery. Bilateral maxillary molar teeth were extracted from rats in the 4W-ML, 1W-ML, and ML groups after being anesthetized with chloral hydrate (350 mg/kg, i.p.). The rats in the C group were anesthetized, but no teeth were extracted. To provide a suitable recovery time after teeth extraction, experimental dentures were fitted to rats. Experimental dentures were produced from an impression made of silicone impression material and a resin tray. Occlusal adjustments were made until maxillomandibular incisor contacts were obtained [27].

2.4. In Vivo Microdialysis and High-Performance Liquid Chromatography. In vivo microdialysis was performed by implanting microdialysis probe into the striatum through the guide cannula by continuously perfusing with artificial cerebrospinal fluid (126 mM NaCl, 2.4 mM KCl, 1.1 mM $CaCl_2$, 0.85 mM $MgCl_2$, 27.5 mM $NaHCO_3$, 0.5 mM Na_2SO_4, and 0.5 mM KH_2PO_4, pH = 7.0) at a flow rate of 2 μL/min driven by a microinjection pump (CMA/100, CMA Microdialysis AB, Stockholm, Sweden). After 90 min, microdialysate in the striatum were collected for 60 minutes; each sample was collected in a 250 μL tubes for 10 min for a total of 6 tubes. Each tube was placed in an ice box containing 15 L of 10 mmol

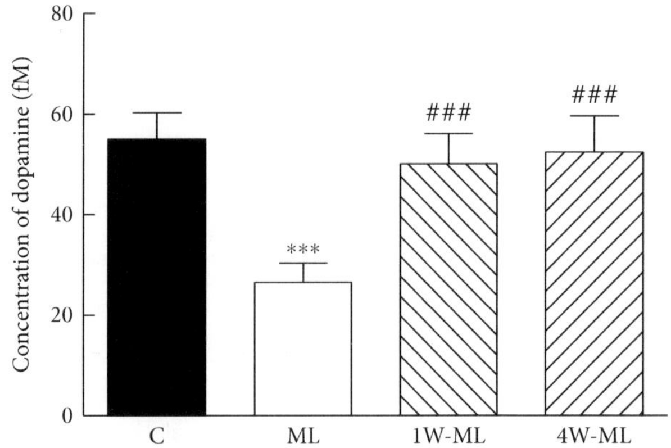

FIGURE 1: Dynamic changes of striatal dopamine level in each group. $^{***}P < 0.01$ compared with C group. $^{###}P < 0.01$ compared with ML group.

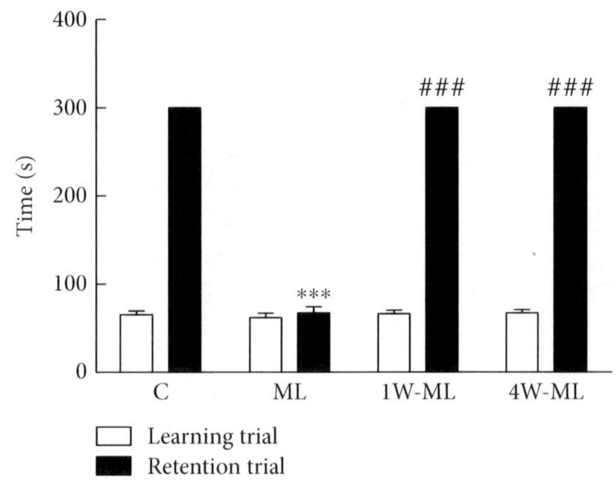

FIGURE 2: The latency time of rats in learning trial and retention trial. $^{***}P < 0.001$ compared with C group. $^{###}P < 0.01$ compared with ML group.

HCL. Then, dopamine level in the samples was measured using HPLC with electrochemical detection. The flow rate of the mobile phase (50 mM NaH_2PO_3, 2 mM decanesulfonic acid, 0.7 mM ethylenediaminetetraacetic acid, 11% *v*/*v* acetonitrile, and 11% *v*/*v* methanol, pH = 6.0) was 1 μL/min.

2.5. Passive Avoidance Test. Cognitive function was assessed by passive avoidance test [28]. After the learning trail, the retention test was measured 24 h after the learning trial. Each animal was put in an illuminated compartment, and the door opened after 2 minutes. Latency to enter the dark compartment was recorded to a maximum of 300 s. Animals that did not enter the dark chamber during the retention test were allotted a latency of 300 s [29].

2.6. Elevated Plus Maze Test. Emotion was assessed by elevated plus maze test [30]. The elevated plus maze was made of plastic and consisted of two white open arms (25 × 8 cm), two black enclosed arms (25 × 8 × 20 cm), and a central platform (8 × 8 × 8 cm) in the form of a cross. The maze was placed 50 cm above the floor. Rats were individually placed in the center with their heads directed toward one of the closed arms. The total time spent in each arm or in the

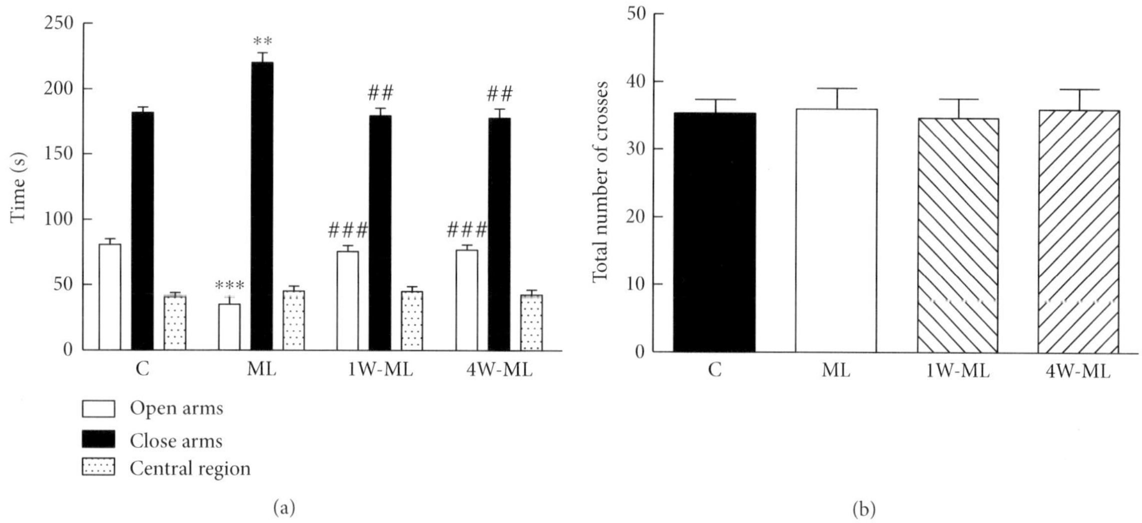

FIGURE 3: (a) Time spent of four rat groups in each arm. $^{***}P < 0.001$ and $^{**}P < 0.01$ compared with C group. $^{\#\#\#}P < 0.001$ and $^{\#\#}P < 0.01$ compared with ML group. (b) Total number of crosses in each group.

center and the total number of entries into each arm were analyzed by video monitoring for 5 min. After 5 min, rats were removed from the maze and returned to their home cage. The maze was then cleaned with a solution of 70% ethyl alcohol and permitted to dry between tests [31].

2.7. Statistical Analysis. Data were analyzed by GraphPad Prism 5. A two-way analysis of variance (ANOVA) was used to analyze the data. The comparison of cognition and emotion was made with two-tailed Student's t test.

3. Results

3.1. Dynamic Changes of Striatal Dopamine Level in Each Group. Figure 1 shows dynamic changes of striatal dopamine level in each group. The dopamine level in C, ML, 1W-ML, and 4W-ML groups was 55.02 ± 9.05 fmol, 26.48 ± 6.67 fmol, 50.01 ± 10.52 fmol, 52.34 ± 12.54 fmol, respectively. Compared with C group, the extracellular dopamine level of ML group significantly decreased ($P < 0.001$). Compared with ML group, the extracellular dopamine level of 1W-ML and 4W-ML group significantly increased ($P < 0.001$). However, the extracellular dopamine level has no significant difference between 1W-ML and 4W-ML groups ($P > 0.05$). The results indicated that 1-week or 4-week volunteer wheel running increased striatum dopamine level after molar loss.

3.2. Passive Avoidance Test. Figure 2 shows that the latency time of passive avoidance test in each group. In learning trial, the time in C, ML, 1W-ML, and 4W-ML group was 65.5 ± 11.89 s, 62 ± 13.41 s, 66.5 ± 8.56 s, and 67.5 ± 10.27 s and 300 s, 67.5 ± 16.69 s, 300 s, and 300 s in retention trial. There was no significant difference in the learning trial for each group ($P > 0.05$). Compared with C group, the retention time of ML group was significantly shorter ($P < 0.001$). Compared with ML group, the retention time of 1W-ML and 4W-ML groups was significantly longer ($P < 0.001$). However, the retention time has no significant difference between 1W-ML and 4W-ML groups ($P > 0.05$). The results indicated that 1-week and 4-week volunteer wheel running can promote cognition after molar loss.

3.3. Elevated Plus Maze Test. Figure 3(a) shows that the time spent of each rat groups in each arm. Compared with C group, the time spent of open arms in the ML group was significantly shorter ($P < 0.001$), adversely close arms ($P < 0.01$). Compared with ML group, the time spent of open arms in the 1W-ML and 4W-ML groups was significantly longer ($P < 0.001$), adversely close arms ($P < 0.01$). However, the time spent in each arm has no difference between 1W-ML and 4W-ML groups ($P > 0.05$). Meanwhile, there was no significant difference in the central region time for each group ($P > 0.05$). Figure 3(b) shows that total number of crosses in three groups. But there was no significant difference in the total number of crosses for each group ($P > 0.05$). The results indicated that 1-week or 4-week volunteer wheel running can promote emotion after molar loss.

4. Discussion

Alzheimer's disease (AD) can be considered as the most common cause of cognitive dysfunction among the aged, and tooth loss might be a risk factor for Alzheimer-type dementia [32–34]. New advances have shown that tooth loss caused the decline of cognition [35–37]. Previous research used passive avoid test to evaluate cognition, which shows that molar loss may cause accumulation of the amyloid cascade in the brain that leads to cognitive impairment [38]. Thus, we chose passive avoidance test to assess cognition in rats. We also choose elevated plus maze test to evaluate emotion. The results show that the cognition and emotion were worse after molar loss. Therefore, we successfully established the rat model of cognitive and emotive dysfunction after molar loss in this experiment. Previous study has shown that molar loss-induced cognitive and emotive impairments are related to neural cell loss [38-39]. In this study, we also demonstrated that molar loss-induced cognitive and emotive impairments are associated with the decrease of striatal dopamine level. Clinical studies have demonstrated that cognitive impairment had pathophysiology of dopamine system by the loss of midbrain neurons that synthesize the neurotransmitter dopamine [40-41]. Animal study also demonstrated that depression and anxiety might be associated with a specific loss of dopamine innervation in the limbic system [42]. Thus, it is reasonable to suggest that the decrease of striatal dopamine level can be one of the important reason of cognitive and emotive impairment after molar loss.

However, therapeutic strategies for the cognitive and emotive impairment after molar loss have not been well established so far. Molecular chemistry and biology highlight the promoted effect of physical exercise on cognition and emotion [43–45]. Some research has shown that exercise increased synaptic plasticity and the level of BGF and promoted cognition [46-47]. Other research also have shown that exercise can enhance cell proliferation, thereby alleviating anxiety-like behavior and improve emotion [48-49]. Especially, studies also indicated that physical exercise, voluntary wheel running in particularly, can be one of the best ways to promote cognition and emotion [50-51]. So, the present study chose voluntary wheel running as intervention approach. Our behavioral data indicated that voluntary wheel running promoted cognitive and emotive recovery after molar loss. As reported previously, physical exercise promoted the new growth of synaptic plasticity and the level of brain glucose and improve cognition and emotion thereafter [52–54]. In our research, we demonstrate that 4-week and 1-week voluntary wheel running promoted cognitive and emotive recovery after molar loss is associated with the increase of striatal dopamine level. Previous studies have demonstrated that physical exercise increased antioxidant defense and dopamine levels [55–57]. The increased dopamine level is related to recovery of cognitive and emotive impairments. Thus, we suggest that the increased of striatal dopamine level can be one of the reasons to induce that voluntary wheel running promotes cognition and emotion after molar loss in rats.

It is worth to mention that there was no difference between 4 weeks and 1 week of physical exercise-promoted cognition and emotion after molar loss in dopamine concentration aspect. Since previous research have found that small amount of physical exercise could be beneficial to cognitive function, it is reasonable that 1 week of physical exercise is enough to promote cognition and emotion after molar loss in dopamine concentration aspect. Although we did not find difference of dopamine level in striatum after 1 week and 4 weeks of physical exercise in our experiment condition, it is still possible that dopamine dynamic change in different brain regions could be induced by different physical exercise processes. In addition, whether there is difference in other aspects, such as other cognitive behavioral models or cellular levels, needs to be studied further.

5. Conclusions

Physical exercise significantly promoted the cognition and emotion in rats of molar loss by increasing the striatal dopamine level. However, it is necessary to further study other neurochemicals related to dopaminergic system to elucidate more underlying mechanisms of physical exercise-promoted cognition and emotion after molar loss.

Acknowledgments

The authors gratefully acknowledge the financial support by NSF of China (Grant no. 21475089), Innovation Platform of Beijing Municipality (PXM2015_014206_000053, PXM 2015_014206_000072, and PXM2015_014206_000051).

References

[1] Q. Pang, X. Hu, X. Li, J. Zhang, and Q. Jiang, "Behavioral impairments and changes of nitric oxide and inducible nitric oxide synthase in the brains of molarless KM mice," *Behavioural Brain Research*, vol. 278, pp. 411–416, 2015.

[2] K. J. Joshipura, C. W. Douglass, and W. C. Willett, "Possible explanations for the tooth loss and cardiovascular disease relationship," *Annals of Periodontology*, vol. 3, no. 1, pp. 175–183, 1998.

[3] J. Luo, B. Wu, Q. Zhao et al., "Association between tooth loss and cognitive function among 3063 Chinese older adults: a community-based study," *PLoS One*, vol. 10, no. 3, article e0120986, 2015.

[4] H. Nilsson, J. Berglund, and S. Renvert, "Tooth loss and cognitive functions among older adults," *Acta Odontologica Scandinavica*, vol. 72, no. 8, pp. 639–644, 2014.

[5] D. Lexomboon, M. Trulsson, I. Wårdh, and M. G. Parker, "Chewing ability and tooth loss: association with cognitive impairment in an elderly population study," *Journal of the American Geriatrics Society*, vol. 60, no. 10, pp. 1951–1956, 2012.

[6] K. Yamazaki, N. Wakabayashi, T. Kobayashi, and T. Suzuki, "Effect of tooth loss on spatial memory and TrkB-mRNA levels in rats," *Hippocampus*, vol. 18, no. 6, pp. 542–547, 2008.

[7] T. Kato, T. Usami, Y. Noda, M. Hasegawa, M. Ueda, and T. Nabeshima, "The effect of the loss of molar teeth on spatial memory and acetylcholine release from the parietal cortex in aged rats," *Behavioural Brain Research*, vol. 83, no. 1-2, pp. 239–242, 1997.

[8] D. Davis, J. Fiske, B. Scott, and D. R. Radford, "The emotional effects of tooth loss: a preliminary quantitative study," *British Dental Journal*, vol. 188, no. 09, pp. 503–506, 2000.

[9] C. H. Hillman, K. I. Erickson, and A. F. Kramer, "Be smart, exercise your heart: exercise effects on brain and cognition," *Nature Reviews Neuroscience*, vol. 9, no. 1, pp. 58–65, 2008.

[10] B. K. Tivadar, "Physical activity improves cognition: possible explanations," *Biogerontology*, vol. 18, no. 4, pp. 477–483, 2017.

[11] Z. Radak, S. Kumagai, A. W. Taylor, H. Naito, and S. Goto, "Effects of exercise on brain function: role of free radicals," *Applied Physiology, Nutrition, and Metabolism*, vol. 32, no. 5, pp. 942–946, 2007.

[12] N. Okudan and M. Belviranli, "Effects of exercise training on hepatic oxidative stress and antioxidant status in aged rats," *Archives of Physiology and Biochemistry*, vol. 122, no. 4, pp. 180–185, 2016.

[13] M. A. Moro, A. Almeida, J. P. Bolaños, and I. Lizasoain, "Mitochondrial respiratory chain and free radical generation in stroke," *Free Radical Biology & Medicine*, vol. 39, no. 10, pp. 1291–1304, 2005.

[14] F. T. A. Pijlman, G. Wolterink, and J. M. Van Ree, "Physical and emotional stress have differential effects on preference for saccharine and open field behaviour in rats," *Behavioural Brain Research*, vol. 139, no. 1-2, pp. 131–138, 2003.

[15] S. Vaynman, Z. Ying, and F. Gomez-Pinilla, "Hippocampal BDNF mediates the efficacy of exercise on synaptic plasticity and cognition," *European Journal of Neuroscience*, vol. 20, no. 10, pp. 2580–2590, 2004.

[16] C. H. Chae, H. C. Lee, S. L. Jung et al., "Swimming exercise increases the level of nerve growth factor and stimulates neurogenesis in adult rat hippocampus," *Neuroscience*, vol. 212, pp. 30–37, 2012.

[17] R. Šumec, P. Filip, K. Sheardová, and M. Bareš, "Psychological benefits of nonpharmacological methods aimed for improving balance in Parkinson's disease: a systematic review," *Behavioural Neurology*, vol. 2015, Article ID 620674, 16 pages, 2015.

[18] S. K. Mittal and C. Eddy, "The role of dopamine and glutamate modulation in Huntington disease," *Behavioural Neurology*, vol. 26, no. 4, pp. 255–263, 2013.

[19] A. Costa, A. Peppe, I. Mazzù, M. Longarzo, C. Caltagirone, and G. A. Carlesimo, "Dopamine treatment and cognitive functioning in individuals with Parkinson's disease: the "cognitive flexibility" hypothesis seems to work," *Behavioural Neurology*, vol. 2014, Article ID 260896, 11 pages, 2014.

[20] A. Venkatraman, B. L. Edlow, and M. H. Immordino-Yang, "The brainstem in emotion: a review," *Frontiers in Neuroanatomy*, vol. 11, p. 15, 2017.

[21] A. Nieoullon, "Dopamine and the regulation of cognition and attention," *Progress in Neurobiology*, vol. 67, no. 1, pp. 53–83, 2002.

[22] A. Nieoullon and A. Coquerel, "Dopamine: a key regulator to adapt action, emotion, motivation and cognition," *Current Opinion in Neurology*, vol. 16, Supplement 2, pp. S3–S9, 2003.

[23] R. A. Wise, "Roles for nigrostriatal—not just mesocorticolimbic—dopamine in reward and addiction," *Trends in Neurosciences*, vol. 32, no. 10, pp. 517–524, 2009.

[24] A. Gröger, R. Kolb, R. Schäfer, and U. Klose, "Dopamine reduction in the substantia nigra of Parkinson's disease patients confirmed by in vivo magnetic resonance spectroscopic imaging," *PLoS One*, vol. 9, no. 1, article e84081, 2014.

[25] D. Wang, X. Liu, and D. Qiao, "Modulatory effect of subthalamic nucleus on the development of fatigue during exhausting exercise: an in vivo electrophysiological and microdialysis study in rats," *Journal of Sports Science & Medicine*, vol. 11, no. 2, pp. 286–293, 2012.

[26] S. Fediuc, J. E. Campbell, and M. C. Riddell, "Effect of voluntary wheel running on circadian corticosterone release and on HPA axis responsiveness to restraint stress in Sprague-Dawley rats," *Journal of Applied Physiology*, vol. 100, no. 6, pp. 1867–1875, 2006.

[27] S. Iida, T. Hara, D. Araki et al., "Memory-related gene expression profile of the male rat hippocampus induced by teeth extraction and occlusal support recovery," *Archives of Oral Biology*, vol. 59, no. 2, pp. 133–141, 2014.

[28] O. Y. Calhan and V. Seyrantepe, "Mice with catalytically inactive cathepsin a display neurobehavioral alterations," *Behavioural Neurology*, vol. 2017, Article ID 4261873, 11 pages, 2017.

[29] M. Tahamtan, M. Allahtavakoli, M. Abbasnejad et al., "Exercise preconditioning improves behavioral functions following transient cerebral ischemia induced by 4-vessel occlusion (4-VO) in rats," *Archives of Iranian Medicine*, vol. 16, no. 12, pp. 697–704, 2013.

[30] L. L. Furlanetti, M. D. Döbrössy, I. A. Aranda, and V. A. Coenen, "Feasibility and safety of continuous and chronic bilateral deep brain stimulation of the medial forebrain bundle in the naïve Sprague-Dawley rat," *Behavioural Neurology*, vol. 2015, Article ID 256196, 13 pages, 2015.

[31] D. B. Pahaye, E. N. Bum, G. S. Taïwé et al., "Neuroprotective and antiamnesic effects of Mitragyna inermis willd (Rubiaceae) on scopolamine-induced memory impairment in mice," *Behavioural Neurology*, vol. 2017, Article ID 5952897, 11 pages, 2017.

[32] C. Jenner, G. Reali, M. Puopolo, and M. C. Silveri, "Can cognitive and behavioural disorders differentiate frontal variant-frontotemporal dementia from Alzheimer's disease at early stages?," *Behavioural Neurology*, vol. 17, no. 2, pp. 89–95, 2006.

[33] S. Sil and T. Ghosh, "Cox-2 plays a vital role in the impaired anxiety like behavior in colchicine induced rat model of Alzheimer disease," *Behavioural Neurology*, vol. 2016, Article ID 1501527, 8 pages, 2016.

[34] B. C. Dickerson and R. A. Sperling, "Large-scale functional brain network abnormalities in Alzheimer's disease: insights from functional neuroimaging," *Behavioural Neurology*, vol. 21, no. 1-2, pp. 63–75, 2009.

[35] X. Xu, B. Cao, J. Wang, T. Yu, and Y. Li, "Decision-making deficits associated with disrupted synchronization between basolateral amygdala and anterior cingulate cortex in rats after tooth loss," *Progress in Neuro-Psychopharmacology and Biological Psychiatry*, vol. 60, pp. 26–35, 2015.

[36] E. J. Yang, U. Mahmood, H. Kim et al., "Alterations in protein phosphorylation in the amygdala of the 5XFamilial Alzheimer's disease animal model," *Journal of Pharmacological Sciences*, vol. 133, no. 4, pp. 261–267, 2017.

[37] M. Onozuka, K. Watanabe, S. Nagasaki et al., "Impairment of spatial memory and changes in astroglial responsiveness following loss of molar teeth in aged SAMP8 mice," *Behavioural Brain Research*, vol. 108, no. 2, pp. 145–155, 2000.

[38] H. Oue, Y. Miyamoto, S. Okada et al., "Tooth loss induces memory impairment and neuronal cell loss in APP transgenic mice," *Behavioural Brain Research*, vol. 252, pp. 318–325, 2013.

[39] S. Sakamoto, T. Hara, A. Kurozumi et al., "Effect of occlusal rehabilitation on spatial memory and hippocampal neurons after long-term loss of molars in rats," *Journal of Oral Rehabilitation*, vol. 41, no. 10, pp. 715–722, 2014.

[40] L. Bäckman, L. Nyberg, U. Lindenberger, S. C. Li, and L. Farde, "The correlative triad among aging, dopamine, and cognition:

current status and future prospects," *Neuroscience & Biobehavioral Reviews*, vol. 30, no. 6, pp. 791–807, 2006.

[41] J. H. Kim, J. M. Auerbach, J. A. Rodríguez-Gómez et al., "Dopamine neurons derived from embryonic stem cells function in an animal model of Parkinson's disease," *Nature*, vol. 418, no. 6893, pp. 50–56, 2002.

[42] P. Remy, M. Doder, A. Lees, N. Turjanski, and D. Brooks, "Depression in Parkinson's disease: loss of dopamine and noradrenaline innervation in the limbic system," *Brain*, vol. 128, no. 6, pp. 1314–1322, 2005.

[43] J. J. Annesi, "Effects of minimal exercise and cognitive behavior modification on adherence, emotion change, self-image, and physical change in obese women," *Perceptual and Motor Skills*, vol. 91, no. 1, pp. 322–336, 2000.

[44] F. Nozariyan, P. Shafiniya, V. Shahvali, and M. A. Makiyani, "Emotion changes during exercise in males' physical education student," vol. 9, 2016.

[45] T. Nozawa, Y. Taki, A. Kanno et al., "Effects of different types of cognitive training on cognitive function, brain structure, and driving safety in senior daily drivers: a pilot study," *Behavioural Neurology*, vol. 2015, Article ID 525901, 18 pages, 2015.

[46] A. S. Aguiar Jr., A. A. Castro, E. L. Moreira et al., "Short bouts of mild-intensity physical exercise improve spatial learning and memory in aging rats: involvement of hippocampal plasticity via AKT, CREB and BDNF signaling," *Mechanisms of Ageing and Development*, vol. 132, no. 11-12, pp. 560–567, 2011.

[47] T. Kobila, Q. R. Liu, K. Gandhi, M. Mughal, Y. Shaham, and H. van Praag, "Running is the neurogenic and neurotrophic stimulus in environmental enrichment," *Learning & Memory*, vol. 18, pp. 605–609, 2011.

[48] S. J. Lee, T. W. Kim, H. K. Park et al., "Postnatal treadmill exercise alleviates prenatal stress-induced anxiety in offspring rats by enhancing cell proliferation through 5-Hydroxytryptamine 1A receptor activation," *International Neurourology Journal*, vol. 20, Supplement 1, pp. S57–S64, 2016.

[49] E. E. Bernstein and R. J. McNally, "Acute aerobic exercise hastens emotional recovery from a subsequent stressor," *Health Psychology*, vol. 36, no. 6, pp. 560–567, 2017.

[50] X. Zhao, J. Aronowski, S. J. Liu et al., "Wheel-running modestly promotes functional recovery after a unilateral cortical lesion in rats," *Behavioural Neurology*, vol. 16, no. 1, pp. 41–49, 2005.

[51] Y. Lin, X. Lu, J. Dong et al., "Involuntary, forced and voluntary exercises equally attenuate neurocognitive deficits in vascular dementia by the BDNF–pCREB mediated pathway," *Neurochemical Research*, vol. 40, no. 9, pp. 1839–1848, 2015.

[52] M. C. Lee, M. Okamoto, Y. F. Liu et al., "Voluntary resistance running with short distance enhances spatial memory related to hippocampal BDNF signaling," *Journal of Applied Physiology*, vol. 113, no. 8, pp. 1260–1266, 2012.

[53] A. C. McKee, D. H. Daneshvar, V. E. Alvarez, and T. D. Stein, "The neuropathology of sport," *Acta Neuropathologica*, vol. 127, no. 1, pp. 29–51, 2014.

[54] X. Xiao, Q. Lin, W. L. Lo et al., "Cerebral reorganization in subacute stroke survivors after virtual reality-based training: a preliminary study," *Behavioural Neurology*, vol. 2017, Article ID 6261479, 8 pages, 2017.

[55] M. Harvey, K. Muir, I. Reeves et al., "Long term improvements in activities of daily living in patients with hemispatial neglect," *Behavioural Neurology*, vol. 23, no. 4, pp. 237–239, 2010.

[56] M. Asghar, L. George, and M. F. Lokhandwala, "Exercise decreases oxidative stress and inflammation and restores renal dopamine D1 receptor function in old rats," *American Journal of Physiology-Renal Physiology*, vol. 293, no. 3, pp. F914–F919, 2007.

[57] L. Pruimboom, C. L. Raison, and F. A. J. Muskiet, "Physical activity protects the human brain against metabolic stress induced by a postprandial and chronic inflammation," *Behavioural Neurology*, vol. 2015, Article ID 569869, 11 pages, 2015.

16

The Effect of Gentle Handling on Depressive-Like Behavior in Adult Male Mice: Considerations for Human and Rodent Interactions in the Laboratory

Caroline Neely,[1] **Christina Lane**,[2] **Julio Torres**,[2] **and Jane Flinn**[1]

[1]*Department of Psychology, George Mason University, 4400 University Drive, Fairfax, VA 22030, USA*
[2]*Interdisciplinary Program in Neuroscience, George Mason University, 4400 University Drive, Fairfax, VA 22030, USA*

Correspondence should be addressed to Caroline Neely; cneely3@masonlive.gmu.edu

Academic Editor: Christopher Grunseich

Environmental factors play a significant role in well-being of laboratory animals. Regulations and guidelines recommend, if not require, that stressors such as bright lighting, smells, and noises are eliminated or reduced to maximize animal well-being. A factor that is often overlooked is handling and how researchers interact with their animals. Researchers, lab assistants, and husbandry staff in animal facilities may use inconsistent handling methods when interacting with rodents, but humans should be considered a part of the animal's social environment. This study examined the effects of different handling techniques on depressive-like behavior, measured by the Porsolt forced swim test, in adult C57BL/6J male mice. The same two researchers handled the mice in a gentle, aggressive, or minimal (control) fashion over approximately two weeks prior to testing. The results demonstrated a beneficial effect of gentle handling: gentle handling reduced swimming immobility in the forced swim test compared to mice that were aggressively or minimally handled. We argue that gentle handling, rather than methodical handling, can foster a better relationship between the handlers and rodents. Although handling is not standardized across labs, consistent gentle handling allows for less challenging behavioral testing, better data collection, and overall improved animal welfare.

1. Introduction

Environmental conditions within an animal facility have great impact on the well-being of rodents used in behavioral experiments and can affect results, especially of tests that measure spontaneous behavior [1]. Regulations at animal facilities are dependent on certifications, institutional requirements, and the needs of individual principal investigators; however, most facilities follow recommendations, such as *The Guide* [2], that enforce ethical, valid, and scientific practices. Measures are taken in order to reduce or eliminate salient, unpleasant factors such as bright lighting [3–6], smells [1, 7–9], and loud noises [10] which negatively affect animal health.

An additional factor that may be considered a random implementation is handling prior to and/or during behavioral testing. Rodents are regarded as social animals [11–13], and social housing is recommended as standard care [2]. Care and handling become an integral part of an animal's routine [14, 15]; for example, rats can recognize humans and prefer to be with those that they know [16], but this has yet to be confirmed in mice. In light of these findings, personnel that perform care-related tasks and interact with laboratory animals should be considered a part of the animal's social experience. Lack of familiarity and relatedness among cagemates has been shown to induce stress [17] and aggression in mice, suggesting that unfamiliar experimenters may also provoke anxious, aggressive, or depressive-like states. Mice become less anxious and more receptive after multiple handling sessions by human caretakers but continue to show signs of escape [18]. What remains underreported is the description of quantity and quality of human-rodent social interactions [19], and how differences in handling affect animal's reactivity to human caretakers and overall behavior.

Lack of description of handling sessions may introduce experimenter error and bias [20]. For example, some experimenters may handle rodents in a gentle manner by permitting freedom of movement in the experimenter's hands or by preventing short-term tail suspension during cage changes. Criteria for what is considered gentle handling can vary from playful tickling of the rodent's back and stomach [21–23] to tapping or moving the homecage to maintain a state of arousal [24–26]. Using a playful handling technique, Costa et al. [23] demonstrated that this method reduced anxiety, improved cognitive behavior, and decreased norepinephrine secretion in rats. This study, however, measured the anxiolytic effects through increased entries into the open arm of an elevated plus maze. Other work has suggested that handling can be used as a substitute for social enrichment for animals that are individually housed due to aggression and/or illness. Cloutier and colleagues [21] demonstrated that social contact in the form of rough-and-tumble play for 2 minutes each day for 21 days reduced anxiety-related behavior and increased positive affective ultrasonic vocalizations of individually housed rats. This effect was also observed when researchers implemented the same rough-and-tumble play (through "tickling") in juvenile rats, which were then injected intraperitoneally with saline 40 to 50 days after play. Handling before and after injections, and especially when implemented during juvenile development, reduced stress calls during injections and increased positive affective ultrasonic vocalizations [22]. Other research groups may handle in a minimally or less gently fashion, and this may explain discrepancies often found in published literature concerning rodent models of anxiety or depression [18, 27–29]. These findings further strengthen the notion that handling procedures need to be standardized, if not reported in published literature, in order to reduce confounds in affective measures.

Anxiety and depression are considered to have relatively high comorbidity in both humans and animals [30–32]; thus, the same handling techniques that decrease anxiety in laboratory animals may also decrease depression. Handling can be short-term, beginning several days prior to or during behavioral testing, or it may begin during neonatal development. Neonatal handling increases maternal behavior in the form of increased licking and grooming of pups, which in turn reduces behavioral fearfulness in offspring postweaning [33–36]. What remains uncertain is whether or not handling beginning in late adulthood and lasting for several days, rather than continuous handling for several weeks/months beginning after weaning, can reduce depression and mimic the same effects observed in neonatal-handling studies. In this experiment, we operationally defined gentle, aggressive, and minimal handling and examined the different handling styles on depressive-like behavior in adult mice by using the forced swim test (FST). The FST is used to measure depressive behaviors in rodents [37]; in addition, it is used to assess manipulations in experimental procedures with the intention of curbing or altogether avoiding depressive states [38]. We conducted the FST in order to examine if aggressive handling caused depressive-like behavior and/or if gentle handling improved an animal's resiliency. We hypothesized that gentle handling of mice would increase latency before immobility and would decrease duration of immobility in the FST compared to the control group. We also hypothesized that aggressive handling would decrease latency before immobility and increase duration of immobility when compared to the control group. This study examined the importance of rodent-human social interactions which can impact an animal's performance across a broad spectrum of behaviors.

2. Methods

All procedures were approved by the George Mason University Institutional Animal Care and Use Committee and were carried out in accordance with the National Institutes of Health Guide for the Care and Use of Laboratory Animals.

2.1. Animals. Twenty-one adult 7.5-month-old ($N = 8$) and 10-month-old ($N = 13$) C57BL/6J male mice (Jackson Laboratories, Bar Harbor, ME) were provided for the study. These mice were excess mice donated from other projects within the testing facility, were raised in homecages for respective periods of time prior to testing, and were naïve to handling and other testing procedures for approximately 3 months. Animals were group-housed by age. Homecages were lined with TEKFresh bedding (Envigo, Indianapolis, IN) and contained a PVC pipe and nylabone as additional forms of enrichment. The colony was maintained on a 12-hour light/dark cycle (lights on at 8:00 a.m.) with unautoclaved 7012 diet feed (Envigo, Indianapolis, IN) and water offered ad libitum. Cages were washed and autoclaved once a week by husbandry staff.

2.2. Handling. Mice were separated into three groups: a gently handled condition, an aggressively handled condition, and a control condition (Table 1). Mice were handled in the housing room under a lit biosafety cabinet by the same two experimenters (C.L. and J.T.). The mice were handled over the course of 13 days, every other day, in the evening hours during the light cycle (12:00–8:00 p.m.). The gently handled and aggressively handled groups were handled for 90 seconds per session, whereas the control group was not handled by the researchers. The gently handled mice were individually removed from their homecages, placed in the palm of the experimenter's hand, and were stroked on the left and right flanks and head for 90 seconds. Researchers carefully but firmly held the base of the tail, permitting movement between their hands. The aggressively handled mice were individually removed from their homecages, grasped at the proximal end of their tails, and suspended in the air approximately 15 cm from the surface of a biosafety cabinet for 90 seconds. Care was taken so that the mice would not latch onto any surrounding equipment or attempt to grasp the experimenter's fingers. The control mice were handled only by husbandry staff during routine cage changes; in addition, the gently and aggressively handled mice were handled by husbandry staff during this time.

TABLE 1: Animal characteristics, by age and group.

Age	Gentle	Aggressive	Control
7.5 months	1	4	3
10 months	5	4	4
Total ($N = 21$)	6	8	7

2.3. Porsolt Forced Swim Test (FST). Mice were individually transported to the testing room where they habituated for 10 minutes prior to testing. Three mice were tested at a time and were separated by an opaque barrier to obstruct viewing of other mice. Mice were removed from their transport cages by the base of their tail and slowly placed into an inescapable transparent Plexiglas cylinder (47 × 38 cm) filled to a depth of 32 cm with tap water (25–27°C). Mice were placed and released into the water at the same time. Each mouse was given a single 6-minute trial. Researchers manually recorded latency until the first period of immobility (seconds) and total duration immobile (seconds). Immobility was defined as the period of time that the mouse was not swimming, when movement was only made in order to keep the body in balance or its head above water [30]. At the end of the 6-minute trial, mice were removed from the cylinders and carefully dried and returned to their transport cages under a heat lamp positioned approximately 30 cm above the cage. Water was changed, and temperature was taken for the next trial. All mice successfully completed the 6-minute trial.

2.4. Statistical Analysis. Data were analyzed using R version 3.3.1 [39]. Latency to first instance of immobility (seconds) and total duration of immobility (seconds) were subjected to Levene's test of equality of variances. Due to unequal, small sample sizes and violations of normality, data were subjected to the nonparametric Mann–Whitney-Wilcoxon rank sum test and Kruskal-Wallis H test using the *FSA* package [40]. Significant Kruskal-Wallis results were followed by Dunn-Bonferroni pairwise comparisons that adjusted for familywise type I error rate. Statistical results are reported as mean ranks. Data points were considered outliers if they were beyond 1.5 times the interquartile range. The results were considered statistically significant if $p < 0.05$ and marginally significant if $p < 0.10$. Original box plots with medians were constructed using *ggplot2* [41] and regraphed in Microsoft Excel (2016) for publication purposes.

3. Results

We first examined any potential differences between the 7.5-month-old mice ($N = 8$) and 10-month-old mice ($N = 13$). A Mann–Whitney-Wilcoxon test yielded no significant differences in duration of immobility, $W = 64.50$, $p = 0.38$, with mean rank durations of 12.56 for the 7.5-month-old mice and 10.04 seconds for the 10-month-old mice. Likewise, latency before immobility was not significantly different, $W = 60.50$, $p = 0.56$, with mean ranks of 12.06 for the 7.5-month-old mice and 10.35 seconds for the 10-month-old mice.

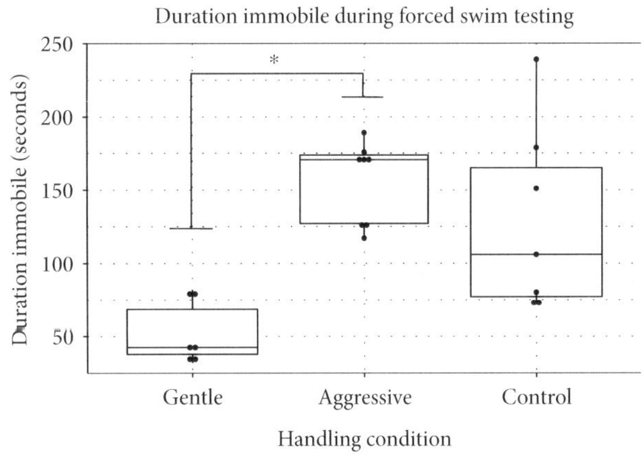

FIGURE 1: Duration immobile by handling group (gentle, aggressive, and control). The results demonstrate significant differences (∗) between the gently handled mice (median = 42.50 s) compared to the aggressively handled mice (median = 170.50 s) and marginally significant differences between the gently handled mice and control mice (median = 106.00 s). No differences were found between the aggressively handled and control mice. Box plots illustrate individual data points (solid dots), lower and upper quartiles (upper and lower sides of box plot), median (dark, middle bar), and lowest and highest values (whiskers).

We then examined the differences among the three handling conditions. A Kruskal-Wallis H test demonstrated a statistically significant difference in duration of immobility, $\chi^2(2) = 10.80$, $p = 0.004$, with a mean rank duration of 4.33, 15.25, and 11.86 seconds for the gentle, aggressive, and control groups, respectively (Figure 1). Pairwise comparisons showed a statistically significant difference between the gently (MR = 4.33 s) and aggressively handled (MR = 15.25 s) groups, $p = 0.003$, and marginally significant difference between the gentle and control (MR = 11.86 s) groups, $p = 0.088$. There were no statistical differences between the aggressive and control groups, $p = 0.872$. The proportion of variability for duration immobile accounted by the handling condition was approximately 54% (eta = 0.54), demonstrating a relatively strong effect of handling on depressive-like behaviors in the FST. Analyses on latency before immobility failed to yield statistically significant results, $\chi^2(2) = 2.071$, $p = 0.355$, with mean rank latencies of 14.00, 9.31, and 10.36 seconds for the gentle, aggressive, and control groups, respectively (Figure 2). The proportion of variability for latency accounted by the handling condition was approximately 10% (eta = 0.10). Overall, these data demonstrated that short-term, gentle handling decreases depressive-like behavior in the FST, in comparison to short-term, aggressive handling and handling by husbandry staff alone.

4. Discussion

The FST is a widely accepted method of examining the effectiveness of antidepressant pharmaceuticals and has been used to study other environmental manipulations. There is a large base of data measuring the effects of different pharmaceuticals on rodents and their performance in the FST [30];

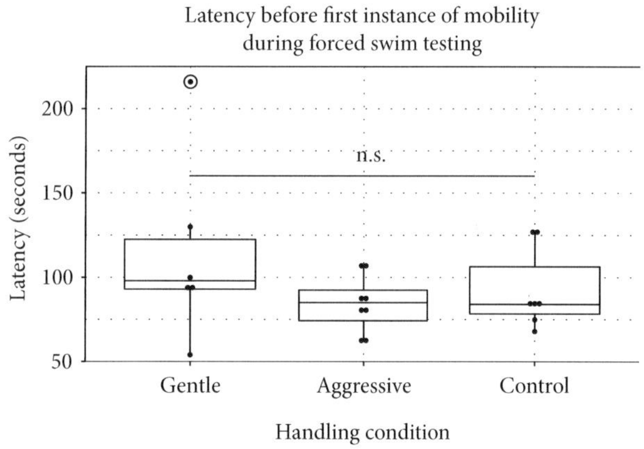

FIGURE 2: Latency prior to the first instance of immobility by the handling groups (gentle, aggressive, and control). There were no significant differences reported among conditions, with the gentle group showing the longest latency to immobility (median = 98.00 s), followed by the aggressive group (median = 85.00 s) and the control group (median = 84.00 s). Box plots illustrate the individual data points (solid dots), lower and upper quartiles (upper and lower sides of boxplot), median (dark, middle bar), and lowest and highest values (whiskers). An outlier is circled in the gently handled group.

however, the amount of data on the effects of handling on FST performance is not nearly as robust. We have demonstrated in this study that short-term gentle handling decreased depressive-like behavior in laboratory mice. The gently handled mice, as an overall group, demonstrated significantly less time immobile, indicating less depressive-like behavior. In comparison, the aggressively handled mice demonstrated the greatest duration immobile, indicating more depressive-like behavior. The control group, which was not handled except during routine husbandry procedures, performed intermediately compared to the gently and aggressively handled groups, showing greater duration immobile compared to the gently handled group. In addition, both methods of handling decreased variability in immobility in comparison to the control group (Figure 1). These data suggest that animals that had not been exposed to researchers prior to testing may react as if challenged by a mild stressor, or in the same way as if they have been aggressively handled.

Husbandry staff members were blind to handling conditions and handled all animals in the same fashion during routine cage changes; therefore, the lack of statistical difference between the aggressively handled and control groups cannot be accounted for by differences in husbandry staff's techniques. Exposure to husbandry staff, rather than exposure to the researcher performing testing, may not suffice for habituation to a human, especially if research concerns behavioral testing and affective-based measures. These results confirm that the way an animal is handled prior to or during behavioral testing can alter affective states. In addition, different handling techniques may be used for different testing procedures: gentle handling may provide a means of testing anxiolytic medications and the effects of stress, whereas aggressive handling may be a better method to detect the effects of antidepressant medications.

Handling has been extensively studied in younger animals, when the developing brain is susceptible to environmental stressors. It is understood that environmental enrichment and juvenile handling produces long-term neurobehavioral effects such as reduced anxiety [18] and improved spatial memory [42]. Handling, especially when implemented in early life and continued through adulthood, acclimatized rodents to human researchers and testing apparatuses. What is not extensively studied is whether handling in older mice can still mimic the benefits of prolonged handling seen in young, weaned mice. A challenge is that older mice may show age-related motor deficits. In this study, the older, 10-month-old mice swam longer (immobile for less time) compared to the 7.5-old mice but this difference was not significant (data not shown). Pooled analyses of 1800 C57BL/6J wild-type mice (independent of handling) showed that 6-7-month-old C57BL/6J mice swam longer than both 4-5-month and 2-3-month old mice in the forced swim test [43]. Other studies, however, have demonstrated an age-related degradation in general locomotion, strength, and endurance domains in mice [44] and swimming and sensitivity to antidepressant treatment in rats [45, 46] which could affect behavioral measures dependent on movement, such as the FST.

In this study, we were limited to the use of male mice, which were excess mice from breeding on other protocols that were kindly donated for behavioral testing. In neuroscientific research, there remains a strong sex bias with estimates suggesting that the use of male rodents in publications outnumber female rodents in a 5.5 to 1 ratio [47]. Research has emphasized that females are no more variable than males [48, 49], but the estrous cycle has been shown to affect responses to antidepressants [50–52]. A weakness of this experiment was that only males were included, which warrants the inclusion of female mice in future studies.

Research tends to favor handling-related behavioral changes in rats but not in mice. Handling in rats has been well studied possibly due to preference for the rat in experimental studies assessing learning and memory, beginning in the 1930s with the purposive behavioral work of Edward Tolman. Attention to mouse behavior has increased more recently due in large part to interest in transgenic mice [53, 54], with behavior often a secondary consideration. Rats have been said to be more sensitive than mice to issues of handling [55]; however, research has demonstrated that mice are also sensitive to types of handling and the presence of a researcher [56–58]. These findings, together with our research, further emphasize that mice should be handled prior to behavioral testing, and in such a way such that potential aggression towards cagemates and/or the researcher during testing does not impact the data obtained.

We handled over a period of two weeks with multiple sessions each week. Some studies do not report if animals were handled, the handling duration, and handling frequency. We note that our handling timeline is short term; however, a duration of two weeks may exceed what other labs consider adequate exposure to a researcher. A follow-up experiment from our lab examined how four consecutive days of gentle handling or husbandry only (i.e., control) handling prior to testing affected FST performance in 2-month-old mice. Although the gently handled mice displayed more resilient and less depressive-like behavior compared to the control group, these results were not significant (data not shown). Although there is no standard for handling, these data suggest that multiple handling sessions may be needed and that shorter time periods (e.g., 24 or 48 hours prior to testing) may not be suitable for habituating animals to researchers.

In conclusion, our study demonstrates the benefits of gentle handling of mice that undergo depression-based testing and shows that a gentle handling technique is effective when interacting with mice prior to and during behavioral testing. If implemented as the standard of care, handling can reduce the depressive symptoms in mice, improve the overall well-being of laboratory animals, produce more reliable data, and raise standards of care when using rodents as models for neuropsychiatric conditions.

Disclosure

At the time of the experiment, Christina Lane and Julio Torres were undergraduate students enrolled in C.N.'s laboratory methods course. Both Christina Lane and Julio Torres have stated that their expectations of their final grades did not influence the execution of the project and data collection. An earlier version of this work was presented as an abstract at the Society for Neuroscience conference in San Diego in November 2016 (see abstract 170.01). The data were also shared at two small George Mason University research symposiums in April and May of 2016.

Acknowledgments

The authors would like to thank the Department of Psychology and Department of Neuroscience for their support, husbandry staff for their assistance and caretaking in the animal facility, and Logan Woodhouse who assisted with data collection. The project was supported by the George Mason University Department of Psychology and the George Mason University Students as Scholars Program.

References

[1] R. M. J. Deacon, "Assessing nest building in mice," *Nature Protocols*, vol. 1, no. 3, pp. 1117–1119, 2006.

[2] National Research Council, *Guide for the Care and Use of Laboratory Animals: Eighth Edition*, National Academies Press, Washington, DC, 2011.

[3] T. A. Bedrosian, C. A. Vaughn, A. Galan, G. Daye, Z. M. Weil, and R. J. Nelson, "Nocturnal light exposure impairs affective responses in a wavelength-dependent manner," *Journal of Neuroscience*, vol. 33, no. 32, pp. 13081–13087, 2013.

[4] L. J. Bertoglio and A. P. Carobrez, "Behavioral profile of rats submitted to session 1-session 2 in the elevated plus-maze during diurnal/nocturnal phases and under different illumination conditions," *Behavioural Brain Research*, vol. 132, no. 2, pp. 135–143, 2002.

[5] E. Igarashi and S. Takeshita, "Effects of illumination and handling upon rat open field activity," *Physiology & Behavior*, vol. 57, no. 4, pp. 699–703, 1995.

[6] A. A. Walf and C. A. Frye, "The use of the elevated plus maze as an assay of anxiety-related behavior in rodents," *Nature Protocols*, vol. 2, no. 2, pp. 322–328, 2007.

[7] R. Hacquemand, N. Choffat, L. Jacquot, and G. Brand, "Comparison between low doses of TMT and cat odor exposure in anxiety- and fear-related behaviors in mice," *Behavioural Brain Research*, vol. 238, pp. 227–231, 2013.

[8] R. E. Sorge, L. J. Martin, K. A. Isbester et al., "Olfactory exposure to males, including men, causes stress and related analgesia in rodents," *Nature Methods*, vol. 11, no. 6, pp. 629–632, 2014.

[9] K. E. A. Wernecke, D. Vincenz, S. Storsberg, W. D'Hanis, J. Goldschmidt, and M. Fendt, "Fox urine exposure induces avoidance behavior in rats and activates the amygdalar olfactory cortex," *Behavioural Brain Research*, vol. 279, pp. 76–81, 2015.

[10] S. L. Uran, L. G. Caceres, and L. R. Guelman, "Effects of loud noise on hippocampal and cerebellar-related behaviors," *Brain Research*, vol. 1361, pp. 102–114, 2010.

[11] H. Arakawa, D. C. Blanchard, K. Arakawa, C. Dunlap, and R. J. Blanchard, "Scent marking behavior as an odorant communication in mice," *Neuroscience & Biobehavioral Reviews*, vol. 32, no. 7, pp. 1236–1248, 2008.

[12] J. L. Silverman, M. Yang, C. Lord, and J. N. Crawley, "Behavioural phenotyping assays for mouse models of autism," *Nature Reviews Neuroscience*, vol. 11, no. 7, pp. 490–502, 2010.

[13] M. L. Terranova and G. Laviola, "Scoring of social interactions and play in mice during adolescence," *Current Protocols in Toxicology*, 2005.

[14] A. M. Claxton, "The potential of the human–animal relationship as an environmental enrichment for the welfare of zoo-housed animals," *Applied Animal Behavior Science*, vol. 133, no. 1-2, pp. 1–10, 2011.

[15] T. C. Krohn, D. B. Sørensen, J. L. Ottesen, and A. K. Hansen, "The effects of individual housing on mice and rats: a review," *Laboratory Animals*, vol. 36, pp. 209–212, 2006.

[16] H. Davis, "Prediction and preparation: Pavlovian implications of research animals discriminating among humans," *ILAR Journal*, vol. 43, no. 1, pp. 19–26, 2002.

[17] A. Bartolomucci, P. Palanza, and S. Parmigiani, "Group housed mice: are they really stressed?," *Ethology Ecology & Evolution*, vol. 14, no. 4, pp. 341–350, 2002.

[18] J. L. Hurst and R. S. West, "Taming anxiety in laboratory mice," *Nature Methods*, vol. 7, no. 10, pp. 825-826, 2010.

[19] E. M. Spangenberg and L. J. Keeling, "Assessing the welfare of laboratory mice in their home environment using animal-based measures – a benchmarking tool," *Laboratory Animals*, vol. 50, no. 1, pp. 30–38, 2015.

[20] M. Bohlen, E. R. Hayes, B. Bohlen, J. D. Bailoo, J. C. Crabbe, and D. Wahlsten, "Experimenter effects on behavioral test scores of eight inbred mouse strains under the influence of ethanol," *Behavioural Brain Research*, vol. 272, pp. 46–54, 2014.

[21] S. Cloutier, J. Panksepp, and R. C. Newberry, "Playful handling by caretakers reduces fear of humans in the laboratory rat," *Applied Animal Behaviour Science*, vol. 140, no. 3-4, pp. 161–171, 2012.

[22] S. Cloutier, K. Wahl, C. Baker, and R. C. Newberry, "The social buffering effect of playful handling on responses to repeated

intraperitoneal injections in laboratory rats," *Journal of the American Association for Laboratory Animal Science*, vol. 53, no. 2, pp. 168–173, 2014.

[23] R. Costa, M. L. Tamascia, M. D. Nogueira, D. E. Casarini, and F. K. Marcondes, "Handling of adolescent rats improves learning and memory and decreases anxiety," *Journal of the American Association for Laboratory Animal Science*, vol. 51, no. 5, pp. 548–553, 2012.

[24] K. Gärtner, D. Büttner, K. Döhler, R. Friedel, J. Lindena, and I. Trautschold, "Stress response of rats to handling and experimental procedures," *Laboratory Animals*, vol. 14, no. 3, pp. 267–274, 1980.

[25] F. Longordo, J. Fan, T. Steimer, C. Kopp, and A. Lüthi, "Do mice habituate to "gentle handling?" A comparison of resting behavior, corticosterone levels and synaptic function in handled and undisturbed C57BL/6J mice," *Sleep*, vol. 34, no. 5, pp. 679–681, 2011.

[26] C. G. Vecsey, L. Peixoto, J. H. K. Choi et al., "Genomic analysis of sleep deprivation reveals translational regulation in the hippocampus," *Physiological Genomics*, vol. 44, no. 20, pp. 981–991, 2012.

[27] J. Burgdorf and J. Panksepp, "Tickling induces reward in adolescent rats," *Physiology and Behavior*, vol. 72, no. 1-2, pp. 167–173, 2001.

[28] M. Meaney, D. H. Aitken, C. van Berkel, S. Bhatnagar, and R. M. Sapolsky, "Effect of neonatal handling on age-related impairments associated with the hippocampus," *Science*, vol. 239, no. 4841, pp. 766–768, 1988.

[29] M. K. Meijer, R. Sommer, B. M. Spruijt, L. F. M. Van Zutphen, and V. Baumans, "Influence of environmental enrichment and handling on the acute stress response in individually housed mice," *Laboratory Animals*, vol. 41, no. 2, pp. 161–173, 2007.

[30] B. N. Gaynes, A. J. Rush, M. H. Trivedi et al., "Major depression symptoms in primary care and psychiatric care settings: a cross-sectional analysis," *The Annals of Family Medicine*, vol. 5, no. 2, pp. 126–134, 2007.

[31] S. H. Kennedy, "Core symptoms of major depressive disorder: relevance to diagnosis and treatment," *Dialogues in Clinical Neuroscience*, vol. 10, no. 3, pp. 271–277, 2008.

[32] D. A. Regier, D. S. Rae, W. E. Narrow, C. T. Kaelber, and A. F. Schatzberg, "Prevalence of anxiety disorders and their comorbidity with mood and addictive disorders," *British Journal of Psychiatry*, vol. 173, no. 34, pp. 24–28, 1998.

[33] C. Caldji, B. Tannenbaum, S. Sharma, D. Francis, P. M. Plotsky, and M. J. Meaney, "Maternal care during infancy regulates the development of neural systems mediating the expression of fearfulness in the rat," *Proceedings of the National Academy of Sciences of the United States of America*, vol. 95, no. 9, pp. 5335–5340, 1998.

[34] V. H. Denenberg, "Commentary: is maternal stimulation the mediator of the handling effect in infancy?," *Developmental Psychobiology*, vol. 34, no. 1, pp. 1–3, 1999.

[35] D. Liu, J. Diorio, B. Tannenbaum et al., "Maternal care, hippocampal glucocorticoid receptors, and hypothalamic-pituitary-adrenal responses to stress," *Science*, vol. 277, no. 5332, pp. 1659–1662, 1997.

[36] A. R. Reis, M. S. de Azevedo, M. A. de Souza et al., "Neonatal handling alters the structure of maternal behavior and affects mother–pup bonding," *Behavioural Brain Research*, vol. 265, pp. 216–228, 2014.

[37] R. D. Porsolt, M. Le Pichon, and M. L. Jalfre, "Depression: a new animal model sensitive to antidepressant treatments," *Nature*, vol. 266, no. 5604, pp. 730–732, 1977.

[38] A. Can, D. T. Dao, M. Arad, C. E. Terrillion, S. C. Piantadosi, and T. D. Gould, "The mouse forced swim test," *Journal of Visualized Experiments*, no. 58, p. e3638, 2011.

[39] R. Core Team, *R: A Language and Environment for Statistical Computing*, R Foundation for Statistical Computing, Vienna, Austria, 2014, http://www.R-project.org/.

[40] D. H. Ogle, *Introductory Fisheries Analyses with R*, vol. 32, CRC Press, Boca Raton, FL, USA, 2016.

[41] H. Wickham, *ggplot2: Elegant Graphics for Data Analysis*, vol. 1, no. 2, 2009, Springer, New York, 2009.

[42] J. C. Bennett, P. A. McRae, L. J. Levy, and K. M. Frick, "Long-term continuous, but not daily, environmental enrichment reduces spatial memory decline in aged male mice," *Neurobiology of Learning and Memory*, vol. 85, no. 2, pp. 139–152, 2006.

[43] H. Shoji, K. Takao, S. Hattori, and T. Miyakawa, "Age-related changes in behavior in C57BL/6J mice from young adulthood to middle age," *Molecular Brain*, vol. 9, no. 1, p. 11, 2016.

[44] J. N. Justice, C. S. Carter, H. J. Beck et al., "Battery of behavioral tests in mice that models age-associated changes in human motor function," *Age*, vol. 36, no. 2, pp. 583–595, 2014.

[45] O. V. Bogdanova, S. Kanekar, K. E. D'Anci, and P. F. Renshaw, "Factors influencing behavior in the forced swim test," *Physiology & Behavior*, vol. 118, pp. 227–239, 2013.

[46] E. Karanges, K. M. Li, C. Motbey, P. D. Callaghan, A. Katsifis, and I. S. McGregor, "Differential behavioural and neurochemical outcomes from chronic paroxetine treatment in adolescent and adult rats: a model of adverse antidepressant effects in human adolescents?," *International Journal of Neuropsychopharmacology*, vol. 14, no. 04, pp. 491–504, 2011.

[47] A. K. Beery and I. Zucker, "Sex bias in neuroscience and biomedical research," *Neuroscience & Biobehavioral Reviews*, vol. 35, no. 3, pp. 565–572, 2011.

[48] P. Palanza, L. Gioiosa, and S. Parmigiani, "Social stress in mice: gender differences and effects of estrous cycle and social dominance," *Physiology and Behavior*, vol. 73, no. 3, pp. 411–420, 2001.

[49] B. J. Prendergast, K. G. Onishi, and I. Zucker, "Female mice liberated for inclusion in neuroscience and biomedical research," *Neuroscience & Biobehavioral Reviews*, vol. 40, pp. 1–5, 2014.

[50] D. Consoli, J. Fedotova, V. Micale, N. S. Sapronov, and F. Drago, "Stressors affect the response of male and female rats to clomipramine in a model of behavioral despair (forced swim test)," *European Journal of Pharmacology*, vol. 520, no. 1-3, pp. 100–107, 2005.

[51] N. Kokras, C. Dalla, A. C. Sideris et al., "Behavioral sexual dimorphism in models of anxiety and depression due to changes in HPA axis activity," *Neuropharmacology*, vol. 62, no. 1, pp. 436–445, 2012.

[52] N. Kokras and C. Dalla, "Sex differences in animal models of psychiatric disorders," *British Journal of Pharmacology*, vol. 171, no. 20, pp. 4595–4619, 2014.

[53] V. Hok, B. Poucet, É. Duvelle, É. Save, and F. Sargolini, "Spatial cognition in mice and rats: similarities and differences in brain and behavior," *Wiley Interdisciplinary Reviews: Cognitive Science*, vol. 7, no. 6, pp. 406–421, 2016.

17

Mechanism of Restoration of Forelimb Motor Function after Cervical Spinal Cord Hemisection in Rats: Electrophysiological Verification

Takumi Takeuchi,[1,2] Masahito Takahashi,[1] Kazuhiko Satomi,[2] Hideaki Ohne,[1] Atsushi Hasegawa,[1] Shunsuke Sato,[1] and Shoichi Ichimura[1]

[1]*Department of Orthopaedic Surgery, Kyorin University, 6-20-2 Shinkawa, Mitaka-shi, Tokyo 181-0004, Japan*
[2]*Department of Orthopaedic Surgery, Kugayama Hospital, 2-14-20 Kitakarasuyama, Setagaya-ku, Tokyo 157-0061, Japan*

Correspondence should be addressed to Takumi Takeuchi; kimotako1107@yahoo.co.jp

Academic Editor: Barbara Picconi

The objective of this study was to electrophysiologically assess the corticospinal tracts of adult rats and the recovery of motor function of their forelimbs after cervical cord hemisection. Of 39 adult rats used, compound muscle action potentials (CMAPs) of the forelimbs of 15 rats were evaluated, before they received left C5 segmental hemisection of the spinal cord, by stimulating the pyramid of the medulla oblongata on one side using an exciting microelectrode. All 15 rats exhibited contralateral electrical activity, but their CMAPs disappeared after hemisection. The remaining 24 rats received hemisection first, and CMAPs of 12 rats were assessed over time to study their recovery time. All of them exhibited electrical activity of the forelimbs in 4 weeks after surgery. The remaining 12 rats received additional right C2 segmental hemisection, and variation of CMAPs between before and after surgery was examined. The right side of the 12 rats that received the additional hemisection exhibited no electrical activity in response to the stimulation of the pyramids on both sides. These results suggest that changes in path between the resected and healthy sides, activation of the ventral corticospinal tracts, and propriospinal neurons were involved in the recovery of motor function after cervical cord injury.

1. Introduction

It is considered that a damaged central nervous system will never be restored [1], but we reported that the once paralyzed motor function of the forelimbs of juvenile rats had been restored due to a significant change that occurred in the corticospinal tract pathways after a brain injury [2]. We also assessed the motor function of the forelimbs of these rats following cervical cord hemisection and reported that restoration of motor function was observed in approximately 60% of the juvenile rats and 40% of the adult rats [3].

In past anatomical verification of experiments in corticospinal tract injury of rodents, it was reported that not only axonal re-elongation and collateral sprouting occurred in the damaged part but also the axons of intact neurons extended new branches in an area apart from the damage, thus allowing the hind limbs to recover better than the forelimbs [4–6]. However, this recovery process has never been electrophysiologically verified over time.

The objective of this research was to electrophysiologically assess the corticospinal tract of adult rats, then electrophysiologically verify the recovery of the forelimb motor function over time after cervical cord hemisection, and lastly, examine the compensation pathways for the recovery of motor function by conducting an additional hemisection.

2. Materials and Methods

2.1. Animals. Of 39 twelve-week-old male Wister rats used as experimental animals, 15 were used for the preliminary experiment prior to segmental hemisection of the cervical cord (group of rats for preliminary experiment), and the remaining 24 received cervical cord hemisection without being subjected to the preliminary experiment (group of rats for hemisection).

2.2. Surgical Procedure. Animals were first anesthetized by intraperitoneal administration of xylazine (10 mg/kg; Bayer HealthCare, Monheim, Germany) and ketamine (90 mg/kg; Daiichi Sankyo, Tokyo, Japan). For monitoring of vital signs during surgery, rectal temperature, arterial oxygen saturation, heart rate, and respiration rate were continuously measured.

The hemisection was performed as follows: the rat was fastened to a brain stereotaxic apparatus, the laminae were exposed by posterior approach between C2 and C5, and laminectomy was performed at C3 and C4. After dissecting the dura mater at that part, cervical cord hemisection at the left C5 segment was performed at a width of 2 mm in the head-to-tail direction, according to the method by coauthor Hasegawa, to prevent readhesion of nerves at the dissected part (Figure 1) [3]. The animals were administered subcutaneous (s.c.) injections of buprenorphine (0.02 mg/kg; Otsuka, Tokyo, Japan) at 12-hour intervals for 3 days as postoperative analgesia, in addition to intramuscular (i.m.) injection of penicillin G (22,000 units/kg; Tsumura & Co., Tokyo, Japan) once every 24 hours for 3 days as an antimicrobial prophylaxis.

An additional hemisection was performed on 12 of the 24 hemisected rats, 6 weeks after the first hemisection. C1 and C2 laminae were exposed by posterior approach, a C2 laminectomy was performed, the dura mater at that part was dissected, and then a right C2 segmental cervical cord hemisection was performed (Figure 2).

2.3. Electrophysiological Procedures. For electrophysiological evaluation, the Neuropack MEB-2200® measuring system (Nihon Kohden, Tokyo, Japan), SS-203J® isolator (Nihon Kohden), and SEN-3401® microstimulator (Nihon Kohden) were used.

To expose the caudal brainstem, a posterior craniotomy was performed, and then an exciting electrode (TK212-048® epoxy-insulated microelectrodes; Unique Medical Co. Ltd., Tokyo, Japan) was installed on the left or the right pyramid of the medulla oblongata by inserting it at a position approximately 1.5 mm closer to the head and 0.5 mm toward the outside, and at an insertion angle of approximately 30° toward the head, with respect to the obex, and a constant current stimulation was provided, respectively [7, 8].

Bipolar recording was performed to examine the electric potential of the flexor and extensor muscles of the forelimbs using needle electrodes. Recording electrodes for the flexor and the extensor were, respectively, installed at positions away from the elbow at an interval of 10 mm to measure compound muscle action potentials (CMAPs) (Figure 2). The recording frequency band was set to fall within a range from 10 Hz to 3 kHz, and stimulation was provided 10 times in total under the following conditions: frequency, 1 Hz; ISI, 1 ms; duration, 0.2 ms; and trains, 3. For the stimulation intensity, the motion threshold which produces waveforms was regarded as 1 T, and the main experiment was performed at 2 T, where latency was stabilized.

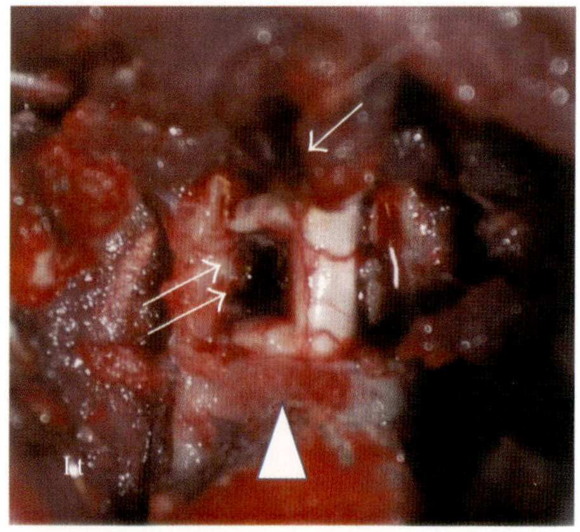

FIGURE 1: Macrographic image of the left C5 segmental hemisection of the cervical cord. Arrows: hemisected part; arrow: C2 spinous process; arrow head: C5 lamina; Lt: left.

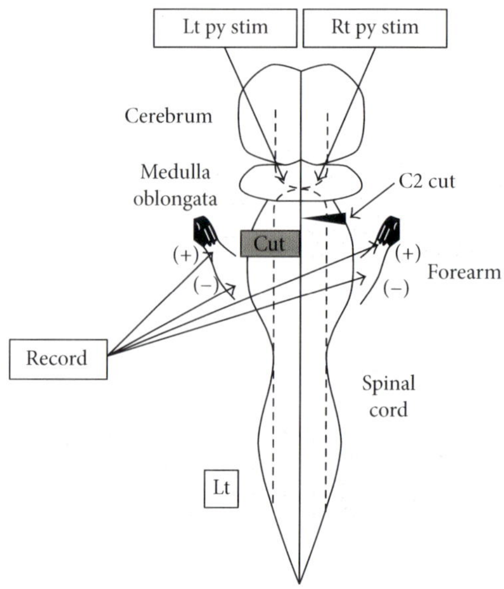

FIGURE 2: Left and right pyramidal tracts and measurement method. The left and right pyramids were stimulated separately, and CMAPs of both forelimbs were recorded. Py: pyramid; stim: stimulation; Lt: left; Rt: right; broken line: pyramidal tracts (plus sign in the medulla oblongata).

2.4. Rats for Preliminary Experiment. Using the 15 rats for preliminary experiment, the motion threshold (1 T) was checked, and then the stimulation intensity was increased from 2 T to 8 T to check the effect of an increase on waveform forming on the stimulated side. The amplitude and latency were recorded at the optimum stimulation intensity, which allowed the latency to stabilize, and then a left C5 segmental hemisection of the cervical cord was performed (Figure 3).

2.5. Rats for Hemisection. Of the 24 rats that received a left C5 segmental hemisection without being subjected to the preliminary experiment, 12 were assessed over time to check the time of their functional recovery, with 3 each, respectively, assessed electrophysiologically at 1, 2, 4, and 6 weeks after the surgery (Figure 3).

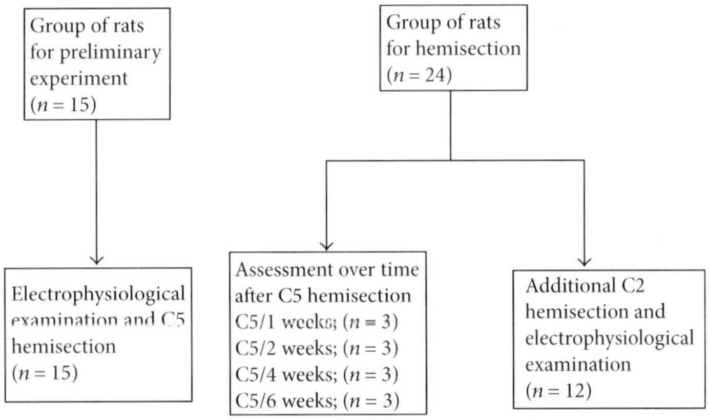

FIGURE 3: Experimental protocol. Group of rats for preliminary experiment: 15. Group of rats for hemisection: 24 (group assessed over time after C5 hemisection: 12; group that received additional C2 hemisection: 12).

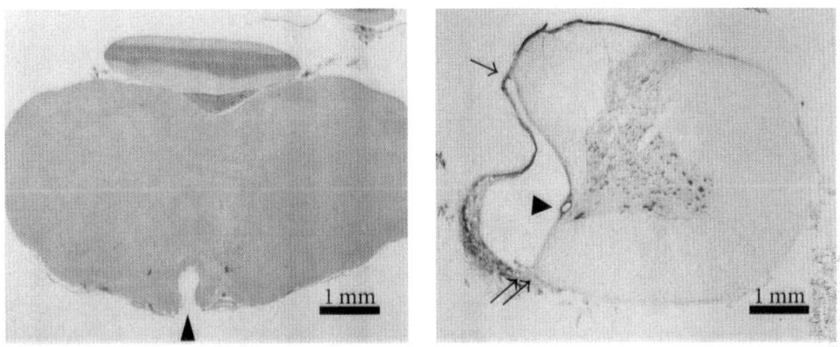

(a) (b)

FIGURE 4: Pathological image of the stimulated part of the pyramid and the hemisected part of the cervical cord. (a) Microscopic image of the stimulated part of the pyramid having undergone burnout process (midbrain level); arrow head: pyramid. (b) Microscopic image of the hemisected part of the cervical cord (C5 segment level) (modification from document 3); arrow head: central canal; arrows: anterior median fissure; arrow: dorsal median sulcus.

The remaining 12 hemisected rats were subjected to an additional C2 segmental hemisection 6 weeks after the first hemisection. They received a right C2 segmental hemisection at the C2 lamina level, and electrophysiological evaluation was performed (Figure 3).

2.6. Evaluation of CMAPs. Peak-to-peak amplitudes were measured for both the flexor and extensor. For the latency, the duration from the first stimulation to the start of a waveform was measured.

2.7. Evaluation of Stimulated and Hemisected Areas. To check the hemisected area of the cervical cord and the stimulated areas of the pyramid, the pyramids of all 39 rats having undergone electrophysiological assessment were burnt out at 20 mA, 50 Hz for 5 minutes. Then, pathological specimens were prepared as follows: under general anesthesia performed by administering 50 mg/kg of pentobarbital sodium into the abdomen, blood was removed using phosphate-buffered saline (PBS), and perfusion fixation was performed using a 4% paraformaldehyde buffer solution. The medulla oblongata and the cervical cord with a width of approximately 10 mm were cut out, with the stimulated area of the pyramid and the damaged area regarded as the center, and embedded by freezing using a 30% sucrose solution. The spinal cord was cut into thin films with a thickness of 20 μm using a microtome, dyed using toluidine blue stain and hematoxylin and eosin stain, and observed under an optical microscope (Figures 4(a) and 4(b)).

2.8. Statistical Analysis. To analyze the CMAP amplitude and latency, three personnel performed the measurement twice, top and bottom outliers were excluded, and the average of the remaining values was used. Statistical analysis was conducted by performing the Mann–Whitney U test for the comparison of two groups and the Steel-Dwass test for the comparison of three or more groups, with the level of significance set to lower than 5%.

3. Results

3.1. Rats for Preliminary Experiment. Before the C5 segmental hemisection, the motion threshold (1 T) of the rats for the preliminary experiment was 110.5 ± 70.5 μA. In response to the stimulation of the right pyramid (at the optimum stimulation intensity of 2 T), all the rats in this group exhibited electric potential on the left side. The average CMAP amplitude of the left forelimb flexor was 780 ± 709 μV and its average latency 8.3 ± 0.95 ms, and the average CMAP amplitude of the left forelimb extensor was 1259 ± 1000 μV and its

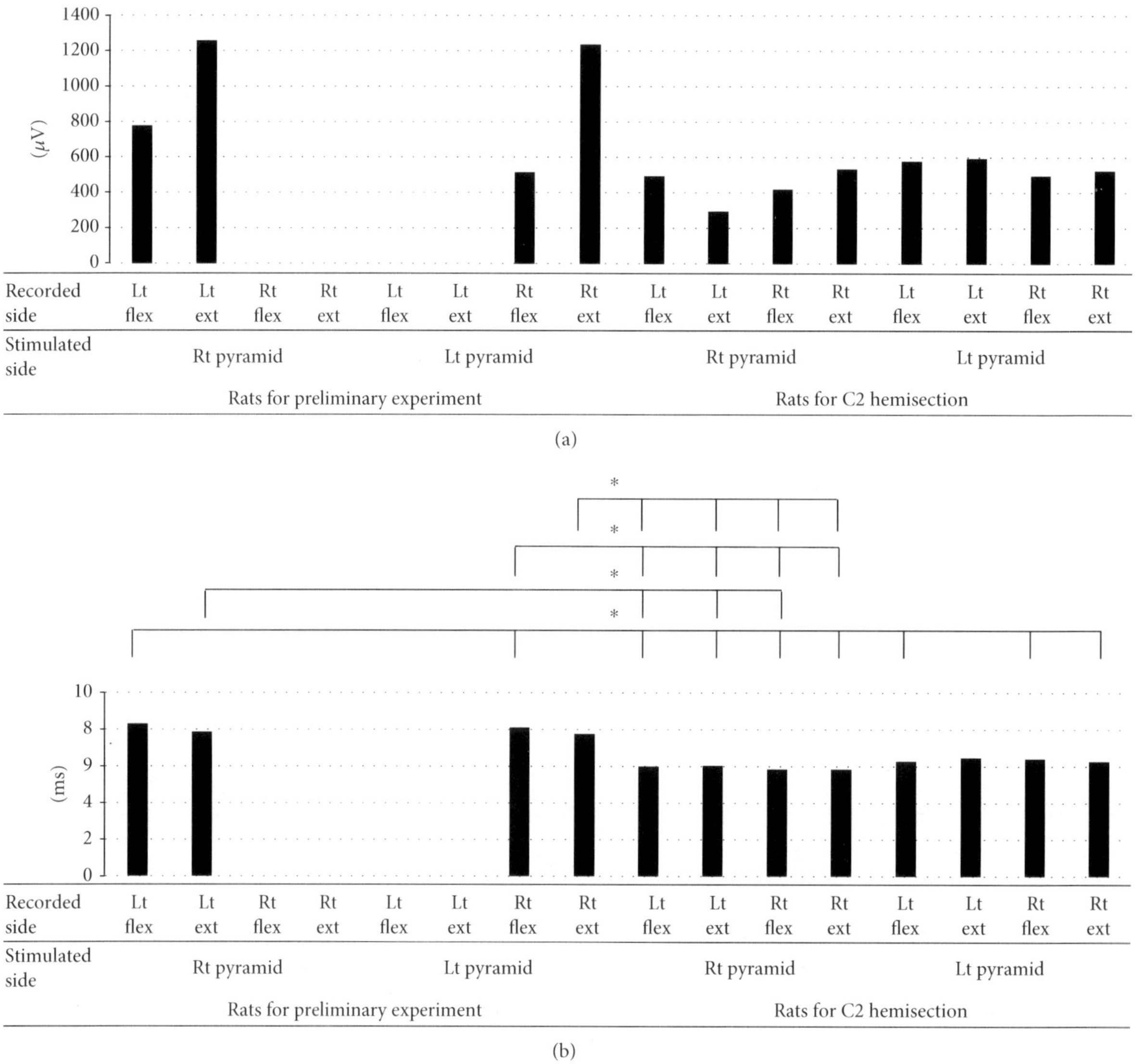

FIGURE 5: Amplitude (a) and latency (b) of CMAPs of the group of rats for preliminary experiment and the group of rats that received additional C2 hemisection. (a) No significant difference was found in the amplitude between the rats for preliminary experiment and the rats that received additional C2 hemisection. (b) Meanwhile, a significant shortening of latency was found in the rats that received C2 hemisection ($^*p < 0.05$). CMAPs: compound muscle action potentials; Rt: right; Lt: left; Flex: flexor; Ext: extensor.

average latency 7.86 ± 0.82 ms. However, neither the flexor nor the extensor on the right side exhibited CMAPs. Likewise, in response to the stimulation of the left pyramid, all the rats exhibited electric potential on the right side. The average CMAP amplitude of the right forelimb flexor was 516 ± 671 μV and its average latency 8.1 ± 0.83 ms, and the average CMAP amplitude of the right forelimb extensor was 1238 ± 1191 μV and its average latency 7.76 ± 0.43 ms. Neither the flexor nor the extensor on the left side exhibited CMAPs (Figures 5(a) and 5(b)).

Then, with the right pyramidal stimulation, the stimulation intensity was increased to 4 T (480 μA) and then to 8 T (960 μA), but no CMAPs were recorded on the stimulated side. Likewise, with the left pyramidal stimulation, the stimulation intensity was increased to 4 T (480 μA) and then to 8 T (960 μA), but no CMAPs were recorded on the stimulated side (Figure 6).

Immediately after the left segmental hemisection, in response to the right pyramidal stimulation, the CMAPs of the left forelimb flexor and that of the extensor were lost (Figure 7).

3.2. Rats for Hemisection. All 6 rats used for the study of functional recovery at 1 to 2 weeks after the surgery exhibited CMAPs of the contralateral forelimb flexor and extensor in response to the right pyramidal stimulation, and two-thirds of them also exhibited CMAPs of the ipsilateral forelimb flexor and extensor. Likewise, in response to the left pyramidal stimulation, all 6 rats exhibited CMAPs of the contralateral forelimb flexor and extensor, and two-thirds of them exhibited CMAPs of the ipsilateral forelimb flexor and extensor. Furthermore, all 6 rats used for the study of functional recovery at 4 to 6 weeks after the surgery exhibited CMAPs on both the right and left

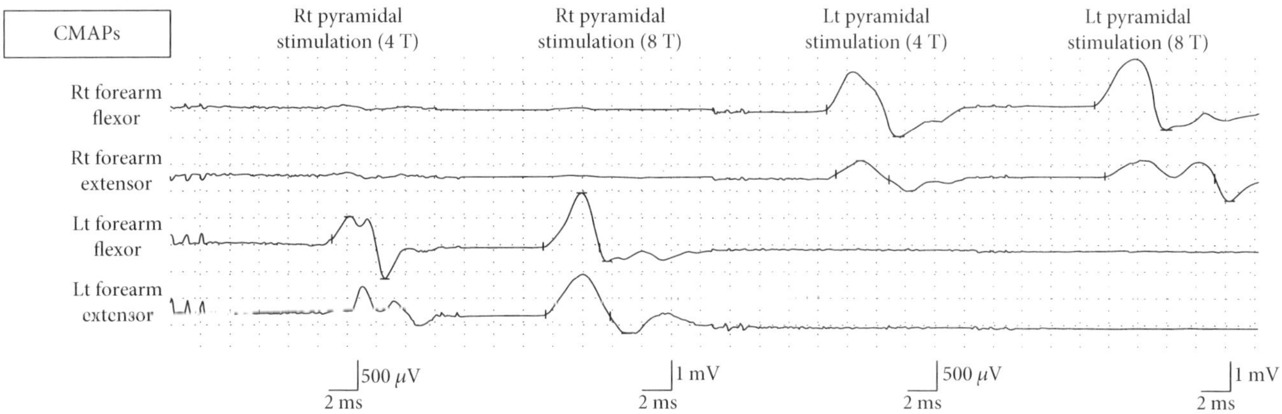

FIGURE 6: CMAPs obtained by stimulating the pyramid of the rats for preliminary experiment. Despite the increase in stimulation intensity from 4 T to 8 T for both the left and right pyramids, no ipsilateral CMAPs were recorded.

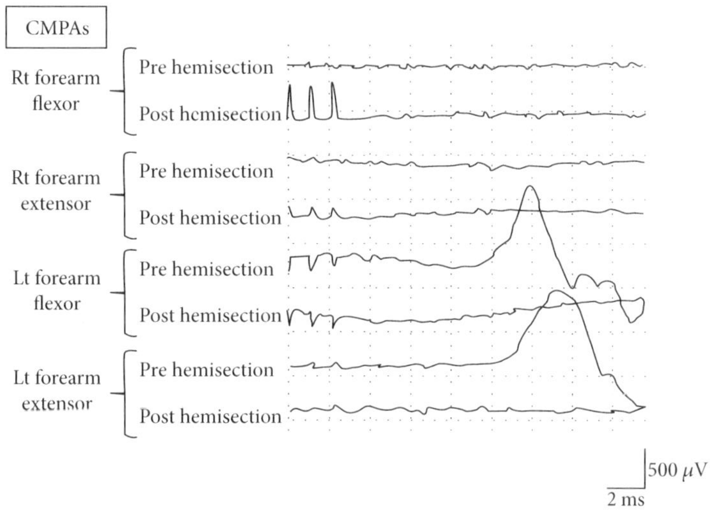

FIGURE 7: CMAPs obtained by stimulating the right pyramid of the rats for preliminary experiment having undergone left C5 segmental hemisection (stimulation intensity: 2 T). Upper row: before hemisection; lower row: after hemisection. No electric potential of the left forelimb flexor/extensor was recorded immediately after the hemisection.

sides in response to the right or left pyramidal stimulation (Table 1).

In response to the right pyramidal stimulation, the group of 12 rats that received an additional right C2 segmental hemisection exhibited the following: an average CMAP amplitude of the left forelimb flexor of 496 ± 784 μV and average latency 6.0 ± 1.02 ms; an average CMAP amplitude of the extensor of 296 ± 207 μV and average latency 6.04 ± 0.95 ms; an average CMAP amplitude of the right forelimb flexor of 420 ± 226 μV and average latency 5.85 ± 1.07 ms; and an average CMAP amplitude of the right forelimb extensor of 536 ± 391 μV and average latency 5.85 ± 1.07 ms. Also, in response to the left pyramidal stimulation, the group exhibited the following: an average CMAP amplitude of the right forelimb flexor of 498 ± 333 μV and average latency 6.42 ± 1.14 ms; an average CMAP amplitude of the right forelimb extensor of 526 ± 350 μV and average latency 6.28 ± 1.29 ms; an average CMAP amplitude of the left forelimb flexor of 580 ± 581 μV and average latency 6.29 ± 1.07 ms; and an average CMAP amplitude of the left forelimb extensor of 569 ± 679 μV and average latency 6.48 ± 1.38 ms (Figures 5(a) and 5(b)).

Comparison of the CMAP amplitude and latency between the group of rats for the preliminary experiment and the group that received the additional C2 segmental hemisection exhibited no significant difference in amplitude, but a significant shortening of latency was found with the group that received the additional C2 segmental hemisection ($^*p < 0.05$) (Figures 5(a) and 5(b)).

With the group that received the additional C2 segmental hemisection, their right pyramid was stimulated, and then a right C2 segmental hemisection was performed. The average CMAP amplitude of their right forelimb flexor, which was 377 ± 195 μV on average before the surgery, changed to 0 μV, and the CMAP amplitude of their right forelimb extensor, which was 573 ± 391 μV on average before the surgery, was also lost. Meanwhile, the average CMAP amplitude of their left forelimb flexor decreased significantly from

TABLE 1: Existence or nonexistence of CMAPs in the group of rats for preliminary experiment and the group of rats for assessment over time after C5 hemisection.

Stimulated side	Recorded side	Rats for preliminary experiment (15 rats)	Assessment over time after C5 hemisection			
			Post hemisection 1 week (3 rats)	Post hemisection 2 weeks (3 rats)	Post hemisection 4 weeks (3 rats)	Post hemisection 6 weeks (3 rats)
Rt pyramid	Rt flex	0/15	2/3	2/3	3/3	3/3
	Rt ext	0/15	2/3	2/3	3/3	3/3
	Lt flex	15/15	3/3	3/3	3/3	3/3
	Lt ext	15/15	3/3	3/3	3/3	3/3
Lt pyramid	Rt flex	0/15	3/3	3/3	3/3	3/3
	Rt ext	0/15	3/3	3/3	3/3	3/3
	Lt flex	15/15	2/3	2/3	3/3	3/3
	Lt ext	15/15	2/3	2/3	3/3	3/3

Number of rats that exhibited electric potential/number of rats measured. All the rats in the group for the preliminary experiment exhibited contralateral electrical potential only in response to stimulation on the opposite side, whereas all the rats assessed over time after the surgery exhibited electric potential on both sides in response to stimulation of the right or left pyramid at 4 to 6 weeks after the surgery. Rt: right; Lt: left; Flex: flexor; Ext: extensor.

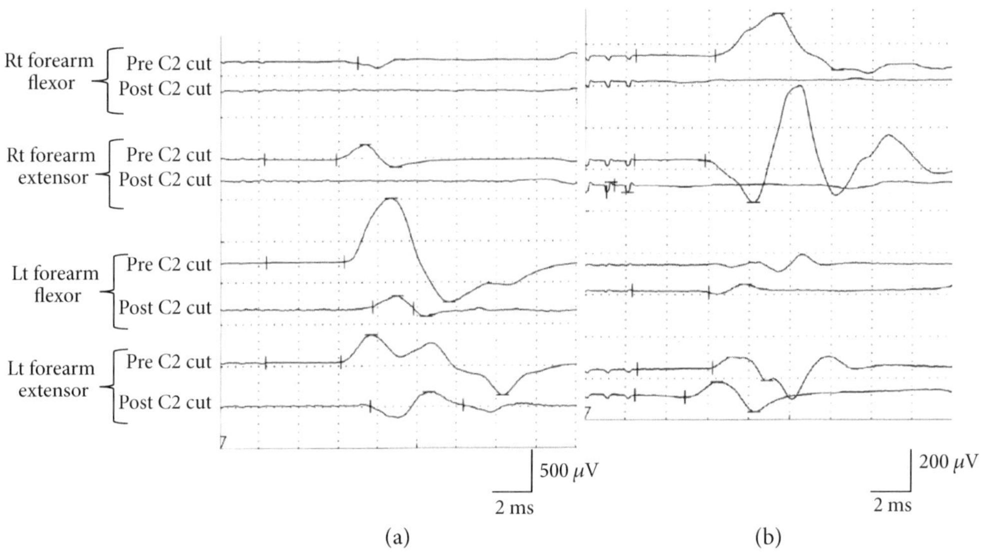

FIGURE 8: CMAPs (stimulation intensity: 2 T) of rats having undergone additional right C2 hemisection. (a) Immediately after right C2 hemisection, electric potential of the right forelimb was lost in response to the stimulation of the right pyramid, whereas the electric potential of the left forelimb was not lost although the waveform amplitude decreased. (b) Immediately after right C2 hemisection, electric potential of the right forelimb was lost in response to the stimulation of the left pyramid, whereas the electric potential of the left forelimb was not lost although the waveform amplitude decreased.

303 ± 254 to 147 ± 94 μV and that of their left forelimb extensor also exhibited a significant decrease from 232 ± 178 to 121 ± 77 μV, but was not lost ($p < 0.05$) (Figures 8(a) and 9(a)). As the result of the left pyramidal stimulation, the average CMAP amplitude of their right forelimb flexor, which was 460 ± 316 μV before the surgery, was lost (0 μV) and also that of their extensor, which was 496 ± 332 μV, was lost (0 μV). Whereas a significant decrease was found in the average CMAP amplitude of their left forelimb flexor, from 545 ± 622 to 227 ± 183 μV, and also in that of their extensor, from 535 ± 721 to 220 ± 219 μV, it was not lost ($^*p < 0.05$) (Figures 8(b) and 9(a)). Significant extension of latency was found in the left forelimb record as the result of the right pyramidal stimulation ($^*p < 0.05$), and significant shortening was found in the left forelimb record as the result of the left pyramidal stimulation ($^*p < 0.05$) (Figure 9(b)).

The results are summarized as follows: all the rats in the group for the preliminary experiment exhibited contralateral CMAPs only as the result of stimulation of the other side before the surgery. All 6 rats used for the study of functional recovery at 4 weeks after the hemisection onward exhibited CMAPs of both forelimb muscles as the result of stimulation of one side. Although no change was found in the amplitude, latency was found to have decreased. As the result of the additional right segmental hemisection at C2 level, which is closer to the head, only the electric potential on the hemisected side was lost (Figure 10).

4. Discussion

In the development process of the corticospinal tract of the rats, the leading axons are at the level of the medulla

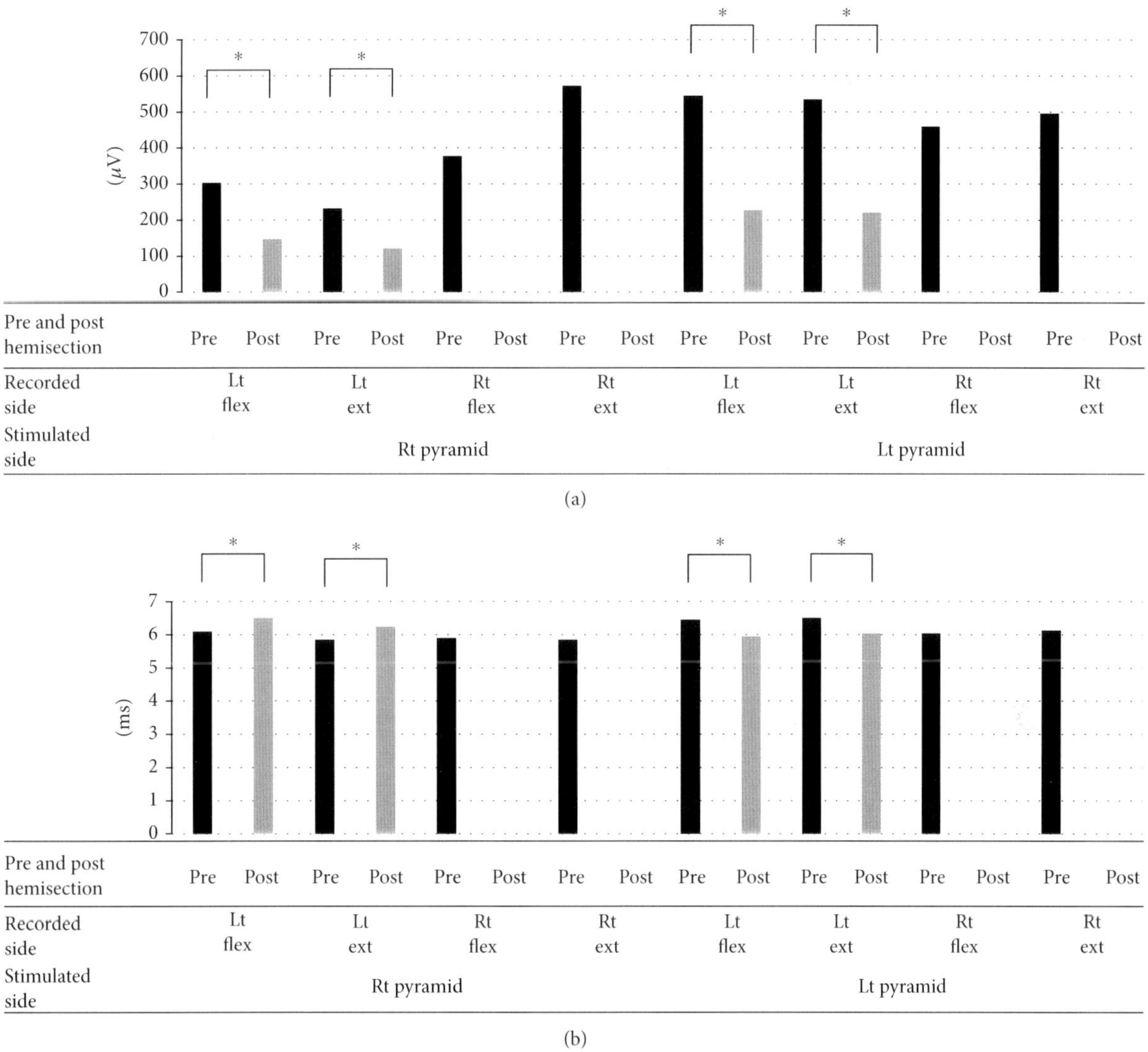

FIGURE 9: Amplitude (a) and latency (b) of CMAPs before and after the additional C2 hemisection performed on the C2 rat group. (a) In response to the stimulation of both the left and right pyramids, CMAPs of the right forelimb were lost after the additional right C2 hemisection, whereas the amplitude of CMAPs of the left forelimb was not lost although it decreased significantly ($^*p < 0.05$). (b) Significant extension of the latency was found in the record of the left forelimb in response to the stimulation of the right pyramid, whereas a significant shortening of latency was found in the record of the left forelimb in response to the stimulation of the left pyramid ($^*p < 0.05$). CMAPs: compound muscle action potentials; Rt: right; Lt: left; Flex: flexor; Ext: extensor.

oblongata immediately after birth and extend toward the lumbosacral cord over a period of approximately 3 weeks, reaching the state of adult rats [9, 10]. Corticofugal projection fibers also form axonal projections on the neurons existing in the red nuclei, vestibular nuclei, bulbar ventral reticular nuclei, and the bulbar raphe nuclei of the brainstem, which is considered to be involved in motor control [11–13]. It has been confirmed using adult rats that unilateral damage in the cerebral hemisphere caused during the juvenile period (when corticospinal tract axons are still forming projections in a caudal direction) allows the corticofugal projection fibers that are descending from the sensorimotor area of the cerebral cortex on the undamaged side to form bilateral axonal projections at each level of the thalamus [14]; striatum [15]; superior colliculus, red nuclei, and pontine nuclei in the midbrain [16]; pyramidal decussation [17]; and spinal cord [18]. We confirmed this bilateral axonal projection by electrophysiological verification [19]. Past studies have reported cases of cervical spinal cord contusion injury and simple selective cutting [20–23], but there have been no reports on a case where segmental cervical cord hemisection was performed to eliminate the possibility of readhesion of the nerve fibers in the hemisected area. The present study adopted this injury method because it allows assessment of the reproducible compensation function by clearly leaving the intact part. Also, regarding electrophysiological evaluation, there have been no reports on a case where the pyramid of one side is selectively subjected to microstimulation to assess functional recovery over time.

		Rats for preliminary experiment (12 rats)	Pre C2 hemisection (12 rats)		Post C2 hemisection (12 rats)
Rt pyramidal stimulation	Rt CMAPs	-	+	Rt C2 hemisection	Disappear
	Lt CMAPs	+	+		+
Lt pyramidal stimulation	Rt CMAPs	+	+		Disappear
	Lt CMAPs	-	+		+

FIGURE 10: Summary of the results of this experiment. All the rats in the group for the preliminary experiment (those that later received the left C5 segmental hemisection) exhibited contralateral electrical activity in response to the stimulation on one side. Also, at 6 weeks after the C5 hemisection surgery, all 12 rats exhibited CMAPs from both forelimb muscles in response to the stimulation on one side before the additional C2 hemisection. With the rats that received the additional C2 hemisection, only the electric potential on the right side was lost. CAMPs: compound muscle action potentials; Rt: right; Lt: left.

The result of electrophysiological assessment of the corticospinal tract of adult rats, which was the first objective of this study, was as follows: only contralateral forelimb compound muscle action potentials (CMAPs) were recorded in response to the stimulation of the pyramid on one side, and no ipsilateral CMAPs were recorded even with stimulation of an intensity 8 times as high as the exercise threshold. The corticospinal tract of the rats originates from the pyramidal neuron of layer V of the sensorimotor cortex of the brain, and the axons descend along the internal capsule, cerebral peduncle, and the pyramid of the ventral medulla oblongata. Axonal projections are formed along two pathways: 90 to 95% of the axons cross the pyramid, extending toward the dorsal funiculus on the opposite side, and the remaining axons extend toward the ventral spinal cord on the same side without crossing the pyramid [24, 25]. The existence of such ipsilateral ventral-descending neural circuit was not confirmed by the electrophysiological assessment of the corticospinal tract of adult rats conducted this time.

Regarding the time of recovery from motor paralysis in the electrophysiological evaluation, which was the second objective of this study, all 12 rats exhibited CMAPs from both the forelimb muscles in response to the stimulation on one side at 4 weeks after the surgery onward. This result was consistent with the results of recovery time in our behavioral assessment [3]. The past reports also indicated similar results: recovery in 4 to 6 weeks [26, 27].

By comparing the CMAP waveform of the rats for the preliminary experiments and that of the rats for the additional hemisection, shortening in latency was observed in the latter (Figure 6, Table 1). Furthermore, as a result of performing the additional right C2 segmental hemisection to confirm the existence of compensation pathways, which was the last objective of the present study, the electric potential on the right side was lost, and a decrease in electric potential was found on the left side. There are various reports on the study of compensation pathways formed after an injury in the central nervous system of rodents. Also, with rodents, even if half of their thoracic cord is cut off, they do not lose their walking ability, and the involvement of serotonin (5-hydroxytryptamine (5-HT)) fibers in this compensation mechanism has been reported [28–30]. In this model, the mechanism of activating motor cells in the circuit for adjusting walking motion patterns (central pattern generator (CPG)) [31–33] and budding of 5-HT fibers at the lumbar cord level after thoracic cord hemisection [29, 30] has been confirmed.

With adult rats that received dissection of the pyramid on one side and were administered mAb, sprouting from the healthy side toward the damaged side was confirmed at the brainstem and spinal cord levels after the functional recovery [34]. Also, with rats whose dorsal funiculi on both sides were cut off completely at a high C3 level, it has been reported that their motor function was restored naturally in approximately 4 weeks; sprouting from the undamaged ventral corticospinal tract was confirmed; and furthermore, when the ventral corticospinal tract was cut, recovery from paralysis was not observed [33]. As described above, also with adult rodents, sprouting across the damaged and healthy sides and that from the ventral corticospinal tract has been confirmed. Meanwhile, as compensation of the forelimb motor function different from these recovery pathways, C3-C4 propriospinal neurons were reported for the first time with cats. They form an indirect corticomotoneuronal pathway together with a direct pathway for direct projection from the brain to the motor neurons [35–38]. The propriospinal neurons have been reported to exist also in primates and rats, and they are considered extremely important for the recovery of the motor function of fingers in particular [39–42]. In this study, the left propriospinal neurons were cut by the C5 segmental

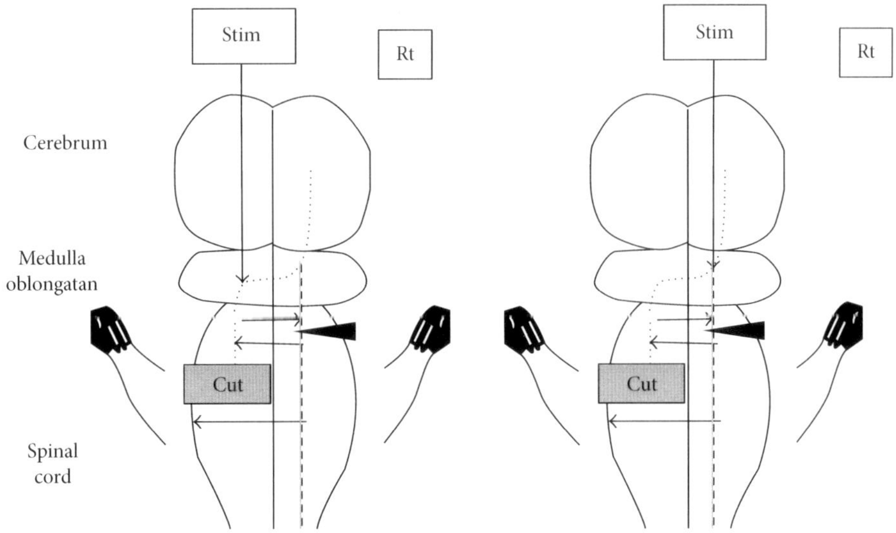

FIGURE 11: Compensation pathway of the corticospinal tract after the recovery of motor function. Stim: stimulation; Rt: right; cut: left C5 segmental hemisection of cervical cord; short broken line: dorsal corticospinal tract (posterior funiculus); long broken line: ventral corticospinal tract; arrow: sprouting; gray line: activation of the ventral corticospinal tract; arrow head: contralateral additional C2 hemisection.

hemisection of the left cervical cord. Meanwhile, since the right propriospinal neurons remained intact, there is a possibility that they were involved in the recovery. However, since the corticospinal tracts on the left and right sides were cut at different levels, the compensation pathways cannot be accounted for without the sprouting across the damaged and healthy sides. Although the extension of latency was thus expected, the opposite result was obtained due to causes such as anesthetic depth and difference in nerve conduction velocity between the dorsal and ventral sides of the corticospinal tract. Technical factors may also have been involved. To identify the exact causes, we consider it necessary to conduct anatomical verification by neuroanatomical tract tracing.

5. Conclusion

These results suggest that sprouting across the damaged and healthy sides, activation of the ventral corticospinal tracts, and propriospinal neurons were complexly involved in the growth of compensation pathways assumed by the electrophysiological verification (Figure 11).

Disclosure

A part of the manuscript was presented in Clinical Neurophysiology as a society proceeding (volume 128, issue 9, September 2017, pages e171–e172).

Acknowledgments

The authors thank Ms. Mizuho Kosuge for her assistance with this study. This work was supported by a grant from the Japan Orthopaedics and Traumatology Foundation, Inc. (no. 252).

References

[1] R. S. Cajal, *Degeneration and Regeneration of the Central Nervous System*, Oxford University Press, Oxford, UK, 1928.

[2] M. Takahashi, A. Vattanajun, T. Umeda, K. Isa, and T. Isa, "Large-scale reorganization of corticofugal fibers after neonatal hemidecortication for functional restoration of forelimb movements," *European Journal of Neuroscience*, vol. 30, no. 10, pp. 1878–1887, 2009.

[3] A. Hasegawa, M. Takahashi, K. Satomi et al., "Mechanism of forelimb motor function restoration after cervical spinal cord hemisection in rats: a comparison of juveniles and adults," *Behavioural Neurology*, vol. 2016, Article ID 1035473, 9 pages, 2016.

[4] L. Filli, B. Zörner, O. Weinmann, and M. E. Schwab, "Motor deficits and recovery in rats with unilateral spinal cord hemisection mimic the Brown-Séquard syndrome," *Brain*, vol. 134, no. 8, pp. 2261–2273, 2011.

[5] A. Ghosh, E. Sydekum, F. Haiss et al., "Functional and anatomical reorganization of the sensory-motor cortex after incomplete spinal cord injury in adult rats," *The Journal of Neuroscience*, vol. 29, no. 39, pp. 12210–12219, 2009.

[6] O. Raineteau and M. E. Schwab, "Plasticity of motor system after incomplete spinal cord injury," *Nature Reviews Neroscience*, vol. 2, pp. 263–273, 2001.

[7] B. Alstermark and J. Ogawa, "In vivo recordings of bulbospinal excitation in adult mouse forelimb motoneurons," *Journal of Neurophysiology*, vol. 92, no. 3, pp. 1958–1962, 2004.

[8] J. Ogawa and B. Alstermark, "C3-C4 propriospinal neuron in rat," *Journal of Functional Diagnosis*, vol. 34, pp. 16–19, 2012.

[9] A. A. Gribnau, E. J. de Kort, P. J. Dederen, and R. Nieuwenhuys, "On the development of the pyramidal tract in the rat. II. An anterograde tracer study of the outgrowth of the corticospinal fibers," *Anatomy and Embryology*, vol. 175, no. 1, pp. 101–110, 1986.

[10] E. A. Joosten, R. L. Schuitman, M. E. Vermelis, and P. J. Dederen, "Postnatal development of the ipsilateral corticospinal component in rat spinal cord: a light and electron microscopic anterograde HRP study," *The Journal of Comparative Neurology*, vol. 324, pp. 133–146, 1992.

[11] B. Alstermark, J. Ogawa, and T. Isa, "Lack of monosynaptic corticomotoneuronal EPSPs in rats: disynaptic EPSPs mediated via reticulospinal neurons and polysynaptic EPSPs via segmental interneurons," *Journal of Neurophysiology*, vol. 91, no. 4, pp. 1832–1839, 2004.

[12] L. T. Brown, "Corticorubral projections in the rat," *The Journal of Comparative Neurology*, vol. 154, no. 2, pp. 149–167, 1974.

[13] S. Nisiike, W. O. Guldin, and J. Bäurle, "Corticofugal connections between the cerebral cortex and the vestibular nuclei in the rat," *The Journal of Comparative Neurology*, vol. 420, pp. 363–372, 2000.

[14] Y. XH, V. Moret, and E. M. Rouiller, "Re-examination of the plasticity of the corticothalamic projection after unilateral neonatal lesion of the sensorimotor cortex in the rat: a phaseolus vulgaris-leucoagglutinin tracing study," *Journal fur Hirnforschung*, vol. 36, pp. 123–133, 1995.

[15] B. Kolb, R. Gibb, and D. V. Kooy, "Cortical and striatal structure and connectivity are altered by neonatal hemidecortication in rats," *The Journal of Comparative Neurology*, vol. 322, no. 3, pp. 311–324, 1992.

[16] W. J. Z'Graggen, K. Fouad, O. Raineteau, G. A. S. Metz, M. E. Schwab, and G. L. Kartje, "Compensatory sprouting and impulse rerouting after unilateral pyramidal tract lesion in neonatal rats," *The Journal of Neuroscience*, vol. 20, pp. 6561–6569, 2000.

[17] K. Ono, Y. Watanabe, C. Ishizuka et al., "Axon ramification following unilateral cortical ablation in neonatal rats," *Brain and Development*, vol. 16, no. 3, pp. 264–266, 1994.

[18] A. Aisaka, Y. Aimi, O. Yasuhara, I. Tooyama, H. Kimura, and M. Shimada, "Two modes of corticospinal reinnervation occur close to spinal targets following unilateral lesion of the motor cortex in neonatal hamsters," *Neuroscience*, vol. 90, no. 1, pp. 53–67, 1999.

[19] T. Umeda, M. Takahashi, K. Isa, and T. Isa, "Formation of descending pathways mediating cortical command to forelimb motoneurons in neonatally hemidecorticated rats," *Journal of Neurophysiology*, vol. 104, no. 3, pp. 1707–1716, 2010.

[20] K. D. Anderson, K. G. Sharp, and O. Steward, "Bilateral cervical contusion spinal cord injury in rats," *Experimental Neurology*, vol. 220, pp. 9–22, 2009.

[21] K. D. Anderson, A. Gunawan, and O. Steward, "Quantitative assessment of forelimb motor function after cervical spinal cord injury in rats: relationship to the corticospinal tract," *Experimental Neurology*, vol. 194, pp. 161–174, 2005.

[22] S. M. Onifer, C. D. Nunn, J. A. Decker et al., "Loss and spontaneous recovery of forelimb evoked potentials in both the adult rat cuneate nucleus and somatosensory cortex following contusive cervical spinal cord injury," *Experimental Neurology*, vol. 207, no. 2, pp. 238–247, 2007.

[23] S. M. Onifer, Y. P. Zhang, D. A. Burke et al., "Adult rat forelimb dysfunction after dorsal cervical spinal cord injury," *Experimental Neurology*, vol. 192, no. 1, pp. 25–38, 2005.

[24] C. Brosamle and M. E. Schwab, "Cells of origin, course and termination patterns of the ventral, uncrossed component of the mature rat corticospinal tract," *The Journal of Comparative Neurology*, vol. 386, no. 2, pp. 293–303, 1997.

[25] E. A. Joosten and D. P. Bar, "Axon guidance of outgrowing corticospinal fibres in the rat," *Journal of Anatomy*, vol. 194, Part 1, pp. 15–32, 1999.

[26] M. Ueno, Y. Hayano, H. Nakagawa, and T. Yamashita, "Intraspinal rewiring of the corticospinal tract requires target-derived brain-derived neurotrophic factor and compensates lost function after brain injury," *Brain*, vol. 135, no. 4, pp. 1253–1267, 2012.

[27] N. Weidner, A. Ner, N. Salimi, and M. H. Tuszynski, "Spontaneous corticospinal axonal plasticity and functional recovery after adult central nervous system injury," *Proceedings of the National Academy of Sciences of the United States of America*, vol. 98, no. 6, pp. 3513–3518, 2001.

[28] T. Hashimoto and N. Fukuda, "Contribution of serotonin neurons to the functional recovery after spinal cord injury in rats," *Brain Research*, vol. 539, no. 2, pp. 263–270, 1991.

[29] Y. Saruhashi and W. Young, "Effect of mianserin on locomotory function after thoracic spinal cord hemisection in rats," *Experimental Neurology*, vol. 129, no. 2, pp. 207–216, 1994.

[30] Y. Saruhashi, W. Young, and R. Pedkins, "The recovery of 5-HT in lumbosacral spinal cord and locomotor function after thoracic hemisection," *Experimental Neurology*, vol. 139, no. 2, pp. 203–213, 1996.

[31] T. G. Deliagina, G. N. Orlovsky, and G. A. Pavliva, "The capacity for generation of rhythmic oscillations is distributed in the lumbosacral spinal cord of the cat," *Experimental Brain Research*, vol. 53, no. 1, pp. 81–90, 1983.

[32] D. Feraboli-Lohnherr, D. Orsal, A. Yakovleff, M. Giménezy Ribotta, and A. Privat, "Recovery of locomotor activity in the adult chronic spinal rat after sublesional transplantation of embryonic nervous cells: specific role of serotonergic neurons," *Experimental Brain Research*, vol. 113, no. 3, pp. 443–454, 1997.

[33] U. Slawinka, H. Majczynski, and R. Djavadian, "Recovery of hindlimb motor functions after spinal cord transection is enhanced by grafts of the embryonic raphe nuclei," *Experimental Brain Research*, vol. 132, pp. 27–38, 2000.

[34] M. Thallmair, G. A. S. Metz, W. J. Z'Graggen, O. Raineteau, G. L. Kartje, and M. E. Schwab, "Neurite growth inhibitors restrict plasticity and functional recovery following corticospinal tract lesions," *Nature Neuroscience*, vol. 1, no. 2, pp. 124–131, 1998.

[35] B. Alstermark and S. Sasaki, "Integration in descending motor pathways controlling the forelimb in the cat. 13. Corticospinal effects in shoulder, elbow, wrist, and digit motoneurones," *Experimental Brain Research*, vol. 59, no. 2, pp. 353–364, 1985.

[36] M. Illert, A. Lundberg, Y. Padel, and R. Tanaka, "Integration in descending motor pathways controlling the forelimb in the cat. 5. Properties of and monosynaptic excitatory convergence on C3-C4 propriospinal neurones," *Experimental Brain Research*, vol. 33, no. 1, pp. 101–130, 1978.

[37] M. Illert, A. Lundberg, and R. Tanaka, "Integration in descending motor pathways controlling the forelimb in the cat. 3. Convergence on propriospinal neurones transmitting

disynaptic excitation from the corticospinal tract and other descending tracts," *Experimental Brain Research*, vol. 29, no. 3-4, pp. 323–346, 1977.

[38] M. Illerat and E. Widemann, "Pyramidal actions in identified radial motornuclei of the cat," *Pflügers Archiv*, vol. 41, pp. 132–142, 1984.

[39] B. Alstermark, T. Isa, Y. Ohki, and Y. Saito, "Disynaptic pyramidal excitation in forelimb motorneurons mediated via C_3–C_4 propriospinal neurons in the *Macaca fuacata*," *Journal of Neurophysiology*, vol. 82, no. 6, pp. 3580–3585, 1999.

[40] B. Alstermark, L. G. Pettersson, Y. Nishimura et al., "Motor command for precision grip in the macaque monkey can be mediated by spinal interneurons," *Journal of Neurophysiology*, vol. 106, no. 1, pp. 122–126, 2011.

[41] Y. Nishimura, Y. Morichika, and T. Isa, "A subcortical oscillatory network contributes to recovery of hand dexterity after spinal cord injury," *Brain*, vol. 132, no. 3, pp. 709–721, 2009.

[42] S. Sasaki, T. Isa, L. G. Pettersson et al., "Dexterous finger movements in primate without monosynaptic corticomotoneuronal excitation," *Journal of Neurophysiology*, vol. 92, no. 5, pp. 3142–3147, 2004.

18

Allergic Rhinitis in Rats is Associated with an Inflammatory Response of the Hippocampus

Shasha Yang,[1] Jing Wu,[2] Qinxiu Zhang,[3] Xinrong Li,[3] Daien Liu,[1] Bin Zeng,[1] Zhiqing Liu,[1] Haoran Kang,[1] and Zhendong Zhong[4]

[1]*Chengdu University of Traditional Chinese Medicine, Chengdu, Sichuan province, China*
[2]*Guiyang College of Traditional Chinese Medicine, Guiyang, Guizhou province, China*
[3]*Department of Otorhinolaryngology, Head and Neck Surgery, Teaching Hospital of Chengdu University of Traditional Chinese Medicine, Chengdu, Sichuan province, China*
[4]*Sichuan Academy of Medical Sciences and Sichuan Provincial People's Hospital, Chengdu, China*

Correspondence should be addressed to Qinxiu Zhang; zhqinxiu@163.com

Academic Editor: Veit Roessner

Allergic rhinitis (AR) is a major concern in personal and public health, which negatively affects emotions and behavior, leading to cognitive deficits, memory decline, poor school performance, anxiety, and depression. Several cellular and molecular mediators are released in the inflammatory process of AR and activate common neuroimmune mechanisms, involving emotionally relevant circuits and the induction of anxiety. Responsiveness of the hypothalamic-pituitary-adrenal (HPA) axis to allergic processes have been reported, which may also include responsiveness of the hippocampus, cortex, and other brain regions. Here, we have used an optimized rat model of AR to explore whether the disease has a relationship with inflammatory responses in the hippocampus. AR was established in adult rats by ovalbumin sensitization, and the expression of various inflammatory substances in the hippocampus was measured by specific assays. Comparison between experimental and various control groups of animals revealed an association of AR with significant upregulation of substance P, microglia surface antigen (CD11b), glial fibrillary acid protein (GFAP), tumor necrosis factor-α (TNF-α), and interleukin 6 (IL-6) in the hippocampus. Thus, we hypothesize that the AR challenge may activate these inflammatory mediators in the hippocampus, which in turn contribute to the abnormal behavior and neurological deficits associated with AR.

1. Introduction

Allergic rhinitis (AR) is an IgE antibody-mediated immune reaction, in which expansion of the type 2 (TH2) subset of T cells [1, 2] causes typical allergy symptoms, consisting of sneezing, itching, nasal congestion, watery rhinorrhea, and even impaired quality of life (QOL) [3–5], affecting sleep, psychomotor functions, and social activities. AR is a highly prevalent chronic disease that affects approximately 40% of the world's population [6]. Consequently, the overall socioeconomic burden and the medical expenses associated with AR have become areas of major concern.

In addition, multiple clinical practitioners have reported behavioral complications associated with the progression of AR, which include cognitive deficits, memory decline, poor school performance, attention deficiency and hyperactivity, anxiety, and depression [7–9], mainly in childhood and adolescent populations. Recent human studies have hinted at a direct relationship between antigen exposure and alteration in brain function that may precipitate high levels of anxiety and emotional reactivity [10, 11]. Several rodent studies have also shown that cellular and molecular mediators are released in the inflammatory process of AR and activate common neuroimmune mechanisms that involve emotionally relevant circuits and the induction of anxiety [12, 13]. Increased anxiety in the open field test and activation of limbic brain regions was reported during the early phase in a mice model of food allergies [14]. In humans, increased brain activity in the prefrontal cortex was observed using functional magnetic resonance during the late phase of an asthma episode [12].

Other hypotheses for the association between allergic diseases and internalizing disorder invoke the role of interleukin 1β in hypersensitivity reactions, which activates the hypothalamic-pituitary-adrenal (HPA) axis, stimulating the release of cortisol that in turn modifies serotonin release, leading to mood disturbances [15]. Moreover, mouse models have proposed a direct relationship between antigen exposure and altered brain function leading to increased anxiety. Production of T helper 2 cytokines in the prefrontal cortex and olfactory bulbs of rats with tree pollen- and ovalbumin-induced AR has also been demonstrated [12].

While these studies provide a foundation in identifying brain regions and behavioral responses associated with allergen challenge, the notion that these allergies may initiate, perpetuate, and exacerbate pathological anxiety remains controversial and largely unstudied. Besides, the relationship between allergic rhinitis and anxiety has been shown to be bidirectional and likely to share genetic and neuroimmune mechanisms that remain undefined. Studies of brain regions and behavioral responses associated with AR mostly focused on the limbic brain and prefrontal cortex, much less on the hippocampus, even though the hippocampus is closely related to learning, memory, and emotion, which appear to be affected in AR [16].

The brain and the immune system interact with each other through neurons [17, 18] and body fluids, and the central nervous system (CNS) regulates the HPA axis that includes the hypothalamus, pituitary gland, and adrenal gland. The HPA axis is in fact an important part of the neuroendocrine system, involved in controlling stress and regulating many physical activities, such as digestion, immune system, mood, emotions, and sexuality, as well as energy storage and consumption. In turn, the immune system transmits signals to the brain through neural and humoral routes. Immune organs are innervated by the sympathetic nervous system, and immune cells express receptors for neurotransmitters, including catecholamines and neuropeptides, and for hormones, including those of the HPA axis.

The nasal mucosa is also innervated by sensory, sympathetic, and parasympathetic nerves. Thus, immune activity in the nasal mucosa may be passed into the brain by the body fluid and neural pathways, such as the afferent of cytokines and the vagus nerve. Sensory neurons transmit signals that generate sensations such as itching and motor reflexes such as sneezing, whereas parasympathetic and sympathetic reflexes regulate the glandular and vascular systems [19]. Moreover, due to inflammation or airborne allergens, the integrity of the nasal epithelium is disrupted, and the exposed sensory nerve endings promptly release substance P (SP), calcitonin gene-related peptide (CGRP), and vasoactive intestinal peptide (VIP). Produced in the cell body of C-fibre neurons, these peptides can be transported in granule structures within the cytoplasm to nerve terminals in the CNS. This leads to "central sensitization," a phenomenon associated with the activation of nociceptive C-fibres [19].

Finally, the glial cells, widely distributed in the CNS, support the blood-brain barrier (BBB) and nourish the neurons; however, their immune function has received increasing attention in recent years, focusing on the microglia (detected as OX42 antibody-reactive) and glial fibrillary acid protein (GFAP) levels. Microglia, in particular, is considered one of the most important immune defenses of the CNS and is also a major source of proinflammatory cytokines in oxidative stress, such as tumor necrosis factor (TNF), nitric oxide, interleukin, and neurotoxic substances. In these conditions, massive proliferation of glial cells results in increased GFAP expression [20]. Additionally, a large number of studies have demonstrated a close association of glial cells with learning, memory, and other cognitive functions [21, 22]. In parallel, a growing body of evidence has implicated a role for cytokines in the normal, nonpathological brain and, hence, in the associated learning and memory behaviors [23]. TNF-α is also important for activity-dependent synaptic scaling within the hippocampus [24]. TNF-α, as well as multiple interleukins (e.g., IL-6, IL-1, and IL-10) and prostaglandins, can markedly influence cognitive function, primarily memory (reviewed in [25]). High-frequency stimulation in the hippocampus also increases IL-6 mRNA expression [26]. Finally, psychological stress has been associated with increased proinflammatory cytokines such as IL-6 and TNF-α in human and animal studies [27].

Together, the brain, the neuroendocrine, and the immune systems appear to be inextricably linked. Based on the accumulated evidence, we hypothesized that AR may activate inflammatory responses of the hippocampus that signals through emotionally relevant circuits and causes anxiety, leading to the abnormal behavior patterns. In the current study, we have used a Sprague-Dawley rat model, optimized in our laboratory, to interrogate whether hypersensitivity reactions and altered behavior in AR are associated with increased glial proliferation and induction of inflammatory response in the hippocampus.

2. Materials and Methods

2.1. Antibodies and Reagents. The OVA antigen was purchased from Sigma (A8040, USA) and aluminum hydroxide as adjuvant was from Kelong chemical factory (lot number 201110328, Chengdu, Sichuan, China). Enzyme-linked immunosorbent assay (ELISA) kits, specific for IgE (sIgE), interleukin 4 (IL-4), interferon-γ (IFN-γ), TNF-α, and IL-6 were purchased from Abcam (England). Antibodies against SP, GFAP, and CD11b (OX42) and rabbit anti-mouse secondary antibody were also purchased from Abcam, England. Where mentioned, biotin-conjugated rat anti-mouse antibodies were purchased from BD Pharmingen, Beijing, China. Sodium citrate buffer (0.01 M, pH 6.0) was prepared for dilution, where needed. The microscopic image acquisition and analysis system were, respectively, from BA200 Digital and Image-Pro Plus 6.0 (Media Cybernetics, USA).

2.2. Animals. Adult, male Sprague-Dawley rats (250–300 g) were obtained from Da Shuo Biological Technology Co. Ltd. (Chengdu, Sichuan, China). Before the experiment began, all rats were adapted for 1 week in the Experimental Animal Center of Chengdu University of TCM. The committee recognized that the proposed experimental procedures complied with the Animal Protection Law. All rats were housed in a temperature-controlled room (22–24°C) under a 12-hour light/dark cycle (7 am–7 pm). Food and water were available ad libitum in home cages.

2.3. Establishment of the AR Model. The AR model was established using an ovalbumin (OVA) sensitization method [14]. Rats were sensitized (days 1–13) with 7 intraperitoneal (i.p.) injections of 0.3 mg OVA (Sigma A8040, USA) as antigen and 30 mg aluminum hydroxide as adjuvant dissolved in 1 ml of saline. Following the i.p. immunization, the nasal antigen challenge (days 14–21) was performed with intranasal dripping of 50 μl of 2% OVA daily for 7 consecutive days. The animals in the control group were administrated with the same volume of saline. All animals were closely observed for development of any nasal responses of sneezing and watery rhinorrhea, and scraping, for 30 min after each challenge. Symptoms and signs of AR were then provoked (days 22–24) with intranasal dripping of 80 μl of 1% OVA daily for 3 consecutive days. Ten minutes after the last instillation of 1% OVA, all animals were subjected to i.p. injection of 1% sodium pentobarbital (50 mg/kg) to collect tail venous blood. Serum levels of cytokines sIgE, IL-4, and IFN-γ were measured by ELISA to evaluate whether AR was successfully established. The sensitization was maintained with intranasal dripping of 50 μl of 1% OVA every other day until the cytokine results confirmed AR. Finally, blood samples and hippocampus tissue were collected for detection of various other parameters by the corresponding methods.

2.4. Assay for Animal Behavior. The number of sneezes, degree of runny nose, and nasal rubbing movements during the 30 min period after the final allergen challenge were recorded in each experimental group. Following superimposition of the recording results, a total score of greater than 5 (>5) was used as the benchmark for successful establishment of AR [24]. In addition, we observed the patterns of emotion-related behavior as external manifestations of the AR, including fur color, physical energy, activity intensity, and food intake.

2.5. Specimen Collection. Animals of all groups ($n = 8$) were sacrificed with i.p. injection of 3% sodium pentobarbital (30 mg/kg) and then transcardially perfused with 350 ml 0.9% saline and fixed in solution containing 2% paraformaldehyde and 1.25% glutaraldehyde phosphate buffer solution (pH = 7.2). Blood collected from the femoral artery was subjected to the measurement of sera sIgE, IL-4, and INF-γ. The nasal mucosa tissues and the hippocampus tissues were quickly removed and separately postfixed in 4% paraformaldehyde for 72 h at 4°C. They were cut in coronal 4-5 μm sections and slide-mounted for microscopic examination.

2.6. Enzyme-Linked Immunosorbent Assay (ELISA). The sIgE, IL-4 and IFN-γ levels in the sera and the TNF-α and IL-6 levels in hippocampus homogenates were measured by solid-phase ELISA in accordance with the manufacturer's instructions. Bound immunoglobulin isotypes were detected with biotin-conjugated secondary antibody.

2.7. Hematoxylin-Eosin (HE) Staining Analysis. Paraffin sections of nasal mucosa tissue were stained with the hematoxylin and eosin method to examine pathological morphology. These sections were immersed in 4% paraformaldehyde for 4 h and transferred to 70% ethanol. Individual lobes of nasal mucosa biopsy material were placed in processing cassettes, dehydrated through a serial alcohol gradient, and embedded in paraffin wax blocks. Before immunostaining, 5 μm thick nasal mucosa tissue sections were dewaxed in xylene, rehydrated through decreasing concentrations of ethanol, and washed in PBS and then stained with hematoxylin and eosin (H&E). After staining, sections were dehydrated through increasing concentrations of ethanol and xylene. The stained sections were observed in mounting media for image acquisition. The pathological morphology were detected by microscopy at 400x magnification.

2.8. Immunohistochemical (IHC) Analysis. Paraffin sections of hippocampus tissue were stained with the streptavidin peroxidase method to examine SP, GFAP, and CD11b expressions. These sections were incubated in 3% hydrogen peroxide (H_2O_2)/methanol for 15 min. After washing three times in PBS (pH 7.2–7.4) for 5 min each, the sections were immersed in 0.01 M citrate buffer (pH 6.0) for 5 min and then washed twice with PBS. Nonspecific binding was blocked by incubation with normal goat serum for 20 min at 37°C. These sections were then incubated with rabbit anti-SP, anti-GFAP, and anti-OX42 antibodies (1 : 200 dilution) overnight at 4°C and then with biotinylated goat anti-rabbit IgG for 30 min. Following incubation with the horseradish peroxidase-labeled streptomycin ovalbumin reagent, sections were colored using a concentrated DAB kit. The stained sections were observed in mounting media for image acquisition. The immunopositive cells were detected by microscopy at 400x magnification, and the GFAP- and OX42-positive cells were quantified by the average number of positively stained cells per field.

2.9. Statistical Analysis. Data are presented as mean ± standard deviation (SD) (SPSS statistical analysis software, version 20.0). All variables indicated approximately normal distribution and parametric testing and were simultaneously subjected to one-way analysis of variance (ANOVA), followed by post hoc analysis using the Student–Newman–Keuls- (SNK-) q test. Differences were considered to be statistically significant at a P value < 0.05 ($P < 0.05$).

3. Results

In order to determine whether the AR model was established in the rat, we resorted to three major kinds of parameter points, namely, AR behavior; objective indicators including serum sIgE, IL-4, and IFN-γ levels; and HE staining. Our measurement of the behavior score satisfies the AR criteria [28]. Moreover, post hoc analysis revealed that AR behavior scores significantly increased in the model group of rats, compared to the control group ($P < 0.01$, Figure 1). Serum sIgE, in particular, is considered a touchstone diagnostic indicator of AR. Additionally, the levels of IL-4 and IFN-γ,

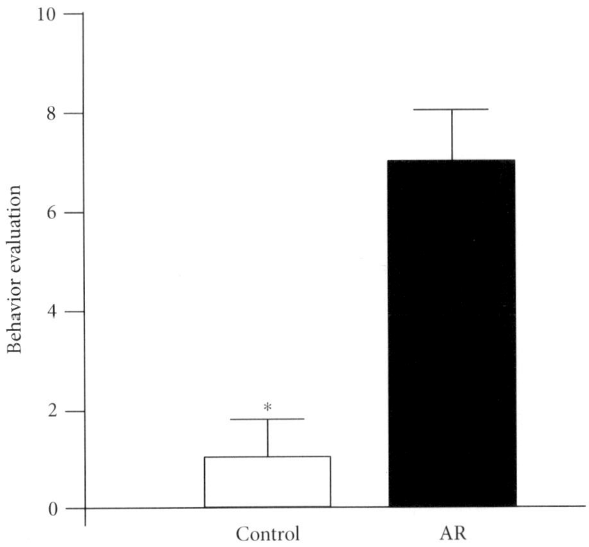

FIGURE 1: Behavior evaluation between the AR model group and the control group of animals. The total scores in AR model group were greater than 5 (>5), which suggested successful establishment of AR. Data are expressed as mean ± SD; $^*P < 0.01$.

TABLE 1: Serum levels of sIgE, IFN-γ, and IL-4.

Group	sIgE (ng/ml)	IFN-γ (mg/ml)	IL-4 (pg/ml)
Control	72.65 ± 9.17	0.59 ± 0.06	10.74 ± 3.05
AR	124.92 ± 15.56*	0.29 ± 0.07$^{\triangle}$	16.04 ± 3.81$^{\#}$

Sera were collected from the control group and the AR model group of rats, and the levels of the indicated molecules were measured as described in Materials and methods. Data are expressed as mean ± SD ($^*P < 0.01$, $^{\triangle}P < 0.01$, $^{\#}P < 0.01$).

respectively, reflect the Th1 and Th2 (T-helper 1and 2) cell populations. Our post hoc analysis revealed that both sIgE and IL-4 significantly increased compared to the control group ($P < 0.01$, Table 1); on the other hand, the levels of IFN-γ significantly decreased in the model group [$F_{(1,\ 14)} = 12.94$, $P < 0.01$]. Nasal mucosa tissues were examined by means of routine HE staining and light microscopy. Results showed that in the AR group of rats, the structural integrity of nasal mucosa tissue was impaired and the ciliated epithelium was irregular with disordered arrangement, exhibiting various degrees of fall-off and edema, and mixed with eosinophils and lymph cells (Figure 2).

Apart from these molecular and cellular indicators of AR, we also observed the emotion-related behavior of the AR and control groups, mostly in external manifestations that specifically included fur color, physical energy, activity intensity, and food intake. Before the sensitization, all rats were normal in daily activities and food intake. However, after the sensitization, the AR group showed external negative manifestations, such as the fur color turned pale or dim, physical energy turned into weakness, activity intensity decreased so that the animals became quiet, and food intake reduced. Overall, the whole body condition was worse than the control group.

In the immunohistochemical (IHC) analysis, we wanted to determine whether inflammation in the hippocampus relates to AR. As shown (Figure 3), the expression of microglial CD11b markers (determined by OX42 antibody staining) and SP in the AR group showed significant increase, compared to the control group ($P < 0.01$, Figures 3(a) and 3(c)). GFAP expression was also significantly higher in the AR group than in the control group [$F_{(1,\ 14)} = 5.46$, $P < 0.05$, Figure 3(b)]. We also observed that the expression of IL-6 in the AR group was higher than in the control group ($P < 0.01$, Figure 4), as determined by ELISA. Finally, TNF-α expression was higher in the AR group compared to the control group ($P < 0.05$; Figure 4). Taken together, the above results show elevated expression of GFAP, SP, IL-6, and TNF-α, as well as a higher number of CD11b$^+$ glial cells under AR conditions. In particular, SP and IL-6 and CD11+ cells showed significantly higher increase compared with GFAP and TNF-α in the AR group. These results clearly indicate that the inflammatory response of the hippocampus correlates with the observed increase of SP and IL-6 and of glial cell activation, which may be affected by nasal hypersensitivity and stimulation. We would like to mention that all rats survived the experiments with no death, and therefore, the observed effects are unlikely due to a general response of severe systemic pathology.

4. Discussion

The results presented here document an inflammatory response of the hippocampus in AR. Simultaneously, we observed higher levels of several proinflammatory mediators, which may relate to behavioral changes. Thus, we postulate that in an AR condition, the activated inflammatory response of the hippocampus may involve emotionally relevant circuits, which would then translate into abnormal behavior and negative emotions, mentioned earlier.

To our knowledge, this is the first study to examine the inflammation mechanisms of hippocampus activity in nasal hypersensitivity of a live animal AR model. In this model, we demonstrated upregulation of a significant cohort of proinflammatory molecular markers that included both cytokines as well as glial surface antigen, namely, GFAP, SP, IL-6, TNF-α, and CD11b. The OX42-reactive CD11b surface marker is characteristic of brain-specific immune cells, specifically the microglia, and thus, its increased expression in AR rats confirms an immune response. In fact, along with SP and IL-6, the CD11b$^+$ microglia population exhibited the most significant increase in the AR group compared to the control group. Moreover, there is a related report that allergy led to a reduced microglia presence and activity and to an elevated level of neurogenesis, such as those of DCX(+) cells and BrdU(+) cells in the hippocampus of allergic mice [29].

Nevertheless, previous studies reported that other brain regions such as the amygdala and hypothalamus are also responsive to respiratory allergies as measured by the expression of c-fos [30, 31]. In addition, functional imaging studies strongly implicated the prefrontal cortex (PFC) in providing inhibitory functions for anxiety and depression [32]. Another study reported Th2 cytokine expression in the brain in response to a peripheral immune challenge [12]. On the other hand, mRNA levels of IL-2 were reported to decrease

Control AR

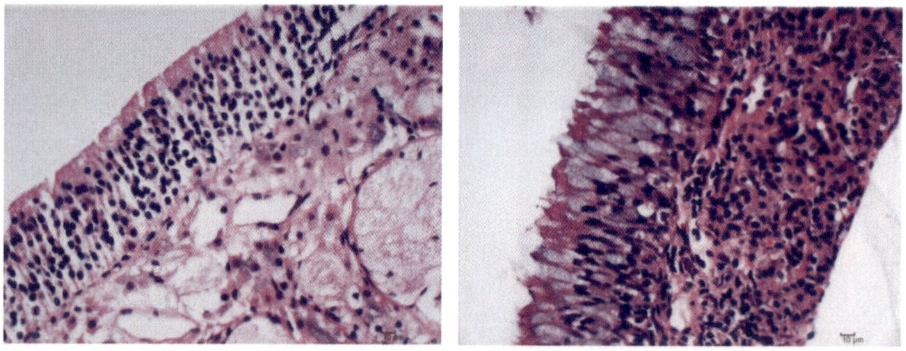

Figure 2

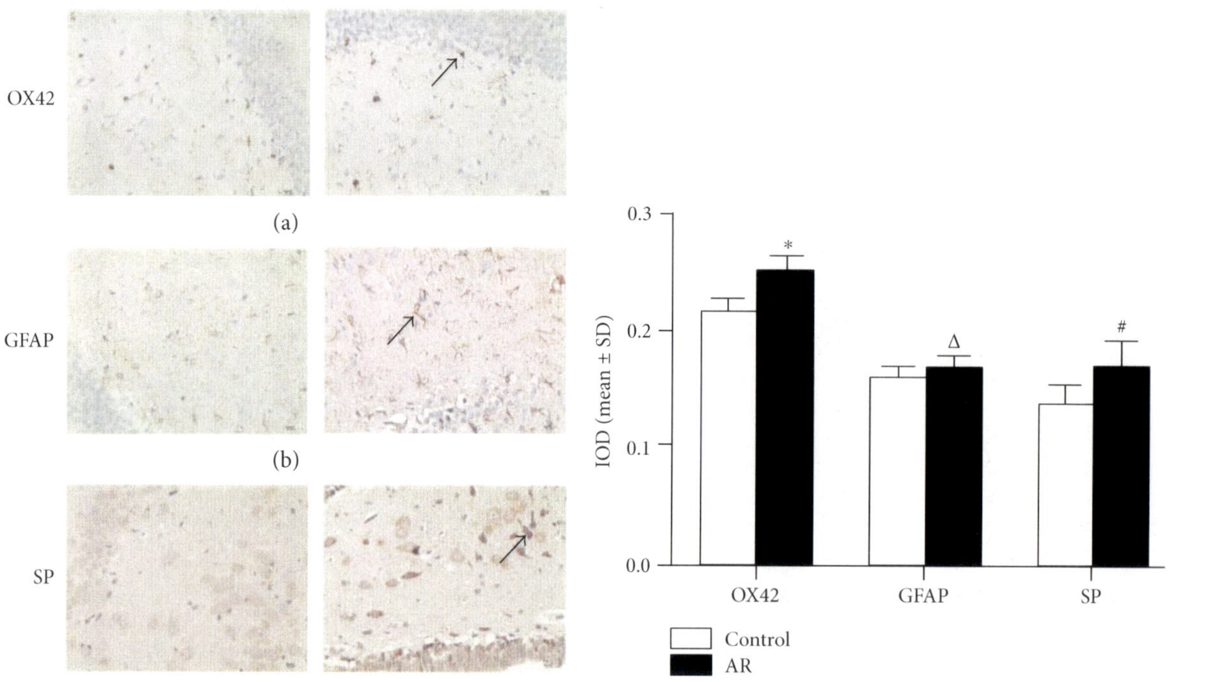

Figure 3: Representative photographs indicating IHC analysis (×400). Expression of (a) CD11b (OX42-stained), (b) GFAP, and (c) SP. (d) shows statistical analysis of the results. Data are expressed as mean ± SD; $^*P < 0.01$, $^{\triangle}P < 0.05$, $^{\#}P < 0.01$; $n = 8$; scale bar = 50 μm).

in the PFC under increased anxiety in the elevated plus maze (EPM) test [33]. As indicated previously, no studies have yet addressed the relationship between behavioral change resulting from AR hypersensitivity and hippocampus activity in a defined laboratory animal model.

While the expression of TNF-α, IL-6, GFAP, and SP, together with microglial activation, follows the pattern of a Th2 cell-dependent allergic reaction, the exact mechanism of their increase or function in the hippocampus is unknown at this time. It is tempting to speculate that increases in these cytokines may provide the link between the hippocampus and behavioral changes. The recognition that AR is a clinical condition, capable of influencing behavioral responses, has far-reaching significance in preventing AR development. If AR is exacerbated or not controlled properly, it may cause brain cognitive and memory dysfunctions or other adverse behaviors such as attention deficit and mental disorders, to name a few. Thus, our study suggests that it is important to reduce the occurrence of AR and manage patients with AR for pathological as well as social and economic reasons.

Although this study provides important new information about the inflammatory response of the hippocampus in the AR process, it has some limitations. First, we did not evaluate emotion-related behavior in view of a lack of objective scores but rather used external manifestations in the AR rats, such as fur color, physical energy, activity, and food intake, none of which may accurately reflect emotion-related behavior. Second, the exact mechanisms underlying the observed hippocampus inflammatory response in the AR rats are likely to be more complex, and possibly other neuroimmune mediators involved in

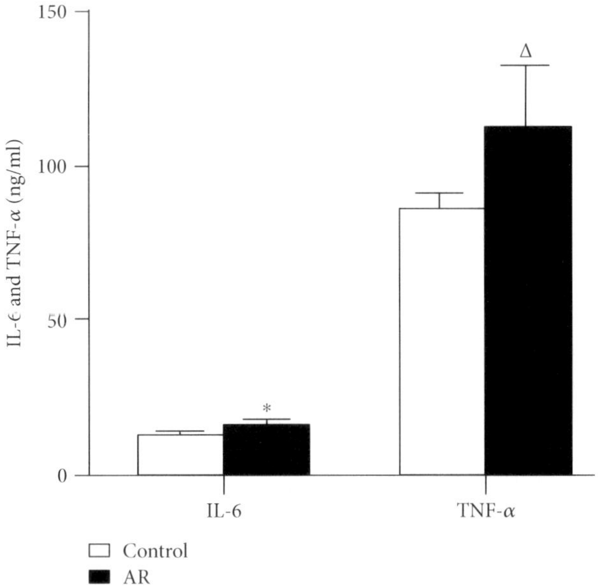

FIGURE 4: Levels of IL-6 and TNF-a, determined by ELISA. Comparing between in the AR model group and the control group. Data are expressed as mean ± SD; $^{*}P < 0.01$, $^{\triangle}P < 0.05$; $n = 8$.

emotional changes remain to be elucidated. In the future, more elaborate and sophisticated experiments need to be considered and designed, such as the use of 24-hour video surveillance and objective assessment methods to monitor AR behavior, in order to further investigate the relationship between the hippocampus and AR. Objective behavioral assessments may include emotional behavior evaluations, including anxiety scores and depression scores. In clinical experiments, we can use multiple detection methods such as functional magnetic resonance imaging (fMRI) and positron emission tomography (PET) to investigate the hippocampus of AR patient-related behavior, for instance, the potential depression- and anxiety-related disorders, memory loss, and cognitive impairment. Nevertheless, our findings open the door to novel insights into the inflammatory response of the hippocampus to allergic rhinitis in the rat model. Additional studies will certainly elucidate the complex neuroimmune relationship between the hippocampus and diverse emotional reactivity disorders. Lastly, our findings emphasize the importance of molecular behavioral studies for comprehensive awareness and prevention of AR. The impact of mental health disorders on society is substantial, especially in children with multiple allergic diseases, and implementing primary prevention activities may be warranted.

Authors' Contributions

Shasha Yang and Jing Wu contributed equally to this work.

Acknowledgments

This work was supported by grants from the National Natural Science Foundation of China (no. 81273985 and no. 81473523) and the National Science and Technology Pillar Program during the Twelfth Five-year Plan Period of China (no. 2015BAI04B00).

References

[1] A. KleinJan, M. Willart, M. van Nimwegen et al., "United airways: circulating Th2 effector cells in an allergic rhinitis model are responsible for promoting lower airways inflammation," *Clinical & Experimental Allergy*, vol. 40, no. 3, pp. 494–504, 2010.

[2] M. Okano, A. R. Satoskar, M. Abe et al., "Interleukin-4-independent production of Th2 cytokines by nasal lymphocytes and nasal eosinophilia in murine allergic rhinitis," *Allergy*, vol. 55, no. 8, pp. 723–731, 2000.

[3] D. I. Bernstein, G. Schwartz, and J. A. Bernstein, "Allergic rhinitis: mechanisms and treatment," *Immunology and Allergy Clinics of North America*, vol. 36, no. 2, pp. 261–278, 2016.

[4] A. Roger, E. Arcalá Campillo, M. C. Torres et al., "Reduced work/academic performance and quality of life in patients with allergic rhinitis and impact of allergen immunotherapy," *Allergy, Asthma & Clinical Immunology*, vol. 12, no. 1, p. 40, 2016.

[5] D. K. Kim, C. S. Rhee, D. H. Han, T. B. Won, D. Y. Kim, and J. W. Kim, "Treatment of allergic rhinitis is associated with improved attention performance in children: the Allergic Rhinitis Cohort Study for Kids (ARCO-Kids)," *PLoS One*, vol. 9, no. 10, article e109145, 2014.

[6] X. D. Wang, M. Zheng, H. F. Lou et al., "An increased prevalence of self-reported allergic rhinitis in major Chinese cities from 2005 to 2011," *Allergy*, vol. 71, no. 8, pp. 1170–1180, 2016.

[7] B. Feng, H. Jin, H. Xiang et al., "Association of pediatric allergic rhinitis with the ratings of attention-deficit/hyperactivity disorder," *American Journal of Rhinology and Allergy*, vol. 31, no. 3, pp. 161–167, 2017.

[8] S. Y. Kim, M. S. Kim, B. Park, J. H. Kim, and H. G. Choi, "Allergic rhinitis, atopic dermatitis, and asthma are associated with differences in school performance among Korean adolescents," *PLoS One*, vol. 12, no. 2, article e0171394, 2017.

[9] M. A. Strom and J. I. Silverberg, "Associations of physical activity and sedentary behavior with atopic disease in United States children," *The Journal of Pediatrics*, vol. 174, pp. 247–253.e3, 2016.

[10] M. A. Rosenkranz, W. W. Busse, T. Johnstone et al., "Neural circuitry underlying the interaction between emotion and asthma symptom exacerbation," *Proceedings of the National Academy of Sciences of the United States of America*, vol. 102, no. 37, pp. 13319–13324, 2005.

[11] F. A. Costa-Pinto, A. S. Basso, L. R. G. Britto, B. E. Malucelli, and M. Russo, "Avoidance behavior and neural correlates of allergen exposure in a murine model of asthma," *Brain, Behavior, and Immunity*, vol. 19, no. 1, pp. 52–60, 2005.

[12] L. H. Tonelli, M. Katz, C. E. Kovacsics et al., "Allergic rhinitis induces anxiety-like behavior and altered social interaction in rodents," *Brain, Behavior, and Immunity*, vol. 23, no. 6, pp. 784–793, 2009.

[13] J. Palermo-Neto and R. K. Guimarães, "Pavlovian conditioning of lung anaphylactic response in rats," *Life Sciences*, vol. 68, no. 6, pp. 611–623, 2000.

[14] A. Bartolomucci, P. Palanza, S. Parmigiani et al., "Chronic psychosocial stress down-regulates central cytokines mRNA," *Brain Research Bulletin*, vol. 62, no. 3, pp. 173–178, 2003.

[15] M. K. Nanda, G. K. LeMasters, L. Levin et al., "Allergic diseases and internalizing behaviors in early childhood," *Pediatrics*, vol. 137, no. 1, article e20151922, 2016.

[16] S. D. Bilbo and J. M. Schwarz, "The immune system and developmental programming of brain and behavior," *Frontiers in Neuroendocrinology*, vol. 33, no. 3, pp. 267–286, 2012.

[17] S. Rivest, "Interactions between the immune and neuroendocrine systems," *Progress in Brain Research*, vol. 181, pp. 43–53, 2010.

[18] A. Marques-Deak, G. Cizza, and E. Sternberg, "Brain-immune interactions and disease susceptibility," *Molecular Psychiatry*, vol. 10, no. 3, pp. 239–250, 2005.

[19] S. Sarin, B. Undem, A. Sanico, and A. Togias, "The role of the nervous system in rhinitis," *Journal of Allergy and Clinical Immunology*, vol. 118, no. 5, pp. 999–1014, 2006.

[20] J. Middeldorp and E. M. Hol, "GFAP in health and disease," *Progress in Neurobiology*, vol. 93, no. 3, pp. 421–443, 2011.

[21] L. Brambilla, F. Martorana, and D. Rossi, "Astrocyte signaling and neurodegeneration: new insights into CNS disorders," *Prion*, vol. 7, no. 1, pp. 28–36, 2014.

[22] G. Ricci, L. Volpi, L. Pasquali, L. Petrozzi, and G. Siciliano, "Astrocyte-neuron interactions in neurological disorders," *Journal of Biological Physics*, vol. 35, no. 4, pp. 317–336, 2009.

[23] J. McAfoose and B. T. Baune, "Evidence for a cytokine model of cognitive function," *Neuroscience & Biobehavioral Reviews*, vol. 33, no. 3, pp. 355–366, 2009.

[24] D. Stellwagen and R. C. Malenka, "Synaptic scaling mediated by glial TNF-α," *Nature*, vol. 440, no. 7087, pp. 1054–1059, 2006, 16547515.

[25] R. Yirmiya and I. Goshen, "Immune modulation of learning, memory, neural plasticity and neurogenesis," *Brain, Behavior, and Immunity*, vol. 25, no. 2, pp. 181–213, 2011.

[26] J. L. Jankowsky, B. E. Derrick, and P. H. Patterson, "Cytokine responses to LTP induction in the rat hippocampus: a comparison of in vitro and in vivo techniques," *Learning & Memory*, vol. 7, no. 6, pp. 400–412, 2000.

[27] K. A. O'Connor, J. D. Johnson, S. E. Hammack et al., "Inescapable shock induces resistance to the effects of dexamethasone," *Psychoneuroendocrinology*, vol. 28, no. 4, pp. 481–500, 2003.

[28] M.S. Miao, L.L. Xiang, and Y.Y. Miao, "Specification for preparation of allergic rhinitis animal model (draft)," *Chinese Traditional and Herbal Drugs*, vol. 49, no. 1, pp. 50–57, 2018.

[29] B. Klein, H. Mrowetz, J. Thalhamer, S. Scheiblhofer, R. Weiss, and L. Aigner, "Allergy enhances neurogenesis and modulates microglial activation in the hippocampus," *Frontiers in Cellular Neuroscience*, vol. 10, p. 169, 2016.

[30] F. A. Costa-Pinto, A. S. Basso, L. C. De Sa-Rocha, L. R. G. Britto, M. Russo, and J. Palermo-Neto, "Neural correlates of IgE-mediated allergy," *Annals of the New York Academy of Sciences*, vol. 1088, no. 1, pp. 116–131, 2006.

[31] F. A. Costa-Pinto, A. S. Basso, and M. Russo, "Role of mast cell degranulation in the neural correlates of the immediate allergic reaction in a murine model of asthma," *Brain, Behavior, and Immunity*, vol. 21, no. 6, pp. 783–790, 2007.

[32] J. D. Bremner, "Brain imaging in anxiety disorders," *Expert Review of Neurotherapeutics*, vol. 4, no. 2, pp. 275–284, 2004.

[33] C. R. Pawlak, R. K. W. Schwarting, and A. Bauhofer, "Cytokine mRNA levels in brain and peripheral tissues of the rat: relationships with plus-maze behavior," *Molecular Brain Research*, vol. 137, no. 1-2, pp. 159–165, 2005.

19

Metabolic Risk Factors of Alzheimer's Disease, Dementia with Lewy Bodies, and Normal Elderly

Chih-Kuang Cheng,[1] **Yu-Chien Tsao**,[2,3,4] **Yuan-Chih Su**,[5,6] **Fung-Chang Sung**,[7] **Hsu-Chih Tai**,[8] **and Woon-Man Kung**[8,9,10]

[1]*Stroke Center and Department of Neurology, Linkou Medical Center, Chang Gung Memorial Hospital and College of Medicine, Chang Gung University, Taoyuan, Taiwan*
[2]*Department of Internal Medicine, Yonghe Cardinal Tien Hospital, Taipei, Taiwan*
[3]*Department of Neurology, Neurological Institute, Taipei Veterans General Hospital, Taipei, Taiwan*
[4]*School of Medicine, National Yang-Ming University, Taipei, Taiwan*
[5]*Management Office for Health Data, China Medical University Hospital, Taichung, Taiwan*
[6]*College of Medicine, China Medical University, Taichung, Taiwan*
[7]*Department of Public Health, China Medical University, Taichung, Taiwan*
[8]*Department of Exercise and Health Promotion, College of Education, Chinese Culture University, Taipei, Taiwan*
[9]*Division of Neurosurgery, Department of Surgery, Taipei Tzu Chi Hospital, Buddhist Tzu Chi Medical Foundation, New Taipei City, Taiwan*
[10]*Department of Surgery, School of Medicine, Buddhist Tzu Chi University, Hualien, Taiwan*

Correspondence should be addressed to Woon-Man Kung; nskungwm@yahoo.com.tw

Academic Editor: Jan Aasly

Background. Alzheimer's disease (AD) and dementia with Lewy bodies (DLB) share many risk factors. Evidence suggests that metabolic risk factors are important to AD; however, their association with DLB is unclear. The risk of cardiovascular diseases (CVD) associated with AD and DLB is also uncertain. Thus, this nationwide, population-based study was designed to evaluate the metabolic and CVD risks in AD and DLB. *Materials and Methods.* Data were obtained from the Taiwan National Health Insurance Research Database. AD patients, DLB patients, and normal control (NC) individuals from 1996 to 2013 were enrolled for risk assessment. *Results.* In total, 7544 NC individuals, 1324 AD patients, and 562 DLB patients were enrolled. Participants with one or more metabolic risk factors had significantly higher odds of AD or DLB. No significant differences in metabolic risk factors were observed between DLB and AD patients. AD patients had a lower risk of CVD (aHR = 0.67, 95% CI = 0.59–0.76, p value < 0.001) and coronary artery disease (CAD) (aHR = 0.59, 95% CI = 0.51–0.69, p value < 0.001) than NC. DLB patients had a higher risk of ischemic stroke (aHR = 2.27, 95% CI = 1.68–3.06, p value < 0.001) than NC. *Conclusion.* Metabolic risk factors are important in AD and DLB. Patients with AD might have a lower risk of CAD and ischemic strokes. Patients with DLB might have a higher risk of ischemic stroke.

1. Introduction

Alzheimer's disease (AD) and dementia with Lewy bodies (DLB) are leading causes of dementia [1]. AD is caused by progressive neurodegeneration in the medial temporal lobe, hippocampus formation, and other brain areas with synergistic amyloid and tau proteinopathy [1, 2]. The risk factors for sporadic AD are complex. Apolipoprotein E $\varepsilon 4$ allele (APOE4) is one of best-known genetic risk factors. Additional risk factors include age, family history of AD, previous stroke, sleep apnea, traumatic brain injury (TBI), and limited education [1]. DLB is characterized by the propagation of aggregated intracellular α-synuclein (Lewy bodies) [3]. Risk factors of DLB overlap with that of AD to some extent; for example, APOE4, previous stroke, and TBI are risk factors of both DLB and AD [1, 4–6].

Emerging evidence suggests that metabolic risk factors contribute not only to cardiovascular diseases (CVD) like coronary artery disease (CAD), and ischemic strokes, such as cerebrovascular accident (CVA), but also to dementia [7–9]. Hypertension, diabetes mellitus (DM), and hyperlipidemia are known risk factors for AD [9, 10]. Moreover, a history of CAD or CVA is associated with accelerated cognitive decline in AD patients [8, 11, 12].

However, it is unclear if metabolic risks are also important risk factors of DLB, and it is unclear if AD and DLB patients are more susceptible to CVD. Hence, we conducted a nationwide, population-based, normal control, risk-adjusted, retrospective cohort study in Taiwan to investigate the metabolic risks and the incidence of CVD in patients with AD and DLB. Our purpose is to determine the modifiable metabolic risk factors in DLB and the risk of CVD in AD and DLB to improve the prevention of dementia and CVD.

2. Materials and Methods

2.1. Study Design. We conducted a retrospective cohort study using health insurance data from the National Health Insurance Research Database (NHIRD), which contained medical information of over 99% of Taiwan citizens. The Longitudinal Health Insurance Database 2000 (LHID2000), a subdataset of the NHIRD, was applied for this study. The LHID2000 contains diagnostic data of the International Classification of Diseases, 9th Revision, Clinical Modification (ICD-9-CM) code, and treatment data from the outpatient visits and hospitalizations from 1996 to 2013 of 1 million random individuals. All participants were encrypted with a dummy number. This study was approved by the Institutional Review Board and the Ethics Committee of China Medical University Hospital, Taiwan (CMUH104-REC2-115 (CR-2)).

This study investigated AD patients, DLB patients, and normal control (NC) individuals who were enrolled. Both AD and DLB patients were identified using specific criteria. AD patients who met any of the following criteria were included: (1) the ICD-9-CM code 331.0 (AD diagnosis date defined as the index date), or (2) having a diagnosis record of dementia (ICD-9-CM: 290.0–290.4, 294.1, and 331.0–331.2) and receiving acetylcholinesterase inhibitors or memantine treatment (dementia diagnosis date defined as the index date). The exclusion criteria for the AD cohort were patients with (1) any records of cognitive impairment (ICD-9-CM: 331.8, 331.83, and 331.9), Huntington's disease (ICD-9-CM: 333.4), Creutzfeldt-Jakob disease (ICD-9-CM: 046.11 and 046.19), and hydrocephalus (ICD-9-CM: 331.3, 331.4, 331.5, 741.0, and 742.3), (2) a history of stroke (ICD-9-CM: 430–435) or CAD (ICD-9-CM: 410–414) before the index date, and (3) Parkinson's disease (PD) or Parkinsonism diagnosis recorded within 1 year after the index date. For DLB patients, the inclusion criteria were (1) the diagnosis of PD and Parkinsonism (ICD-9-CM: 332, 332.0, 332.1, 333, 333.0, and 333.9) 1 year after diagnosis of dementia (ICD-9-CM: 290.0–290.3, 294.1, and 331.0) (dementia diagnosis date defined as the index date), (2) diagnosis of dementia within 1 year after diagnosis of PD and Parkinsonism (dementia diagnosis date defined as the index date), and (3) ICD-9-CM code 331.82 (DLB diagnosis date defined as the index date). The exclusion criteria for DLB patients included a history of stroke, CAD, head injury (ICD-9-CM: 850–854 and 959.01), or hydrocephalus. Patients with the diagnosis of both AD and DLB were excluded from the study cohorts. The NC population was defined as patients without the diagnosis of AD, DLB, other dementias, or Parkinson's disease. The NC population excluded individuals with a history of stroke or CAD. The study population selection procedure is shown in Figure 1.

2.2. Statistical Analysis. The main outcomes of this study were stroke (ICD-9-CM: 430–435) and CAD (ICD-9-CM: 410–414) after the index date. Only inpatient records were used to identify patients with stroke. A history of hypertension (ICD-9-CM: 401–405), diabetes mellitus (ICD-9-CM: 250), and hyperlipidemia (ICD-9-CM: 272) were included as comorbidities. All comorbidities were considered to be significant after at least one inpatient visit or two outpatient visits. In addition, we investigated the use of aspirin, clopidogrel, and warfarin before the index date. Demographic characteristics of sex and age were considered as covariates. We combined the AD and DLB cohorts and matched them with the NC population according to sex and age in a 1 : 4 ratio by propensity score matching. This study compared the risk of the main outcomes, that is, CAD and stroke, among the three cohorts. The risk factors for AD and DLB were also evaluated. The baseline characteristics among the three groups were tested using the chi-square test and ANOVA. Logistic regression was used to evaluate the probable risk factors of AD and DLB. We examined whether the risk of stroke and CAD increases among AD and DLB patients using the Cox proportional hazard regression. A p value less than 0.05 was significant. All the statistical analyses were conducted using the statistical software package, SAS, version 9.4 (SAS Institute Inc., Cary, NC).

3. Results

The final study population consisted of 7544 NC individuals, 1324 AD patients, and 562 DLB patients (Table 1). The number of female participants was higher than male participants in the AD cohort. Contrarily, the DLB cohort included a higher number of male participants. The difference in the average ages among the three cohorts was insignificant (p value = 0.26). Participants under 65 years were less than 20% in each cohort. The distributions of baseline comorbidities differed among the NC, AD, and DLB groups (p value < 0.001). The medication status was also significantly different (p value < 0.01) among the cohorts. The proportions of diabetes mellitus and hyperlipidemia were higher in AD patients than in DLB patients. There were 58.4% and 60.5% hypertensive individuals in the AD group and the DLB group, respectively.

Between AD and NC, compared to participants without any metabolic risk factors, the participants with one or more metabolic risk factors had significantly higher odds of AD

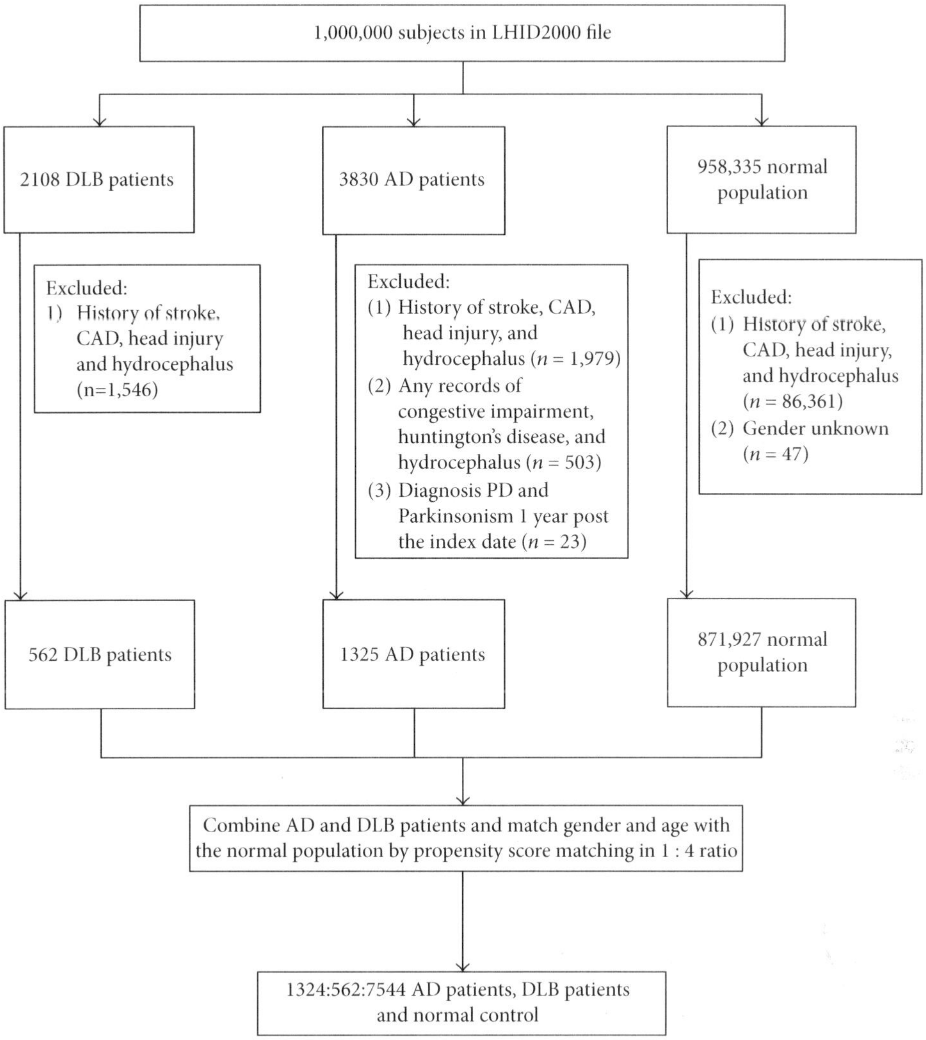

Figure 1: Enrollment flow chart for the study population.

Table 1: Demographic and background characteristics of NC, AD, and DLB patients.

	NC	AD	DLB	p value
N	7544	1324	562	
Sex, f/m	3758/3786	768/556	242/320	<0.001
Age				
<50	216 (2.9)	39 (2.9)	15 (2.7)	
50–64	939 (12.4)	188 (14.2)	50 (8.90)	
≥65	6389 (84.7)	1097 (82.9)	497 (88.4)	
Mean (SD)	74.5 (11.1)	74.2 (11.4)	75.1 (10.3)	0.26*
Comorbidity				
Hypertension	2777 (36.8)	773 (58.4)	340 (60.5)	<0.001
Diabetes mellitus	1132 (15.0)	387 (29.2)	142 (25.3)	<0.001
Hyperlipidemia	1201 (15.9)	466 (35.2)	146 (26.0)	<0.001
Drug				
Aspirin	1139 (15.1)	468 (35.3)	186 (33.1)	<0.001
Clopidogrel	21 (0.28)	18 (1.36)	7 (1.25)	<0.001
Warfarin	45 (0.6)	20 (1.51)	5 (0.89)	0.002

Chi-square test; *ANOVA. NC, normal control; AD, Alzheimer's disease; DLB, dementia with Lewy bodies; SD, standard deviation.

TABLE 2: Risk factors for AD and DLB patients.

Risk factors	Multivariable ORs (95% CI) AD versus NC	DLB versus NC	DLB versus AD
Sex			
Female	1 (reference)	1 (reference)	1 (reference)
Male	0.82 (0.72–0.92)**	1.42 (1.19–1.69)***	1.75 (1.43–2.15)***
Age, per year	1.0 (0.99–1.0)	1.0 (0.99–1.01)	1 (0.99–1.01)
Combination of metabolic risk factors (hypertension, diabetes, and hyperlipidemia)			
(− − −)	1 (reference)	1 (reference)	1 (reference)
(+ − −)	2.29 (1.95–2.69)***	2.74 (2.2–3.42)***	1.16 (0.89–1.52)
(− + −)	2.28 (1.64–3.18)***	2.23 (1.38–3.62)***	0.91 (0.52–1.6)
(− − +)	3.7 (2.78–4.93)***	2.66 (1.65–4.29)***	0.66 (0.39–1.11)
(+ + −)	3.08 (2.42–3.92)***	3.6 (2.6–4.99)***	1.18 (0.81–1.73)
(+ − +)	3.63 (2.94–4.49)***	3.25 (2.37–4.46)***	0.88 (0.62–1.26)
(− + +)	3.58 (2.48–5.17)***	2.14 (1.1–4.17)*	0.62 (0.3–1.28)
(+ + +)	4.9 (4.01–5.99)***	3.64 (2.65–5)***	0.7 (0.5–0.99)

+, presence; −, absence; CI, confidential interval; OR, odds ratio; NC, normal control; AD, Alzheimer's disease; DLB, dementia with Lewy bodies. Adjusted sex and age in logistic regression. *$p < 0.05$, **$p < 0.01$, and ***$p < 0.001$.

(Table 2). The odds ratio of AD was 4.9 (95% CI = 4.01–5.99, p value < 0.001) in patients with three metabolic risk factors. For DLB and NC, the logistic regression showed an odds ratio of 3.64 for DLB (95% CI = 2.65–5, p value < 0.001) in patients with three metabolic risk factors. Between DLB and AD, there were no significant odds of DLB in patients with any metabolic risk factors. The male patients had low odds of AD (OR = 0.82, 95% CI = 0.72–0.92, p value < 0.01), but high odds of DLB (OR = 1.42, 95% CI = 1.19–1.69, p value < 0.001).

The results of the Cox model indicated that the AD patients had a lower risk of outcomes (aHR = 0.67, 95% CI = 0.59–0.76, p value < 0.001) than the NC population (Table 3). Separated, the risks of CAD and stroke were 0.59-fold (95% CI = 0.51–0.69, p value < 0.001) and 1.02-fold (95% CI = 0.8–1.3, p value > 0.05), respectively, in AD patients. Compared with the NC cohort, there was a higher stroke risk in the DLB group (aHR = 2.08, 95% CI = 1.58–2.73, p value < 0.001). The risk of both outcomes combined was also higher (aHR = 1.23, 95% CI = 1.06–1.44, p value < 0.01). However, the risk of CAD alone was negligible (aHR = 1.04, 95% CI = 0.86–1.24, p value > 0.05) among DLB patients. The risk of outcomes in males was higher than that in females (aHR = 1.14, 95% CI = 1.06–1.23, p value < 0.001). The risk of outcomes increased 1.03-fold per year with increasing age (95% CI = 1.03–1.04, p value < 0.001). The aHR outcomes of hypertension and diabetes mellitus were 1.39 (95% CI = 1.28–1.51, p value < 0.001) and 1.2 (95% CI = 1.09–1.34, p value < 0.001), respectively. Hyperlipidemia reduced the risk of stroke (aHR = 0.7, 95% CI = 0.55–0.9, p value < 0.01), but did not affect the risk of outcomes (aHR = 0.9, 95% CI = 0.81–1, p value > 0.05) and CAD (aHR = 0.96, 95% CI = 0.86–1.09, p value > 0.05). There was no significant effect on the risk of outcomes with aspirin (aHR = 0.98, 95% CI = 0.89–1.09, p value > 0.05), clopidogrel (aHR = 1.25, 95% CI = 0.72–2.16, p value > 0.05), and warfarin (aHR = 0.66, 95% CI = 0.38–1.13, p value > 0.05). Additionally, we divided stroke outcome into ischemic and hemorrhagic stroke. The ischemic stroke risk was insignificant among AD patients (aHR = 1.01, 95% CI = 0.77–1.33, p value > 0.05) when compared to the NC population (Table 4). In contrast, the DLB group had a higher ischemic stroke risk (aHR = 2.27, 95% CI = 1.68–3.06, p value < 0.001). The aHRs of hemorrhagic stroke among AD and DLB patients were insignificant (for AD: aHR = 1.04, 95% CI = 0.61–1.77, p value > 0.05; for DLB: aHR = 1.4, 95% CI = 0.7–2.8, p value > 0.05).

4. Discussion

In this retrospective cohort study, female patients were more likely to have AD, while male patients were more likely to have DLB. Patients with any one of the metabolic risk factors considered, had an increased risk of having AD or DLB. Patients who had three comorbid risk factors (hypertension, diabetes mellitus, and hyperlipidemia) simultaneously were at higher risk of having AD or DLB than patients with a single risk factor. The consequences of metabolic risk factors for AD are similar to those for DLB. Patients with AD had a lower risk, while patients with DLB had a higher risk of all CVD outcomes than the NC population. When outcomes were separated, patients with AD had a lower risk of CAD, and patients with DLB had a higher risk of ischemic stroke than the NC population. Patients with AD or DLB had no increased risk of hemorrhagic stroke.

We found that AD was more prevalent among female patients, while DLB was more prevalent among male patients. Sex differences between AD and DLB have been reported [13]. The age at onset of AD may be lower in women than in men with the same copies of the APOE $\varepsilon4$ allele [14]. Male sex is a known risk factor for DLB [3, 5].

TABLE 3: Multivariable analysis of risk of CAD and stroke in Cox proportional hazard regression.

Risk factors	All outcomes Adjusted HR (95% CI)	CAD Adjusted HR (95% CI)	Stroke Adjusted HR (95% CI)
NC	1 (reference)	1 (reference)	1 (reference)
AD	0.67 (0.59–0.76)***	0.59 (0.51–0.69)***	1.02 (0.8–1.3)
DLB	1.23 (1.06–1.44)**	1.04 (0.86–1.24)	2.08 (1.58–2.73)***
Sex			
Female	1 (reference)	1 (reference)	1 (reference)
Male	1.14 (1.06–1.23)***	1.11 (1.02–1.21)*	1.26 (1.07–1.49)**
Age, per year	1.03 (1.03–1.04)***	1.03 (1.02–1.03)***	1.05 (1.04–1.06)***
Hypertension (yes versus no)	1.39 (1.28–1.51)***	1.39 (1.27–1.53)***	1.37 (1.14–1.64)***
Diabetes mellitus (yes versus no)	1.2 (1.09–1.34)***	1.15 (1.02–1.29)*	1.43 (1.15–1.78)**
Hyperlipidemia (yes versus no)	0.9 (0.81–1)	0.96 (0.86–1.09)	0.7 (0.55–0.9)**
Aspirin (yes versus no)	0.98 (0.89–1.09)	0.95 (0.85–1.07)	1.1 (0.89–1.37)
Clopidogrel (yes versus no)	1.25 (0.72–2.16)	1.29 (0.69–2.41)	1.14 (0.36–3.58)
Warfarin (yes versus no)	0.66 (0.38–1.13)	0.6 (0.31–1.15)	0.84 (0.31–2.27)

HR, hazard ratio; CI, confidence interval; NC, normal control; AD, Alzheimer's disease; DLB, dementia with Lewy bodies. Adjusted sex, age, hypertension, diabetes mellitus, hyperlipidemia, aspirin, clopidogrel, and warfarin in Cox proportional hazards regression. $^{*}p < 0.05$, $^{**}p < 0.01$, and $^{***}p < 0.001$.

TABLE 4: Multivariable analysis of the risk of ischemic stroke and hemorrhagic stroke in Cox proportional hazard regression.

Risk factors	Ischemic stroke Adjusted HR (95% CI)	Hemorrhage stroke Adjusted HR (95% CI)
NC	1 (reference)	1 (reference)
AD	1.01 (0.77–1.33)	1.04 (0.61–1.77)
DLB	2.27 (1.68–3.06)***	1.4 (0.7–2.8)
Sex		
Female	1 (reference)	1 (reference)
Male	1.16 (0.97–1.4)	1.74 (1.21–2.49)**
Age, per year	1.05 (1.04–1.06)***	1.05 (1.03–1.07)***
Hypertension (yes versus no)	1.34 (1.09–1.64)**	1.5 (1.03–2.19)*
Diabetes mellitus (yes versus no)	1.48 (1.16–1.88)**	1.25 (0.76–2.06)
Hyperlipidemia (yes versus no)	0.75 (0.57–0.98)*	0.52 (0.29–0.95)*
Aspirin (yes versus no)	1.21 (0.95–1.53)	0.76 (0.46–1.27)
Clopidogrel (yes versus no)	0.91 (0.22–3.68)	2.36 (0.32–17.36)
Warfarin (yes versus no)	1.05 (0.39–2.82)	

HR, hazard ratio; CI, confidence interval; NC, normal control; AD, Alzheimer's disease; DLB, dementia with Lewy bodies. Adjusted sex, age, hypertension, diabetes mellitus, hyperlipidemia, aspirin, clopidogrel, and warfarin in Cox proportional hazards regression. $^{*}p < 0.05$, $^{**}p < 0.01$, and $^{***}p < 0.001$.

The cause of these sex differences remains uncertain and need to be clarified.

We found that hypertension significantly increased the risk of both AD (OR = 2.29, 95% CI = 1.95–2.69) and DLB (OR = 2.74, 95% CI = 2.20–3.42). Hypertension is a risk factor for dementia [9]. Studies have shown that hypertension increases the risk of AD, and that antihypertensive treatment can reduce the risk of AD [10]. The relationship between hypertension and DLB is less understood. In a neuropathological study, patients with DLB pathology were found to have a significantly higher incidence of hypertension [15].

We also found that diabetes mellitus increased the risk of AD (OR = 2.28, 95% CI = 1.64–3.18) and DLB (OR = 2.23, 95% CI = 1.38–3.62). Diabetes mellitus is a risk factor for cognitive decline [10]. Insulin insufficiency increases the risk of AD [10]. Either an excessive glucose level or an insulin dysfunction may play a role in AD [10]. There is limited information about the effect of diabetes on DLB. Although diabetes was a risk factor for DLB in our study, it did not alter the risk of DLB in another study [5]. This conflicting result may have arisen because of the different diagnostic criteria for diabetes in different populations, and further studies are warranted to clarify if diabetes causes DLB.

Hyperlipidemia was another risk factor that increased AD (OR = 3.70, 95% CI = 2.78–4.93) and DLB (OR = 2.66, 95% CI = 1.65–4.29). Dysfunction of lipid metabolism plays an important role in dementia. High total serum cholesterol levels are associated with dementia and AD [10]. APOE is an important class of lipoprotein in lipid metabolism, and APOE4, an allele of APOE, is implicated in AD. APOE4 is also more frequent in DLB patients than in controls [5]. Nevertheless, the mechanism by which lipid disorders affect DLB is obscure. Considering its close association with dementia and that it is a modifiable risk factor, we suggest that studies focus more on lipid disorders in future DLB studies.

Having three metabolic risk factors simultaneously further increased the risk of AD (OR = 4.90, 95% CI = 4.01–5.99) and DLB (OR = 3.64, 95% CI = 2.65–5.00). The hazard of metabolic risk factors is similar in AD and DLB. AD and DLB share many similar risk factors such as depression, smoking, and the APOE $\varepsilon4$ allele [5]. Cerebrovascular lesions are also frequent in both AD and DLB [16, 17]. AD and DLB show clinical and pathological similarity, and metabolic risk factors may have similar roles in the risk of developing AD and DLB. Summarizing, better lifestyle modifications and medication for the treatment of metabolic risk factors may not only prevent stroke and CAD but also AD and DLB.

In a risk-adjusted long-term follow-up, we found that AD had a decreasing risk of CAD (aHR = 0.59, 95% CI = 0.51–0.69), while DLB had an increasing risk of ischemic stroke (aHR = 2.27, 95% CI = 1.68–3.06). AD is associated with atherosclerosis [18]. Evidence has shown that cerebral atherosclerosis, involving extracranial or intracranial arteries, contributes to the cognitive decline in AD [19, 20]. Coronary atherosclerosis also worsens cognitive function in AD [11]. These facts reflect the hemodynamic compromise or hypoperfusion of the brain which correlates with AD deterioration [21–23]. However, AD itself does not necessarily increase the risk of CAD. In fact, a recent study showed that APOE $\varepsilon4$ does not interact with CAD [24]. Interestingly, our results implied that patients with AD might have protective factors to CAD, with the underdiagnosis of CAD or ischemic stroke in AD having been one possible explanation. However, we did not find a similar effect in DLB, making it less likely. A change in eating behaviour in AD was another possible explanation. Anorexia and weight loss, which are common in advanced AD [25], may reduce blood sugar or lipid level and decrease the risk of atherosclerosis. A change in amyloid β (Aβ) metabolism may affect the risk of CAD in AD. Extracellular deposition of Aβ in the brain is the pathological hallmark of AD [26]. A dysfunction of Aβ production and clearance in the central nervous system may contribute to the accumulation of cerebral Aβ in late onset AD [27, 28]. Higher plasma Aβ also correlates with cerebral white matter lesions and ischemic heart disease [29]. In short, the change in the Aβ metabolic pathway in AD may be associated with cerebrovascular and cardiovascular risks, and further investigations are warranted.

A history of stroke is more frequently observed in patients with DLB [5]. White matter hyperintensities on cerebral T2-weighted magnetic resonance imaging are higher in DLB than in AD patients [17]. DLB usually shows hypoperfusion in the striatum and the visual cortex [3]. All these studies suggest that DLB correlates with the function of cerebral small vessels. Postural hypotension is commonly seen in DLB [3], and is also a potential risk factor for ischemic stroke. Intracellular α-synuclein aggregation is characteristic of DLB [1]. Studies also show a potential role for α-synuclein in ischemic stroke modulation [30]. Further studies are required to determine the mechanism of stroke in DLB.

Cerebral microbleeds are small hemosiderin deposits in the brain and are not unusual in AD or DLB [31, 32]. The gradual spreading of the intracellular aggregation of hyperphosphorylated tau (P-tau) in the brain is associated with AD progression [1]. Studies also reveal the association between cerebral microbleeds and P-tau [33, 34]. Interestingly, our data did not reveal increased hemorrhagic stroke in both AD and DLB patients when compared to NC individuals. This may imply that the pathological processes for intracerebral hemorrhage and cerebral microbleeds may differ in AD and DLB.

Limitations were inevitable in this study. First, subjects were classified based on the main clinical diagnosis and bias from misclassification was possible. Dementia is a complex syndrome and accurate diagnosis is challenging because of the overlapping clinical presentation. Although we used multiple methods during the inclusion process to identify the diagnosis and to minimize misclassification, a few atypical cases may still present difficulties in classification. Second, the severity of metabolic risk factors and their different treatment methods can potentially affect the risk of CAD or stroke. Third, this was a Taiwan-based study, and the influence of risk may vary among different racial groups. Fourth, this was a retrospective study, and selection and information biases cannot be completely excluded.

5. Conclusions

Hypertension, diabetes mellitus, and hyperlipidemia are risk factors of AD and DLB. Multiple metabolic risk factors, when simultaneously present, might aggravate the risk of AD and DLB. The control of metabolic risk factors is crucial for the prevention of AD and DLB. Patients with AD might have a lower risk of CAD, while patients with DLB might have a higher risk of ischemic stroke. Our study suggests that better lifestyle modifications and medications for the treatment of metabolic risk factors may lower the risk of AD and DLB. Furthermore, stroke prevention is important in patients with DLB. Further studies to understand the mechanism of stroke in DLB are warranted.

Acknowledgments

This work was supported by grants from the Ministry of Health and Welfare, Taiwan (MOHW107-TDU-B-212-123004), China Medical University Hospital, Academia Sinica Stroke Biosignature Project (BM10701010021), MOST

Clinical Trial Consortium for Stroke (MOST 106-2321-B-039-005), Tseng-Lien Lin Foundation, Taichung, Taiwan, and Katsuzo and Kiyo Aoshima Memorial Funds, Japan.

References

[1] F. M. Elahi and B. L. Miller, "A clinicopathological approach to the diagnosis of dementia," *Nature Reviews Neurology*, vol. 13, no. 8, pp. 457–476, 2017.

[2] B. V. Zlokovic, "Neurovascular pathways to neurodegeneration in Alzheimer's disease and other disorders," *Nature Reviews Neuroscience*, vol. 12, no. 12, pp. 723–738, 2011.

[3] Z. Walker, K. L. Possin, B. F. Boeve, and D. Aarsland, "Lewy body dementias," *The Lancet*, vol. 386, no. 10004, pp. 1683–1697, 2015.

[4] I. G. McKeith, B. F. Boeve, D. W. Dickson et al., "Diagnosis and management of dementia with Lewy bodies: fourth consensus report of the DLB Consortium," *Neurology*, vol. 89, no. 1, pp. 88–100, 2017.

[5] B. P. Boot, C. F. Orr, J. E. Ahlskog et al., "Risk factors for dementia with Lewy bodies: a case-control study," *Neurology*, vol. 81, no. 9, pp. 833–840, 2013.

[6] R. E. Mrak and W. S. Griffin, "Dementia with Lewy bodies: definition, diagnosis, and pathogenic relationship to Alzheimer's disease," *Neuropsychiatric disease and treatment*, vol. 3, no. 5, pp. 619–625, 2007.

[7] T. B. Chen, S. Y. Yiao, Y. Sun et al., "Comorbidity and dementia: a nationwide survey in Taiwan," *PLoS One*, vol. 12, no. 4, article e0175475, 2017.

[8] S. Kaffashian, A. Dugravot, A. Elbaz et al., "Predicting cognitive decline: a dementia risk score vs the Framingham vascular risk scores," *Neurology*, vol. 80, no. 14, pp. 1300–1306, 2013.

[9] F. W. Unverzagt, L. A. McClure, V. G. Wadley et al., "Vascular risk factors and cognitive impairment in a stroke-free cohort," *Neurology*, vol. 77, no. 19, pp. 1729–1736, 2011.

[10] C. Y. Santos, P. J. Snyder, W. C. Wu, M. Zhang, A. Echeverria, and J. Alber, "Pathophysiologic relationship between Alzheimer's disease, cerebrovascular disease, and cardiovascular risk: a review and synthesis," *Alzheimer's & Dementia: Diagnosis, Assessment & Disease Monitoring*, vol. 7, pp. 69–87, 2017.

[11] M. Bleckwenn, L. Kleineidam, M. Wagner et al., "Impact of coronary heart disease on cognitive decline in Alzheimer's disease: a prospective longitudinal cohort study in primary care," *British Journal of General Practice*, vol. 67, no. 655, pp. e111–e117, 2017.

[12] J. Attems and K. A. Jellinger, "The overlap between vascular disease and Alzheimer's disease—lessons from pathology," *BMC Medicine*, vol. 12, no. 1, p. 206, 2014.

[13] S. A. Vann Jones and J. T. O'Brien, "The prevalence and incidence of dementia with Lewy bodies: a systematic review of population and clinical studies," *Psychological Medicine*, vol. 44, no. 4, pp. 673–683, 2014.

[14] S. C. Neu, J. Pa, W. Kukull et al., "Apolipoprotein E genotype and sex risk factors for Alzheimer disease: a meta-analysis," *JAMA Neurology*, vol. 74, no. 10, pp. 1178–1189, 2017.

[15] J. De Reuck, V. Deramecourt, C. Cordonnier, D. Leys, F. Pasquier, and C. A. Maurage, "Prevalence of small cerebral bleeds in patients with a neurodegenerative dementia: a neuropathological study," *Journal of the Neurological Sciences*, vol. 300, no. 1-2, pp. 63–66, 2011.

[16] K. A. Jellinger, "Prevalence and impact of cerebrovascular lesions in Alzheimer and Lewy body diseases," *Neurodegenerative Diseases*, vol. 7, no. 1-3, pp. 112–115, 2010.

[17] L. Sarro, N. Tosakulwong, C. G. Schwarz et al., "An investigation of cerebrovascular lesions in dementia with Lewy bodies compared to Alzheimer's disease," *Alzheimer's & Dementia*, vol. 13, no. 3, pp. 257–266, 2017.

[18] A. Hofman, A. Ott, M. M. B. Breteler et al., "Atherosclerosis, apolipoprotein E, and prevalence of dementia and Alzheimer's disease in the Rotterdam Study," *The Lancet*, vol. 349, no. 9046, pp. 151–154, 1997.

[19] A. E. Roher, S. L. Tyas, C. L. Maarouf et al., "Intracranial atherosclerosis as a contributing factor to Alzheimer's disease dementia," *Alzheimer's & Dementia*, vol. 7, no. 4, pp. 436–444, 2011.

[20] M. Silvestrini, B. Gobbi, P. Pasqualetti et al., "Carotid atherosclerosis and cognitive decline in patients with Alzheimer's disease," *Neurobiology of Aging*, vol. 30, no. 8, pp. 1177–1183, 2009.

[21] A. E. Roher, Z. Garami, S. L. Tyas et al., "Transcranial Doppler ultrasound blood flow velocity and pulsatility index as systemic indicators for Alzheimer's disease," *Alzheimer's & Dementia*, vol. 7, no. 4, pp. 445–455, 2011.

[22] A. Salminen, A. Kauppinen, and K. Kaarniranta, "Hypoxia/ischemia activate processing of amyloid precursor protein: impact of vascular dysfunction in the pathogenesis of Alzheimer's disease," *Journal of Neurochemistry*, vol. 140, no. 4, pp. 536–549, 2017.

[23] L. Qiu, G. Ng, E. K. Tan, P. Liao, N. Kandiah, and L. Zeng, "Chronic cerebral hypoperfusion enhances Tau hyperphosphorylation and reduces autophagy in Alzheimer's disease mice," *Scientific Reports*, vol. 6, no. 1, article 23964, 2016.

[24] D. M. Lyall, J. Ward, S. J. Ritchie et al., "Alzheimer disease genetic risk factor *APOE* e4 and cognitive abilities in 111,739 UK Biobank participants," *Age and Ageing*, vol. 45, no. 4, pp. 511–517, 2016.

[25] S. Gillette-Guyonnet, F. Nourhashémi, S. Andrieu et al., "Weight loss in Alzheimer disease," *The American Journal of Clinical Nutrition*, vol. 71, no. 2, pp. 637S–642S, 2000.

[26] F. L. Heppner, R. M. Ransohoff, and B. Becher, "Immune attack: the role of inflammation in Alzheimer disease," *Nature Reviews Neuroscience*, vol. 16, no. 6, pp. 358–372, 2015.

[27] A. Ramanathan, A. R. Nelson, A. P. Sagare, and B. V. Zlokovic, "Impaired vascular-mediated clearance of brain amyloid beta in Alzheimer's disease: the role, regulation and restoration of LRP1," *Frontiers in Aging Neuroscience*, vol. 7, p. 136, 2015.

[28] H. J. Ahn, D. Zamolodchikov, M. Cortes-Canteli, E. H. Norris, J. F. Glickman, and S. Strickland, "Alzheimer's disease peptide β-amyloid interacts with fibrinogen and induces its oligomerization," *Proceedings of the National Academy of Sciences of the United States of America*, vol. 107, no. 50, pp. 21812–21817, 2010.

[29] S. Janelidze, E. Stomrud, S. Palmqvist et al., "Plasma β-amyloid in Alzheimer's disease and vascular disease," *Scientific Reports*, vol. 6, no. 1, article 26801, 2016.

[30] T. H. Kim and R. Vemuganti, "Mechanisms of Parkinson's disease-related proteins in mediating secondary brain damage after cerebral ischemia," *Journal of Cerebral Blood Flow & Metabolism*, vol. 37, no. 6, pp. 1910–1926, 2017.

[31] A. A. Sepehry, D. Lang, G. Y. Hsiung, and A. Rauscher, "Prevalence of brain microbleeds in Alzheimer disease: a systematic review and meta-analysis on the influence of neuroimaging techniques," *American Journal of Neuroradiology*, vol. 37, no. 2, pp. 215–222, 2016.

[32] S. W. Kim, S. J. Chung, Y.-S. Oh et al., "Cerebral microbleeds in patients with dementia with Lewy bodies and Parkinson disease dementia," *American Journal of Neuroradiology*, vol. 36, no. 9, pp. 1642–1647, 2015.

[33] T. Poliakova, O. Levin, A. Arablinskiy, E. Vasenina, and I. Zerr, "Cerebral microbleeds in early Alzheimer's disease," *Journal of Neurology*, vol. 263, no. 10, pp. 1961–1968, 2016.

[34] G. C. Chiang, J. C. Cruz Hernandez, K. Kantarci, C. R. Jack, M. W. Weiner, and for the Alzheimer's Disease Neuroimaging Initiative, "Cerebral microbleeds, CSF p-Tau, and cognitive decline: significance of anatomic distribution," *American Journal of Neuroradiology*, vol. 36, no. 9, pp. 1635–1641, 2015.

Glucose Metabolic Brain Network Differences between Chinese Patients with Lewy Body Dementia and Healthy Control

Danyan Chen,[1] Jiaying Lu,[2] Hucheng Zhou,[1] Jiehui Jiang,[1,3] Ping Wu,[2] Qihao Guo,[4] Jingjie Ge,[2] Huiwei Zhang,[2] Kuangyu Shi,[5] and Chuantao Zuo[2,6]

[1]*Shanghai Institute for Advanced Communication and Data Science, Shanghai University, Shanghai, China*
[2]*PET Center, Huashan Hospital, Fudan University, Shanghai, China*
[3]*Institute of Biomedical Engineering, Shanghai University, Shanghai, China*
[4]*Department of Neurology, Huashan Hospital, Fudan University, Shanghai, China*
[5]*Department of Nuclear Medicine, Technische Universität München, Munich, Germany*
[6]*Institute of Functional and Molecular Medical Imaging, Fudan University, Shanghai, China*

Correspondence should be addressed to Jiehui Jiang; jiangjiehui@shu.edu.cn and Ping Wu; pwu001@163.com

Academic Editor: Cheng-Yu Wei

Dementia with Lewy bodies (DLB) is the second most common degenerative dementia of the central nervous system. The technique ^{18}F-fluorodeoxyglucose positron emission tomography (^{18}F FDG PET) was used to investigate brain metabolism patterns in DLB patients. Conventional statistical methods did not consider intern metabolism transforming connections between various brain regions; therefore, most physicians do not understand the underlying neuropathology of DLB patients. In this study, ^{18}F FDG-PET images and graph-theoretical methods were used to investigate alterations in whole-brain intrinsic functional connectivity in a Chinese DLB group and healthy control (HC) group. This experimental study was performed on 22 DLB patients and 22 HC subjects in Huashan Hospital, Shanghai, China. Experimental results indicate that compared with the HC group, the DLB group has severely impaired small-world network. Compared to those of the HC group, the clustering coefficients of the DLB group were higher and characteristic path lengths were longer, and in terms of global efficiencies, those of the DLB group was also lower. Moreover, four significantly altered regions were observed in the DLB group: Inferior frontal gyrus, opercular part (IFG.R), olfactory cortex (OLF.R), hippocampus (HIP.R), and fusiform gyrus (FFG.L). Amongst them, in the DLB group, betweenness centrality became strong in OLF.R, HIP.R, and FFG.L, whereas betweenness centrality became weaker in IFG.R. Finally, IFGoperc.R was selected as a seed and a voxel-wise correlation analysis was performed. Compared to the HC group, the DLB group showed several regions of strengthened connection with IFGoperc.R; these regions were located in the prefrontal cortex and regions of weakened connection were located in the occipital cortex. The results of this paper may help physicians to better understand and characterize DLB patients.

1. Introduction

Dementia with Lewy bodies (DLB) is the second most common degenerative dementia of the central nervous system. Its clinical symptoms include fluctuating levels of cognition, cognitive impairment, parkinsonism, and visual hallucination [1]. Because clinical, neuropsychological, and pathological features of DLB are similar to those of Parkinson's disease (PD) and other dementia subtypes, such as Alzheimer's disease (AD), the rate of misdiagnosis has increased despite the publication of refined clinical criteria for DLB [2]. In clinical practice, it is necessary to have an exact diagnosis and identification of DLB.

In recent years, in order to better understand and characterize DLB patients, few scholars have used functional imaging techniques to elucidate brain metabolism patterns in DLB patients. Amongst them, ^{18}F fluorodeoxyglucose positron emission tomography (^{18}F- FDG PET) is considered as the gold standard [3] due to its high accuracy. Recently, ^{18}F-FDG PET imaging has been used to identify different disease-specific patterns [4] that disrupt metabolic connectivity (MC). Moreover, it is being increasingly used in routine clinical practice [5].

Many research studies have described the advantages of ^{18}F-FDG PET technique. O'Brien et al. conducted an experimental research study to compare the accuracy with which ^{18}F-FDG PET and (hexamethylpropyleneamine oxime (HMPAO)) SPECT cerebral perfusion could diagnose DLB. They found that both modalities showed broadly similar patterns: parietal and temporal lobes of dementia patients showed reduced levels of activity. Moreover, DLB patients showed reduced uptake in the occipital lobe. Nevertheless, ^{18}F-FDG PET was significantly superior to cerebral blood flow SPECT [6]. There is consistent evidence to prove that DLB patients develop a specific dysfunctional pattern, characterized by significant hypometabolism in the occipital and parietotemporal lobes. In the frontal cortex of DLB patients, metabolism is reduced to a lesser extent [2]. For instance, DLB patients showed posterior brain hypometabolism primarily involving parietooccipital regions [7]. In particular, cingulate island sign (CIS), which refers to sparing of the posterior cingulate relative to the precuneus and cuneus, has been proposed as an FDG-PET imaging biomarker of DLB [8].

Although some initial findings can be found in previous research, more evidences are needed to validate these findings. As a complex integrative system in which billions of neurons are connected with each other, the human brain continuously processes and transmits information between spatially distributed but functionally linked regions [9]. However, such connections between functionally linked regions are not considered in traditional statistical methods. Therefore, scholars seed a new method to optimize current findings.

Brain network analysis may be a good alternative for addressing such issues. Presently, abnormal topology of different diseases can be determined with this method. Thus, the pathological mechanism of different diseases, such as Alzheimer's disease or schizophrenia, may be understood by a new perspective. Thus, it is possible to have an early diagnosis and evaluation of diseases with brain network imaging biomarkers [10]. For instance, using resting-state functional magnetic resonance imaging (rs-fMRI), researchers performed brain network analysis to assess brain network organization in patients diagnosed with DLB (22 patients) and Alzheimer's disease (24 patients). They found that global brain network measures of DLB patients were significantly different from those of Alzheimer's patients and healthy controls. By studying the metabolic network of DLB patients, researchers gained important insights into the link between local vulnerabilities, long-range disconnection, and neuropathological differences. For instance, Caminiti et al. studied fMRI images of 42 DLB patients and 42 healthy controls (HC) using sparse inverse covariance estimation method and graph theory. These methods revealed substantial alterations in connectivity indexes, brain modularity, and hub configuration. Compared to healthy controls, local metabolic connectivity was significantly decreased within the occipital cortex, thalamus, and cerebellum of DLB patients. However, local metabolic connectivity was significantly increased in the frontal, temporal, parietal, and basal ganglia regions of DLB patients. There were also long-range disconnections between these brain regions. This implies that the functional hierarchy of a normal brain was disrupted in DLB patients [11]. However, these studies were mainly conducted on Western subjects. These results may not be applicable to Chinese subjects.

The two main objectives of this study are therefore as follows: (1) to explore the differences in glucose metabolism of Chinese patients with DLB and to compare related parameters with HC and (2) to identify altered hubs of brain networks and to locate regions significantly correlated with altered hubs of brain networks in DLB patients. Finally, clear evidences on the differences between ^{18}F-FDG PET images of DLB and HC subjects are expected to be presented from the aspect of brain connectome.

Table 1: Statistical information of all participants.

Info	HC ($n = 22$)	DLB ($n = 22$)	p value
Male : female	5 : 17	21 : 1	$p < 0.001^a$
Age	63.5 ± 5.6	66.9 ± 8.4	$p = 0.126^b$
MMSE	28.9 ± 1.3	20.0 ± 5.0	$p < 0.001^b$

Age and MMSE are given as mean ± standard deviation. $^a\chi^2$ test, HC, and DLB. ^{b}Analysis of variance, HC, and DLB.

2. Experimental Procedure

2.1. Subjects. In this study, the experimental data were obtained from the PET Center of Huashan Hospital in Shanghai, China. All participants were right-handed, including 22 normal subjects and 22 DLB patients. Standardized uptake value ratios (SUVR) of FDG were calculated by dividing the cerebellar cortex-standardized uptake values. Three days before or after PET image acquisition, we obtained basic information of these subjects, including age, gender, and Mini-Mental State Examination (MMSE) values. Table 1 displays statistical information of all participants.

2.2. PET Image Acquisition and Preprocessing. Whole brain PET images of 44 participants were acquired using Siemens Biograph 64 PET/CT machine, which was present in the PET Center of Huashan Hospital in Shanghai, China. The spatial resolution of the PET scanner was 5.9 mm full width at half maximum (FWHM) in the transaxial plane and 5.5 mm FWHM in axial plane. All subjects were intravenously injected with 185 MBq FDG in a dimly lit, quiet room. They were asked to keep their eyes closed for 60 min in order to minimize the confounding effects of any activity. Thereafter, static emission scans were continued for 10 min. Using a Shepp–Logan filter, we implemented a filtered back projection algorithm to reconstruct transaxial images of the following dimensions: $168 \times 168 \times 148$ matrices and a size of $2.0 \times 2.0 \times 1.5$ mm. The institutional review board of Huashan Hospital approved the acquisition of PET images

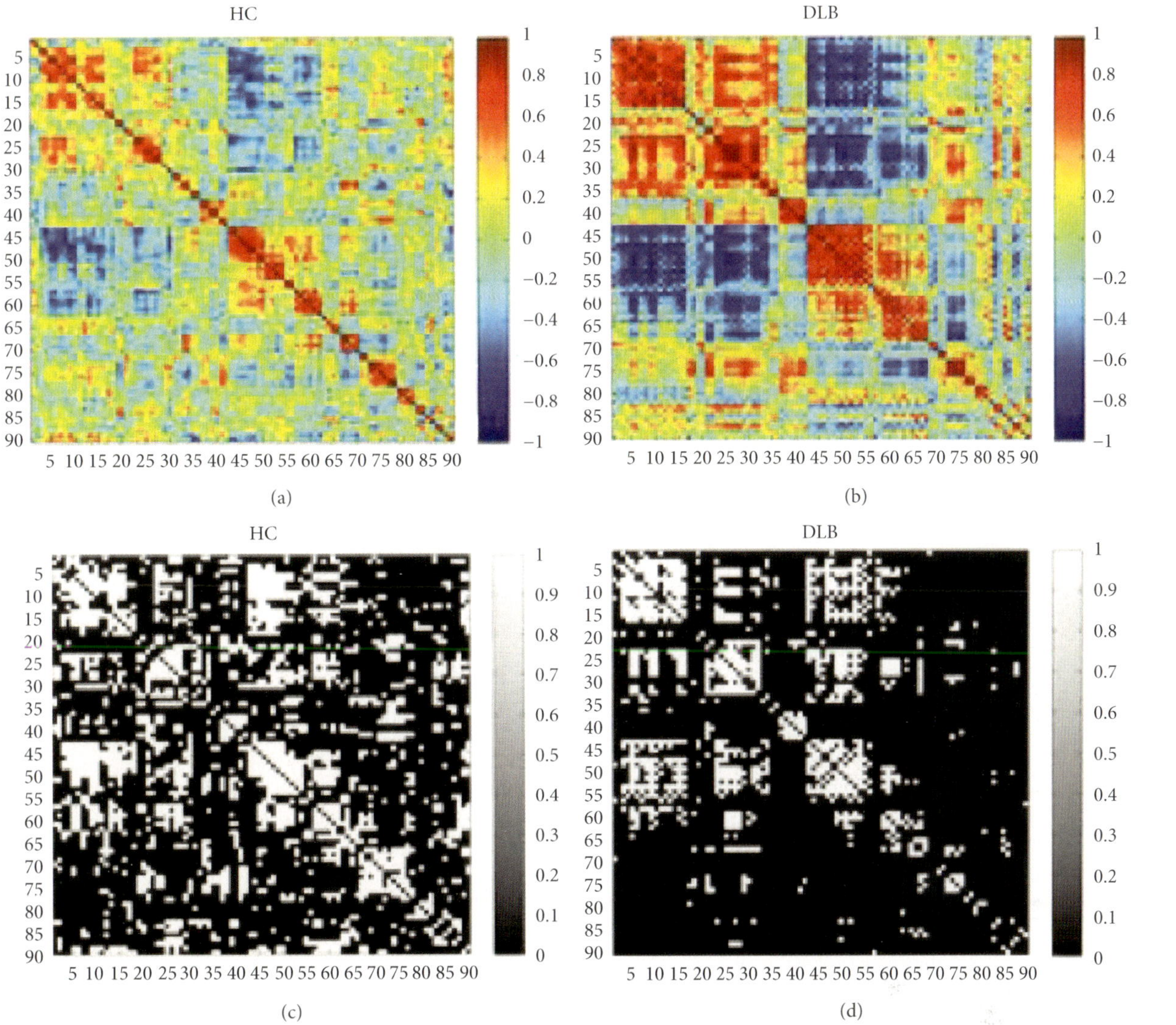

Figure 1: The partial correlation coefficient matrices and the binary matrices of the two groups. (a) The partial correlation coefficient matrix of the HC group. (b) The partial correlation coefficient matrix of the DLB group. (c) The binary matrix of the HC group in sparsity 21%. (d) The binary matrix of the DLB group in sparsity 21%.

[11]. The informed consent form was signed by all participants of this study.

All the original images were obtained in Digital Imaging and Communications in Medicine (DICOM) format. They were converted to NIfTI format using DCM2NII software (https://www.nitrc.org/projects/dcm2nii/). For preprocessing converted images, Statistical Parametric Mapping 8 (SPM8) software was implemented in MATLAB 2014a. Firstly, PET images were spatially normalized to the Montreal Neurological Institute (MNI, McGill University, Montreal, Canada) space. In this step, individual images were spatially warped to a reference PET template using SPM software. Spatial warping is a completely automated procedure based on 12-parameter affine transformation. Then, normalized images were smoothed by convolution using an isotropic Gaussian kernel with $10 \times 10 \times 10\,mm^{*}3$ FWHM. Finally, these images were transformed into gray level images with a grayscale of [0,255].

2.3. Brain Network Construction. Two networks of the HC and DLB groups were built based on two datasets, based on the definition of the network in graph theory [12]. The standardized AAL template contains 90 brain regions and 45 hemispheres, all of which are used to divide brain regions [13]. This AAL template was used to split all FDG-PET images into 90 nodes; each node implied a brain region. To further calculate the value of the node in the network, the average value of the intensity of each brain area was estimated. Then, we considered the value of each node as a whole and normalized it as a whole. Each node was normalized to zero-mean and unit-variance. It was obtained by subtracting the average value of the individual's whole brain and then dividing it by the standard deviation of the individual's whole brain. In previous studies, the partial correlation coefficient between each group of nodes was calculated, generating a partial correlation matrix of (90×90) samples. Figures 1(a) and 1(b) illustrate the partial correlation matrix of the HC and DLB groups, respectively.

In this study, a sparse threshold method was used [12]. The covariance correlation matrix represents an undirected weighted graph. Then, the partial correlation coefficient values of each two brain regions were calculated, which represented the connection strengths of the two brain regions. A larger partial correlation coefficient value indicated a stronger correlation between these two brain regions, which meant that the transform of glucose metabolism in these brain regions was more obvious. Furthermore, in this study, a binary comparison-weighted graph was used. A strategy was used to get the binary matrix and to set the sparsity of the connection matrix. In particular, the data was sorted in the connection matrix in terms of absolute value. Then, the sparsity was set to 21%, implying that the first 21% of the sequence was converted to 1. This indicates that a connection exists between two regions, vice versa, behind which the value would be converted to 0. This implies that there was no connection. With increasing sparsity, the connection matrix becomes sparser. Conversely, the greater the sparsity, the higher would be the density of the connected graph. Network topology is significantly impacted by the choice of sparse threshold. Instead of selecting a single sparse value randomly and subjectively, sparse values from sparsity (min = 0.06) to sparsity (max = 0.40) are considered. The two groups of subjects are connected with the lower limit. The choice of cap satisfies the strongly suppressed contribution of pseudocorrelation, ensuring that the resulting graph has a small world. What needs to be clarified is the fact that in the academic community, it is difficult to deal with negative correlations at the time of binarization. In our experiment, the negative correlation was converted to 1 once the absolute value of the negative correlation was greater than sparsity 21% [10].

Subsequently, the binarized network matrix can be generated. As shown in Figures 1(c) and 1(d), an element of 1 and 0 stands for "connection" and "no connection" in the binary matrix.

2.4. Network Parameter Analysis. To further investigate the differences between two sets of network parameters, the following parameters were considered: clustering coefficient (C), characteristic path length (L), local E, global E, γ, lambda, sigma, and node agent center (BC). All parameters were obtained from open-source toolkit GRETNA (https://www.nitrc.org/projects/gretna/) [14] and Brain Connectivity Toolkit (BCT, http://www.nitrc.org/projects/bct/) [15].

Based on graph theory, clustering coefficient C (i) was defined as the network that expressed a local connection probability, that is, the probability of connecting any two nodes around the node i [16]. The clustering coefficient C of the entire network was defined as the average of clustering coefficients of all nodes in the network, and it was a measure of the degree to which nodes in the graph tend to be clustered together [17]. In topology, the shortest path length was defined as the shortest path distance from node i to node j. In practice, it represents the minimum number of points connecting node i with node j. The shortest path lengths of all the nodes was calculated. The characteristic path length L was defined as the average of these path lengths. A network was formed with high global network efficiency [18]. If there was no connection between two points, then, path lengths between them was infinite.

If the network satisfies the clustering coefficient, then, it also satisfies the corresponding random network clustering coefficient ratio, $\gamma = C/C\_r$. Moreover, it was determined using the characteristic path length; the clustering coefficient $\gg 1$ satisfies the characteristic path length and the corresponding stochastic network. The average path length was greater than $\lambda = L/L\_\text{rand} = 1$. For the comprehensive parameter $\sigma = \gamma/\lambda > 1$, it can be explained that the network had all the characteristics of a small world [16]. Random networks were obtained by randomly reattaching the original brain network between node edges. Meanwhile, the same number of nodes, edges, and degrees was preserved. To achieve statistical significances, we repeated 200 times random networks.

Global efficiency (global E) and local sales (local E) were also worked out to intuitively express transmission efficiency of the network at global and local levels. Global E is the average of shortest paths between nodes, reflecting the efficiency of the global network [19]. Local E is the average of the shortest paths between different connecting nodes, reflecting the efficiency of information exchange between subgraphs [20].

To further explore the nodes of this network, the concept of betweenness centrality was used. Betweenness centrality Bi of node i was defined as the number of shortest paths from all vertices to all others passing through node i. The betweenness centrality of the entire network was defined as the average of Bi from each node. In general, the Bi value was standardized while the normalized betweenness centrality of node i was defined by the expression: bi = Bi/B. From this definition, it can be inferred that the bi value was influenced by node i that transmits information in the entire network. Higher the bi value, stronger would be the regional centrality of the node. According to Seo et al. [21], hub regions of brain networks were proposed as nodes who have high bi values (bi > 1.5). To identify the hub region significantly altered, the results of the DLB group were compared with those of the HC group. A nonparametric permutation test was performed 1000 times. Statistical results were used to identify altered hubs ($p < 0.05$). Table 2 summarizes all the parameters defined in this study.

2.5. Seed Correlation Analysis. Once altered hubs were determined for each of the two groups, they were considered as seed points and the relationship between them and rest voxels of the individual's brain was calculated. This step was to validate the significances of altered hubs. Pearson correlation coefficient method was used firstly. Then, Fisher's r-to-z transformation was used to convert Pearson's correlation coefficients to z values. Thus, an

TABLE 2: The definitions of network parameters used in this study.

Parameters	Abbreviation	Equations	Meaning
Clustering coefficient	C	$C = (1/N)\sum_{i=1}^{N}((2E(i))/(k_i(k_i-1)))$ N: number of nodes K_i: number of nodes connected with node i $E(i)$: actual connection edges among k_i	A measure of the degree to nodes in a network which tend to cluster together
Characteristic path length	L	$L = 1/((1/N(N-1))(\Sigma_{i,j\in V,i\neq j}(1/d_{ij})))$ N: number of nodes in a network d_{ij}: the shortest path between node i and j	A measure of the efficiency of the information or mass transport on a network
Gamma	Gamma	$\text{Gamma} = C/C_{\text{rand}}$ C_{rand}: clustering coefficient of the corresponding random network	A network could be defined as small-world network when gamma $\gg 1$, lambda$\sim$1, and sigma > 1
Lambda	Lambda	$\text{Lambda} = L/L_{\text{rand}}$ L_{rand}: path length of the corresponding random network	
Small-world coefficient	Sigma	Sigma = gamma/lambda	
Global efficiency	Global E	$\text{Global E} = (1/N(N-1))\sum_{i,j\in V,i\neq j}(1/d_{ij})$	Measures how efficiently the network exchanges information
local efficiency	Local E	$\text{Local E} = (1/N)\sum_{k\in V}((1/(N_{vk}(N_{vk}-1)))\sum_{i,j\in V,i\neq j}(1/d_{ij}))$ N_{vk}: subgraph of node k	
Betweenness centrality	BC	$BC_k = \sum_{i,j\in V,i\neq j}((n_{ij}(k))/n_{ij})$ $n_{ij}(k)$: shortest path pass between nodes i and j through node k	An indicator of a node's centrality in a network

approximated Gaussian distribution was calculated using the following formula:

$$z_i = \frac{1}{2} \times \log\left[\frac{1+r_i}{1-r_i}\right]. \quad (1)$$

Here, r_i refers to correlation coefficients and z_i refers to the transformed z value. Finally, Z test was used to compare z values between groups, whose expression is mentioned as follows:

$$z = \frac{z_1 - z_2}{\sqrt{(1/(n_1-3)) + (1/(n_2-3))}}. \quad (2)$$

Here, n_1 and n_2 refer to samples of two groups [22]. To adjust variations associated with multiple comparison, a false discovery rate (FDR) method was performed at q value of 0.05.

2.6. Statistical Analysis. To confirm statistical significance of network parameters representing the DLB group and HC group, 2000 nonparametric permutation tests were performed [22].

To determine if the observed subject difference occurred accidentally (null hypothesis), we conducted further statistical analysis. The PET images of 44 participants were randomly assigned to the HC and DLB groups and then, the partial correlation matrix was calculated again according to Section 2.3. A set of binary matrices was obtained. The network parameters were also calculated for each network separately. The above process was repeated 1000 times, and the 95 percentile score for each differential distribution was considered as a cutoff ($p < 0.05$, one tailed). This meant that when the original results were within the first 5% of the random results, our results were considered to have significant differences.

3. Results

3.1. Network Parameters. As shown in Figures 1(a) and 1(b), partial correlation coefficient matrices of four groups were calculated using partial correlation analysis. Figure 1 illustrates that color distribution was not uniform for different groups; therefore, partial correlation coefficient was inconsistent. The DLB group exhibited a deep colored distribution; its partial correlation coefficient had the highest absolute value. As shown in Figures 1(c) and 1(d), the threshold for binary matrices of two groups was at a fixed sparsity of 21% (refer to Section 3.2 for threshold selection).

Figure 2 illustrates network parameters of gamma, lambda, and sigma for the DLB group and HC group. As shown in Figure 2, the entire threshold was ranging 6–40%. For both the DLB and HC groups, network parameters were as follows: gamma $\gg 1$, lambda ≈ 1, and sigma > 1. A small-world network was observed in this study. Compared to the DLB group, this property was more obvious and noticeable in the HC group. At sparsity 18%, the value of sigma was 1.625 and 1.244 for the HC group and DLB group, respectively. By performing further permutation tests, it was found that over the entire threshold range, the gamma and sigma values in the DLB group were significantly smaller than those in the HC group.

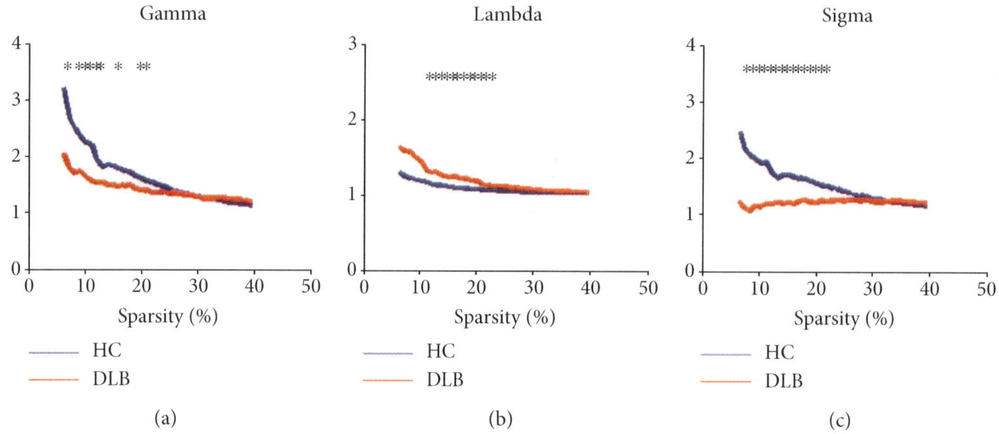

Figure 2: Gamma, lambda, and sigma values in the two groups. The asterisk refer to significant differences between the HC and DLB groups at the sparsity threshold ($p < 0.05$).

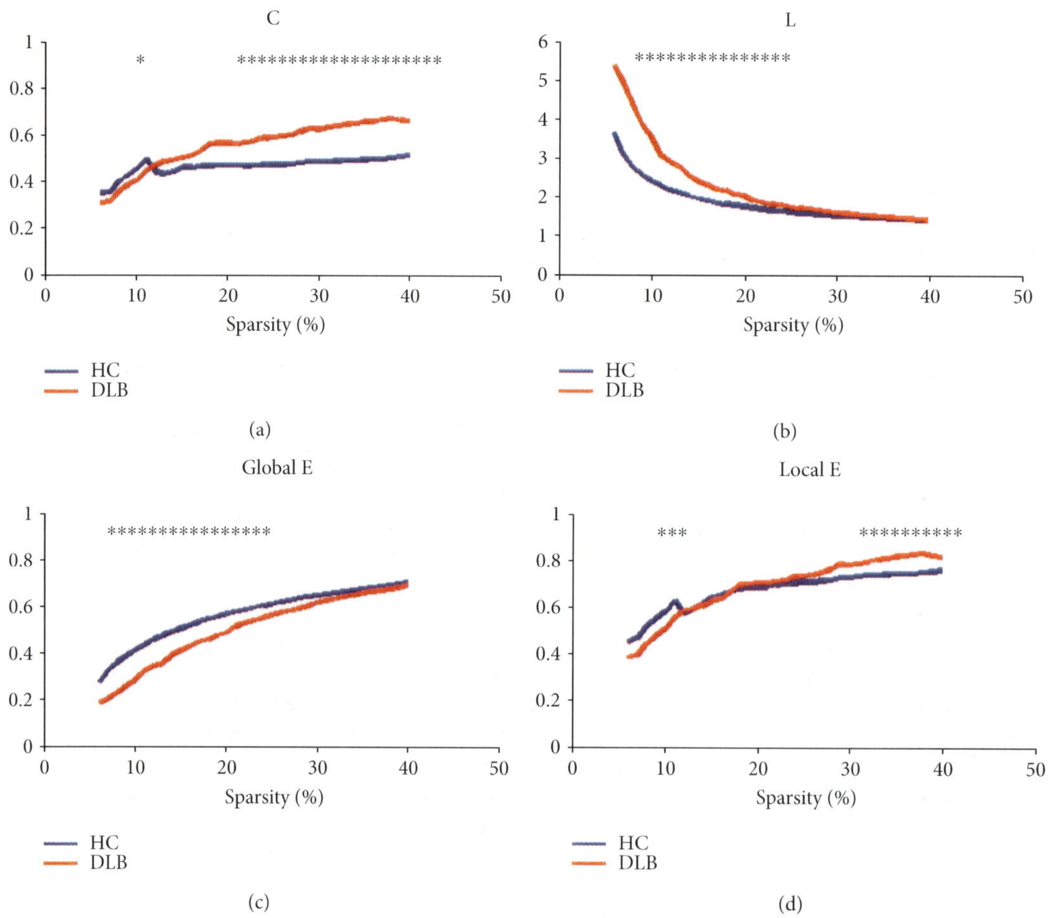

Figure 3: C, L, local E, and global E values in the two groups. The asterisk refer to significant differences between the HC and DLB groups at the sparsity threshold ($p < 0.05$).

On the other hand, the lambda value was higher in the DLB group than in the HC group ($p < 0.05$).

As shown in Figure 3, network parameters C, L, global E, and local E were completely different for both the two groups. To compare the DLB group with the HC group, a nonparametric permutation test was performed to display statistical significance of differences between the two groups ($p = 0.05$).

3.2. Hub Regions. In a complex network, the normalized betweenness centrality (bi) was an important indicator of regional characteristics. These characteristics were used

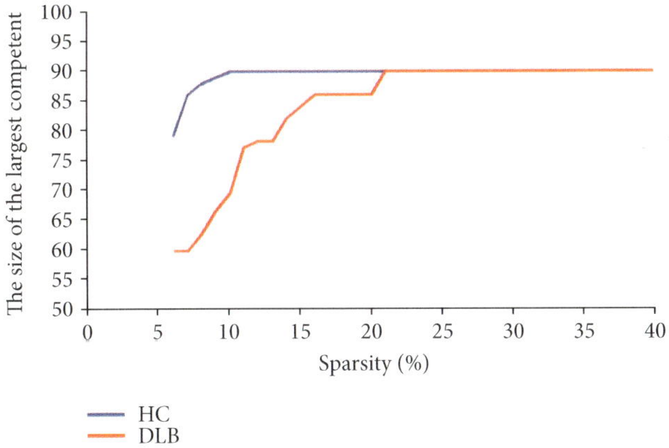

Figure 4: Different component of sizes of the two networks.

to determine the relative importance of network nodes and to identify key nodes in the network. These key nodes are defined as hubs in this study. To identify hubs in two groups, bi was calculated at a fixed sparsity of 21%. At the lowest sparsity of 21%, the component size was largest at 90. To guarantee >50 component size of the two networks, minimum sparsity thresholds were found to be 9% and 21% for the HC and DLB groups, respectively. At these thresholds, no node could be isolated from the remaining network. Figure 4 shows different component sizes of two networks with a different sparsity threshold. As a result, sparsity 21% was chosen as the threshold and bi values were calculated for each node in the two networks [21].

At sparsity of 21%, 16 hubs and 21 hubs were identified for the HC and DLB groups, respectively. bi values and functional classification of hub regions were also presented in Tables 3 and 4, respectively. Functionally, hubs were primarily located in association areas for HC and DLB groups. Figure 5 illustrates the results for hub nodes in the axial view. In the HC group, hubs are primarily located in the prefrontal and occipital cortices. In the DLB group, hubs are located in prefrontal, occipital, and subcortical cortices of the brain. (Figure 5 was drawn by BrainNet Viewer package [23]).

For comparing different groups, statistical analysis was done with permutation test. It was found that the DLB group showed significantly altered regions in the four brain regions ($p < 0.05$), including pars opercularis (IFGoperc.R), right lingual gyrus (LING.R), fusiform gyrus (FFG.L), and olfactory cortex (OLF.R). Amongst them, betweenness centrality in the DLB group became strong in OLF.R, HIP.R, and FFG.L compared to that in the HC group, whereas betweenness centrality became weak in IFG.R. Table 5 shows betweenness centrality values and p values of these four hubs.

3.3. Seed Correlation. To further investigate connectivity between hubs in two groups, the right inferior frontal gyrus and pars opercularis (IFGoperc.R) were selected as the seed. The region was selected because of two primary reasons: IFGoperc.R is the hub's node in the HC group (bi > 1.5), but it is not targeted for hubs in DLB groups. The values of normalized bi were 1.83 and 0.08 in the HC group and DLB group, which has the smallest bi value in the DLB among hubs in the HC group. Compared with the HC group, IFGoperc.R status was different for DLB groups. Second, statistical analysis was conducted by conducting permutation test; it shows that for IFGoperc.R, bi values of DLB groups were significantly different from those of the HC group (p value = 0.0295). As shown in Figure 6, the results of voxel-wise correlation analysis were obtained with IFGoperc.R seed. Figure 6 illustrates the correlation coefficient map (R-map) associated with IFGoperc.R seed in the HC and DLB groups. (Figure 6 was drawn by the REST Slice Viewer [24]). In the HC group, the R-map shows that areas, which present positive connections with IFGoperc.R seed, were focused on the following components of parietal cortex: the bilateral postcentral gyrus (PoCG.R and PoCG.L), right middle frontal gyrus (MFG.R), and right angular gyrus (ANG.R). The weakened regions of the brain were mainly located in the following areas: the right and left cuneus (CUN.R and CUN.L), left insula (INS.L), and right parahippocampal gyrus (PHG.R).

In the DLB group, the prefrontal cortex showed enhanced brain activity in the following areas: the bilateral middle frontal gyrus (MFG.R and MFG.L), bilateral inferior frontal gyrus, pars triangularis (IFGtriang.R and IFGtriang.L), bilateral inferior frontal gyrus, and pars orbitalis (ORBinf.R and ORBinf.L). Weakened brain regions were mainly located in the occipital cortex, including the left calcarine sulcus (CAL.L), left middle occipital gyrus (MOG.L), parietal cortex left postcentral gyrus (PoCG.L), and right inferior parietal lobule (IPL.R).

Table 3: The hub regions of the HC group.

Hubs	Anatomical classification	Bi (>1.5)	p with DLB value
IFGoperc.R	*Prefontal*	*1.83*	*0.0295*[a]
SMA.L	Frontal	1.70	0.058
SFGmed.L	Prefontal	2.09	0.218
SFGmed.R	Prefontal	1.69	0.059
ORBsupmed.R	Prefontal	1.61	0.3265
INS.L	Subcortical	1.51	0.109
INS.R	*Subcortical*	*2.50*	*0.037*[a]
DCG.R	Frontal	1.55	0.108
AMYG.L	Temporal	2.02	0.1035
CUN.L	Occipital	3.01	0.1065
CUN.R	*Occipital*	*2.62*	*0.041*[a]
LING.R	*Occipital*	*1.59*	*0.135*[a]
PUT.R	*Subcortical*	*2.71*	*0.138*[a]
PAL.R	Subcortical	2.62	0.2475
ITG.L	*Temporal*	*1.70*	*0.0155*[a]
ITG.R	*Temporal*	*2.18*	*0.0260*[a]

Hub is defined as the brain region with a bi value > 1.5; class represents the functional classification of the corresponding brain regions; bi represents the normalized betweenness centrality; and the p with DLB value represents the statistical p value of the permutation test between the DLB and HC groups. [a]Statistically significant difference ($p < 0.05$).

Table 4: The hub regions of DLB group.

Hubs	Anatomical classification	Bi (>1.5)	*p* value
ORBsup.L	Prefontal	1.51	0.2185
ORBmid.L	Prefontal	1.73	0.23
ORBinf.R	Prefontal	1.92	0.0955
ROL.L	Frontal	2.59	0.173
OLF.L	Prefontal	3.83	0.134
OLF.R	*Prefontal*	*4.02*	*0.015*[a]
ORBsupmed.L	Prefontal	1.96	0.3045
REC.L	Prefontal	1.55	0.374
INS.L	Subcortical	3.67	0.109
HIP.R	*Temporal*	*5.19*	*0.008*[a]
CUN.L	Occipital	1.63	0.1065
SOG.R	Occipital	2.23	0.1375
MOG.R	Occipital	2.69	0.115
IOG.L	Occipital	1.68	0.2235
IOG.R	Occipital	2.04	0.204
FFG.L	*Temporal*	*2.65*	*0.0135*[a]
IPL.L	Parietal	2.26	0.128
ANG.R	Parietal	1.54	0.28
PCUN.L	Parietal	2.27	0.0895
PAL.R	Subcortical	1.82	0.2475
THA.R	Subcortical	3.88	0.0675

Hub is defined as the brain region with a bi value > 1.5; class represents the functional classification of the corresponding brain regions; bi represents the normalized betweenness centrality; and p value indicates statistic meaning. [a]Statistically significant difference ($p < 0.05$).

In this study, the DLB group was used as a reference for further analysis. Z-statistical mapping was performed in the IFGoperc.R region of the brain of the HC group. Figure 7 illustrates the results obtained by Z-statistical test (z-map).

Compared to the HC group, the results of Z-statistics indicated brain regions that had strengthened connections with IFGoperc.R in the DLB group. These regions were located in the prefrontal cortex, which included the right middle frontal gyrus (MFG.R), bilateral inferior frontal gyrus, pars triangularis (IFGtriang.R and IFGtriang.L), right middle frontal gyrus, orbital part (ORBmid.R), and right medial frontal gyrus (SFGmed.R) ($p < 0.05$, FDR corrected).

4. Discussion

In this study, we found that the functional brain network of DLB patients was significantly different from that of healthy controls. Firstly, network alterations were broad in the DLB group. Secondly, divergent network alterations were manifested in the LDB group. Compared to the HC group, the DLB group suffered very severe dementia due to loss of characteristics of the small-world network. To perform seed correlation analysis, the brain region IFGoperc.R was selected as a seed in this study. Compared to the HC group, the results of z-map showed regions of strengthened connection with IFGoperc.R in the DLB group; these regions were located in the prefrontal cortex, and regions of weakened connection were located in the occipital cortex.

The physiological and pathological meanings of the above findings were discussed below.

4.1. Network Parameters. As shown in Figure 3, parameter C gradually becomes larger as the sparsity increases. When the HC group increases from 0.349 to 0.517, the DLB group increases from 0.305 to 0.668 over an entire threshold range. Statistical analysis based on permutation test showed that C was significantly higher in the DLB group than in the HC group at sparsity 10–14% and 21% ($p < 0.05$). Moreover, parameter L in the DLB group was significantly greater than that in the HC group when sparsity values were in the range of 21–40% ($p < 0.05$). At sparsity values of 31–40%, local E in the DLB group was significantly greater than that in the HC group. Global E in the DLB group was significantly lower than that in the HC group when sparsity values were in the range 7–22% ($p < 0.05$). Sigma in the DLB group was significantly smaller than that in the HC group when sparsity values were in the range 7–21% ($p < 0.05$). Finally, the local E values in the DLB group and HC group were approximately equal over the entire threshold range.

By accurately performing quantitative analysis, a small-world network was constructed. This network showed high global efficiency and optimal organizational structure, which better supported distributed information processing and extremely complex computation. In this study, small-world network was observed in both groups. The results of network parameters indicate that many changes were observed in the DLB group. Compared to the HC group, the characteristic path length was longer for the DLB group. Because characteristic path length was greater for observed points, the organization of the brain network was altered and network efficiency was lowered. In the DLB group brain network, the greater the clustering coefficient of the brain network, the longer would be the characteristic path length of the brain network in the DLB group. This network change tends to be a regular network, which has obvious shortcomings in communication and synchronization abilities of the signal when compared to a small-world network. Many diseases caused by disconnection of the nervous system were associated with loss of global characteristics of a small-world network, and they tend to form a regular network. A previous study had proved that in the DLB group [11], there was a significant loss in small-world network. This might be associated with presynaptic dysfunction, which is caused by α-synuclein aggregates present in the brain cortex, even at early stages of the disease. This finding was also confirmed in our research study.

4.2. Hubs of the Brain Network. Many studies have used fMRI and graph-based analysis method to investigate the functional network of the brain, revealing attributes such as small-world attributes [25, 26]. An important finding was that the networks governing the function of the human brain contained a small number of hubs, which were disproportionately associated with numerous connections. These hubs

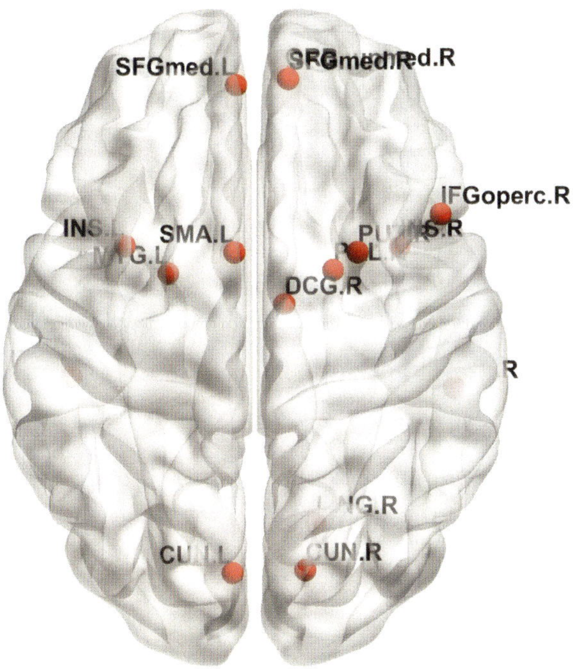

(a)

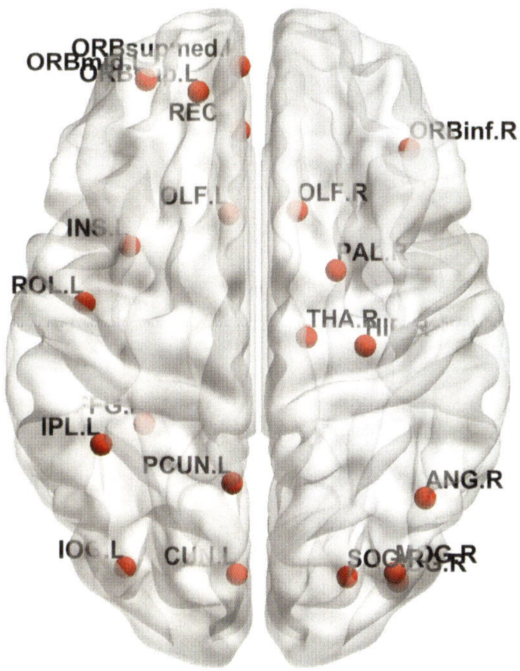

(b)

FIGURE 5: Hub nodes of two groups. (a) 16 hub nodes in the HC group. (b) 21 hub nodes in the DLB group.

TABLE 5: The significantly altered hubs in the DLB group compared to those in the HC group.

Hubs	Anatomical classification	Bi in HC	Bi in DLB	p value
IFGoperc.R	Prefontal	**1.83**	0.008	0.0295[a]
OLF.R	Prefontal	0.24	**4.02**	0.015[a]
HIP.R	Temporal	0.85	**5.19**	0.008[a]
FFG.L	Temporal	0.58	**2.65**	0.0135[a]

Compared with the HC group, the DLB group showed significantly different hubs. [a]Statistically significant difference ($p < 0.05$).

act as way stations for information processing by connecting distinct, functional specialized systems [27]. These brain hubs, which are mainly located in medial and lateral sections of frontal and parietal cortices, have higher rates of the following functions: cerebral blood flow, aerobic glycolysis, and oxidative glucose metabolism. They play vital roles in supporting fast communication across various brain regions [28]. In the present study, most brain hubs were located in the prefrontal and frontal cortices of the HC group. In the DLB group, brain hubs underwent significant changes, because normal hubs were attacked by dementia.

In present experiments, four significantly altered regions in the DLB groups were identified as hubs, including IFGoperc (IFG.R), olfactory cortex (OLF.R), hippocampus (HIP.R), and fusiform gyrus (FFG.L). This result could be proven in previous literature.

In a previous study conducted by Blanc et al., a significant variation in AAL brain regions was observed in the DLB group of patients. They found that in the DLB group, cortical thinning was found predominantly in the right temporoparietal junction, insula, cingulate, orbitofrontal, and lateral occipital cortices [29].

In a study conducted by Laura et al., significant changes were observed in the olfactory cortex and Lewy body pathology. In future studies, the metamorphosis of the olfactory cortex must be investigated to further elucidate the pathophysiology of DLB patients [30].

In DLB patients, major changes occur in the hippocampus of the human brain. Many studies have recorded the unique response of hippocampal CA2/3 in patients with Lewy body disease. By characterizing dystrophy in HIC hippocampal CA2/3 neurites, one may clarify how lesions lead to the development of dementia in DLB patients [31].

In a study conducted by Kosaka et al., a significant change was observed in the hippocampal gyri and fusiform gyri of a patient suffering from DLB. This disease was predominantly observed in the left region of the brain. This finding completely agrees with the conclusion of our current study [32, 33]. Thus, our experimental results have been validated with these findings.

4.3. Seed Correlation Analysis. The significantly altered region IFGoperc.R was selected as a seed. The results indicate that in the HC group, regions of strengthened connection were detected with IFGoperc.R seed. These regions were mainly located in the parietal cortex, including PoCG.R, PoCG.L, and MFG.R. Functional connection strength between prefrontal cortex and FGoperc.R seed was deep in the DLB group (its distribution was demarcated with a deep color.). In DLB patients, there were differences in the intrinsic functional connectivity of brains. Based on the

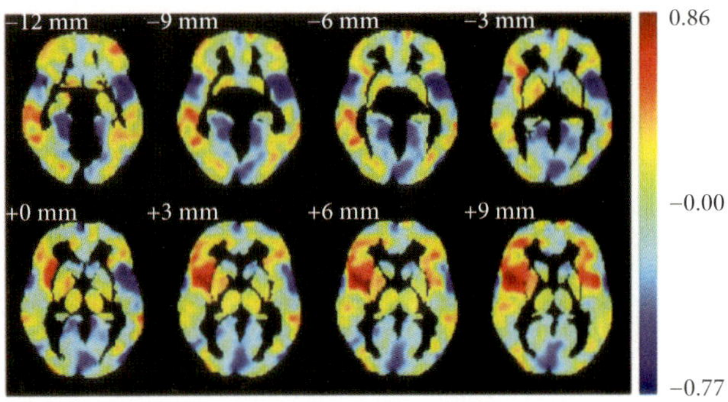

FIGURE 6: Seed correlation associated with the IFGoperc.R seed. (a) Correlation coefficient map with IFGoperc.R in the HC group; (b) correlation coefficient map with IFGoperc.R in the DLB group.

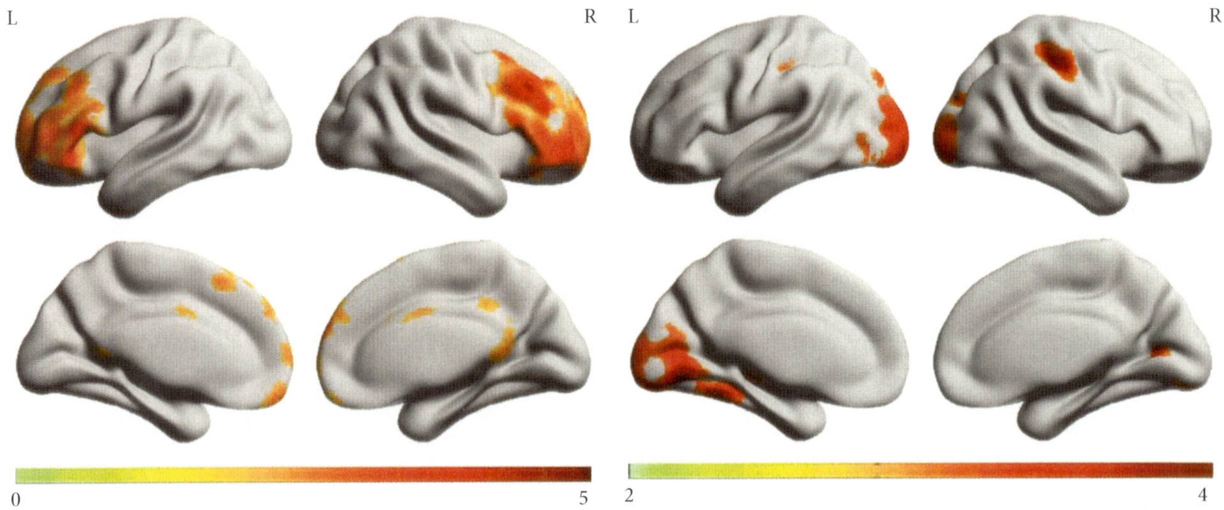

FIGURE 7: Z-statistics map. (a) Z-statistics map showing the brain regions that had strengthened connection with the IFGoperc.R region in the DLB group when compared to the HC group ($p < 0.05$, FDR corrected); (b) Z-statistics map showing the brain regions that had weakened connection with the IFGoperc.R region in the DLB group when compared to the HC group ($p < 0.1$, FDR corrected);

TABLE 6: Comparison of the DLB network parameters between the present study and Western studies.

	Experimental image	N	C	L	Sigma	E	Gamma
Our study	FDG-PET	22	0.59	1.95	1.23	0.55	1.36
Western study [34]	fMRI	22	~0.52	~1.9	~1.35	~0.6	—

N: the number of subjects participating in the experiment.

differences in this connectivity, a new biomarker, IFGoperc.R, was obtained for precisely diagnosing DLB. In the DLB group of patients, there was also a significant decrease in the functional connectivity between extraordinary regions (LING.L, PoCG.R, SMG.R, and SOG.R) and IFGoperc.R seed. These findings were useful for neuroscientists to further understand the pathology of DLB.

4.4. Comparison between Chinese and Western Patients with DLB. Not many studies have investigated the parameters of the brain function network on DLB patients. For the first time, Peraza et al. conducted a representative study on the brain function network parameters [34] to understand the impact of fMRI in 22 DLB patients; however, this study was conducted on Western subjects with DLB. To further explore similar treatment processes for DLB patients in China, the relationship between DLB brain network changes and race was explored. By comparing experimental results with current results in Table 6, broadly similar results were obtained. However, the differences between Chinese and Western DLB people were as follows: larger C and L values and smaller values would be sigma and global efficiencies.

This is an important point to consider because a change between these parameters was same as the difference between DLB and HC groups. To a certain extent, the parameter results of Chinese DLB patients were more serious than those of Western DLB patients. However, we cannot yet identify specific reasons for this difference. They also need to be studied further.

4.5. Limitations. In this study, there are still several limitations that need to be considered. Firstly, the gender distribution of the participants in the DLB group was extremely uneven (M : F = 21 : 1) in this study. The influences of gender for brain region analysis in the DLB group need be studied in the future. Secondly, the AAL template with 90 regions was used in this study. However, other templates with more regions could also be applied [35], and differences of brain region analysis amongst different templates need be studied. Thirdly, an unweighted and binary network was constructed in this study. Fourthly, partial correlation matrices were used to calculate network parameters and Pearson correlation was used for performing correlation analysis in this study. This may introduce bias in results. Differences of using various correlation matrices need be studied in the future.

5. Conclusion

By performing brain network analysis for FDG-PET images, this study systematically explored glucose metabolic brain network differences in HC and DLB groups in China. As a whole, a small-world topology was demonstrated by both groups. We found that the small-world network was severely impaired in the DLB group, implying that "small-world network" can be used as a biomarker for DLB. Based on seed ROI-based correlation analysis, the differences in brain functional connectivity were observed in DLB groups. One could obtain further insights into pathoetiological mechanisms of this condition. For better understanding and characterizing DLB patients and its triggering mechanisms, more relevant studies must be conducted. An accurate clinical diagnosis of DLB would then be possible.

Acknowledgments

This study was supported by the National Natural Science Foundation of China (nos. 61603236, 81671239, 81401135, 81771483, and 81361120393), the National Key Research and Development Program of China (nos. 2016YFC1306305 and 2016YFC1306500) from the Ministry of Science and Technology of China, Science and Technology Commission of Shanghai Municipality (17JC1401600), Shanghai Sailing Program (no. 16YF1415400), and Scientific and Technological Innovation Project of Traditional Chinese Medicine in Shanghai (ZYKC201602002).

References

[1] J. Calderon, R. J. Perry, S. W. Erzinclioglu, G. E. Berrios, T. R. Dening, and J. R. Hodges, "Perception, attention, and working memory are disproportionately impaired in dementia with Lewy bodies compared with Alzheimer's disease," *Journal of Neurology, Neurosurgery & Psychiatry*, vol. 70, no. 2, pp. 157–164, 2001.

[2] I. G. McKeith, D. W. Dickson, J. Lowe et al., "Diagnosis and management of dementia with Lewy bodies third report of the DLB consortium," *Neurology*, vol. 65, no. 12, pp. 1863–1872, 2005.

[3] S. Minoshima, N. L. Foster, A. A. F. Sima, K. A. Frey, R. L. Albin, and D. E. Kuhl, "Alzheimer's disease versus dementia with Lewy bodies: cerebral metabolic distinction with autopsy confirmation," *Annals of Neurology*, vol. 50, no. 3, pp. 358–365, 2001.

[4] D. Titov, J. Diehl-Schmid, K. Shi et al., "Metabolic connectivity for differential diagnosis of dementing disorders," *Journal of Cerebral Blood Flow & Metabolism*, vol. 37, no. 1, pp. 252–262, 2017.

[5] L. K. Teune, A. L. Bartels, and K. L. Leenders, "FDG-PET imaging in neurodegenerative brain diseases," in *Functional Brain Mapping and the Endeavor to Understand the Working Brain*, InTech, 2013.

[6] J. T. O'Brien, M. J. Firbank, C. Davison et al., "^{18}F-FDG PET and perfusion SPECT in the diagnosis of Alzheimer and Lewy body dementias," *Journal of Nuclear Medicine*, vol. 55, no. 12, pp. 1959–1965, 2014.

[7] L. Mosconi, W. H. Tsui, K. Herholz et al., "Multicenter standardized ^{18}F-FDG PET diagnosis of mild cognitive impairment, Alzheimer's disease, and other dementias," *Journal of Nuclear Medicine*, vol. 49, no. 3, pp. 390–398, 2008.

[8] J. Graff-Radford, M. E. Murray, V. J. Lowe et al., "Dementia with Lewy bodies basis of cingulate island sign," *Neurology*, vol. 83, no. 9, pp. 801–809, 2014.

[9] M. P. van den Heuvel, C. J. Stam, R. S. Kahn, and H. E. Hulshoff Pol, "Efficiency of functional brain networks and intellectual performance," *Journal of Neuroscience*, vol. 29, no. 23, pp. 7619–7624, 2009.

[10] M. Göttlich, T. F. Münte, M. Heldmann, M. Kasten, J. Hagenah, and U. M. Krämer, "Altered resting state brain networks in Parkinson's disease," *PLoS One*, vol. 8, no. 10, article e77336, 2013.

[11] S. P. Caminiti, M. Tettamanti, A. Sala et al., "Metabolic connectomics targeting brain pathology in dementia with Lewy bodies," *Journal of Cerebral Blood Flow & Metabolism*, vol. 37, no. 4, pp. 1311–1325, 2017.

[12] E. Bullmore and O. Sporns, "Complex brain networks: graph theoretical analysis of structural and functional systems," *Nature Reviews Neuroscience*, vol. 10, no. 3, pp. 186–198, 2009.

[13] J. Wang, L. Wang, Y. Zang et al., "Parcellation-dependent small-world brain functional networks: a resting-state fMRI study," *Human Brain Mapping*, vol. 30, no. 5, pp. 1511–1523, 2009.

[14] J. Wang, X. Wang, M. Xia, X. Liao, A. Evans, and Y. He, "GRETNA: a graph theoretical network analysis toolbox for imaging connectomics," *Frontiers in Human Neuroscience*, vol. 9, p. 386, 2015.

[15] M. Rubinov and O. Sporns, "Complex network measures of brain connectivity: uses and interpretations," *NeuroImage*, vol. 52, no. 3, pp. 1059–1069, 2010.

[16] D. J. Watts and S. H. Strogatz, "Collective dynamics of 'small-world' networks," *Nature*, vol. 393, no. 6684, pp. 440–442, 1998.

[17] H. Inoue and Y.-Y. Liu, "Revealing the intricate effect of collaboration on innovation," *PLoS One*, vol. 10, no. 3, article e0121973, 2015.

[18] Y. He, Z. J. Chen, and A. C. Evans, "Small-world anatomical networks in the human brain revealed by cortical thickness from MRI," *Cerebral Cortex*, vol. 17, no. 10, pp. 2407–2419, 2007.

[19] V. Latora and M. Marchiori, "Efficient behavior of small-world networks," *Physical Review Letters*, vol. 87, no. 19, article 198701, 2001.

[20] S. Achard and E. Bullmore, "Efficiency and cost of economical brain functional networks," *PLoS Computational Biology*, vol. 3, no. 2, article e17, 2007.

[21] E. H. Seo, D. Y. Lee, J.-M. Lee et al., "Influence of APOE genotype on whole-brain functional networks in cognitively normal elderly," *PLoS One*, vol. 8, no. 12, article e83205, 2013.

[22] Y. He, Z. Chen, and A. Evans, "Structural insights into aberrant topological patterns of large-scale cortical networks in Alzheimer's disease," *Journal of Neuroscience*, vol. 28, no. 18, pp. 4756–4766, 2008.

[23] M. Xia, J. Wang, and Y. He, "BrainNet Viewer: a network visualization tool for human brain connectomics," *PLoS One*, vol. 8, no. 7, article e68910, 2013.

[24] X.-W. Song, Z.-Y. Dong, X.-Y. Long et al., "REST: a toolkit for resting-state functional magnetic resonance imaging data processing," *PLoS One*, vol. 6, no. 9, article e25031, 2011.

[25] Z. Dai, C. Yan, K. Li et al., "Identifying and mapping connectivity patterns of brain network hubs in Alzheimer's disease," *Cerebral Cortex*, vol. 25, no. 10, pp. 3723–3742, 2015.

[26] Y. He and A. Evans, "Graph theoretical modeling of brain connectivity," *Current Opinion in Neurology*, vol. 23, no. 4, pp. 341–350, 2010.

[27] D. Tomasi and N. D. Volkow, "Functional connectivity density mapping," *Proceedings of the National Academy of Sciences of the United States of America*, vol. 107, no. 21, pp. 9885–9890, 2010.

[28] S. N. Vaishnavi, A. G. Vlassenko, M. M. Rundle, A. Z. Snyder, M. A. Mintun, and M. E. Raichle, "Regional aerobic glycolysis in the human brain," *Proceedings of the National Academy of Sciences of the United States of America*, vol. 107, no. 41, pp. 17757–17762, 2010.

[29] F. Blanc, S. J. Colloby, N. Philippi et al., "Cortical thickness in dementia with Lewy bodies and Alzheimer's disease: a comparison of prodromal and dementia stages," *PLoS One*, vol. 10, no. 6, article e0127396, 2015.

[30] L. Silveira-Moriyama, J. L. Holton, A. Kingsbury et al., "Regional differences in the severity of Lewy body pathology across the olfactory cortex," *Neuroscience Letters*, vol. 453, no. 2, pp. 77–80, 2009.

[31] D. W. Dickson, M. L. Schmidt, V. M.-Y. Lee, M.-L. Zhao, S.-H. Yen, and J. Q. Trojanowski, "Immunoreactivity profile of hippocampal CA2/3 neurites in diffuse Lewy body disease," *Acta Neuropathologica*, vol. 87, no. 3, pp. 269–276, 1994.

[32] K. Kosaka, S. Oyanagi, M. Matsushita, A. Hori, and S. Iwase, "Presenile dementia with Alzheimer-, Pick- and Lewy-body changes," *Acta Neuropathologica*, vol. 36, no. 3, pp. 221–233, 1976.

[33] E. L. Dennis and P. M. Thompson, "Functional brain connectivity using fMRI in aging and Alzheimer's disease," *Neuropsychology Review*, vol. 24, no. 1, pp. 49–62, 2014.

[34] L. R. Peraza, J. P. Taylor, and M. Kaiser, "Divergent brain functional network alterations in dementia with Lewy bodies and Alzheimer's disease," *Neurobiology of Aging*, vol. 36, no. 9, pp. 2458–2467, 2015.

[35] A. Zalesky, A. Fornito, I. H. Harding et al., "Whole-brain anatomical networks: does the choice of nodes matter?," *NeuroImage*, vol. 50, no. 3, pp. 970–983, 2010.

21

Cerebral Responses to Acupuncture at GV24 and Bilateral GB13 in Rat Models of Alzheimer's Disease

Shaoyang Cui,[1,2] Mingzhu Xu,[2] Jianting Huang,[2,3] Qing Mei Wang,[2] Xinsheng Lai,[3] Binbin Nie,[4] Baoci Shan,[4] Xun Luo,[5] John Wong,[6,7] and Chunzhi Tang[3]

[1]*Department of Rehabilitation, Shenzhen Hospital of Guangzhou University of Chinese Medicine, Shenzhen, China*
[2]*Stroke Biological Recovery Laboratory, Spaulding Rehabilitation Hospital, Harvard Medical School, Charlestown, MA 02129, USA*
[3]*Clinical Medical College of Acupuncture and Rehabilitation, Guangzhou University of Chinese Medicine, Guangzhou, China*
[4]*Key Laboratory of Nuclear Analysis Techniques, Beijing Engineering Research Center of Radiographic Techniques and Equipment, Institute of High Energy Physics, Chinese Academy of Sciences, Beijing, China*
[5]*Kerry Rehabilitation Medicine Research Institute, Shenzhen, China*
[6]*School of Nursing, MGH Institute of Health Professions, Boston, MA 02129, USA*
[7]*Department of Occupational Therapy, MGH Institute of Health Professions, Boston, MA 02129, USA*

Correspondence should be addressed to John Wong; jwong1@mghihp.edu and Chunzhi Tang; jordan664@163.com

Academic Editor: Péter Klivényi

Acupuncture has been widely used in China to treat neurological diseases including Alzheimer's disease (AD). However, its mechanism remains unclear. In the present study, eighty healthy Wistar rats were divided into a normal control group ($n = 15$) and premodel group ($n = 65$). Forty-five rats that met the criteria for the AD model were then randomly divided into the model group (MG), the nonacupoint group (NG), and the acupoint group (AG). All rats received positron emission tomography (PET) scanning, and the images were analyzed with Statistical Parametric Mapping 8.0. MG exhibited hypometabolism in the olfactory bulb, insular cortex, orbital cortex, prelimbic cortex, striatum, parietal association cortex, visual cortex, cingulate gyrus, and retrosplenial cortex. AG exhibited prominent and extensive hypermetabolism in the thalamus, hypothalamus, bed nucleus of the stria terminalis, cerebral peduncle, midbrain tegmentum, and pontine tegmentum compared to NG. These results demonstrated that acupuncturing at GV24 and bilateral GB13 acupoints may improve the learning and memory abilities of the AD rats, probably via altering cerebral glucose metabolism (CGM) in the hypothalamus, thalamus, and brain stem. The observed effects of acupuncture may be caused by regulating the distribution of certain kinds of neurotransmitters and enhancing synaptic plasticity.

1. Introduction

Alzheimer's disease (AD) is a neurodegenerative brain disease and the most common type of dementia in the elderly [1], accounting for approximately 40–50% of the total cases of dementia [2]. The symptoms of AD inevitably worsen progressively and lead to fatality [3]. At present, over 40 million people worldwide suffer from AD [4], including approximately 700,000 Americans aged 65 years or older in the United States, where it costs $259 billion in 2017 [5].

The main neuropathological features of AD are senile plaques and neurofibrillary tangles [6], which gradually accumulate in the brain. As the disease progresses, these features damage brain circuits involved in cognition. The diagnosis of AD is mainly based on the clinical manifestation of symptoms, including progressive cognitive deficit, initially confined to episodic memory systems [7].

Recently, noninvasive neuroimaging has also been used increasingly in the diagnosis of AD [8], as cerebral glucose metabolism (CGM) is a consistent feature of AD [9]. ^{18}F-2-Fluoro-deoxy-D-glucose (^{18}F-FDG) positron emission tomography (PET) allows the observation of metabolic processes by monitoring positron-emitting radioactive tracers [7] as a marker of neuronal activity [10] and synaptic density

Table 1: Reagents and instruments.

Reagents and instruments	Source
D-Galactose	Shanghai No. 2 Reagent Company, China
$A\beta 1-40$	Sigma Co. Ltd., USA
Sodium pentobarbital	Beijing Chemical Reagents Company, China
Sodium benzylpenicillin	Harbin Pharmaceutical Group Co. Ltd., China
Sterile normal saline	Guangdong Dazhong Pharmaceutical Co. Ltd., China
Isoflurane	Hebei Jiupai Pharmaceutical Co. Ltd., China
Stereotaxic apparatus	Xi'an Northwest Photoelectric Instrument Factory, China
MicroPET imaging system	Siemens, Germany
ECAT EXACT HR + PET imaging system	Siemens, Germany
Matrx animal anaesthesia machine	Midmark Corporation, USA
Y-Maze	Yuanyang Zhenhua Teaching Instrument, Hebei, China
Acupuncture needles	Suzhou Acupuncture & Moxibustion Appliance Co. Ltd., China

[11]. As previous studies have shown that the metabolic changes of the extensive functional networks of the brain are associated with AD [12], some researchers have accepted FDG-PET as a suitable technique for the early and differential diagnosis of dementia [13], with a sensitivity of 94% and specificity of 73% [14].

Acupuncture has been used as a kind of traditional Chinese medicine (TCM) therapy to treat senile dementia including AD in the past decades. Satisfactory and promising effects have been reported in clinical trials and animal experiments [15–19]. Shenting (GV24) and bilateral Benshen (GB13), belonging to the Governing Vessel and Foot Shaoyang Gall Bladder Channel, respectively, are commonly used in treating memory impairment and cognitive deficits [20–22]. However, the mechanism is uncertain. According to the TCM theory, the therapeutic effect of acupuncture is mainly related to the selected acupoints for acupuncture manipulation [23]. Therefore, the acupoint is a breakthrough in understanding the mechanism of acupuncture.

With the integration of acupuncture and modern imaging techniques, research has been conducted based on PET to observe the brain responses of acupuncture [24–26]. We hypothesized that the efficacy of acupuncture is achieved by stimulating specific acupoints, initially targeting certain parts of the brain and subsequently causing neurohumoral interactions to rebalance body homeostasis. In our study, Shenting (GV24) and bilateral Benshen (GB13) were selected to explore the effects of acupuncture in the brain of a rat model of AD.

2. Materials and Methods

2.1. Animals. Eighty adult Wistar rats (40 females and 40 males) weighing 200–250 g were obtained from the China Academy of Chinese Medical Sciences. All rats were housed in standard rodent laboratory cages with a temperature of $20 \pm 2^{\circ}C$, relative humidity of $55 \pm 10\%$, and lights on from 6 am to 6 pm each day. Sterilized drinking water and standard diet were supplied ad libitum. All rats were allowed to have seven days acclimation before any experimentation. The experimental protocols were in strict accordance with the guidelines of the care and use of laboratory animals of the Ministry of Science and Technology of the People's Republic of China and were approved by the Animals Research Ethics Committee of Guangzhou University of Chinese Medicine (20110032SPF). All efforts were made to minimize the animals' suffering.

2.2. Reagents and Instruments. Reagents and instruments used in this study are listed in Table 1.

2.3. Modeling Procedures. All rats were randomly divided into a premodel group (PMG) ($n = 65$, including 32 males and 33 females) and a control group (CG) ($n = 15$, including 8 males and 7 females). First, the PMG received intraperitoneal D-galactose injections (10 mg in 1 ml 0.9% saline) each day for 6 weeks. Then after intraperitoneal injection of pentobarbital anesthesia (50 mg/kg), the rat's scalp was cut open to expose the skull and put in a stereotaxic frame. A microinjection needle was placed in the hippocampal CA1 regions, 3.5 mm lateral and 2 mm posterior to the brain bregma and 2.7 mm deep under the skull surface [27]. $A\beta 1-40$ was injected at a rate of $0.4\,\mu l/min$. After that, the brain scalp was sutured. Gluteus intramuscular injection of penicillin (40,000 U/day) was performed for three days. At the same time, CG received an intraperitoneal injection of sterile normal saline for 6 weeks. The Y-maze task was used to gauge the success of modeling two weeks after the $A\beta 1-40$ injection. The criteria of the AD model, based on the Y-maze result from the control group, is described below. Rats in PMG that met the criteria of the AD model were included in the next step. Eleven rats (6 females and 5 males) died during D-gal and $A\beta 1-40$ administration. Nine rats (5 females and 4 males) did not meet the model criteria. Therefore, 45 rats (23 males and 22 females) from PMG were included, and they were then randomly divided into three groups: the model group (MG) including 8 females and 7 males, the nonacupoint group (NG) including 8 females and 7 males, and the acupoint group (AG) including 7 females and 8 males. All rats underwent micro-PET scanning.

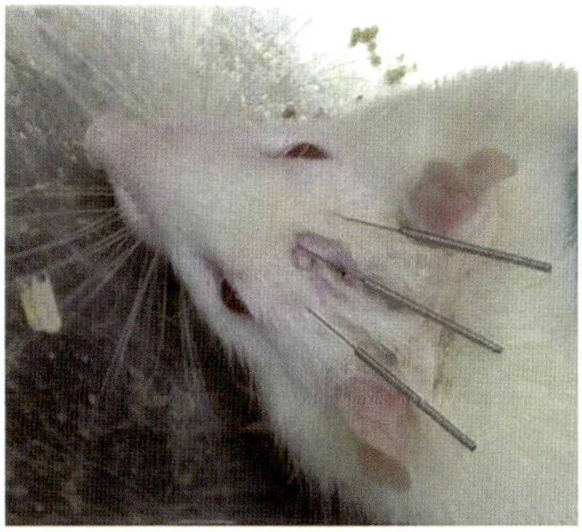

(a)

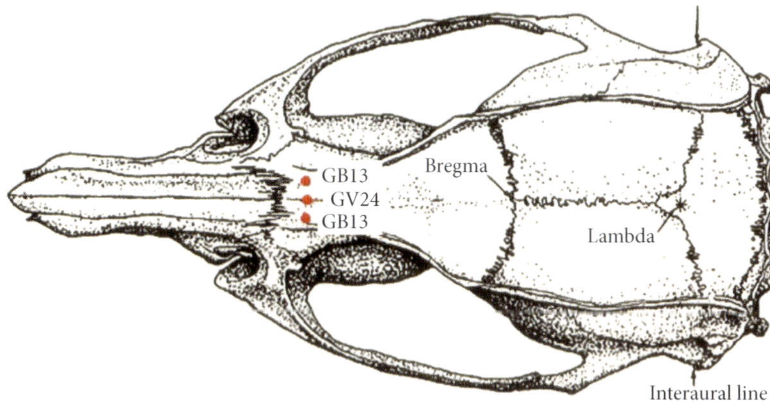

(b)

FIGURE 1: Acupuncture points GV24 and bilateral GB13.

2.4. Acupoint and Nonacupoint Locations. GV24 is located 2 mm directly above the midpoint of the rat's eyes, while GB13 is located 3 mm lateral to GV24, both of which are in the scalp of the frontal pole (Figure 1) [28]. The nonacupoints are located under the bilateral costal arch regions, 10 mm above the crista iliaca, which are not true acupoints and do not belong to any meridians in the theory of TCM.

2.5. Acupuncture. Acupuncture manipulation was performed in both AG and NG. Each rat was needled once per day, 5 days a week for a total of 4 weeks. A sterilized, disposable, stainless steel acupuncture needle (25 mm in length and 0.2 mm in diameter) was inserted obliquely as deep as 4-5 mm into the acupoints or the nonacupoints. The needles were mildly twirled, lifted, and thrusted to equally reinforce and reduce. The twisting was performed at a range of 90–180° and a rate of 100–150 times/min. The lifting and thrusting were performed at a range of approximately 2-3 mm and a rate of 60–90 times/min. Lasting about 15 minutes per rat, the manipulation process was performed by the same acupuncturist during the experiment from 8 a.m. to 12 a.m. every day.

2.6. Y-Maze Task. Fourteen days after the Aβ1–40 injection, the Y-maze task was conducted in a quiet, dark environment from 2 p.m. to 6 p.m. every day. The task was administered by two specially assigned workers who were blinded to the experimental groups and the interventions. The Y-maze was a dark, opaque plexiglass cage, with a conductive grid floor consisting of three identical arms (I-II-III, 40 L × 25H × 10 W cm each) positioned at equal angles. One light bulb was fixed on top of each arm. The grid floor and light bulbs were connected to an electric controller. The arm of the Y-maze with a light represented the safety zone, while the other dark arms were nonsafety zones where grid floor shocks were applied [29].

2.7. Pretreatment and Posttreatment Memory Test. After 5 minutes of adaptation to the Y-maze, rats were trained to learn that the arm with the light was the safe direction by changing the safety zone and the electric shock zone. The electric stimulation parameters were set to 50 V with 5 seconds of delay. If the rat could run to the safety zone directly in 10 seconds after receiving an electric shock on its feet, it was considered the correct reaction; otherwise, it was considered incorrect. The training was repeated 20 times everyday. The pretreatment memory test was performed on day 4, while the posttreatment memory test was performed 4 weeks after acupuncture treatment. The total reaction time (TRT) was recorded to reflect spatial working memory. The test was performed as follows: the safety zone was changed in the order of arm I-II-III-I. The light would be kept on for 10 seconds after the rat ran into the safety zone. After the lights were turned off, one test was completed. After a break of 20–30 seconds, another test would commence. A statistically significant difference between an experimental group and CG was set as the criteria for the AD model. The maze was cleaned with 0.9% sodium chloride solution and dried with a cloth before the next rat was tested.

2.8. Brain ^{18}F-FDG Micro-PET Imaging. After the Y-maze task, all rats received micro PET scanning in batches. First, the initial blood glucose level was determined, and the rats were then allowed to rest for 20 minutes in a darkroom. Then ^{18}F-FDG (a dose of 0.11 mci per kg) was injected intravenously through the tail vein. After that, they were kept in a quiet environment to allow ^{18}F-FDG uptake which lasted about 40 minutes [30]. Then, each rat received a brain scan under anesthesia using 1% isoflurane inhalation. During the scanning, the rat was placed on the scanner bed in a prone position with a plastic stereotactic head holder in place for 10 minutes. ^{18}FDG-PET imaging was performed at the PET Center of China PLA General Hospital with a micro-PET/CT imaging system (Explore Vista CT, GE, USA). A 1.0 mm full width at half maximum (FWHM) at the center of the field of view (FOV) was set as the radial spatial resolution. All the images were reconstructed on a 175 × 175 × 61 matrix, with the voxel size equals 0.39 × 0.39 × 0.77 mm through a 3D ordered set expectation maximization (3D-OSEM) algorithm. All scans were saved in the Analyze format.

2.9. Statistical Analysis and Image Processing. All Y-maze test data were analyzed using IBM SPSS Statistics 21.0 and presented as mean ± standard deviation. Differences between groups were determined by one-way analysis of variance (ANOVA) using the least significant difference (LSD) method for post hoc tests. Statistical significance referred to P value < 0.05.

The PET imaging data analysis was performed using spmratIHEP [31, 32] based on Statistical Parametric Mapping 8.0 (SPM8). First, we removed body tissues and background of rat images by MRIcro, and repositioned the original image at D3V which corresponded to the standard template. Then, data sets were processed automatically in spmratIHEP as follows: (1) Individual brain images were spatially normalized to Paxinos and Watson space, and then the voxel size was scaled up four times in the analysis header, registering to the FDG-PET template, removing extracranial tissues, and shearing matrix to delete background. (2) All the normalized images were smoothed through a Gaussian kernel of $2 \times 2 \times 4\,mm^3$ FWHM. Then based on the framework of the general linear model (GLM), the preprocessed brain images were analyzed. An independent sample t-test was used to determine differences in FDG signals between two groups. Finally, the brain regions with significant changes in FDG were valued by a voxel-level height threshold of $P < 0.001$ (uncorrected) and a cluster size ≥ 50 voxels.

3. Results

3.1. Y-Maze Task. There was a statistically significant difference in the TRT of pretreatment memory among the different groups ($F(3,56) = 3.366$; $P = 0.025$): the TRT of pretreatment memory was much longer in MG ($P = 0.028$), NG ($P = 0.026$), and AG ($P = 0.010$) compared with CG (Figure 2). After 4 weeks of acupuncture stimulation, there was a statistically significant difference in the TRT of pretreatment memory among the different groups ($F(3,56) = 17.459$; $P < 0.001$): the TRT of posttreatment memory in AG was shorter than that of both MG ($P < 0.001$) and NG ($P < 0.001$).

3.2. PET Imaging. MG exhibited hypometabolism in the olfactory bulb, insular cortex, orbital cortex, prelimbic cortex, striatum, parietal association cortex, visual cortex, cingulate gyrus, and retrosplenial cortex (Table 2 and Figure 3(a)). AG exhibited hypermetabolism in the bed nucleus of the stria terminalis, lateral and midline nucleus group of the dorsal thalamus, mammillary, supraoptic, and tuberal regions of the hypothalamus, cerebral peduncle, midbrain tegmentum, and pontine tegmentum after 4 weeks (Table 3 and Figure 3(b)). NG showed hypermetabolism in the lateral and midline nucleus group of the dorsal thalamus and mammillary and tuberal regions of the hypothalamus after 4 weeks (Table 4 and Figure 3(c)).

4. Discussion

AD begins with impaired memory, gradually leading to total cognitive dysfunction [33]. To date, evidence supports the idea that dysfunction in learning and memory abilities due to structural and functional damage to specific brain regions

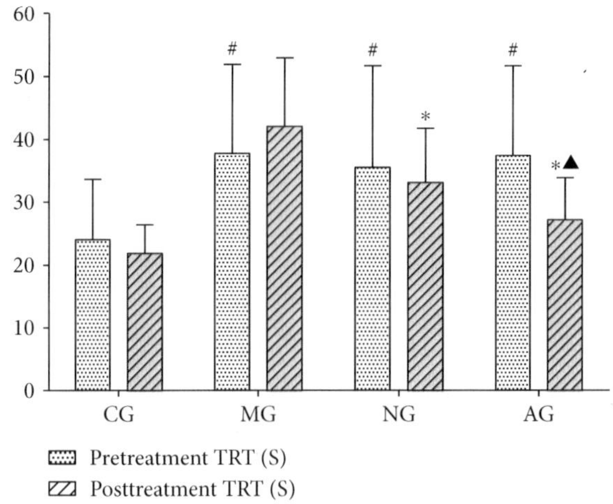

FIGURE 2: The total reaction time (TRT) of pretreatment memory and posttreatment memory in the Y-maze task. Pretreatment: TRT on the 4th day; posttreatment: TRT on the 29th day. #$P < 0.05$ compared with CG. *$P < 0.05$ compared with the MG. ▲$P < 0.05$ compared with NG.

is associated with AD [34]. It has been demonstrated that hypometabolism, representing synaptic abnormality or neuronal injury, may be also a part of the pathophysiology of AD [14, 35, 36].

In our study, we observed decreased CGM in many areas of the brain, consistent with published findings. People with AD have reduced activity in the retrosplenial cortex [37]. Evidence has shown that the retrosplenial cortex, which is involved in forming and retrieving associations following neutral stimuli, contributes to hippocampal-dependent forms of learning and memory [38], and it connects the hippocampus to the visual cortex and other brain regions. A large amount of amyloid deposits have been found in the retrosplenial cortex of AD patients [39], suggesting that this may be an important area in the development of AD. The parietal association cortex involved with spatial navigation and memory is associated with different sensory modalities [40]. The reduced CGM in this area that we and others have observed may be an important trigger for the onset of AD [41]. Previous studies have reported that AD patients exhibit hypometabolism in the cingulate gyrus from an early stage [42]. The Papez circuit enables the connection between the cingulate gyrus and hippocampus, and it plays an important role in memory function [43]. Recently, the hypometabolism of the olfactory bulb has served as a potential marker of the diagnosis of AD and is related to memory deficits [44, 45]. Although some studies suggested that Aβ deposits in this area may promote AD pathology [46, 47], another study has found that the deposition of the TAR DNA-binding protein of 43 kDa (TDP-43) in the olfactory bulb was associated with AD and associated symptoms including episodic memory loss and hippocampal atrophy [48, 49]. Consistent with the previous finding, metabolic decline was observed in the striatum, probably due to the loss of synaptic contacts [50]. MRI analysis has shown that the atrophy of the striatum may also be involved in the development of AD [51]. Therefore, our rat model could reliably

TABLE 2: Areas with higher PET signals (control group versus model group).

Area	Size (voxels)	Local maximum t value	Talairach coordinates (mm) x	y	z	Side	Related brain region	Panel in Figure 3(a)
1	8804	7.27	1.64	0.47	−3.48	Right	Parietal association cortex	A1
2	8804	7.81	0.49	1.51	2.28	Right	Cingulate gyrus	A1
3	8804	8.51	1.80	0.63	−5.16	Right	Visual cortex	A1
4	8804	8.19	−0.22	0.41	−3.96	Left	Retrosplenial cortex	A2
5	1733	5.63	0.88	3.63	3.24	Right	Prelimbic cortex	A3
6	1733	4.87	2.50	6.15	2.28	Right	Striatum	A3
7	1733	6.47	3.15	4.77	3.48	Right	Insular cortex	A4
8	1733	6.21	2.88	4.75	1733	Right	Orbital cortex	A4
9	605	8.48	0.83	3.88	7.08	Right	Olfactory bulb	A1

reproduce glucose hypometabolism characteristic of AD, and we speculate that the association between hypometabolism in these brain areas and memory deficits may reflect disease-related dysfunction in these brain regions.

Our results demonstrated that the activated brain regions in AG were much more prominent and extensive compared to NG in AD rats. Taking our Y-maze data into consideration, we speculate that acupuncture at GV24 and bilateral GB13 may improve a memory deficit through activating the thalamus, hypothalamus, and brain stem. The midline group nuclei of the thalamus have close connections with the hippocampus, and previous studies have showed that stimulation of the midline group may activate CA1 and improve acquisition memory and short-term memory by enhancing synaptic plasticity and altering A-beta clearing in rat models of the AD model [52]. The right ventrolateral thalamus has also been demonstrated to contribute more to memory recall while the left side to memory encoding [53]. Recent studies have found volume atrophy and functional degeneration in the thalamus and hippocampus in AD [54, 55]. Neurodegeneration in these structures may lead to further degeneration of the connected regions [56]. It has also been suggested that AD-related memory loss is contributed by the impairment of connections between the anterior thalamus and hippocampus [57]. Lai et al. hypothesized that acupuncture can prevent atrophy and degeneration of AD-related regions by increasing regional glucose metabolism to postpone the progress of the disease and further improve memory and learning abilities [58]. The hypothalamus is highly interconnected with the brainstem and its reticular formation, other limbic structures including the amygdala and septum, and areas of the autonomous nervous system. The hypothalamus can influence the hippocampus-dependent memory function through the limbic response by the activation of the fornix [57]. The brainstem contains many nuclei which are interconnected with the higher cortical or limbic association areas [59]. It regulates cognitive, autonomic, and behavioral functions via its wildly distributed norepinephrine, dopamine, and serotonin neurotransmitter projections to modulate the cortical circuits [60]. Lee et al. postulated that cognitive symptoms such as memory impairment may be related to the morphological alterations of the brainstem in AD patients, as regionally contracted areas were observed in the upper midbrain areas and posterior portion of the brainstem [59].

Acupuncture stimulation may alter brain metabolism by affecting the structure, function, and signaling pathways in the brain. Previous studies have shown that acupuncture on specific acupoints can modulate the cerebral blood flow and strengthen the hippocampal connectivity [61, 62]. Recently, it was also reported that phosphorylated adenosine monophosphate-activated protein kinase (AMPK) and AKT serine/threonine kinase were two critical metabolic homeostatic factors for glucose metabolism, and several studies have demonstrated that acupuncture can activate the expression of AMPK and AKT in rat models of AD [63, 64] and decrease the accumulation of Aβ in the cortex and hippocampus by inhibiting the phosphorylation level of the mammalian target of rapamycin (mTOR) [65]. Other possible effects of acupuncture may also be related to its ability to decrease the level of cytokines in the hippocampus [66], reverse the decreased acetylcholine neurotransmission [67], and reduce oxidative damage by increasing the activity of superoxide dismutase (SOD) [68]. The inhibition of nerve apoptosis and necrosis and suppression of oxidative stress are the main signaling pathways to be considered [69].

We also observed hypermetabolism in the bed nucleus of the stria terminalis, which has been shown to be associated with anxiety [70] and with behavioral responses to unfamiliar things [71]. However, we are not sure whether this is caused by the fear of acupuncture, and this postulation still needs to be further confirmed. In our study, we chose distant nonacupoints mainly because the rat's head was too small, so needling at completely different sites could exert a better perspective of the brain regional effects.

There are other limitations in this study: (1) the AD model was induced by the intraperitoneal injection of D-gal and the bilateral hippocampus injection of Aβ1–40, which could mimic some symptoms of AD, but it was difficult to fully demonstrate the characteristics of AD patients. This model was established according to the previous studies [72–74]. (2) We simply used the Y-maze to test the progression of AD rats, but it may be better for us to analyze some biochemical markers at the same time. (3) We were unable to explain why acupuncture did

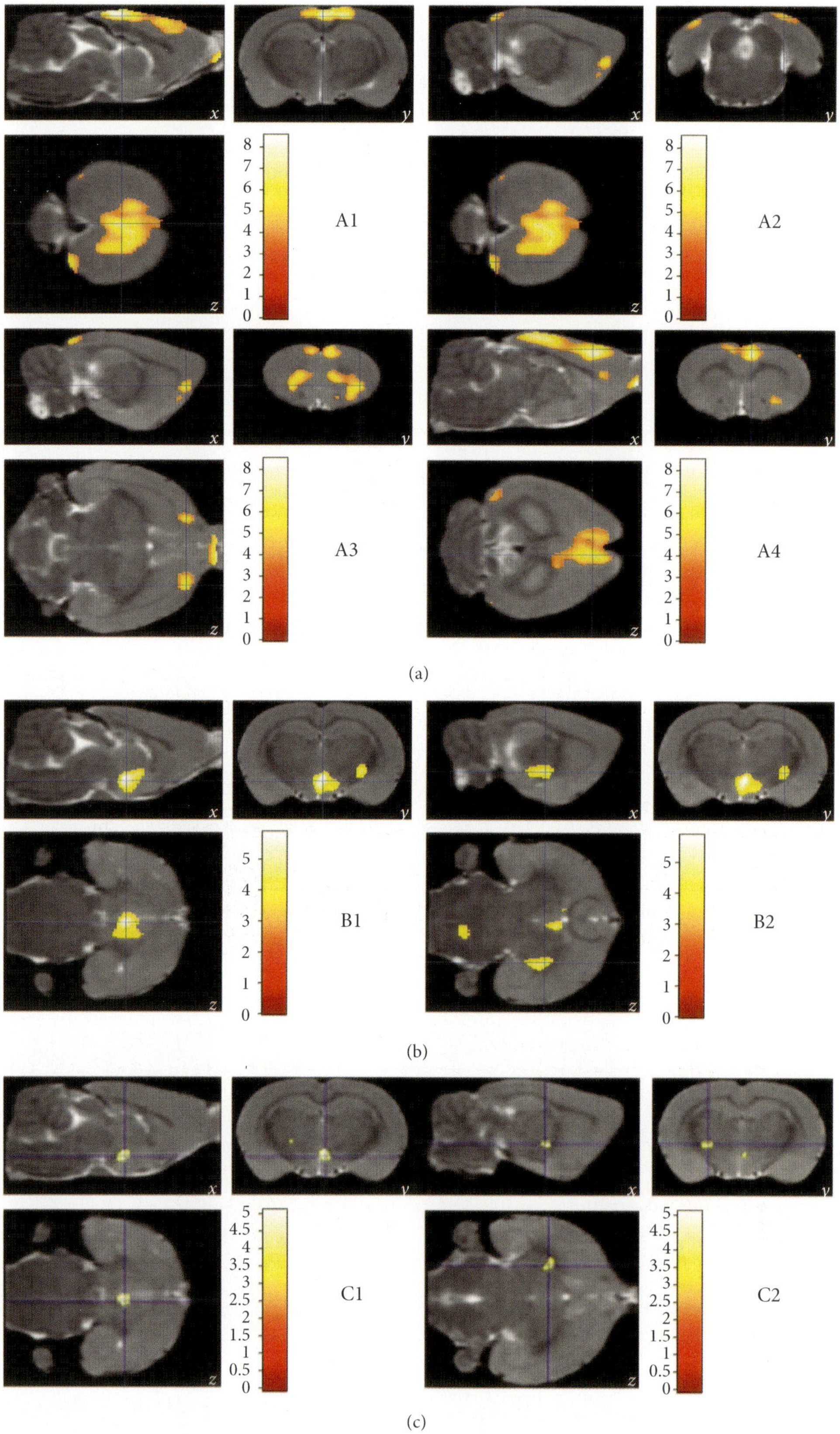

FIGURE 3: Cerebral areas with decreased (a) or increased (b and c) glucose uptake. The areas with significantly different FDG-PET signals in CG versus MG (a), AG versus MG (b), and NG versus MG (c) ($P < 0.05$) identified in Tables 2, 3, and 4 are shown in these FDG-PET three-dimensional (3D) images. All the data were analyzed with a 2-tailed t-test for independent samples.

Table 3: Areas with higher PET signals (acupoint group versus model group).

Area	Size (voxels)	Local maximum t value	Talairach coordinates (mm) x	y	z	Side	Related brain region	Panel in Figure 3(b)
1	1608	3.93	−1.20	6.21	−0.84	Left	Bed nucleus of stria terminalis	B1
2	1608	4.84	0.29	6.59	−2.52	Right	Dorsal thalamus-lateral nucleus group	B1
3	1608	5.85	0.03	7.03	−2.76	Right	Dorsal thalamus-midline nucleus group	B1
4	1608	5.34	0.03	7.22	−3.24	Right	Hypothalamus-mammillary region	B1
5	1608	3.71	0.28	7.57	−2.04	Right	Hypothalamus-supraoptic region	B1
6	1608	5.24	−0.24	7.58	−2.52	Left	Hypothalamus-tuberal region	B1
7	482	4.50	3.65	6.60	−3.72	Right	Midbrain-cerebral peduncle	B2
8	482	3.76	0.70	7.26	−3.24	Right	Midbrain tegmentum	B2
9	259	3.99	1.22	7.44	−11.64	Right	Pontine tegmentum	B1

Table 4: Areas with higher PET signals (nonacupoint group versus model group).

Area	Size (voxels)	Local maximum t value	Talairach coordinates (mm) x	y	z	Side	Related brain region	Panel in Figure 3(c)
1	172	4.99	0.16	7.06	−3.00	Right	Dorsal thalamus-midline nucleus group	C1
2	172	4.64	0.17	7.23	−3.24	Right	Hypothalamus-mammillary region	C1
3	172	4.14	0.30	7.51	−3.00	Right	Hypothalamus-tuberal region	C1
4	108	3.97	−3.19	5.62	−2.04	Left	Dorsal thalamus-lateral nucleus group	C2

not target the corresponding pathological brain areas in AD rats. Future research should also explore the relationship between the brain areas in AD rats that exhibit hypometabolism and the brain areas where acupuncture activates hypermetabolism.

5. Conclusion

This study demonstrated that acupuncture at GV24 and bilateral GB13 acupoints could improve learning and memory abilities of the AD rats and increase the CGM in the thalamus, hypothalamus, and brain stem. These findings suggest that the neuromodulatory mechanism of acupuncture may be achieved by enhancing synaptic plasticity and regulating the production of certain kinds of neurotransmitters, but longitudinal studies might be needed to confirm this explanation. These preclinical findings will undoubtedly enhance the understanding of the pathophysiological mechanisms of AD. The improved perspectives on brain functional neurocognition will be helpful in understanding the mechanism of acupuncture and may also serve as a fundamental basis to diagnose and develop efficient treatment to improve the quality of life of AD patients and their families.

Authors' Contributions

Shaoyang Cui and Mingzhu Xu are joint first authors and contributed equally.

Acknowledgments

This work was conducted in China and was supported by the National Natural Science Foundation of China (No. 81173350) and Shenzhen Special Fund for Introducing High-Level Medical Team Project (2015).

References

[1] R. S. Wilson, E. Segawa, P. A. Boyle, S. E. Anagnos, L. P. Hizel, and D. A. Bennett, "The natural history of cognitive decline in Alzheimer's disease," *Psychology and Aging*, vol. 27, no. 4, pp. 1008–1017, 2012.

[2] K. Narazaki, Y. Nofuji, and S. Kumagai, "Association between middle- to late-life physical performance and incident Alzheimer's disease: recent findings and potential mechanisms," *The Journal of Physical Fitness and Sports Medicine*, vol. 6, no. 4, pp. 191–200, 2017.

[3] R. Mayeux, "Clinical practice. Early Alzheimer's disease," *The New England Journal of Medicine*, vol. 362, no. 23, pp. 2194–2201, 2010.

[4] A. Uflacker and P. M. Doraiswamy, "Alzheimer's disease: an overview of recent developments and a look to the future," *Focus*, vol. 15, no. 1, pp. 13–17, 2017.

[5] Alzheimer's Association, "2017 Alzheimer's disease facts and figures," *Alzheimer's & Dementia*, vol. 13, no. 4, pp. 325–373, 2017.

[6] C. Duyckaerts, B. Delatour, and M. C. Potier, "Classification and basic pathology of Alzheimer disease," *Acta Neuropathologica*, vol. 118, no. 1, pp. 5–36, 2009.

[7] L. P. Schilling, E. R. Zimmer, M. Shin et al., "Imaging Alzheimer's disease, pathophysiology with PET," *Dementia & Neuropsychologia*, vol. 10, no. 2, pp. 79–90, 2016.

[8] C. Marcus, E. Mena, and R. M. Subramaniam, "Brain PET in the diagnosis of Alzheimer's disease," *Clinical Nuclear Medicine*, vol. 39, no. 10, pp. e413–e426, 2014.

[9] G. E. Gibson, J. Elder, R. Cirio, P. Fonzetti, J. Hirsch, and B. Jordan, "Glucose metabolism as a therapeutic target in Alzheimer's disease," *Alzheimer's & Dementia*, vol. 13, no. 7, article P611, 2017.

[10] L. Sokoloff, M. Reivich, C. Kennedy et al., "The [^{14}C]deoxyglucose method for the measurement of local cerebral glucose utilization: theory, procedure, and normal values in the conscious and anesthetized albino rat," *Journal of Neurochemistry*, vol. 28, no. 5, pp. 897–916, 1977.

[11] A. B. Rocher, F. Chapon, X. Blaizot, J. C. Baron, and C. Chavoix, "Resting-state brain glucose utilization as measured by PET is directly related to regional synaptophysin levels: a study in baboons," *NeuroImage*, vol. 20, no. 3, pp. 1894–1898, 2003.

[12] R. A. Sperling, B. C. Dickerson, M. Pihlajamaki et al., "Functional alterations in memory networks in early Alzheimer's disease," *Neuromolecular Medicine*, vol. 12, no. 1, pp. 27–43, 2010.

[13] L. Mosconi, W. H. Tsui, K. Herholz et al., "Multicenter standardized ^{18}F-FDG PET diagnosis of mild cognitive impairment, Alzheimer's disease, and other dementias," *The Journal of Nuclear Medicine*, vol. 49, no. 3, pp. 390–398, 2008.

[14] D. H. S. Silverman, G. W. Small, C. Y. Chang et al., "Positron emission tomography in evaluation of dementia: regional brain metabolism and long-term outcome," *JAMA*, vol. 286, no. 17, pp. 2120–2127, 2001.

[15] B. Lee, B. Sur, J. Shim, D. H. Hahm, and H. Lee, "Acupuncture stimulation improves scopolamine-induced cognitive impairment via activation of cholinergic system and regulation of BDNF and CREB expressions in rats," *BMC Complementary and Alternative Medicine*, vol. 14, no. 1, pp. 338–338, 2014.

[16] Z. Wang, B. Nie, D. Li et al., "Effect of acupuncture in mild cognitive impairment and Alzheimer disease: a functional MRI study," *PLoS One*, vol. 7, no. 8, article e42730, 2012.

[17] W. Li, L. H. Kong, H. Wang et al., "High-frequency electroacupuncture evidently reinforces hippocampal synaptic transmission in Alzheimer's disease rats," *Neural Regeneration Research*, vol. 11, no. 5, pp. 801–806, 2016.

[18] Y. Cao, L. W. Zhang, J. Wang et al., "Mechanisms of acupuncture effect on Alzheimer's disease in animal-based researches," *Current Topics in Medicinal Chemistry*, vol. 16, no. 5, pp. 574–578, 2016.

[19] H. Y. Cheng and D. Q. Cheng, "Progress in research on acupuncture treatment of senile dementia," *Journal of Traditional Chinese Medicine*, vol. 29, no. 3, pp. 224–233, 2009.

[20] J. B. Huang, H. F. Cao, J. Hu, L. H. Liu, Z. Wang, and H. Lin, "Clinical research on children mental retardation treated with acupuncture," *Zhongguo Zhen Jiu*, vol. 33, no. 8, pp. 682–685, 2013.

[21] Y. Watanabe, T. Urakami, S. Hongo, and T. Ohtsubo, "Frontal lobe function and social adjustment in patients with schizophrenia: near-infrared spectroscopy," *Human Psychopharmacology*, vol. 30, no. 1, pp. 28–41, 2015.

[22] D. Y. Kimberg and M. J. Farah, "A unified account of cognitive impairments following frontal lobe damage: the role of working memory in complex, organized behavior," *Journal of Experimental Psychology: General*, vol. 122, no. 4, pp. 411–428, 1993.

[23] F. Li, T. He, Q. Xu et al., "What is the acupoint? A preliminary review of acupoints," *Pain Medicine*, vol. 16, no. 10, pp. 1905–1915, 2015.

[24] F. Zeng, L. Lan, Y. Tang et al., "Cerebral responses to puncturing at different acupoints for treating meal-related functional dyspepsia," *Neurogastroenterology & Motility*, vol. 27, no. 4, pp. 559–568, 2015.

[25] M. Yang, J. Yang, F. Zeng et al., "Electroacupuncture stimulation at sub-specific acupoint and non-acupoint induced distinct brain glucose metabolism change in migraineurs: a PET-CT study," *Journal of Translational Medicine*, vol. 12, no. 1, p. 351, 2014.

[26] F. Zeng, L. Lan, X. Liu et al., "PP-061: acupuncture for functional dyspepsia at acupoints on stomach meridian: a PET–CT study protocol," *European Journal of Integrative Medicine*, vol. 2, no. 4, p. 244, 2010.

[27] G. Paxinos, *The Rat Brain in Stereotaxic Coordinates: Compact, Sixth Edition*, Academic Press, London, 2007.

[28] Z. Li, *Experimental Acupuncture Science*, China Press of Traditional Chinese Medicine, China, 2010.

[29] M. Nobakht, S. M. Hoseini, P. Mortazavi et al., "Neuropathological changes in brain cortex and hippocampus in a rat model of Alzheimer's disease," *Iranian Biomedical Journal*, vol. 15, no. 1-2, pp. 51–58, 2011.

[30] A. Matsumura, S. Mizokawa, M. Tanaka et al., "Assessment of microPET performance in analyzing the rat brain under different types of anesthesia: comparison between quantitative data obtained with microPET and ex vivo autoradiography," *NeuroImage*, vol. 20, no. 4, pp. 2040–2050, 2003.

[31] B. Nie, K. Chen, S. Zhao et al., "A rat brain MRI template with digital stereotaxic atlas of fine anatomical delineations in Paxinos space and its automated application in voxel-wise analysis," *Human Brain Mapping*, vol. 34, no. 6, pp. 1306–1318, 2013.

[32] B. Nie, H. Liu, K. Chen, X. Jiang, and B. Shan, "A statistical parametric mapping toolbox used for voxel-wise analysis of FDG-PET images of rat brain," *PLoS One*, vol. 9, no. 9, article e108295, 2014.

[33] K. Ishii, "PET approaches for diagnosis of dementia," *AJNR American Journal of Neuroradiology*, vol. 35, no. 11, pp. 2030–2038, 2014.

[34] G. H. Weissberger, R. J. Melrose, T. A. Narvaez, D. Harwood, M. A. Mandelkern, and D. L. Sultzer, "^{18}F-Fluorodeoxyglucose positron emission tomography cortical metabolic activity associated with distinct agitation behaviors in Alzheimer disease," *The American Journal of Geriatric Psychiatry*, vol. 25, no. 6, pp. 569–579, 2017.

[35] K. P. Ng, T. A. Pascoal, S. Mathotaarachchi et al., "Neuropsychiatric symptoms predict hypometabolism in preclinical Alzheimer disease," *Neurology*, vol. 88, no. 19, pp. 1814–1821, 2017.

[36] L. Rice and S. Bisdas, "Review. The diagnostic value of FDG and amyloid PET in Alzheimer's disease—a systematic

review," *European Journal of Radiology*, vol. 94, pp. 16–24, 2017.

[37] D. Mao, S. Kandler, B. L. McNaughton, and V. Bonin, "Sparse orthogonal population representation of spatial context in the retrosplenial cortex," *Nature Communications*, vol. 8, no. 1, p. 243, 2017.

[38] T. P. Todd and D. J. Bucci, "Retrosplenial cortex and long-term memory: molecules to behavior," *Neural Plasticity*, vol. 2015, Article ID 414173, 9 pages, 2015.

[39] F. Torrealba and J. L. Valdés, "The parietal association cortex of the rat," *Biological Research*, vol. 41, no. 4, pp. 369–377, 2008.

[40] X. Lai, G. Zhang, Y. Huang et al., "A cerebral functional imaging study by positron emission tomography in healthy volunteers receiving true or sham acupuncture needling," *Neuroscience Letters*, vol. 452, no. 2, pp. 194–199, 2009.

[41] E. Bruner and H. I. Jacobs, "Alzheimer's disease: the downside of a highly evolved parietal lobe?," *Journal of Alzheimer's Disease*, vol. 35, no. 2, pp. 227–240, 2013.

[42] P. J. Nestor, T. D. Fryer, P. Smielewski, and J. R. Hodges, "Limbic hypometabolism in Alzheimer's disease and mild cognitive impairment," *Annals of Neurology*, vol. 54, no. 3, pp. 343–351, 2003.

[43] N. Murayama, K. Ota, K. Kasanuki et al., "Cognitive dysfunction in patients with very mild Alzheimer's disease and amnestic mild cognitive impairment showing hemispheric asymmetries of hypometabolism on ^{18}F-FDG PET," *International Journal of Geriatric Psychiatry*, vol. 31, no. 1, pp. 41–48, 2016.

[44] N.-A. Xiao, J. Zhang, M. Zhou et al., "Reduction of glucose metabolism in olfactory bulb is an earlier Alzheimer's disease-related biomarker in 5XFAD mice," *Chinese Medical Journal*, vol. 128, no. 16, pp. 2220–2227, 2015.

[45] A. V. Masurkar and D. P. Devanand, "Olfactory dysfunction in the elderly: basic circuitry and alterations with normal aging and Alzheimer's disease," *Current Geriatrics Reports*, vol. 3, no. 2, pp. 91–100, 2014.

[46] D. W. Wesson, E. Levy, R. A. Nixon, and D. A. Wilson, "Olfactory dysfunction correlates with amyloid-β burden in an Alzheimer's disease mouse model," *The Journal of Neuroscience*, vol. 30, no. 2, pp. 505–514, 2010.

[47] D. W. Wesson, A. H. Borkowski, G. E. Landreth, R. A. Nixon, E. Levy, and D. A. Wilson, "Sensory network dysfunction, behavioral impairments, and their reversibility in an Alzheimer's β-amyloidosis mouse model," *The Journal of Neuroscience*, vol. 31, no. 44, pp. 15962–15971, 2011.

[48] K. A. Josephs and D. W. Dickson, "TDP-43 in the olfactory bulb in Alzheimer's disease," *Neuropathology and Applied Neurobiology*, vol. 42, no. 4, pp. 390–393, 2016.

[49] K. A. Josephs, J. L. Whitwell, S. D. Weigand et al., "TDP-43 is a key player in the clinical features associated with Alzheimer's disease," *Acta Neuropathologica*, vol. 127, no. 6, pp. 811–824, 2014.

[50] D. J. Selkoe, "Alzheimer's disease is a synaptic failure," *Science*, vol. 298, no. 5594, pp. 789–791, 2002.

[51] E. Micotti, A. Paladini, C. Balducci et al., "Striatum and entorhinal cortex atrophy in AD mouse models: MRI comprehensive analysis," *Neurobiology of Aging*, vol. 36, no. 2, pp. 776–788, 2015.

[52] I. Arrieta-Cruz, C. Pavlides, and G. M. Pasinetti, "Deep brain stimulation in midline thalamic region facilitates synaptic transmission and short-term memory in a mouse model of Alzheimer's disease," *Translational Neuroscience*, vol. 1, no. 3, pp. 188–194, 2010.

[53] G. A. Ojemann, K. I. Blick, and A. A. Ward Jr., "Improvement and disturbance of short-term verbal memory with human ventrolateral thalamic stimulation," *Brain*, vol. 94, no. 2, pp. 225–240, 1971.

[54] I. Štěpán-Buksakowska, N. Szabó, D. Hořínek et al., "Cortical and subcortical atrophy in Alzheimer disease: parallel atrophy of thalamus and hippocampus," *Alzheimer Disease & Associated Disorders*, vol. 28, no. 1, pp. 65–72, 2014.

[55] S.-J. Son, J. Kim, and H. Park, "Structural and functional connectional fingerprints in mild cognitive impairment and Alzheimer's disease patients," *PLoS One*, vol. 12, no. 3, article e0173426, 2017.

[56] T.-F. Yuan and B. M. Slotnick, "Roles of olfactory system dysfunction in depression," *Progress in Neuro-Psychopharmacology and Biological Psychiatry*, vol. 54, pp. 26–30, 2014.

[57] C. Hamani, M. P. McAndrews, M. Cohn et al., "Memory enhancement induced by hypothalamic/fornix deep brain stimulation," *Annals of Neurology*, vol. 63, no. 1, pp. 119–123, 2008.

[58] X. Lai, J. Ren, Y. Lu et al., "Effects of acupuncture at HT7 on glucose metabolism in a rat model of Alzheimer's disease: an ^{18}F-FDG-PET study," *Acupuncture in Medicine*, vol. 34, no. 3, pp. 215–222, 2016.

[59] J. H. Lee, J. Ryan, C. Andreescu, H. Aizenstein, and H. K. Lim, "Brainstem morphological changes in Alzheimer's disease," *Neuroreport*, vol. 26, no. 7, pp. 411–415, 2015.

[60] R. A. Hurley, L. A. Flashman, T. W. Chow, and K. H. Taber, "The brainstem: anatomy, assessment, and clinical syndromes," *The Journal of Neuropsychiatry and Clinical Neurosciences*, vol. 22, no. 1, pp. iv–i7, 2010.

[61] Z. Wang, P. Liang, Z. Zhao et al., "Acupuncture modulates resting state hippocampal functional connectivity in Alzheimer disease," *PLoS One*, vol. 9, no. 3, article e91160, 2014.

[62] S. Kim, Y. I. Kim, R. S. Sin et al., "Study on cerebral blood flow regulatory features of acupuncture stimulation at various acupoints," *Medical Acupuncture*, vol. 28, no. 6, pp. 316–324, 2016.

[63] W. Dong, W. Guo, X. Zheng et al., "Electroacupuncture improves cognitive deficits associated with AMPK activation in SAMP8 mice," *Metabolic Brain Disease*, vol. 30, no. 3, pp. 777–784, 2015.

[64] A. Tominaga, N. Ishizaki, Y. Naruse, H. Kitakoji, and Y. Yamamura, "Repeated application of low-frequency electroacupuncture improves high-fructose diet-induced insulin resistance in rats," *Acupuncture in Medicine*, vol. 29, no. 4, pp. 276–283, 2011.

[65] W. Liu, P. Zhuo, L. Li et al., "Activation of brain glucose metabolism ameliorating cognitive impairment in APP/PS1 transgenic mice by electroacupuncture," *Free Radical Biology & Medicine*, vol. 112, pp. 174–190, 2017.

[66] Y. Fang and R. Sui, "Electroacupuncture at the Wangu acupoint suppresses expression of inflammatory cytokines in the hippocampus of rats with vascular dementia," *African Journal of Traditional, Complementary and Alternative Medicines*, vol. 13, no. 5, pp. 17–24, 2016.

[67] Z.-B. Liu, W. M. Niu, X. H. Yang, X. M. Niu, and Y. Wang, "Effect of "Xiusanzhen" on learning-memory ability and

hippocampal ChAT and AChE activity in Alzheimer disease rats," *Zhen Ci Yan Jiu*, vol. 34, no. 1, pp. 48–51, 2009.

[68] C.-Z. Liu and B. Lei, "Effect of acupuncture intervention on learning-memory ability and cerebral superoxide dismutase activity and malonaldehyde concentration in chronic fatigue syndrome rats," *Zhen Ci Yan Jiu*, vol. 38, no. 6, pp. 478–481, 2013.

[69] K.-Y. Huang, S. Liang, M. L. Yu, S. P. Fu, X. Chen, and S. F. Lu, "A systematic review and meta-analysis of acupuncture for improving learning and memory ability in animals," *BMC Complementary and Alternative Medicine*, vol. 16, no. 1, p. 297, 2016.

[70] K. Luyck, T. Tambuyzer, M. Deprez, J. Rangarajan, B. Nuttin, and L. Luyten, "Electrical stimulation of the bed nucleus of the stria terminalis reduces anxiety in a rat model," *Translational Psychiatry*, vol. 7, no. 2, article e1033, 2017.

[71] A. S. Fox, S. E. Shelton, T. R. Oakes, A. K. Converse, R. J. Davidson, and N. H. Kalin, "Orbitofrontal cortex lesions alter anxiety-related activity in the primate bed nucleus of stria terminalis," *The Journal of Neuroscience*, vol. 30, no. 20, pp. 7023–7027, 2010.

[72] T. Yue, G. Shanbin, M. Ling, W. Yuan, X. Ying, and Z. Ping, "Sevoflurane aggregates cognitive dysfunction and hippocampal oxidative stress induced by β-amyloid in rats," *Life Sciences*, vol. 143, pp. 194–201, 2015.

[73] N. Chen, S. Dong, T. Yan, N. Yan, Y. Ma, and C. Yu, "High-frequency stimulation of anterior nucleus thalamus improves impaired cognitive function induced by intra-hippocampal injection of Aβ1–40 in rats," *Chinese Medical Journal*, vol. 127, no. 1, pp. 125–129, 2014.

[74] B. Wan, X. Hu, J. Nie et al., "Effects of triptolide on degeneration of dendritic spines induced by $A\beta_{1-40}$ injection in rat hippocampus," *Neurological Sciences*, vol. 35, no. 1, pp. 35–40, 2014.

Screening for Emotional Expression in Frontotemporal Dementia

Andrew R. Carr,[1,2] Mark M. Ashla,[2] Elvira E. Jimenez,[1,2] and Mario F. Mendez[1,2,3]

[1]*VA Greater Los Angeles Healthcare System, Los Angeles, CA, USA*
[2]*Department of Neurology, David Geffen School of Medicine, University of California at Los Angeles, Los Angeles, CA, USA*
[3]*Department of Psychiatry & Biobehavioral Sciences, David Geffen School of Medicine, University of California at Los Angeles, Los Angeles, CA, USA*

Correspondence should be addressed to Mario F. Mendez; mmendez@ucla.edu

Academic Editor: Luigi Trojano

Objective. Although emotional blunting is a core feature of behavioral variant frontotemporal dementia (bvFTD), there are no practical clinical measures of emotional expression for the early diagnosis of bvFTD. *Method.* Three age-matched groups (bvFTD, Alzheimer's disease (AD), and healthy controls (HC)) of eight participants each were presented with real-life vignettes varying in emotional intensity (high versus low) with either negative or positive outcomes. This study evaluated verbal (self-reports of distress) and visual (presence or absence of facial affect) measures of emotional expression during the vignettes. *Results.* The bvFTD patients did not differ from the AD and HC groups in reported distress or in the amount of facial affect during vignettes with high emotional intensity or type of outcome. However, the bvFTD patients reported significantly less distress and had correspondingly few facial affective expressions when compared on vignettes of low intensity. *Conclusions.* Patients with bvFTD require a high intensity of emotional stimulus and are significantly hyporesponsive to low-intensity stimuli. Simple screening or observations of verbal and facial responsiveness to mildly arousing stimuli may aid in differentiating bvFTD from normal subjects and patients with other dementias. Future studies can investigate whether delivering information with high emotional intensity can facilitate communication with patients with bvFTD.

1. Introduction

Behavioral variant frontotemporal dementia (bvFTD) results in socioemotional changes including abnormalities in context-appropriate behavior and personality [1]. These changes manifest as apathy or abulia, loss of empathy or sympathy, and disinhibition or poor impulse control, as well as other behaviors [2, 3]. Numerous studies demonstrate prominent impairments in socioemotional processing suggesting generalized emotional blunting may underlie many of these disturbed behaviors in bvFTD [4–6].

BvFTD patients generally fail to report distress and demonstrate decreased reactivity to emotional stimuli [7, 8]. Decreased verbal and facial expressions of emotion may result from an impaired ability to correctly recognize emotions [9–12], evident in decreased recognition of facial affect [9, 13–15]. Patients with bvFTD are especially impaired in the recognition of negative emotions [11, 16, 17], with relative preservation of the recognition of pleasant emotions such as happiness [10, 11, 15, 18]. Thus, while bvFTD patients demonstrate deficits in recognizing most emotions, and a striking paucity of emotional reactions [14, 19], they are not entirely devoid of emotional recognition.

There is a relationship of decreased emotional reactivity, manifest as decreased verbal and visual emotional expression, and decreased empathic behavior. The lack of verbal or visual emotional expression, operationalized as "emotional blunting" or "callous-unemotional" traits, is correlated not only with lack of empathy in bvFTD [4, 7] but also with decreased cognitive and affective empathy, affective perspective taking, and psychopathic traits in other populations [20, 21]. Empathy in bvFTD is a complex multidimensional construct and may correspond more directly to decreased emotional expressivity rather than with more traditional measures of emotion in bvFTD, such as the ability to identify facial expressions [22, 23]. To date, there has been little work on this relationship.

The lack of emotional expressivity may be a major clinical clue to the presence of bvFTD and, as such, could serve as the basis for a clinical test. Such a test is needed because the differentiating of bvFTD from other dementias, psychiatric conditions, and even normal subjects is important for management and prognosis [24, 25]. For example, there are patients with the behavioral criteria of bvFTD who prove to have Alzheimer's disease (AD) [26–28] and there are patients with bvFTD who have prominent memory deficits as in AD [29, 30]. In most clinical situations, there are no readily available and definitive biomarkers for screening these patients, again emphasizing the need for a practical screening test for bvFTD.

This study investigated screening for verbal and visual emotional expressions during video and audio presentation of real-life vignettes among patients with bvFTD compared with those with AD and healthy control (HC) subjects. Emotional expressions may vary depending on the emotional intensity of the eliciting stimuli [31, 32], and psychophysiological studies indicate a lowering of basic sympathetic tone in bvFTD, with reactivity to more intense stimuli [7]. Accordingly, this study compares self-reports of emotional distress and degree of facial expressivity on a standardized facial coding system during viewing of emotional vignettes of both high and low emotional intensity having either negative or positive outcomes.

2. Methods

2.1. Participants. Among patients in a university subspecialty clinic, this study recruited participants diagnosed with probable bvFTD per International Consensus Criteria [1], all of whom met criteria for loss of sympathy or empathy, and comparably impaired patients with clinically probable AD per National Institute on Aging–Alzheimer Association criteria [33]. The AD patients were age matched with the bvFTD patients within three years. Additionally, age-matched HC participants were recruited from volunteers in the community. Exclusion criteria included the presence of medical or psychiatric comorbidities save those of hypertension and diabetes. The dementia patients completed a screening interview, a standard neurological examination, and cognitive screening. The UCLA Institutional Review Board (IRB) approved this study, and each participant provided informed consent.

2.2. Procedures. The presentation of vignettes and the recording of facial affect were conducted in a quiet testing room. On entering the room, the participants were instructed to sit in a comfortable chair situated three feet in front of a computer screen and given instructions on the vignettes. They were asked to monitor the screen for a prompt indicating the onset of a vignette. During the vignette presentations, they were told to take note of their levels of distress. They were also informed that, during the viewing of the vignette, a video camera would be recording their visual gaze for purposes of assuring their attention to the vignettes and to later evaluate their facial responses. Finally, the participants were informed that their level of distress and recollection of the vignette would be queried immediately after each vignette.

2.2.1. Video Vignettes. The study involved 16 emotional vignettes of 30 seconds or less duration presented in a randomized order in three different counterbalanced presentation sequences. All vignettes were performed by the same actor looking directly into the camera and presented through SuperLab Pro 4.0 with audio through headphones. There were four basic vignette scenarios: (1) relating the results of a test for cancer, (2) reporting on an automobile accident involving the presenter's grandfather, (3) informing on the status of a missing child, and (4) discussing the military deployment of the presenter's brother. These four scenarios were each presented with high intensity (delivered with prominent vocal prosody and facial affect) or low intensity (delivered with a flat and static voice and facial image) and with a final (last few seconds) negative outcome or a positive outcome, for a total of 16 vignettes. During development, an independent group of 10 HC participants analyzed the emotional intensity of these vignettes on a five-point scale, where "1"—not intense and "5"—very intense, and reliability agreed on emotional intensity content ($k = 0.91$). The items resulted in a bimodal distribution consistent with our classification of 8 "high-intensity" versus 8 "low-intensity" vignettes.

2.2.2. Verbal Distress Ratings. Immediately after each vignette presentation, participants were queried on their comprehension of the vignettes and asked to rate their degree of distress on a Likert scale responding to the question, "How do you feel at the end of the story?" On the scale, "1" anchored to "no distress" and "5" anchored to "very distressed." In order to assure understanding as well as attention to the vignettes, participants were also asked to describe each vignette's content in their own words and their responses recorded for the presence of understanding of the essence of each vignette.

2.2.3. Facial Coding. Two independent raters coded the videos of the participants for facial expression using an established coding system for facial affect, the Facial Action Coding System (FACS) [34]. Both were FACS-certified raters who had previously practiced facial coding on a group of 7 normal subjects who watched the vignettes while being videotaped. For this study, the raters coded the participants' facial expressions (e.g., furrowed brow, angry) during the vignettes and determined whether they expressed any identifiable emotion, as defined by the FACS system. During viewing of each 30-second vignette, the raters coded each for the presence or absence of any observable facial expressions with "1" and no identifiable facial expressions with "0" with summary scores for the higher intensity and the lower intensity vignettes. The two raters demonstrated substantial interrater reliability, $k = 0.80$.

2.3. Statistical Analyses. This study utilized SPSS 23.0 software for statistical analysis. Chi-square and F-tests were used to evaluate group differences, and analyses of variance (ANOVA) were used for formal hypothesis testing. Pearson correlations assessed the relations between the distress scores and the number of facial expressions for each vignette. Post hoc analyses of pairwise comparisons were done with Fisher's least significant difference (LSD) and Tukey tests.

3. Results

3.1. Basic Group Comparisons. There were no significant group differences on demographic variables of age, sex, years of education, or handedness (see Table 1). The two dementia groups did not differ on the Montreal Cognitive Assessment scale [35].

3.2. Vignette General Results. The participants' attention and understanding of the vignettes were adequate for the study. On the videotapes, they maintained their eye gaze on the screen during the vignettes. After each vignette, all subjects demonstrated understanding of the vignettes by relating the essence of each vignette's content.

3.3. Reported Distress Levels. The bvFTD group reported less distress than the other two groups when listening and viewing lower intensity vignettes ($\eta^2 = 0.41$, $F(2, 19) = 9.85$, $p = 0.003$; see Figure 1). Post hoc analysis for lower intensity vignettes reviewed significant pairwise differences for the bvFTD group versus the AD group and for the bvFTD group versus the HC group (both LSD and Tukey $p < 0.05$) but not between the AD group and HC group. In contrast, the groups reported no differences in level of distress among higher intensity vignettes. Additionally, there were no significant group differences in reported distress between vignettes with negative (high or low intensity) or positive (high or low intensity) outcomes.

3.4. Facial Coding. Facial affect scores for the two raters were summed for the 8 higher intensity vignettes ($n = 16$) and the 8 lower intensity vignettes ($n = 16$). There were no differences in the presence of facial expression between groups on the higher intensity vignettes, but the bvFTD patients demonstrated significantly fewer facial expressions on the lower intensity vignettes ($\eta^2 = 0.49$, $F(2, 19) = 16.84$, $p < 0.001$; see Figure 2). Post hoc analysis for lower intensity vignettes reviewed significant pairwise differences for the bvFTD group versus the AD group and for the bvFTD group versus the HC group (both LSD and Tukey $p < 0.05$) but not between the AD group and HC group. Similar to the verbal distress scores, there were no significant facial affect score differences between groups based on negative or positive outcomes.

3.5. Correlations between Self-Report Distress and Facial Affect. Across all three groups, the overall level of self-reported distress correlated with the total number of facial expressions across the vignettes (i.e., the participants' level of distress increased correspondingly to more facial affective expressions to the stimuli), $r(24) = 0.76, p = 0.002$. Within the bvFTD group, the total level of distress also correlated to the instances of facial affect, such that they frequently responded to high-intensity content with some type of facial expression but lacked responsiveness to low-intensity content, $r(8) = 0.54$, $p = 0.021$. Likewise, within the AD and HC groups, the reported distress level positively correlated with instances of facial affect (AD: $r(8) = 0.62$, $p = 0.008$; HC: $r(8) = 0.77$, $p = 0.002$).

4. Discussion

In this preliminary study, bvFTD and AD, the two most common early-onset neurodegenerative dementias, are easily distinguished on verbal and facial measures of emotional reactivity. This study examines emotional reactivity by comparing self-reported levels of distress and observing facial expressions to emotional vignettes of varying emotional intensity. When the vignettes were of high emotional intensity, the bvFTD patients did not differ from the AD and HC participants in self-reported level of distress or the amount of facial affect. However, when the emotional stimuli were of low intensity, the bvFTD participants significantly differed from the AD and HC participants, reporting less distress and showing fewer facial expressions of affect. Observing the lack of verbal and visual emotional responses to mild-moderate intensity, emotional stimuli in bvFTD suggests a promising method for distinguishing these patients from those with other dementias and from normal subjects.

The correct recognition and diagnosis of bvFTD is important for clinical management, clinical trial enrollment, genetic analysis, and the understanding of these disorders [24, 25]. Clinicians may misdiagnose bvFTD as AD if there are deficits in episodic declarative memory [29, 30] or if the patient does not meet established criteria for bvFTD [1]. In contrast, clinicians may misdiagnose AD as bvFTD in the presence of early neuropsychiatric features [27, 28] or in the presence of the frontal or "behavioral/dysexecutive" variant of AD [26]. Clinically accessible tests, such as positron emission tomography (PET) scans, could mitigate the number of misdiagnoses; however, even fluorodeoxyglucose PET scans can be normal in early bvFTD [36], and amyloid or tau PET imaging are not readily or economically available for AD.

The use of diagnostic measures of emotional expression in bvFTD is a good alternative, not only because of clinical availability but also because of the neuroanatomical foci of this disease. Compared to AD, where brain regions for emotional processing are relatively intact [37], bvFTD affects multiple neuroanatomical regions involved in emotion. Their lack of empathy and connectedness corresponds to atrophy of frontal regions, such as the anterior cingulate cortex (ACC) and ventromedial prefrontal cortex (VMPFC) [38, 39], and of the anterior temporal lobes [40, 41]. Symptoms of apathy and the tendency to respond to emotional situations with disinterest most often associate with frontal dysfunction, especially of the ACC and VMPFC [39, 42], and symptoms involving emotion processing, including

TABLE 1: Characteristics between behavioral variant frontotemporal dementia (bvFTD), Alzheimer's disease (AD), and healthy control (HC) groups.

	BvFTD M (SD; range) or %	AD M (SD; range) or %	HC M (SD; range) or %	Sig.
Age (years)	61.3 (10.1; 42–78)	60.0 (4.9; 49–65)	59.0 (5.1; 49–66)	n.s.
Sex (% male)	50%	38%	38%	n.s.
Education (years)	15.9 (2.4; 12–20)	16.3 (2.0;12–18)	16.1 (3.1;12–18)	n.s.
Handedness (% right)	88%	88%	100%	n.s.
Montreal Cognitive Assessment	17.4 (6.3; 11–29)	16.9 (5.8; 11–23)	—	n.s.

M = mean; SD = standard deviation; % = percentage.

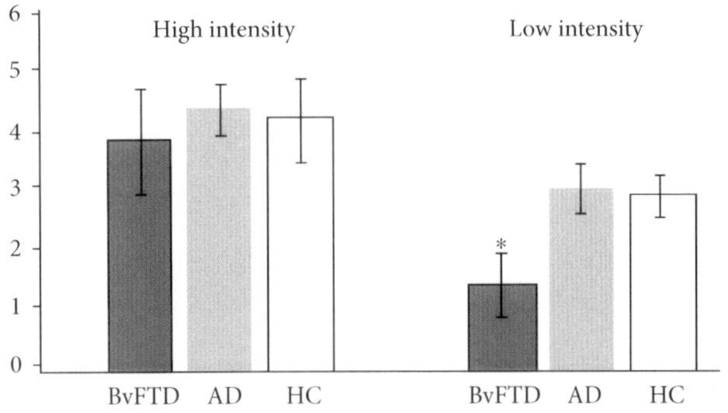

FIGURE 1: Group distress by level of vignette intensity among behavioral variant frontotemporal dementia (bvFTD), Alzheimer's disease (AD), and healthy control (HC) groups. The bvFTD group reported less distress ($M = 1.40$, SD = 1.05) than the other two groups when listening and viewing lower intensity vignettes ($M_{AD} = 3.01$, $SD_{AD} = 0.95$; $M_{HC} = 2.88$, $SD_{HC} = 0.71$). The groups reported no differences in the level of distress among higher intensity vignettes ($M_{bvFTD} = 3.81$, $SD_{bvFTD} = 1.75$; $M_{AD} = 4.34$, $SD_{AD} = 0.95$; $M_{HC} = 4.15$, $SD_{HC} = 1.38$). Asterisk indicates post hoc significance of the bvFTD group from the other groups.

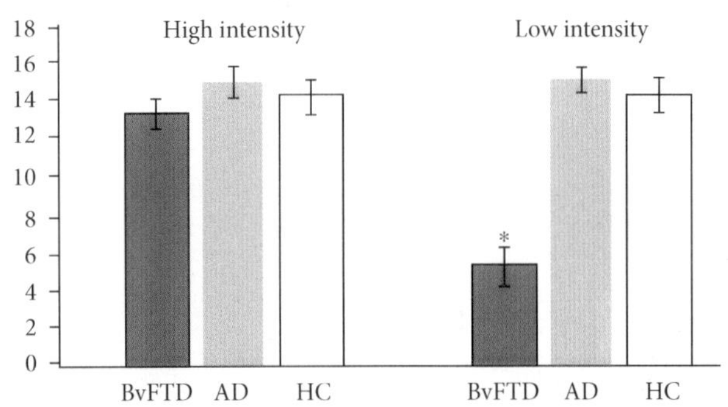

FIGURE 2: Group occurrences of facial affect by vignette intensity among behavioral variant frontotemporal dementia (bvFTD), Alzheimer's disease (AD), and healthy control (HC) groups. There were no differences in the presence of facial expression between the groups on the higher intensity vignettes ($M_{bvFTD} = 13.13$, $SD_{bvFTD} = 1.61$; $M_{AD} = 15.01$, $SD_{AD} = 1.66$; $M_{HC} = 14.20$, $SD_{HC} = 1.79$; $p = 0.169$), but the bvFTD patients demonstrated significantly fewer facial expressions on the lower intensity vignettes ($M_{bvFTD} = 5.20$, $SD_{bvFTD} = 2.01$; $M_{AD} = 15.00$, $SD_{AD} = 1.25$; $M_{HC} = 14.20$, $SD_{HC} = 1.78$). Asterisk indicates post hoc significance of the bvFTD group from the other groups.

emotional blunting and emotion recognition, additionally correlate with the right anterior temporal region [14]. Patients with bvFTD may fail to recognize or misinterpret emotional stimuli such as facial affect [10, 13, 43]. These patients may be unable to understand the context of the emotional stimuli, extract its meaning, experience interoceptive emotional awareness, or intentionally express emotions [44–48]. Furthermore, bvFTD patients have decreased physiological reactivity to emotional stimuli suggesting the need for a higher threshold of intensity to react to emotions [7].

In this study, the intensity of the emotional stimuli differentially affects the elicitation of self-reported distress and corresponding facial affect among the bvFTD participants compared to the other groups. Tasks varying in emotional intensity may be especially sensitive in detecting impairments in emotion recognition [49], regardless of the presence of a negative or a positive outcome. The results of this study suggests that bvFTD patients require a high intensity of emotional stimulus in order to elicit distress and affective expression. It is also possible that the relative preservation of happiness and surprise in some studies of bvFTD could indicate a greater experience of intensity for these emotions [10, 15]. In addition, in normal socioemotional settings, low levels of emotional intensity are the norm, so bvFTD patients may appear as if they have total affective blunting. Finally, the findings of this preliminary study suggest an approach to interactions and interventions for caregivers and others through the use of a higher intensity of emotional expression as a way to facilitate communication [20].

There are several methodological concerns with this study. First, the study has a relatively small sample size per group and may be underpowered. Nevertheless, in this pilot study, the number of participants per group is sufficient to disclose significant group differences. A future study with larger numbers can further investigate these findings. Second, the study used a Likert scale of distress, which only accounts for ratings from very upset to not very upset without assessing different individual emotions. Third, the lack of differential results based on negative or positive outcome could be based on the experimental design, as only the last few seconds of the vignette involved different outcomes. Finally, there could be concerns with the facial coding, and as with the verbal self-reports, this study did not specifically analyze the different types of emotions or the participants' recognition of specific emotions. This procedure, however, is an established technique for determining the presence or absence of facial affect, and this methodology lends itself to evaluation of specific emotions in future studies.

In summary, clinicians and investigators may observe and document the emotional blunting in bvFTD as a relative absence of verbal and facial emotional expression to mild-moderate emotional stimuli that routinely elicit emotional responses in others. Further systematic research on how to observe and record emotional expression in bvFTD, for example, as responses to simple picture stimuli in the clinic, may help better recognize, diagnose, and eventually manage these patients.

Authors' Contributions

Andrew R. Carr contributed to the design of the study, performed statistical analysis, analyzed the data, and helped write the article. Mark M. Ashla was responsible for the stimulus production and some of the data collection as well as assisting in writing the article. Elvira E. Jimenez assisted with formulating the research question, designing the study, and analyzing the data. Mario F. Mendez formulated the research question, designed the study, and assisted with analyzing the data and writing the article.

Acknowledgments

Dr. Mario F. Mendez is supported by NIA Grants R01AG034499-05 and R01AG050967.

References

[1] K. Rascovsky, J. R. Hodges, D. Knopman et al., "Sensitivity of revised diagnostic criteria for the behavioural variant of frontotemporal dementia," *Brain*, vol. 134, no. 9, pp. 2456–2477, 2011.

[2] M. F. Mendez and J. S. Shapira, "Loss of emotional insight in behavioral variant frontotemporal dementia or "frontal anosodiaphoria"," *Consciousness and Cognition*, vol. 20, no. 4, pp. 1690–1696, 2011.

[3] D. Robertson, J. Snarey, O. Ousley et al., "The neural processing of moral sensitivity to issues of justice and care," *Neuropsychologia*, vol. 45, no. 4, pp. 755–766, 2007.

[4] A. Joshi, J. P. Barsuglia, M. J. Mather, E. E. Jimenez, J. Shapira, and M. F. Mendez, "Evaluation of emotional blunting in behavioral variant frontotemporal dementia compared to Alzheimer's disease," *Dementia and Geriatric Cognitive Disorders*, vol. 38, no. 1-2, pp. 79–88, 2014.

[5] G. J. Lee, P. H. Lu, M. J. Mather et al., "Neuroanatomical correlates of emotional blunting in behavioral variant frontotemporal dementia and early-onset Alzheimer's disease," *Journal of Alzheimer's Disease*, vol. 41, no. 3, pp. 793–800, 2014.

[6] M. F. Mendez, S. S. Fong, J. S. Shapira et al., "Observation of social behavior in frontotemporal dementia," *American Journal of Alzheimer's Disease &Other Dementias*, vol. 29, no. 3, pp. 215–221, 2014.

[7] A. Joshi, M. F. Mendez, N. Kaiser, E. Jimenez, M. Mather, and J. S. Shapira, "Skin conductance levels may reflect emotional blunting in behavioral variant frontotemporal dementia," *The Journal of Neuropsychiatry and Clinical Neurosciences*, vol. 26, no. 3, pp. 227–232, 2014.

[8] P. D. Fletcher, J. M. Nicholas, T. J. Shakespeare et al., "Dementias show differential physiological responses to salient sounds," *Frontiers in Behavioral Neuroscience*, vol. 9, 2015.

[9] F. Kumfor, M. Irish, J. R. Hodges, and O. Piguet, "Discrete neural correlates for the recognition of negative emotions: insights from frontotemporal dementia," *PLoS One*, vol. 8, no. 6, article e67457, 2013.

[10] S. Lough, C. M. Kipps, C. Treise, P. Watson, J. R. Blair, and J. R. Hodges, "Social reasoning, emotion and empathy in frontotemporal dementia," *Neuropsychologia*, vol. 44, no. 6, pp. 950–958, 2006.

[11] I. Lavenu, F. Pasquier, F. Lebert, H. Petit, and M. V. der Linden, "Perception of emotion in frontotemporal dementia and Alzheimer disease," *Alzheimer Disease & Associated Disorders*, vol. 13, no. 2, pp. 96–101, 1999.

[12] H. J. Rosen, K. Pace-Savitsky, R. J. Perry, J. H. Kramer, B. L. Miller, and R. W. Levenson, "Recognition of emotion in the frontal and temporal variants of frontotemporal dementia," *Dementia and Geriatric Cognitive Disorders*, vol. 17, no. 4, pp. 277–281, 2004.

[13] H. J. Rosen, S. C. Allison, G. F. Schauer, M. L. Gorno-Tempini, M. W. Weiner, and B. L. Miller, "Neuroanatomical correlates of behavioural disorders in dementia," *Brain*, vol. 128, no. 11, pp. 2612–2625, 2005.

[14] C. M. Kipps, P. J. Nestor, J. Acosta-Cabronero, R. Arnold, and J. R. Hodges, "Understanding social dysfunction in the behavioural variant of frontotemporal dementia: the role of emotion and sarcasm processing," *Brain*, vol. 132, no. 3, pp. 592–603, 2009.

[15] F. Kumfor, L. Miller, S. Lah et al., "Are you really angry? The effect of intensity on facial emotion recognition in frontotemporal dementia," *Social Neuroscience*, vol. 6, no. 5-6, pp. 502–514, 2011.

[16] B. Bediou, I. Ryff, B. Mercier et al., "Impaired social cognition in mild Alzheimer disease," *Journal of Geriatric Psychiatry and Neurology*, vol. 22, no. 2, pp. 130–140, 2009.

[17] J. Keane, A. J. Calder, J. R. Hodges, and A. W. Young, "Face and emotion processing in frontal variant frontotemporal dementia," *Neuropsychologia*, vol. 40, no. 6, pp. 655–665, 2002.

[18] D. Fernandez-Duque and S. E. Black, "Impaired recognition of negative facial emotions in patients with frontotemporal dementia," *Neuropsychologia*, vol. 43, no. 11, pp. 1673–1687, 2005.

[19] V. E. Sturm and R. W. Levenson, "Alexithymia in neurodegenerative disease," *Neurocase*, vol. 17, no. 3, pp. 242–250, 2011.

[20] J. H. L. Lui, C. T. Barry, and D. F. Sacco, "Callous-unemotional traits and empathy deficits: mediating effects of affective perspective-taking and facial emotion recognition," *Cognition and Emotion*, vol. 30, no. 6, pp. 1049–1062, 2016.

[21] R. E. Kahn, A. L. Byrd, and D. A. Pardini, "Callous-unemotional traits robustly predict future criminal offending in young men," *Law and Human Behavior*, vol. 37, no. 2, pp. 87–97, 2013.

[22] L. A. Miller, S. Hsieh, S. Lah, S. Savage, J. R. Hodges, and O. Piguet, "One size does not fit all: face emotion processing impairments in semantic dementia, behavioural-variant frontotemporal dementia and Alzheimer's disease are mediated by distinct cognitive deficits," *Behavioural Neurology*, vol. 25, no. 1, pp. 53–60, 2012.

[23] J. Diehlschmid, C. Pohl, C. Ruprecht, S. Wagenpfeil, H. Foerstl, and A. Kurz, "The Ekman 60 Faces Test as a diagnostic instrument in frontotemporal dementia," *Archives of Clinical Neuropsychology*, vol. 22, no. 4, pp. 459–464, 2007.

[24] O. Piguet, M. Hornberger, E. Mioshi, and J. R. Hodges, "Behavioural-variant frontotemporal dementia: diagnosis, clinical staging, and management," *The Lancet Neurology*, vol. 10, no. 2, pp. 162–172, 2011.

[25] M. F. Mendez, J. S. Shapira, A. McMurtray, and E. Licht, "Preliminary findings: behavioral worsening on donepezil in patients with frontotemporal dementia," *The American Journal of Geriatric Psychiatry*, vol. 15, no. 1, pp. 84–87, 2007.

[26] R. Ossenkoppele, Y. A. L. Pijnenburg, D. C. Perry et al., "The behavioural/dysexecutive variant of Alzheimer's disease: clinical, neuroimaging and pathological features," *Brain*, vol. 138, no. 9, pp. 2732–2749, 2015.

[27] M. F. Mendez, A. Joshi, K. Tassniyom, E. Teng, and J. S. Shapira, "Clinicopathologic differences among patients with behavioral variant frontotemporal dementia," *Neurology*, vol. 80, no. 6, pp. 561–568, 2013.

[28] H. W. Querfurth and F. M. LaFerla, "Alzheimer's disease," *The New England Journal of Medicine*, vol. 362, no. 4, pp. 329–344, 2010.

[29] M. Hornberger, S. Wong, R. Tan et al., "*In vivo* and post-mortem memory circuit integrity in frontotemporal dementia and Alzheimer's disease," *Brain*, vol. 135, no. 10, pp. 3015–3025, 2012.

[30] C. M. Pleizier, A. E. van der Vlies, E. Koedam et al., "Episodic memory and the medial temporal lobe: not all it seems. Evidence from the temporal variants of frontotemporal dementia," *Journal of Neurology, Neurosurgery, & Psychiatry*, vol. 83, no. 12, pp. 1145–1148, 2012.

[31] S. Baez, F. Manes, D. Huepe et al., "Primary empathy deficits in frontotemporal dementia," *Frontiers in Aging Neuroscience*, vol. 6, p. 262, 2014.

[32] R. W. Levenson and B. L. Miller, "Loss of cells—loss of self: frontotemporal lobar degeneration and human emotion," *Current Directions in Psychological Science*, vol. 16, no. 6, pp. 289–294, 2007.

[33] G. M. McKhann, D. S. Knopman, H. Chertkow et al., "The diagnosis of dementia due to Alzheimer's disease: recommendations from the National Institute on Aging-Alzheimer's Association workgroups on diagnostic guidelines for Alzheimer's disease," *Alzheimer's & Dementia*, vol. 7, no. 3, pp. 263–269, 2011.

[34] R. Buck, "Using fags vs. communication scores to measure spontaneous facial expression of emotion in brain-damaged patients: a reply to Mammucari et al. (1988)," *Cortex*, vol. 26, no. 2, pp. 275–280, 1990.

[35] Z. S. Nasreddine, N. Phillips, and H. Chertkow, "Normative data for the Montreal Cognitive Assessment (MoCA) in a population-based sample," *Neurology*, vol. 78, no. 10, pp. 765-766, 2012.

[36] B. J. Kerklaan, B. N. M. van Berckel, K. Herholz et al., "The added value of 18-fluorodeoxyglucose-positron emission tomography in the diagnosis of the behavioral variant of frontotemporal dementia," *American Journal of Alzheimer's Disease & Other Dementias*, vol. 29, no. 7, pp. 607–613, 2014.

[37] G. B. Karas, E. J. Burton, S. A. R. B. Rombouts et al., "A comprehensive study of gray matter loss in patients with Alzheimer's disease using optimized voxel-based morphometry," *NeuroImage*, vol. 18, no. 4, pp. 895–907, 2003.

[38] P. J. Eslinger and A. R. Damasio, "Severe disturbance of higher cognition after bilateral frontal lobe ablation Patient EVR," *Neurology*, vol. 35, no. 12, pp. 1731–1741, 1985.

[39] F. Peters, D. Perani, K. Herholz et al., "Orbitofrontal dysfunction related to both apathy and disinhibition in frontotemporal dementia," *Dementia and Geriatric Cognitive Disorders*, vol. 21, no. 5-6, pp. 373–379, 2006.

[40] S. M. Brambati, N. C. Renda, K. P. Rankin et al., "A tensor based morphometry study of longitudinal gray matter contraction in FTD," *NeuroImage*, vol. 35, no. 3, pp. 998–1003, 2007.

[41] H. J. Rosen, J. H. Kramer, M. L. Gorno-Tempini, N. Schuff, M. Weiner, and B. L. Miller, "Patterns of cerebral atrophy in primary progressive aphasia," *The American Journal of Geriatric Psychiatry*, vol. 10, no. 1, pp. 89–97, 2002.

[42] W. Liu, B. L. Miller, J. H. Kramer et al., "Behavioral disorders in the frontal and temporal variants of frontotemporal dementia," *Neurology*, vol. 62, no. 5, pp. 742–748, 2004.

[43] F. Kumfor, M. Irish, C. Leyton et al., "Tracking the progression of social cognition in neurodegenerative disorders," *Journal of Neurology, Neurosurgery, & Psychiatry*, vol. 85, no. 10, pp. 1076–1083, 2014.

[44] A. R. Carr, P. Paholpak, M. Daianu et al., "An investigation of care-based vs. rule-based morality in frontotemporal dementia, Alzheimer's disease, and healthy controls," *Neuropsychologia*, vol. 78, pp. 73–79, 2015.

[45] M. F. Mendez, A. K. Chen, J. S. Shapira, and B. L. Miller, "Acquired sociopathy and frontotemporal dementia," *Dementia and Geriatric Cognitive Disorders*, vol. 20, no. 2-3, pp. 99–104, 2005.

[46] K. A. Gola, T. Shany-Ur, P. Pressman et al., "A neural network underlying intentional emotional facial expression in neurodegenerative disease," *NeuroImage: Clinical*, vol. 14, pp. 672–678, 2017.

[47] A. Ibanez, E. Gleichgerrcht, and F. Manes, "Clinical effects of insular damage in humans," *Brain Structure and Function*, vol. 214, no. 5-6, pp. 397–410, 2010.

[48] A. Ibáñez, M. M. Velásquez, M. M. Caro, and F. Manes, "Implicit emotional awareness in frontotemporal dementia," *Cognitive Neuroscience*, vol. 4, no. 3-4, pp. 204–206, 2013.

[49] I. Chiu, O. Piguet, J. Diehl-Schmid et al., "Dissociation in rating negative facial emotions between behavioral variant frontotemporal dementia and major depressive disorder," *The American Journal of Geriatric Psychiatry*, vol. 24, no. 11, pp. 1017–1027, 2016.

23

Mediational Model of Multiple Sclerosis Impairments, Family Needs, and Caregiver Mental Health in Guadalajara, Mexico

Melody N. Mickens,[1,2] Paul B. Perrin,[1] Adriana Aguayo,[3,4] Brenda Rabago,[3] Miguel A. Macías-Islas,[3] and Juan Carlos Arango-Lasprilla[5,6]

[1]*Department of Psychology, Virginia Commonwealth University, Richmond, VA, USA*
[2]*Department of Physical Medicine & Rehabilitation, Virginia Commonwealth University School of Medicine, Richmond, VA, USA*
[3]*Department of Neuroscience, CUCS, University of Guadalajara, Guadalajara, JAL, Mexico*
[4]*Department of Psychology, Enrique Diaz de Leon University, Guadalajara, JAL, Mexico*
[5]*BioCruces Health Research Institute, Cruces University Hospital Barakaldo, Bizkaia, Spain*
[6]*IKERBASQUE, Basque Foundation for Science, Bilbao, Spain*

Correspondence should be addressed to Juan Carlos Arango-Lasprilla; jcalasprilla@gmail.com

Academic Editor: Mary H. Kosmidis

Individuals with multiple sclerosis (MS), especially those living in Latin America, often require assistance from family caregivers throughout the duration of the disease. Previous research suggests that family caregivers may experience positive and negative outcomes from providing care to individuals with MS, but few studies have examined the unmet needs of individuals providing care to family members with MS and how these unmet needs may mediate the relationship between MS symptoms and caregiver mental health. The current study examined the relationships among MS impairments (functional, neurological, cognitive, behavioral, and emotional), unmet family needs (household, informational, financial, social support, and health), and caregiver mental health (satisfaction with life, anxiety, burden, and depression) in a sample of 81 MS caregivers from Guadalajara, Mexico. A structural equation model demonstrated the mediational effect of unmet family needs on the relationship between MS impairments and caregiver mental health. These findings suggest that intervention research on MS caregivers in Latin America may consider focusing on caregiver mental health problems by addressing unmet family needs and teaching caregivers ways to manage the impairments of the individual with MS.

1. Introduction

Multiple sclerosis (MS) is a chronic neurological illness that eventually results in physical disability and cognitive impairments which limit an individual's ability to function independently [1]. Approximately 2.5 million people have been diagnosed with MS worldwide [2], and research demonstrates that worldwide prevalence rates are increasing [3]. As with other countries, researchers have observed that MS prevalence rates may be higher than previously reported in Latin American countries such as Mexico, where current prevalence rates vary by region and range from 7 to 30 cases per 100,000 people [4, 5].

In Latin America, where rates of MS are increasing but disparities still exist in its diagnosis and treatment [6, 7], sociocultural values such as allocentrism, familism, and filial obligation [8, 9] increase the likelihood that family members will serve as informal caregivers to individuals with MS. When compared to other racial/ethnic groups, Latino caregivers often report limited use of formal support services [10, 11], larger informal social networks [8], increased role strain [12], lower rates of institutionalization [10], and higher rates of depression [13]. However, very few studies have examined MS caregiving in Latin America [14, 15], and associations in this region among MS impairments, needs of family members providing care, and caregiver mental health remain largely unknown. Because of this major gap in the research literature, there is a great need for research addressing the process of MS caregiving in Latin America, as well as the impact of MS impairments on family needs and caregiver mental health in this region.

International research has established that compared to noncaregivers, MS caregivers report higher levels of depression [16], anxiety [17], and decreased social support [18]. Patient factors such as level of disability [19–21], cognitive impairments [22–25], behavioral changes [22, 23], incontinence, and fatigue [26] contribute to increased caregiver depression, strain, and burden. Although many of the findings on MS caregiver functioning emphasize the negative aspects of caregiving, the literature also demonstrates that MS caregivers report salubrious outcomes such as personal growth, role fulfillment, positive emotions, and satisfaction as a result of caregiving [11, 27].

MS caregiving can be understood using Pearlin et al.'s [28] conceptual model of caregiver stress. This model identifies three domains of caregiving stress: (a) background and context of the caregiving situation (i.e., caregiver age, gender, ethnicity, socioeconomic status, relationship with the patient, and family and social network composition), (b) primary stressors (i.e., cognitive functioning of patient, behavioral changes, problematic behaviors of the patient, activities of daily living (ADLs), and instrumental ADLs), and (c) secondary stressors (i.e., unmet needs for information, reduced access to employment or need for financial assistance, limited social support, family conflict, conflict with occupational and social role fulfillment, economic strain, changes in self-concept, loss of self, role captivity, mastery, competence, and gain). The model identifies physical and emotional outcomes associated with stressors and alleviated by mediators of stress (i.e., coping strategies and social support). Moreover, Pearlin et al. indicate that stressors, mediators, and outcomes often interact and individually or collectively influence caregiver mental health in a direct, indirect, or cyclical pattern [28]. Because unmet family needs can comprise both background (i.e., affecting family prior to involvement in caregiving roles) variables and stressors associated with the caregiving experience (i.e., lack of knowledge about disease process or need for specific care information), clinicians and providers have increased interest in studying the role of unmet needs on caregiver psychological functioning.

Findings from studies of MS caregivers demonstrate that primary stressors (i.e., patient functioning) have been associated with depression and burden. Although these studies have examined aspects such as the patient's cognitive functioning, psychological functioning, physical disability, and ADL impairments, few have examined unmet family needs in the context of these patient-related stressors. Within the framework of Pearlin et al.'s model [28], family needs (i.e., household needs, informational needs, financial needs, health needs, and social support) are an extension of the background/context and secondary stressor domains. Findings from a previous study demonstrate that unmet family needs are also are a central determinant of caregiver adjustment, as they have been associated with increased burden and depression among MS caregivers [14].

Given the often significant impairments documented in individuals with MS, the unknown levels of unmet family needs, and the generally poor mental health that MS caregivers report, many questions remain regarding the specific connections among these sets of variables, especially in Latin America. As such, the objective of the present study is to examine unmet family needs as a mediator of the established relationship between the care recipients' MS impairments (primary stressor) and caregivers' mental health (outcome). Based on prior research which suggests strong associations between patients' MS symptoms and their caregivers' psychosocial distress [16, 17, 19, 22, 24], it is hypothesized that the relationship between MS impairments and caregiver mental health will be significantly mediated by unmet family needs. At present, no studies in the MS caregiver literature have examined this possible effect, but based on Pearlin et al.'s [28] model, primary stressors (e.g., patient functioning) should be associated with reduced caregiver mental health outcomes. Secondary stressors such as family needs should be associated with both primary stressors (MS impairments) and negative caregiver mental health outcomes and could possibly account for the connection between these two sets of constructs.

2. Method

2.1. Participants. Participants ($n = 81$) were a convenience sample of self-identified MS caregivers recruited from The Mexican Foundation for Multiple Sclerosis and the Department of Neurosciences of the University Center for Health Sciences, University of Guadalajara, Mexico. In order to participate in the study, caregivers had to (a) be the primary caregiver of an individual with a diagnosis of MS who was at least six months past the date of diagnosis, (b) have provided care to the person with MS for a minimum of six months, and (c) have had no history of a cognitive, serious psychiatric, or neurological disorder themselves. Initially, 86 participants were approached, but after screening, five declined or did not meet study criteria. Data were collected from a final sample of 81 caregivers. Demographic information for the caregiver sample is provided in Table 1 and for the patient sample in Table 2.

2.2. Measures. Eligible caregivers completed a battery of questionnaires in Spanish that assessed the following domains: demographic information, MS-related impairments as observed by the caregiver, family needs, and mental health. Measures of depression, anxiety, caregiver burden, satisfaction with life, and caregiver needs had been previously translated to Spanish and validated in Spanish-speaking samples prior to their use in this study. Spanish-speaking norms were used for scoring and interpreting these measures where available. The measure of MS impairments was translated (forward and backward) into Spanish and then English using methods published by Chapman and Carter [29] and Guillemin et al. [30] to ensure cross-cultural equivalence. Both translations were compared by a

Table 1: Characteristics of MS caregivers ($n = 81$).

Demographic variable	Value
Age, years, mean (SD)	43.37 (15.32)
Sex, %	
Female ($n = 54$)	66.7%
Male ($n = 26$)	33.3%
Years of education, mean (SD)	11.74 (4.42)
Marital status, %	
Married or partnered ($n = 55$)	67.9%
Single ($n = 19$)	23.5%
Widowed ($n = 4$)	4.9%
Divorced or separated ($n = 3$)	3.7%
Relationship to individual with MS, %	
Parent ($n = 37$)	45.7%
Spouse/romantic partner ($n = 26$)	32.1%
Sibling ($n = 10$)	12.3%
Child ($n = 5$)	6.2%
Friend ($n = 1$)	1.2%
Professional caregiver ($n = 1$)	1.2%
Other ($n = 1$)	1.2%
Duration of caregiving	
Number of months, mean (SD)	52.31 (59.29)
Hours per week of care, mean (SD)	70.96 (60.66)
Current occupation, %	
Homemaker ($n = 25$)	30.9%
Full-time employment ($n = 21$)	25.9%
Part-time employment ($n = 19$)	23.5%
Student ($n = 7$)	8.6%
Unemployed ($n = 4$)	4.9%
Retired ($n = 3$)	3.7%
Other ($n = 2$)	2.5%
Monthly household income, %	
Less than minimum wage ($n = 1$)	1.2%
Minimum wage ($n = 6$)	7.4%
1-2 times minimum wage ($n = 11$)	13.6%
2-3 times minimum wage ($n = 10$)	12.3%
3-4 times minimum wage ($n = 7$)	8.6%
4-5 times minimum wage ($n = 11$)	13.6%
More than 5 times minimum wage ($n = 35$)	43.2%

Table 2: Characteristics of individuals with MS as reported by caregivers ($n = 81$).

Demographic variable	Value
Age, years, mean (SD)	33.25 (10.78)
Sex, %	
Female ($n = 56$)	69.1%
Male ($n = 25$)	30.9%
Years of education, mean (SD)	13.34 (3.97)
Marital status, %	
Single ($n = 40$)	49.4%
Married or partnered ($n = 36$)	44.4%
Divorced or separated ($n = 5$)	6.2%
MS clinical course, %	
Relapse remitting ($n = 64$)	79.0%
Secondary progressive ($n = 16$)	19.8%
Primary progressive ($n = 1$)	1.2%
Age of symptom onset, mean (SD)	26.29 (9.76)
Age at diagnosis, mean (SD)	28.17 (10.17)
Current occupation, %	
Full-time employment ($n = 22$)	27.2%
Homemaker ($n = 19$)	23.5%
Part-time employment ($n = 15$)	18.5%
Student ($n = 11$)	13.6%
Unemployed ($n = 6$)	7.4%
Receiving disability ($n = 7$)	8.6%
Other ($n = 1$)	1.2%

monolingual psychologist from Mexico and a bilingual psychologist living in Spain. No discrepancies were identified. The final version was reviewed by the monolingual psychologist from Mexico. Participants completed a demographic form created by the investigators. On this form, household income in Mexico was calculated by monthly salary, where the monthly minimum wage at the time of data collection was 2018.70 pesos or approximately 155.40 USD per month [31].

2.2.1. MS Impairments. Caregivers completed the MS Impairment Questionnaire (MS-IQ) [26], a 30-item checklist of common MS impairments. Assessed impairments are grouped into five subscales: cognitive, emotional, behavioral, neurological, and functional. Caregivers completed this measure by reporting "yes" for the specific impairments that their care recipient experienced and "no" for the impairments that the care recipient did not experience. Item scores are summed (yes = 1, no = 0) so that subscale scores with higher values indicate domains with a larger number of impairments. Although it is possible to calculate a total score, only the subscale scores were used in the current study in order to generate a latent construct.

2.2.2. Anxiety. Caregivers completed the Spielberger State-Trait Anxiety Inventory (STAI) [32] as a measure of anxiety. The STAI is a 40-item self-report measure with a two-factor structure. The S-anxiety subscale measures anxiety as a temporary emotional state, while the T-anxiety subscale assesses anxiety as a fixed personality trait [32, 33]. Both subscales can be combined to create a total scale which was used in the current study. Total scale scores range from 40 to 160, with higher scores indicating increased anxiety. The Spanish version of the STAI [34] was used in this study and has demonstrated very good construct validity and internal consistency in samples of male (state $\alpha = 0.93$, trait $\alpha = 0.96$) and female (state $\alpha = 0.88$, trait $\alpha = 0.82$) Spanish speakers [35, 36].

2.2.3. Burden. Caregivers completed the Zarit Burden Inventory (ZBI) [37]. Item scores are summed, and total scores range from 0 to 88 with higher scores indicating greater burden [38]. The ZBI has been validated and used in numerous neurological caregiver populations including TBI caregivers [39], dementia caregivers [37], and Parkinson's caregivers [40]. The Spanish version of the ZBI has demonstrated excellent construct validity and internal reliability ($\alpha = 0.92$) in samples of Spanish-speaking individuals [41].

2.2.4. Depression. Caregivers completed the Patient Health Questionnaire-9 (PHQ-9) [42] as a measure of depressive symptoms experienced within a two-week period. Total scores range from 0 to 27 with higher scores reflecting more severe symptoms of depression. The Spanish version has demonstrated strong construct and criterion validity, as well as excellent internal consistency and convergent validity in Spanish-speaking validation samples [43–45].

2.2.5. Satisfaction with Life. Participants completed the Satisfaction with Life Scale (SWLS) [46]. Higher total scores represent higher life satisfaction [47]. Participants completed the Spanish version of the SWLS, which has high internal consistency ($\alpha = 0.88$) and good construct validity in Spanish-speaking samples [48, 49].

2.2.6. Family Needs. The Family Needs Assessment Tool (FNAT) [50] assesses the degree to which needs are met in family caregivers of individuals with neurological conditions in Latin America. The FNAT is comprised of 14 items and has five unmet needs subscales: household (two items), informational (three items), financial (three items), health (four items), and social support (two items). Higher scores indicate greater areas of unmet needs. As with the MS-IQ, although it is possible to calculate a total score on the FNAT, only the subscale scores were used in the current study in order to generate a latent construct.

2.3. Procedure. Prior to recruitment, the Institutional Review Board of the Mexican Foundation of Multiple Sclerosis reviewed and approved the study protocol. Staff at the Mexican Foundation for Multiple Sclerosis and the Department of Neurosciences of the University Center for Health Sciences, University of Guadalajara recruited prospective study participants from a neurology clinic using verbal and written advertisements. Interested participants contacted the research staff and were screened for eligibility. Eligible caregivers completed informed consent forms prior to data collection. During a 40-minute appointment at the Mexican Foundation for Multiple Sclerosis, a staff psychologist collected sociodemographic information and administered a battery of questionnaires to caregivers using a structured interview format to ensure that the participants understood the item content and did not skip any items.

2.4. Data Analysis

2.4.1. Preliminary Analyses. Frequencies and descriptive statistics were run to summarize MS impairments reported by caregivers, frequently reported unmet family needs, and clinically significant caregiver mental health problems.

2.4.2. Hypothesis Testing. A structural equation model (SEM) was created with three latent variables: MS impairments, family needs, and caregiver mental health. MS impairments was comprised of shared variance from the five impairment variables: functional, cognitive, behavioral, emotional, and physical. Family needs were comprised of shared variance from the five types of family needs: household, informational, financial, health, and social needs. Caregiver mental health was comprised of shared variance from the four mental health variables: depression, burden, anxiety, and satisfaction with life. This SEM was conducted using AMOS 20 [51]. Because most traditional SEMs in rehabilitation research are run with at least 200 participants [52], and the sample size in the current study is 81 participants, estimates of model fit are likely to be inaccurate; we report indices of model fit solely for reference. Instead, the focus of this analysis was on the size and significance level of the standardized β weight for the indirect effect of MS impairments on caregiver mental health through family needs.

3. Results

Participants reported patient impairments in all five domains, as seen in Table 3. Of the neurological impairments reported, more than 75% of participants reported tiring easily, while over half reported paralysis, poor eyesight, loss of sensation, and clumsiness. More than half of the sample reported the following emotional symptoms: depression, easily upset, irritability, and mood changes. Commonly reported functional and cognitive impairments were difficulty walking, doing things slowly, forgetfulness, and difficulty concentrating. Less than half of participants reported behavioral symptoms but endorsed acting impulsively as the most commonly observed behavioral symptom. Caregivers' item responses to the FNAT were ranked (identifying the top five) by the percentage of unmet need endorsements. As illustrated in Table 4, a majority of the unmet needs identified were from the informational domain, while the remaining needs were from the social support domain.

Total scores on the PHQ-9 ranged from 0 to 21 out of a possible maximum score of 27. The sample mean of 5.92 (SD = 5.27) indicated frequent endorsement of mild symptoms of depression. As seen in Table 5, nearly half of the sample reported clinically significant levels of depression, with 26% reporting mild symptoms, 16% reporting moderate symptoms, and 1.2% reporting severe symptoms of depression. Both total and subscale scores (e.g., state and trait) of the STAI were examined. Participants' total scores ranged from 11 to 93 out of a maximum score of 160. Nearly one-third of participants reported clinically significant symptoms of state or trait anxiety with 32% reporting moderate symptoms on the state subscale and 2.5% reporting severe symptoms on the state subscale of the measure. Responses on the trait subscale demonstrated that 31% of participants reported moderate symptoms on the trait subscale, while 3.7% reported severe symptoms. Total scores on the ZBI ranged from 0 to 62 out of a maximum score of 88. The sample mean of 22.02 (SD = 14.72) indicated that on average participants reported mild to moderate symptoms of burden.

TABLE 3: Summary of MS impairments reported by caregivers ($n = 81$).

Impairment domain	Impairments endorsed	% endorsing impairment	Number of patients with observed impairments
Neurological	Tiring easily	79%	64
	Paralysis	69%	56
	Poor eyesight	62%	50
	Loss of sensation	54%	44
	Clumsiness	52%	42
	Pain	36%	29
	Incontinence	27%	22
	Seizures	14%	11
Emotional	Depression	68%	55
	Easily upset	68%	55
	Irritability	58%	47
	Mood changes	58%	47
	Anxiety	49%	40
	Loss of interest	33%	27
Functional	Difficulty walking	69%	56
	Doing things slowly	56%	45
	Trouble reading	33%	27
	Difficulty writing	32%	26
	Difficulty talking	27%	22
	Difficulty eating	22%	18
	Difficulty hearing	20%	16
Cognitive	Forgetfulness	62%	50
	Difficulty concentrating	53%	43
	Difficulty thinking	38%	31
	Poor decision making	30%	24
	Difficulty learning	27%	22
	Denying problems	27%	22
Behavioral	Acting impulsively	35%	28
	Upsetting other people	28%	23
	Not being reliable	12%	10

Further review of clinically significant scores revealed that 29.6% reported mild to moderate symptoms, 12.3% reported moderate to severe symptoms, and 1.2% reported severe symptoms of burden. Total scores on the SWLS ranged from 10 to 35 out of a maximum score of 35. The sample mean of 23.43 (SD = 6.35) indicated an overall feeling of general satisfaction.

Two structural equation models (SEMs) were created to examine whether unmet family needs mediated the relationship between MS impairments and caregiver mental health. Both models included three latent variables: MS impairments, family needs, and caregiver mental health. MS impairments was comprised of the following five manifest variables (i.e., subscale scores from the MS-IQ): neurological, cognitive, functional, behavioral, and emotional symptoms. Family needs was created using the five manifest variables (i.e., subscale scores from the FNAT) of financial, informational, household, health, and social support needs. Caregiver mental health was created using four manifest variables of depression (PHQ-9 total score), anxiety (total STAI score), burden (total ZBI score), and satisfaction with life (total SWLS score). In total, the models were comprised of 33 variables, of which 14 were observed, 16 were unique, and 3 were factors. The manifest variables are directly measured by a total score or subscale score, represented in Figure 1 (the second, structural model) by rectangles. The latent variables are measured indirectly and inferred mathematically from the shared variance of the manifest variables. In Figure 1, the latent variables are represented by ovals.

Normality tests revealed that the distributions of the measured variables were all normal in a univariate sense in terms of skewness (all coefficients $\leq$ an absolute value of 0.93) and kurtosis (all coefficients $\leq$ an absolute value of 1.17). Similarly, a Mardia's coefficient of 2.23 suggested that the variables were not multivariate kurtotic. It was further found by the calculation of Mahalanobis distance that no single observation was meaningfully far from the multivariate centroid (all $ps \geq 0.01$), and therefore there were no multivariate outliers.

The first measurement model SEM examined correlations (e.g., bidirectional paths) between each of the latent variables as opposed to directional paths. In this model, only one statistically significant correlation emerged between MS impairments and caregiver mental health at $r = -0.64$ ($p < 0.01$). The bivariate relationships between MS impairments and family needs ($r = 0.34$, $p = 0.39$) and family needs and caregiver mental health ($r = -0.55$, $p = 0.37$) were not statistically significant. Although two of these correlations were not statistically significant, all three were in the expected direction and were at least medium sized.

In the second SEM (Figure 1), MS impairments were specified to lead directly to caregiver mental health, as well as to have an indirect effect on caregiver mental health through family needs. In this model, MS impairments was significantly associated with caregiver mental health ($\beta = -0.51$, $p = 0.003$). MS impairments were not significantly associated with family needs ($\beta = 0.34$, $p = 0.39$), nor was family needs associated with caregiver mental health ($\beta = -0.38$, $p = 0.39$). However, again all three directional paths were in the hypothesized direction. The indirect effect of MS impairments on caregiver mental health through family needs was statistically significant ($\beta = 0.13$, $p = 0.008$), suggesting the presence of an indirect effect. The following fit indices are presented only for reference: the ratio of the χ^2 statistic to the degrees of freedom in the model was 1.59; the goodness of fit index (GFI) was 0.85; the adjusted goodness of fit index (AGFI) and the normed fit index (NFI) were 0.78 and 0.72, respectively; the incremental fit index (IFI), Tucker-Lewis index (TLI), and comparative fit index (CFI) were 0.87, 0.84, and 0.87, respectively; and the root mean square error of approximation (RMSEA) was 0.09.

TABLE 4: Summary of unmet family needs ($n = 81$).

Family need	% endorsed as unmet	Number of caregivers reporting need	Domain
I need complete information.	71.6%	58	Information
I need specialized information about the patient.	70.3%	57	Information
I get help from the community (reverse coded).	65.5%	53	Social support
I get support from my church (reverse coded).	61.7%	50	Social support
I need to discuss my feelings with someone who has been through the same experience.	45.7%	37	Information

TABLE 5: Summary of caregiver mental health variables.

Variable	Value
PHQ-9 total score, mean (SD)	5.92 (5.27)
Mild depression (%)	26%
Moderate depression (%)	16%
Moderate–severe depression (%)	3.7%
Severe depression (%)	1.2%
STAI total score, mean (SD)	47.01 (21.40)
STAI state, mean (SD)	22.67 (11.82)
STAI trait, mean (SD)	24.34 (10.97)
State moderate anxiety (%)	32%
State severe anxiety (%)	2.5%
Trait moderate anxiety (%)	31%
Trait severe anxiety (%)	3.7%
ZBI total score, mean (SD)	22.02 (14.72)
Mild to moderate burden (%)	29.6%
Moderate to severe burden (%)	12.3%
Severe burden (%)	1.2%
SWLS total score, mean (SD)	23.43 (6.35)
Life dissatisfaction (%)	26%
Neutral (%)	7%
Life satisfaction (%)	67%

4. Discussion

The present study examined the caregiving experiences of MS caregivers living in Guadalajara, Mexico, with a specific emphasis on identifying unmet family needs as a possible mediator of the relationship between MS impairments and caregiver mental health. As hypothesized, this study's findings supported that unmet family needs mediated the relationship between MS impairments and caregiver mental health.

Prior to this study, several researchers had identified a very strong relationship between patients' clinical symptoms and their caregivers' psychosocial functioning. However, few, if any, researchers have been able to identify specific mechanisms or correlates that account for this relationship. The statistically significant indirect effect of MS impairments on caregiver mental health through unmet family needs is the first time this finding has emerged in the research literature. One possible interpretation of this finding is that as patients experience impairments in multiple domains, family caregivers may need additional support or may have new needs that they did not have when the patient's health was more stable [53]. When these needs are unmet, the family has fewer coping resources to draw upon and family members may experience greater distress. Previous research on caregivers of individuals with moderate to severe MS impairments has consistently identified increased needs for social, informational, and financial support, as well as higher rates of burden, strain, and depression [22, 54–57].

Findings from this study suggest that parents are providing the majority of the care for their children. This expands the definition of MS caregiver often seen in previous studies from a singular perspective that includes a spouse or romantic partner to a broader definition that can include parents, siblings, or other individuals providing care to the patient within their family system. As such, health care providers may need to focus on the impact of the patient and their illness on family overall. Consideration for the needs of the family system is particularly warranted in this sample as the overall health of the family unit is an important part of Mexican and Latino American cultures. Because unmet family needs were identified as a mediator of the relationship between MS impairments and caregiver mental health, health care providers may also want to assess the psychosocial functioning of family members in the household and target interventions toward the family system. There is the potential for a multifamily group intervention that informs caregivers about the effects of caregiving on families. Such an intervention may help bring together families within the community and could help normalize feelings of burden, disappointment, guilt, and fear that caregivers may be too guarded to share with others.

With regard to primary unmet needs identified in this study, a large number of participants reported unmet informational needs, which included specific requests for "specialized information about the patient," "complete information," and "to share [their] feelings with someone who has been in the same situation." Caregivers in this sample may benefit from general education about MS (e.g., disease course, symptom types, and treatments), as well as specific information about behavioral and emotional impairments (e.g., psychoeducation, resource identification, and symptom management strategies). Data from caregivers of individuals with Alzheimer's disease [58] and Parkinson's disease [59] have demonstrated decreased burden and caregiver stress among individuals who complete psychoeducational programs for management of symptoms associated with these

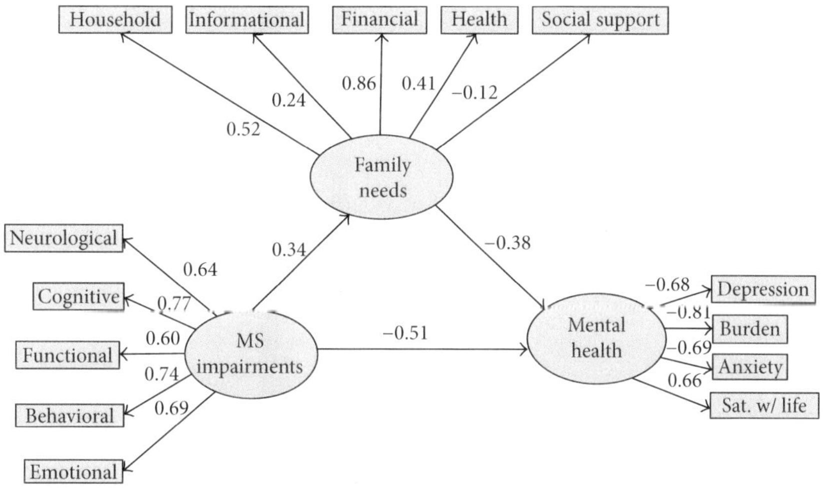

FIGURE 1: SEM of the mediation of family needs on the relationship between MS impairments and caregiver mental health.

illnesses [60]. Likewise, because of the specific interest identified by these caregivers, MS caregivers could possibly benefit from education that assists with daily care needs or helps caregivers understand and anticipate possible sequelae of the disease.

Additionally, the caregivers may have had informational needs that were not assessed. As such, a focus group or follow-up survey to assess the type of information that caregivers need is a feasible way to help meet the needs of caregivers in this sample or other samples as different caregiver cohorts will likely have different needs dependent on the patient's course, family composition, and family's access to medical resources. Moreover, although caregivers were requesting information in this study, they indicated a need to speak with other caregivers and to receive social support in addition to pragmatic suggestions, recommendations, and information. Interventions designed to facilitation dissemination of information through peer support, mentoring, and support groups offered in person or via telephone or internet have demonstrated efficacy in other caregiver populations [61] and could provide MS caregivers with increased access to these resources as well.

Interventions designed to help caregivers determine how to meet financial and household needs could help alleviate the negative mental health outcomes that caregivers in this sample experienced. Addressing these needs may include education about resources in the community (e.g., grants, supplemental income, and respite care services) that are available to families in the region or education about how to delegate household tasks. Addressing these needs may also require education about when to seek support outside of the family (e.g., respite care) and ways to overcome cultural barriers to accepting and accessing care outside of a kinship network.

In addition to this key finding, mental health outcomes reported by this sample differed somewhat from other studies of MS caregivers and individuals in Mexico. Epidemiological data from Mexico suggest a lifetime prevalence of 7.2% for major depressive disorder [62], which demonstrates that reported rates of depression in the current study are higher than those generally reported in the Mexican population. Although few studies have examined anxiety among MS caregivers, Argyriou et al. [63] reported mean scores that reflected mild anxiety in their sample, while the scores in the current study demonstrated subclinical mean values for state and trait anxiety, even though one-third of the sample endorsed moderate symptoms of anxiety. When comparing this sample's scores to epidemiological lifetime prevalence data for anxiety in Mexico, participants in this sample reported higher than expected anxiety (i.e., 14.3% prevalence rate as reported by Medina-Mora et al. [62]). A comparison with other studies of MS caregivers demonstrates that the current sample's percentages of MS caregivers experiencing mild, moderate, and severe burden are much lower than rates reported in other samples. For example, in another sample of MS caregivers, Akkus [18] reported a mean ZBI score of 36.42 (SD = 18.41), while Buchanan and Huang [64] found that 40% of their sample described caregiving as burdensome some of the time and 11.4% reported that caregiving was burdensome all of the time. These findings suggest the need for health care providers to continuously assess the mental health of caregivers and to provide them with access to services that can include emotional support (e.g., support groups, volunteer organizations, nursing care, spiritual/religious leaders, and communities) throughout the disease's duration.

4.1. Limitations and Future Research. The findings of this study should be viewed in light of several limitations, which can be considered potential areas for future research. Unlike many samples of MS caregivers, caregivers in the current study were predominately women who were mothers of the care recipients. This is indeed a rarity in the MS literature, as generally caregivers are male spouses providing care for their wives with MS. Future studies should examine the influence of gender roles prominent in Latino cultures on caregiving behaviors in both women and men MS caregivers and how these roles might play out in same-gender and opposite-gender caregiving relationships.

Because of the strong cultural values of familism and the stigma associated with neurological illness, caregivers within this sample may have underreported symptoms of burden, depression, and anxiety. Given the desire to fulfill cultural roles, Latina women, especially mothers, may not perceive caregiving as burdensome or they may be reluctant to disclose feelings of strain, anxiety, and sadness. By contrast, in other countries where male spouses or romantic partners typically fulfill MS caregiving roles, perceptions of burden may be stronger, as caregiving is a new skill set for them.

Additionally, the reported household incomes of the families in this sample may be higher than other caregivers who do not receive subsidized care and who are not employed while providing care. This study's participants were recruited from an urban university medical center and a local chapter of the MS foundation. As such, this sample's utilization of care and access to resources may be greater than most caregivers, especially those living in rural areas or individuals living in underdeveloped societies where health care is not as accessible. The findings in this sample may overlook or underestimate the true needs and psychosocial functioning of caregivers who do not have adequate resources and thus cannot acquire medical care for their loved ones and are not as well connected with community-based organizations.

Unmet family needs was one of the most important constructs assessed in the current study. At present, there are few empirically validated neurological-specific family needs assessments for use in Latin America other than that used in the current study. As such, the FNAT was used because the measure had been validated in a sample of caregivers of individuals with neurological conditions in Latin America [50]. Despite this strength, this measure's limitations include a narrow assessment of additional possible family needs which may or may not be MS-specific. As administered in the current study, only one individual in the family completed the questionnaire. However, in order to truly assess family needs, administration of the measure should include reports from all family members of the individual receiving care. As the measure is currently written and administered, the results only offer the perspective of one reporter but attribute this variance to the perspectives of others within the family unit. By including multiple reporters, researchers can then differentiate between variance observed within reporters (unique reporter variance) and across reporters (e.g., shared variance).

Another way to improve the measure is to increase the comprehensiveness and specificity of the constructs being assessed. Although the items in the current measure come from an aggregate of items from needs assessments of caregivers of individuals with MS and other neurological disorders, the current measure does not include items that assess potentially important aspects such as the need for respite care, the specific types of information that caregivers need, assistance with obtaining medical equipment, and the need for holistic or nontraditional medical practices that may be common and useful in Latin America. Including these items may come from additional focus groups and surveys with MS caregivers in other communities, especially communities of individuals who are hard to reach or who do not regularly access medical care. As such, the literature could greatly benefit from an MS-specific measure of family needs that has been developed using a Spanish-speaking sample and has been empirically validated in similar samples.

Similarly, the current study used the MS Impairments Questionnaire, a 30-item checklist of MS symptoms developed by Knight et al. [26] to assess the types of symptoms that patients experience. Although this questionnaire assesses the general clusters of symptoms shown to be common in individuals with MS, the measure itself has not gone through extensive psychometric evaluation. Additionally, several of the items comprising this questionnaire are vague and may not translate well into Spanish (e.g., "being unreliable"). Because of the importance of accurate assessment of MS symptoms, this measure should undergo further revision and evaluation in an attempt to assess additional symptoms of MS, as some of the common symptoms such as sexual dysfunction, attention problems, and heat sensitivity were omitted. A revised version should also include a factor analysis of items, as well as measure of disease severity or disability since the presence of a symptom does not necessarily indicate its functional impact or severity. As with the FNAT, a measure of MS symptoms should include multiple raters and/or a review of medical records to support self-reported and caregiver-reported data. Relying on the caregiver's perspective may overlook symptoms that the caregiver is unaware of (e.g., sexual dysfunction) and result in an incomplete assessment of patient functioning.

Finally, although the assumptions of normality were met for the SEM in the current study, the sample size was too small to generate accurate fit indices. Though they were presented for reference, they likely lack the stability that would occur with sample sizes greater than 200. As a result, these fit indices should be interpreted with extreme caution, and similar models should be run with larger samples in order to more accurately assess whether the current model or other models better fit the patterns in the data.

5. Conclusions

This study provided empirical support for the mediational role of unmet family needs in the relationship between MS impairments and caregiver mental health in Guadalajara, Mexico. These findings suggest that MS impairments may affect both the individual caregiver and the family unit. As a result, MS rehabilitation interventions, especially in Mexico and other Latin American countries, should comprehensively assess and target the patient's functioning, the family's unmet needs, and the caregiver's mental health functioning. Doing so—if supported by future research—could improve services for a population that has faced marginalization and a dearth of care within traditional rehabilitation settings.

Disclosure

The present work was developed as part of the Ph.D. dissertation of Dr. Melody N. Mickens, presented and approved at Virginia Commonwealth University in 2014 [65].

References

[1] R. Dutta and B. Trapp, "Pathogenesis of axonal and neuronal damage in multiple sclerosis," *Neurology*, vol. 68, no. 22, Supplement 3, pp. S22–S31, 2007.

[2] National Multiple Sclerosis Society, "Multiple sclerosis: just the facts, general information. (No. ER6007)," March 2016, http://www.nationalmssociety.org/downlad.aspx?id=22.

[3] N. Koch-Henriksen and P. SØrenson, "The changing demographic pattern of multiple sclerosis epidemiology," *Lancet Neurology*, vol. 9, no. 5, pp. 520–532, 2010.

[4] M. De la Maza Flores and G. Arrambide García, "Prevalencia de esclerosis multiple en el municipio de San Pedro Garza García," *Nuevo León Avances*, vol. 3, pp. 7–10, 2006.

[5] M. Veláquez-Quintana, M. A. Macías-Islas, V. Rivera-Olmos, and J. Lozano-Zárate, "Multiple sclerosis in Mexico: a multicentre study," *Revista de Neurologia*, vol. 36, pp. 1019–1022, 2003.

[6] A. Carrá, M. Á. Macías-Islas, A. A. Gabbai et al., "Optimizing outcomes in multiple sclerosis: consensus guidelines for the diagnosis and treatment of multiple sclerosis in Latin America," *Therapeutic Advances in Neurological Disorders*, vol. 4, no. 6, pp. 349–360, 2011.

[7] V. M. Rivera, "Multiple sclerosis in Latin America: reality and challenge," *Neuroepidemiology*, vol. 32, no. 4, pp. 294-295, 2009.

[8] M. S. Hinojosa, B. Zsembik, and M. R. Rittman, "Patterns of informal care among Puerto Rican, African American and white stroke survivors," *Ethnicity & Health*, vol. 14, pp. 591–606, 2009.

[9] M. C. Zea, T. Quezada, and F. Belgrave, "Cultural values and adjustment to disability among Latinos," *Journal of Social Behavior and Personality*, vol. 199, no. 9, pp. 185–200, 1994.

[10] P. Dilworth-Anderson, I. C. Williams, and B. E. Gibson, "Issues of race, ethnicity, and culture in caregiving research: A 20-Year Review (1980–2000)," *The Gerontologist*, vol. 42, pp. 237–272, 2002.

[11] M. Pinquart and S. Sörenson, "Ethnic differences in stressors, resources, and psychological outcomes of family caregiving: a meta-analysis," *The Gerontologist*, vol. 45, no. 1, pp. 90–106, 2005.

[12] C. Cox and A. Monk, "Strain among caregivers: comparing the experiences of African American and Hispanic caregivers of Alzheimer's relatives," *The International Journal of Aging and Human Development*, vol. 43, no. 2, pp. 93–105, 1996.

[13] K. E. Covinsky, R. Newcomer, P. Fox et al., "Patient and caregiver characteristics associated with depression in caregivers of patients with dementia," *Journal of General Internal Medicine*, vol. 18, no. 12, pp. 1006–1014, 2003.

[14] J. C. Arango-Lasprilla, P. Premuda, A. Aguayo, K. Francis, M. A. Macias, and T. Villaseñor, "Needs and psychosocial outcomes of caregivers of individuals with multiple sclerosis in Guadalajara, Mexico," *International Journal of MS Care*, vol. 12, no. 2, pp. 71–80, 2010.

[15] T. Lehan, J. C. Arango-Lasprilla, M. Á. Macias, A. Aguayo, and T. Villaseñor, "Distress associated with patients' symptoms and depression in a sample of Mexican caregivers of individuals with MS," *Rehabilitation Psychology*, vol. 57, no. 4, pp. 301–307, 2012.

[16] M. Buhse, "Assessment of caregiver burden in families of persons with multiple sclerosis," *Journal of Neuroscience Nursing*, vol. 40, no. 1, pp. 25–31, 2008.

[17] K. I. Pakenham, "Couple coping and adjustment to multiple sclerosis in care receiver-carer dyads," *Family Relations*, vol. 47, no. 3, pp. 269–277, 1998.

[18] Y. Akkus, "Multiple sclerosis patient caregivers: the relationship between their psychological and social needs and burden levels," *Disability and Rehabilitation*, vol. 33, no. 4, pp. 326–333, 2011.

[19] K. J. Aronson, G. Cleghorn, and E. Goldenberg, "Assistance arrangements and use of services among persons with multiple sclerosis and their caregivers," *Disability and Rehabilitation*, vol. 18, no. 7, pp. 354–361, 1996.

[20] M. Finlayson and C. Cho, "A descriptive profile of caregivers of older adults with MS and the assistance they provide," *Disability and Rehabilitation*, vol. 30, no. 24, pp. 1848–1857, 2008.

[21] K. M. Myhr, T. Riise, C. Vedeler et al., "Disability and prognosis in multiple sclerosis: demographic and clinical variables important for the ability to walk and awarding of disability pension," *Multiple Sclerosis Journal*, vol. 7, no. 1, pp. 59–65, 2001.

[22] S. Y. Chipchase and N. B. Lincoln, "Factors associated with carer strain in carers of people with multiple sclerosis," *Disability and Rehabilitation*, vol. 23, pp. 768–776, 2001.

[23] J. Dunn, "Impact of mobility impairment on the burden of caregiving in individuals with multiple sclerosis," *Expert Review of Pharmaeconomics & Outcomes Research*, vol. 10, pp. 433–440, 2010.

[24] M. Figved, K. Myhr, J. Larsen, and D. Aarsland, "Caregiver burden in multiple sclerosis: the impact of neuropsychiatric symptoms," *Journal of Neurology, Neurosurgery & Psychiatry*, vol. 78, pp. 1097–1102, 2007.

[25] F. Khan, J. Pallant, and C. Brand, "Caregiver strain and factors associated with caregiver self-efficacy and quality of life in a community cohort with multiple sclerosis," *Disability and Rehabilitation*, vol. 29, no. 16, pp. 1241–1250, 2007.

[26] R. G. Knight, R. C. Devereux, and H. P. Godfrey, "Psychosocial consequences of caring for a spouse with multiple sclerosis," *Journal of Clinical and Experimental Neuropsychology*, vol. 19, pp. 7–19, 1997.

[27] K. I. Pakenham, "Relations between coping and positive and negative outcomes in carers of persons with multiple sclerosis (MS)," *Journal of Clinical Psychology in Medical Settings*, vol. 12, no. 1, pp. 25–38, 2005.

[28] L. I. Pearlin, J. T. Mullan, S. J. Semple, and M. Skaff, "Caregiving and the stress process: an overview of concepts and their measures," *The Gerontologist*, vol. 30, no. 5, pp. 583–594, 1990.

[29] D. W. Chapman and J. F. Carter, "Translation procedures for the cross cultural use of measurement instruments,"

Educational Evaluation and Policy Analysis, vol. 1, no. 3, pp. 71–76, 1979.

[30] F. Guillemin, C. Bombardier, and D. Beaton, "Cross-cultural adaptation of health-related quality of life measures: literature review and proposed guidelines," *Journal of Clinical Epidemiology*, vol. 46, no. 12, pp. 1417–1432, 1993.

[31] M. Schiaffino and R. Espiritu Santo, "Mexico approves an increase to the minimum wage for 2014 for geographic zones "A" and "B"," August 2015, http://www.littler.com/files/press/pdf/2014_1_Mexico_Approves_Increase_Minimum_Wage_2014_Geographic_Zones_A_B_.pdf.

[32] C. D. Spielberger, R. L. Gorsuch, R. E. Lushene, R. E. Vagg, and G. A. Jacobs, *Manual for the State-Trait Anxiety Inventory (STAI)*, Consulting Psychologists Press, Palo Alto, CA, USA, 1983.

[33] C. D. Spielberger, "State-trait anxiety inventory," in *Corsini Encyclopedia of Psychology*, I. B. Weiner and W. E. Craighead, Eds., p. 1, Wiley, New York, NY, USA, 4th edition, 2010.

[34] C. D. Spielberger and R. Diaz-Guerrero, *IDARE, Inventario de ansiedad*, Rasgo-Estado [State-Trait Anxiety Inventory], Mexico: El Manual Moderno, S.A, 1975.

[35] D. M. Novy, D. V. Nelson, K. G. Smith, P. A. Rogers, and R. D. Rowzee, "Psychometric comparability of the English-and Spanish-language versions of the state-trait anxiety inventory," *Hispanic Journal of Behavioral Sciences*, vol. 17, no. 2, pp. 209–224, 1995.

[36] B. Virella, C. Arbona, and D. M. Novy, "Psychometric properties and factor structure of the Spanish version of the state-trait anxiety inventory," *Journal of Personality Assessment*, vol. 63, no. 3, pp. 401–412, 1994.

[37] S. H. Zarit, K. E. Reever, and J. Bach-Peterson, "Relatives of the impaired elderly: correlates of feelings of burden," *The Gerontologist*, vol. 20, no. 6, pp. 649–655, 1980.

[38] G. Karlikaya, G. Yukse, F. Varlibas, and H. Tireli, "Caregiver burden in dementia: a study in the Turkish population," *The Internet Journal of Neurology*, vol. 4, pp. 12–26, 2005.

[39] R. Siegert, D. M. Jackson, A. Tennant, and L. Turner-Stokes, "Factor analysis and Rasch analysis of the Zarit burden interview for acquired brain injury carer research," *Journal of Rehabilitation Medicine*, vol. 42, no. 4, pp. 302–309, 2010.

[40] P. Martínez-Martín, M. J. Forjaz, B. Frades-Payo et al., "Caregiver burden in Parkinson's disease," *Movement Disorders*, vol. 22, no. 7, pp. 924–931, 2007.

[41] M. Martín-Carrasco, I. Salvadó, S. Nadal et al., "Adaptación para nuestro medio de la Escala de Sobrecarga del Cuidador (Caregiver Burden Interview) de Zarit," *Review of Gerontology*, vol. 6, pp. 338–346, 1996.

[42] K. Kroenke, R. L. Spitzer, and J. B. W. Williams, "The PHQ-9: validity of a brief depression severity measure," *Journal of General Internal Medicine*, vol. 16, no. 9, pp. 606–613, 2001.

[43] C. Diez-Quevedo, T. Rangil, L. Sanchez-Planell, K. Kroenke, and R. L. Spitzer, "Validation and utility of the patient health questionnaire in diagnosing mental disorders in 1003 general hospital Spanish inpatients," *Psychosomatic Medicine*, vol. 63, no. 4, pp. 679–686, 2001.

[44] W. Donlan and J. Lee, "Screening for depression among indigenous Mexican migrant farmworkers using the patient health questionnaire-9," *Psychological Reports*, vol. 106, no. 2, pp. 419–432, 2010.

[45] L. W. Wulsin, E. Somoza, and J. Heck, "The feasibility of using the Spanish PHQ-9 to screen for depression in primary care in Honduras," *Primary Care Companion Journal of Clinical Psychiatry*, vol. 4, no. 05, pp. 191–195, 2002.

[46] E. Diener, R. A. Emmons, R. J. Larsen, and S. Griffin, "The satisfaction with life scale," *Journal of Personality Assessment*, vol. 49, no. 1, pp. 71–75, 1985.

[47] W. Pavot and E. Diener, "Review of the satisfaction with life scale," *Psychological Assessment*, vol. 5, no. 2, pp. 164–172, 1993.

[48] F. L. Atienza, D. Pons, I. Balaguer, and M. L. Garcia-Merita, "Satisfaction with life scale: analysis of factorial invariance for adolescents and elderly persons," *Perceptual and Motor Skills*, vol. 91, pp. 62–68, 2000.

[49] C. Vázquez, A. Duque, and G. Hervás, "Satisfaction with life scale in a representative sample of Spanish adults: validation and normative data," *The Spanish Journal of Psychology*, vol. 16, article E82, 2013.

[50] D. Rivera, P. B. Perrin, H. Senra et al., "Development of the family needs assessment tool for caregivers of individuals with neurological conditions in Latin America," *Psicología desde el Caribe*, vol. 3, pp. 1–20, 2013.

[51] J. L. Arbuckle, *Amos 20 User's Guide*, SPSS, Chicago, IL, USA, 2011.

[52] R. Weston, P. Gore, F. Chan, and D. Catalano, "An introduction to using structural equation models in rehabilitation psychology," *Rehabilitation Psychology*, vol. 53, pp. 340–356, 2009.

[53] K. I. Pakenham and S. Cox, "Development of the benefit finding in multiple sclerosis (MS) caregiving scale: a longitudinal study of relations between benefit finding and adjustment," *British Journal of Health Psychology*, vol. 13, no. 4, pp. 583–602, 2008.

[54] H. Carton, R. Loos, J. Pacolet, K. Versieck, and R. Vlietnck, "A quantitative study of unpaid caregiving in multiple sclerosis," *Multiple Sclerosis*, vol. 6, no. 4, pp. 274–279, 2000.

[55] M. Corry and A. While, "The needs of carers of people with multiple sclerosis: a literature review," *Scandinavian Journal of Caring Sciences*, vol. 23, no. 3, pp. 569–588, 2009.

[56] L. J. Kristjanson, S. M. Aoun, and L. Oldham, "Palliative care and support for people with neurodegenerative conditions and their carers," *International Journal of Palliative Nursing*, vol. 12, pp. 368–377, 2005.

[57] K. I. Pakenham, "The nature of caregiving in multiple sclerosis: development of the caregiving tasks in multiple sclerosis scale," *Multiple Sclerosis Journal*, vol. 13, no. 7, pp. 929–938, 2007.

[58] N. Beinart, J. Weinman, D. Wade, and R. Brady, "Caregiver burden and psychoeducational interventions in Alzheimer's disease: a review," *Dementia and Geriatric Cognitive Disorders Extra*, vol. 2, no. 1, pp. 638–648, 2012.

[59] M. Martín-Carrasco, M. F. Martín, C. P. Valero et al., "Effectiveness of a psychoeducational intervention program in the reduction of caregiver burden in Alzheimer's disease patients' caregivers," *International Journal of Geriatric Psychiatry*, vol. 24, no. 5, pp. 489–499, 2009.

[60] M. Y. Savundranayagam, R. J. Montgomery, K. Kosloski, and T. D. Little, "Impact of a psychoeducational program on the three types of caregiver burden among spouses," *International Journal of Geriatric Psychiatry*, vol. 26, pp. 338–396, 2011.

[61] L. N. Gitlin, S. H. Belle, L. D. Burgio et al., "Effect of multicomponent interventions on caregiver burden and depression: the

REACH multisite initiative at 6-month follow-up," *Psychology and Aging*, vol. 18, pp. 361–374, 2003.

[62] M. E. Medina-Mora, G. Borges, C. Benjet, C. Lara, and P. Berglund, "Psychiatric disorders in Mexico: lifetime prevalence in a nationally representative sample," *The British Journal of Psychiatry*, vol. 190, pp. 521–528, 2007.

[63] A. A. Argyriou, P. Karanasios, A. A. Ifanti et al., "Quality of life and emotional burden of primary caregivers: a case-control study of multiple sclerosis patients in Greece," *Quality of Life Research*, vol. 20, no. 10, pp. 1663–1668, 2011.

[64] R. Buchanan and C. Huang, "Informal caregivers assisting people with multiple sclerosis: factors associated with the strength of the caregiver/care recipient relationship," *International Journal of MS Care*, vol. 13, no. 4, pp. 177–187, 2011.

[65] M. N. Mickens, *Todo en la familia: Examining the Relationships Among MS Impairments, Family Needs, and Caregiver Mental Health in Guadalajara, Mexico, [Ph.D. thesis]*, Virginia Commonwealth University, Richmond, VA, USA, 2014.

24

Age- and Gender-based Differences in Nest-Building Behavior and Learning and Memory Performance Measured using a Radial Six-Armed Water Maze in C57BL/6 Mice

Xiang-Dong Xiong[1,2] **Wei-Dong Xiong**[1,3] **Shang-Shen Xiong**[1,3] **and Gui-Hai Chen**[1,4]

[1]*Department of Neurology, The First Affiliated Hospital of Anhui Medical University, Hefei, 230022 Anhui, China*
[2]*Lu'an Affiliated Hospital of Anhui Medical University, People's Hospital of Lu'an City, Lu'an, 237005 Anhui, China*
[3]*Hefei National Level High and New Technology Development Zone, Hefei, 230088 Anhui, China*
[4]*Department of Neurology, The Affiliated Chaohu Hospital of Anhui Medical University, Chaohu, 238000 Anhui, China*

Correspondence should be addressed to Gui-Hai Chen; doctorcgh@163.com

Academic Editor: Antonio Orlacchio

Background. Understanding age-based and gender-based behavioral changes is becoming more important as a greater percentage of people lives longer worldwide. In this study, a C57BL/6 mouse animal model was used to study age-based and gender-based behavioral differences using nest building and radial six-armed water maze (RAWM) testing. *Methods.* In C57BL/6 mice, nest-building behavior was recorded as nesting scores, while spatial learning and memory behaviors were assessed using RAWM platform search errors and latencies. *Results.* In the nest-building test, nest building significantly declined in nineteen 25-month-old mice compared to that of twenty-three 7-month-old mice. Meanwhile, nest building in 25-month-old mice was lower for eight male mice than for eleven female mice, while no significant gender differences were observed in nest building of 7-month-old mice. RAWM performance also declined in aged versus nonaged adult mice, while no significant gender differences were observed in average RAWM performance regardless of age. *Conclusions.* In adult C57BL/6 mice, nest building is a sensitive indicator for detecting both age- and gender-based behavioral declines, while RAWM performance, an assessment of spatial learning and memory behaviors, is not sensitive to gender but significantly declines with aging. Therefore, for a C57BL/6 mouse model of aging, both nest building and RAWM should be useful to further study mechanisms involved in behavioral decline with aging.

1. Introduction

Understanding age-based and gender-based behavioral changes is becoming more important as the elderly population grows. Memory behavioral impairment with advancing years not only reduces the quality of life for the elderly but also increases the costs of healthcare for society. In order to understand the mechanisms that give rise to behavioral decline with aging and gender-based behavioral differences, animal models are needed to unravel the complex changes that disrupt brain function of the aging brain.

In mice, although species' typical behaviors include nest building [1, 2], age- and gender-related nest-building behavioral differences in adult mice have not been reported. Similar age-based and gender-based spatial and memory behavioral studies in radial six-armed water maze (RAWM) spatial cognitive test in adult mice have not yet been reported even though C57BL/6 mouse strain possesses advantages as an animal model. Aside from the fact that C57BL/6 is one of the most commonly used laboratory mouse strains, these mice are also excellent swimmers (useful in water maze tests) and have a short lifespan. It is well known that there are about 30,000 genes in mice similar to detected gene numbers of humans. The interest in C57BL/6 mice and other mouse strains is because of their frequent use in transgenic research. It is well known that there are gender- and age-based differences on cognitive tasks that require the use of spatial learning and memory tests in mice. The only novelty is the use of the radial six-armed water maze test. Moreover, aged C57BL/6 mice (25-month-old) have been shown to exhibit impaired spatial memory relative to nonaged adult mice (five-month-old, but not nonaged adult 17-month-old) using the Morris water maze (MWM) spatial cognitive test, but no significant gender differences were detected by MWM testing [3]. Thus, for the aforementioned reasons, C57BL/6 mice may serve as a preferred animal model to study human aging. Using this animal model, we tested the following: (1) nest-building behavior would be sensitive to both age and gender differences in adult C57BL/6 mice; (2) spatial memory behavior measured using RAWM would detect age- and gender-based spatial memory behavioral changes in adult C57BL/6 mice; (3) behavioral differences measured by nest building and RAWM would show similar trends for aged versus nonaged adult C57BL/6 mice. All of these initiatives were experimentally addressed, and results reported here should encourage future use of this animal model for research to investigate mechanisms of human memory decline with aging.

2. Materials and Methods

2.1. Animals and General Protocols. C57BL/6 mice were purchased from the Experimental Animal Center of the University of Science and Technology of China (Hefei) and were maintained as an inbred strain and bred under specific pathogen-free conditions. Mice were transferred to conventional housing conditions at two months of age, housed in groups of 4 to 6 same-gender mice per cage in $25.5 \times 15 \times 14$ cm plastic cages with wood shavings. Mice were allowed free access to a standard rodent diet and tap water during a 12 h light-dark cycle, with lights turned on at 7:30 AM and off at 7:30 PM. Mice were housed at a constant temperature of 21-22°C and humidity of 55% (±5%). Mice were preselected for overall health and normal behavioral attributes, and animals with gross defects (tumors outside trunk, motor incapacitation, or overt blindness) were excluded from experimentation. A total of 42 C57BL/6 mice comprised two groups: twenty-three 7-month-old (nonaged adult) mice, including ten males and thirteen females, and nineteen 25-month-old (aged) mice, including eight males and eleven females. The body weight of aged mice was similar to that of nonaged adult mice. One hour prior to testing, the mice were transferred to the experimental room for acclimatization. The nest-building test was performed during the dark phase of the light-dark cycle, and remaining tests were performed during the light phase. The order of completed tests was as follows: days 1-2 nest building, day 3 MWM cued learning, and days 4–10 RAWM. The Ethics Committee of The First Affiliated Hospital of Anhui Medical University approved this study, and all experimental protocols were approved by the hospital's Institutional Review Committee using procedures in compliance with the National Institutes of Health Guide for Care and Use of Laboratory Animals.

2.2. Nest-Building Test and Nesting Scores. As previously described [1, 2], mice were individually housed overnight with food, water, and new sawdust bedding. Six pieces of $5 \times 5\ cm^2$ white paper (which mice use to make nests) were placed in each cage. After the overnight nest-building test, nests typically contained with a shallow crater of sawdust spread, surrounded by, or covered with shredded or whole paper. The mice were scored according to the following nesting score scale: 0 = no visible crater of sawdust and no paper; 1 = sawdust crater alone and no shredded paper; 2 = sawdust crater with shredded or whole paper gathered around and in the crater; 3 = sawdust crater with shredded or whole paper gathered around and in the crater forming a cup-shaped nest; 4 = shredded paper forming a ball-shaped nest covering the mouse.

2.3. Cued Learning Using a MWM. A circular black tank 150 cm in diameter and 30 cm in height [4–6] was used. The initial water temperature of 20-21°C [6] was decreased by 1-2°C in the MWM as compared to the temperature of 21-22°C in the RAWM in order to increase aversion to swimming and decrease floating tendency. The tank was situated in an identical orientation to that of the RAWM, with a distance of 75 cm from the tank wall to the white cloth curtain. Cued learning tests were used to evaluate swimming ability, visual acuity, nonspatial learning ability, and motor or sensorimotor function. A black escape platform with diameter 10 cm and height 24 cm was raised 1.0 cm above the water surface, and a 7 cm diameter plastic ball with black and white stripes was attached to the top of the platform with a short rod. The platform position was different for each trial, but the release point was identical for each of five consecutive trials performed on a single day. Latency in finding the visible platform was recorded for a maximum of 60 s. After finding the visible platform, a mouse was allowed to stay there for a 30 s rest. Mice that failed to find the visible platform were guided there and allowed to remain there for 30 s.

2.4. Apparatus and Procedure for RAWM Testing. As described previously [4, 5], a RAWM was constructed using a circular black water tank 100 cm in diameter and 21 cm in depth placed atop a 30 cm high steel rack and filled with 21-22°C water to a depth of 16 cm. A white cloth curtain surrounded the tank at a distance of 150 cm from the tank wall. Three black cardboard pieces, either a circle, triangle, or square (each 30 cm in height), were hung on the curtain equidistantly from the edges of the curtain, and these pieces served as spatial cues. Four 100 W evenly spaced floodlights were placed on the ground around the curtain. The tank contained six $30.5 \times 19 \times 21\ cm^3$ swimming alleys which radiated out from the 40 cm diameter center area. A black escape platform (10 cm in diameter) was submerged 1.0 cm below the water surface and was placed at the peripheral end of one alley a distance of 4.5 cm from the walls. During testing, both the platform and the experimenter remained at a constant position for seven consecutive days. On each day, four consecutive acquisition trials (defined as RAWM learning phase) followed 30 minutes later by one memory retention trial (defined as RAWM memory phase) were completed.

On the first day, each mouse was first placed on the submerged platform for 30 s. From trial 1 to trial 4, the mouse was individually released into the water from four random entry alleys (except from the alley containing the platform and its opposite alley, to avoid the effect of innate direction bias) [7]. In each trial, the mouse was able to find the submerged platform within 60 s and allowed to rest on the platform. After 30 s of rest, it was taken off the platform. Upon entering an incorrect alley with its entire body, or if the mouse failed to select an alley within 10 s, the mouse was gently placed at the start alley; thus, this attempt was defined as an error. After the acquisition trials were completed, the mouse was towel-dried and placed in the home cage under a 150 W floodlight for 30 minutes. The mouse was then returned to the maze to complete trial 5 with the start alley identical to trial 4. Latency was defined as the time from the mouse's entry into the water to the time of finding the submerged platform. Due to the daily changing of sequences of starting points for trials 1–4 and innate swimming direction bias, spatial learning performance of each mouse did not always improve from trial 1 to trial 4. The number of errors and latencies in the daily trials during the 1-to-4-day period was averaged for statistical analysis.

2.5. Statistical Analyses. All results were expressed as the mean ± standard error of the mean (mean ± SEM) values. The Kruskal-Wallis test was used to verify effects of age and gender for the nonparametric data of nest building. For RAWM, analysis of variance (ANOVA) was used, using the statistical design of an age × gender × testing day-mixed ANOVA, with age and gender serving as between-subject factors and testing day as a repeated measure. A value of $P < 0.05$ was considered statistically significant. All analyses were conducted using SPSS 16.0 for Windows.

3. Results

3.1. Nesting Scores. For all C57BL/6 mice, nesting scores and nest building significantly declined in aged mice compared to results of nonaged adult mice [$x^2_{(1,40)} = 10.113$, $P = 0.001$ (<0.01)]. Moreover, age had a significant effect on both male and female mice [$x^2_{(1,16)} = 7.155$, $^{**}P = 0.007$ (<0.01); $x^2_{(1,22)} = 4.345$, $^{*}P = 0.037$ (<0.05)] (Figure 1). Nesting scores significantly declined for aged male mice as compared to scores of aged females [$x^2_{(1,15)} = 4.770$, $^{*}P = 0.029$ (<0.05)] (Figure 1). However, no significant gender differences in nesting scores and nest building were observed for 7-month-old nonaged adult mice [$x^2_{(1,21)} = 0.217$, $Ps = 0.641$ (>0.05)] (Figure 1).

3.2. Latencies in MWM Cued Learning. Latencies (time taken to find the visible platform after entering the water) were progressively and significantly decreased with higher trial number [$F_{(4,116)} = 11.718$, $P < 0.001$] (Figure 2). Latencies significantly decreased either from trial 2 onward or from trials 3 to 5 onward compared to latencies for trial 1 ($P < 0.01$ or $P < 0.001$). In general, during MWM cued learning latency, periods are known to depend on factors that include nonspatial learning ability, visual acuity, and motor or sensorimotor function. In this work, no significant differences were observed in latency between aged and nonaged adult C57BL/6 mice [$F_{(4,132)} < 1$, $Ps > 0.05$] (Figure 2) and no significant gender differences were observed in aged versus nonaged adult mice ($Ps > 0.05$) (Figure 3). By virtue of the constant swimming distance of 100 cm to the visible platform for each of the five consecutive trials, latencies could be reflected by variations in swimming speeds. However, with regard to swimming speeds during latency during MWM cued learning, no significant differences between aged and nonaged adult mice ($Ps > 0.05$) were observed and no significant gender-based differences were observed regardless of age ($Ps > 0.05$). Furthermore, no increased tendency to float was observed in aged mice versus nonaged mice during MWM cued learning.

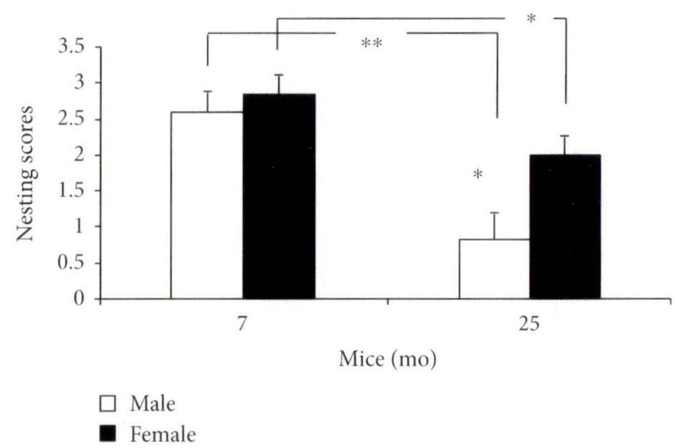

FIGURE 1: Nesting scores in 7- and 25-month-old C57BL/6 male and female mice (mean ± SEM). $^{*}P < 0.05$; $^{**}P < 0.01$.

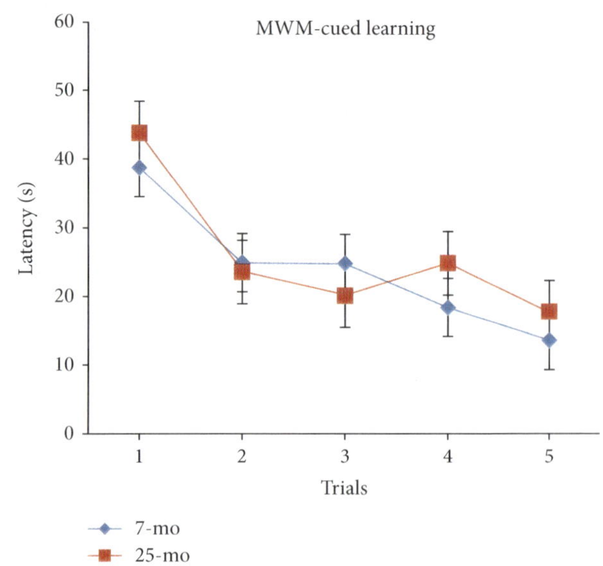

FIGURE 2: Latencies of 7- and 25-month-old C57BL/6 mice in cued learning of MWM (s, mean ± SEM).

3.3. Errors and Latencies during the Learning Phase of RAWM. Overall, the number of errors committed while finding the submerged platform progressively and significantly

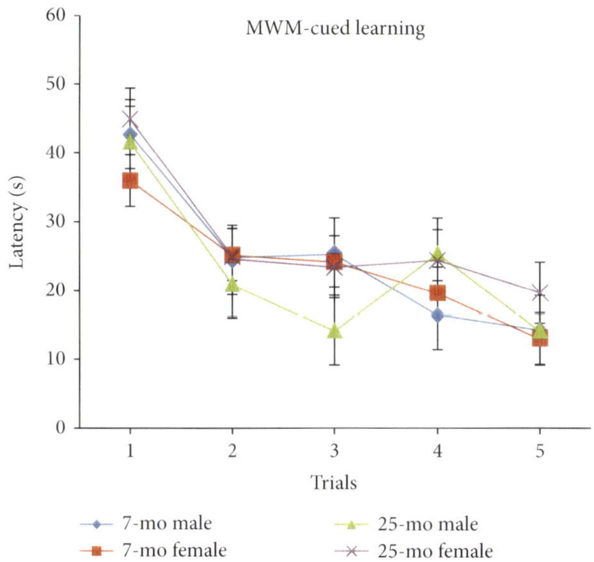

FIGURE 3: Latencies of 7- and 25-month-old C57BL/6 male and female mice in cued learning of MWM (s, mean ± SEM).

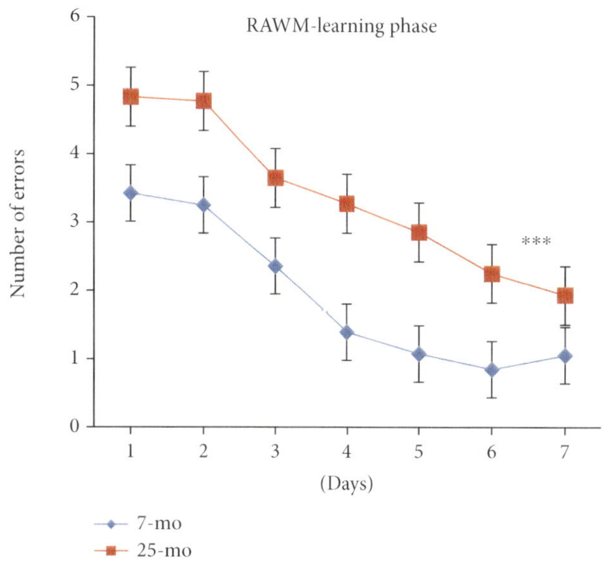

FIGURE 4: Number of errors of 7- and 25-month-old C57BL/6 mice in learning phase of RAWM (mean ± SEM). $^{***}P < 0.001$.

decreased with day [$F_{(6,180)} = 28.375$, $P < 0.001$] (Figure 4). For mice overall, the number of errors significantly decreased by day 3 compared to error numbers on day 1 ($P < 0.01$) or day 2 ($P < 0.05$) and error numbers still significantly decreased on days 5 and 6 compared to numbers on day 4 ($P < 0.05$). Errors continued to reach significantly decreased levels on day 7 relative to day 5 ($P < 0.05$). In aged mice, the number of errors significantly increased, mirroring significant decline in spatial learning performance observed during the RAWM learning phase relative to performance of nonaged adult mice [$F_{(1,34)} = 38.01$, $^{***}P < 0.001$] (Figure 4). Nonaged adult mice exhibited a decreasing trend in error numbers, with an average on day 4 of only one error, while aged mice exhibited an average of two errors at day 7. No significant gender-based differences were observed in error numbers, reflecting absence of gender influences on spatial learning performance during the RAWM learning phase for either aged or nonaged adult mice ($Ps > 0.05$) (Figure 5).

As observed for errors, latencies for all mice progressively and significantly decreased with day [$F_{(6,180)} = 51.753$, $P < 0.001$] (Figure 6) and significantly decreasing on day 2 versus day 1 ($P < 0.01$) and even more significantly by day 3 relative to day 1 ($P < 0.001$) or day 2 ($P < 0.01$); latencies significantly decreased on day 4 relative to day 1 ($P < 0.001$), day 2 ($P < 0.001$), or day 3 ($P < 0.05$) and continued to significantly decrease by day 7 relative to latencies on day 4 ($P < 0.001$), day 5 ($P < 0.001$), or day 6 ($P < 0.05$). Latencies during the RAWM learning phase in aged mice were significantly higher than for nonaged adult mice, indicating decline in spatial learning ability with old age [$F_{(1,34)} = 38.413$, $^{***}P < 0.001$] (Figure 6), but no significant gender-based latency differences were observed ($Ps > 0.05$) (Figure 7). Thus differences in spatial learning performance during the RAWM learning phase were observed between aged mice relative to nonaged adult mice, but no gender-based differences were observed. Finally, no increased floating tendency was observed in aged mice relative to nonaged mice during the RAWM learning phase.

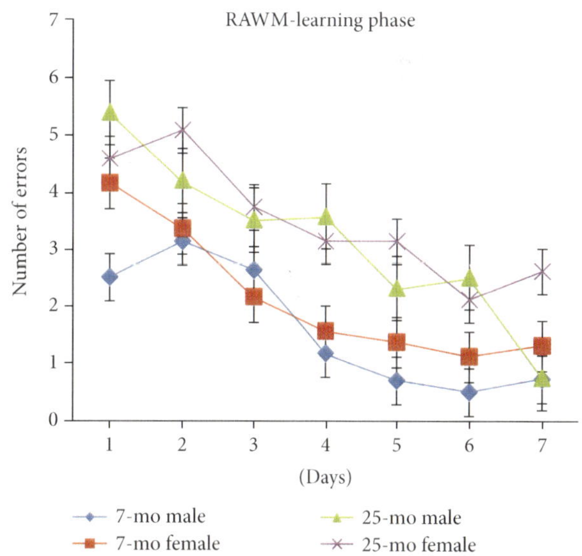

FIGURE 5: Number of errors of 7- and 25-month-old C57BL/6 male and female mice in learning phase of RAWM (mean ± SEM).

3.4. Errors and Latencies during the RAWM Memory Phase. For all mice, numbers of errors committed while searching for the submerged platform progressively and significantly decreased with day [$F_{(6,180)} = 4.461$, $P < 0.001$] (Figure 8) and no significant differences in the number of errors on day 2 or day 3 were observed compared to error numbers on day 1 ($Ps > 0.05$). Numbers of errors continued to significantly decrease by day 4 compared to numbers on day 1 or 2 ($P < 0.01$ or $P < 0.05$), reaching significantly decreased levels on day 4 or 6 compared to those on day 2 ($P < 0.05$ or

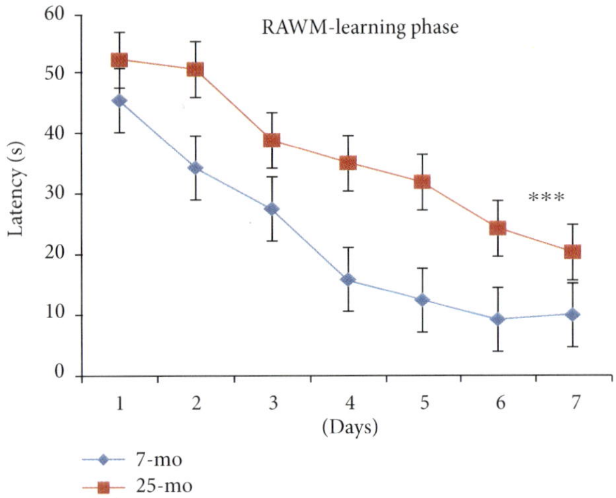

FIGURE 6: Latencies of 7- and 25-month-old C57BL/6 mice in learning phase of RAWM (s, mean ± SEM). $^{***}P < 0.001$.

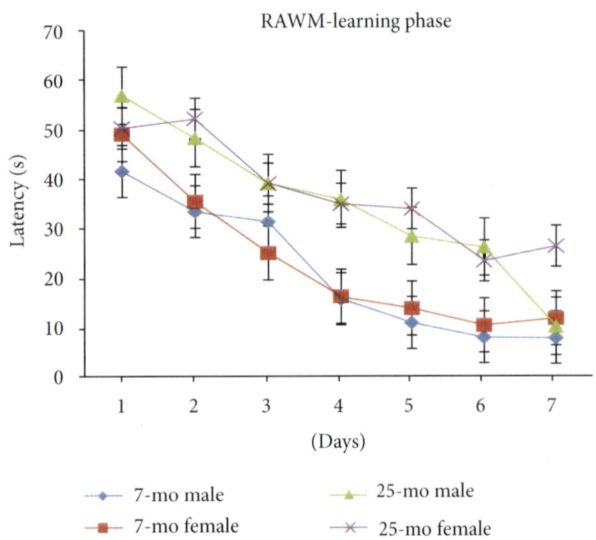

FIGURE 7: Latencies of 7- and 25-month-old C57BL/6 male and female mice in learning phase of RAWM (s, mean ± SEM).

$P < 0.01$). Numbers of errors on day 7 were similar to those on day 5 or 6 ($Ps > 0.05$). For aged mice, numbers of errors significantly increased relative to the error numbers for nonaged adult mice, reflecting significant decline in spatial memory ability with advanced age as measured during the RAWM memory phase [$F_{(1,34)} = 12.440$, $^{**}P = 0.001$ (<0.01)] (Figure 8). No significant gender-based effects were observed in the RAWM memory phase ($Ps > 0.05$) (Figure 9). In Figure 9, the 25-month-old male mice show a dip in error number at day 4 and unstable spatial memory performance.

For all mice, latencies progressively and significantly decreased with day [$F_{(6,180)} = 9.968$, $P < 0.001$] (Figure 10) and were similar on day 1 to day 2 ($P > 0.05$) and on days 3 to 5 ($P > 0.05$). Latencies on days 3 to 7 were significantly lower than latencies on day 1 ($P < 0.05$, $P < 0.001$, $P < 0.01$, $P < 0.001$, and $P < 0.001$). Latencies significantly decreased

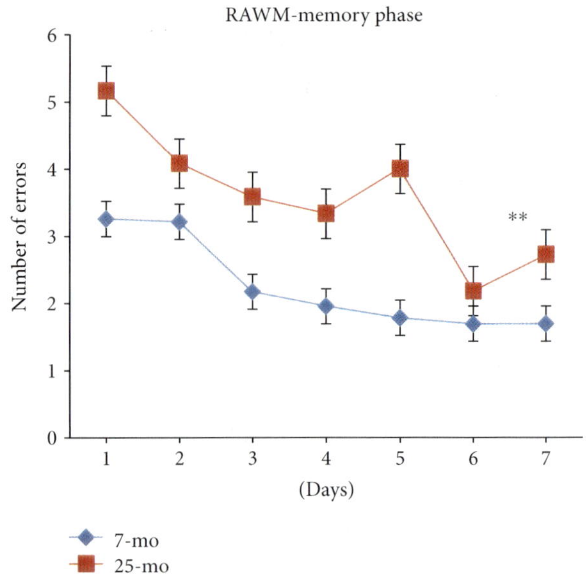

FIGURE 8: Number of errors of 7- and 25-month-old C57BL/6 mice in memory phase of RAWM (mean ± SEM). $^{**}P < 0.01$.

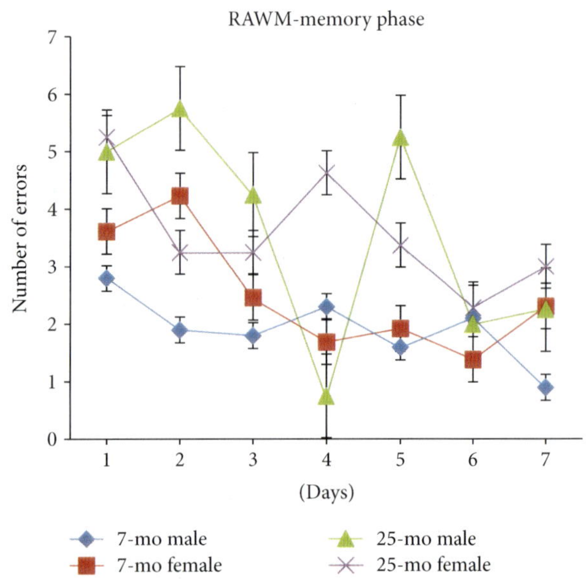

FIGURE 9: Number of errors of 7- and 25-month-old C57BL/6 male and female mice in memory phase of RAWM (mean ± SEM).

on day 4 or day 6 relative to day 2 ($P < 0.01$ or $P < 0.001$), and latencies on day 3 or day 5 were similar to those on day 2 ($Ps > 0.05$). On day 7, latencies were significantly decreased relative to latencies on days 1, 2, 3, and 5 ($P < 0.001$, $P < 0.01$, $P < 0.01$, and $P < 0.05$) but were similar to those on day 4 or 6 ($Ps > 0.05$). Latencies significantly declined more during the RAWM memory phase in nonaged adult mice versus aged mice [$F_{(1,34)} = 13.613$, $^{**}P = 0.001$ (<0.01)] (Figure 10). Overall, no significant gender differences were observed for latencies, reflecting the absence of gender differences in spatial memory performance during the RAWM memory phase regardless of

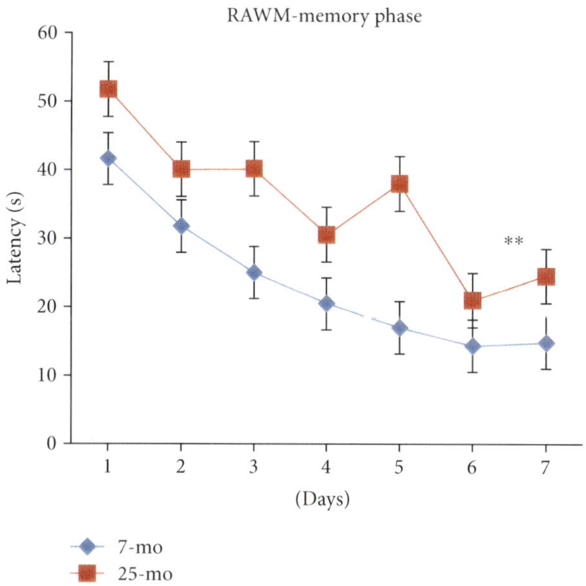

FIGURE 10: Latencies of 7- and 25-month-old C57BL/6 mice in memory phase of RAWM (s, mean ± SEM). $^{**}P < 0.01$.

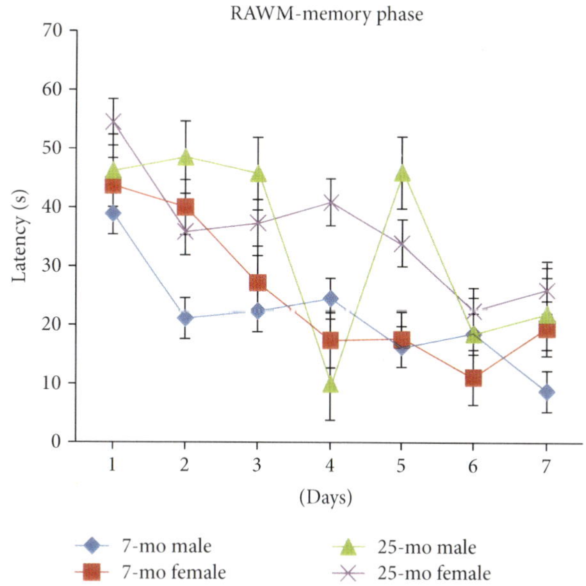

FIGURE 11: Latencies of 7- and 25-month-old C57BL/6 male and female mice in memory phase of RAWM (s, mean ± SEM).

age ($Ps > 0.05$) (Figure 11). Furthermore, no increased floating tendency was observed in aged mice versus nonaged adult mice during the RAWM memory phase. In Figure 11, the 25-month-old male mice show a dip in latency at day 4 and unstable spatial memory performance.

3.5. Correlation of Nest Building and RAWM. There were no significant correlations among nesting scores in nest building and number of errors and latencies in RAWM in aged and nonaged adult male or female C57BL/6 mice ($Ps > 0.05$).

4. Discussion

Age-based and gender-based behavioral differences in nest building and RAWM performance were evaluated for aged and nonaged adult C57BL/6 mice. Significant age and gender differences were observed in nest building, while only age effects were observed in RAWM performance. With regard to nesting behavior, within each age group, significant gender-based nesting score differences were observed and differences were more pronounced for the 25-month-old (aged) group than for the 7-month-old (nonaged adult) group.

In MWM cued learning tests, latencies due to differences in swimming speed, nonspatial learning ability, visual acuity, and motor or sensorimotor functions in aged mice were similar to latencies in nonaged adult mice. Notably, swimming speeds, nonspatial learning ability, visual acuity, and movement capabilities of aged mice did not decline relative to those characteristics for younger adults; therefore, the abovementioned results suggest that significantly increased RAWM latencies in aged C57BL/6 mice were due to significant declines in spatial learning and memory (short-term memory, such as working memory and reference memory) abilities.

Successful completion of nest building in mice depends on hippocampal integrity and an intact medial prefrontal cortex [1, 2]. Here, nest building and RAWM spatial learning and memory capabilities significantly declined in aging C57BL/6 mice. Such behavioral declines may be related to serological, histochemical, and/or morphological changes in specific brain regions. Morphological changes previously associated with aging include changes in hippocampal subregions [8], altered serotonergic, dopaminergic, or cholinergic innervation, changes in dendritic arborization, altered dendritic spines, or altered adult neurogenesis, any or all of which may be responsible for observed behavioral changes in aged C57BL/6 mice and memory impairment in elderly humans.

We explored age- and gender-related behavioral differences in nest building and RAWM performance between aged and nonaged adult C57BL/6 mice in order to evaluate C57BL/6 mice as an aging mouse model. The results of this study provide evidence and add novel data demonstrating behavioral differences in nest building and RAWM performance between aged and nonaged adult wild-type C57BL/6 mice.

5. Conclusions

In C57BL/6 mice, nest building significantly declined in aged mice relative to nonaged adult mice, with greater declines in male versus female aged mice. Therefore, nest building is useful for detecting age-based and gender-based behavioral decline in C57BL/6 mice. In addition, RAWM results reported here demonstrate that spatial learning and memory significantly declined in aged C57BL/6 mice relative to these capabilities in younger adult mice. However, no significant gender differences were detected by RAWM testing regardless of age. In conclusion, both nest building and RAWM tests are sensitive tests for evaluation of age-related behavioral decline using C57BL/6 mouse animal model. This animal model and behavioral tests described here should be useful to further investigate mechanisms responsible for human age-related memory decline and to evaluate treatments or other ways to maintain aging brain function.

Authors' Contributions

Xiang-Dong Xiong, Wei-Dong Xiong, and Shang-Shen Xiong equally contributed to this work.

Acknowledgments

The authors thank all persons very much who provided help in conducting the study.

References

[1] R. M. J. Deacon, A. Croucher, and J. N. P. Rawlins, "Hippocampal cytotoxic lesion effects on species-typical behaviours in mice," *Behavioural Brain Research*, vol. 132, no. 2, pp. 203–213, 2002.

[2] R. M. J. Deacon, C. Penny, and J. N. P. Rawlins, "Effects of medial prefrontal cortex cytotoxic lesions in mice," *Behavioural Brain Research*, vol. 139, no. 1-2, pp. 139–155, 2003.

[3] K. M. Frick, L. A. Burlingame, J. A. Arters, and J. Berger-Sweeney, "Reference memory, anxiety and estrous cyclicity in C57BL/6NIA mice are affected by age and sex," *Neuroscience*, vol. 95, no. 1, pp. 293–307, 1999.

[4] G. W. Arendash, D. L. King, M. N. Gordon et al., "Progressive, age-related behavioral impairments in transgenic mice carrying both mutant amyloid precursor protein and presenilin-1 transgenes," *Brain Research*, vol. 891, no. 1-2, pp. 42–53, 2001.

[5] D. Morgan, D. M. Diamond, P. E. Gottschall et al., "Aβ peptide vaccination prevents memory loss in an animal model of Alzheimer's disease," *Nature*, vol. 408, no. 6815, pp. 982–985, 2000.

[6] A. L. Markowska, E. L. Spangler, and D. K. Ingram, "Behavioral assessment of the senescence-accelerated mouse (SAM P8 and R1)," *Physiology & Behavior*, vol. 64, no. 1, pp. 15–26, 1998.

[7] C. Andrade, M. Alwarshetty, S. Sudha, and J. Suresh Chandra, "Effect of innate direction bias on T-maze learning in rats: implications for research," *Journal of Neuroscience Methods*, vol. 110, no. 1-2, pp. 31–35, 2001.

[8] X. D. Xiong and G. H. Chen, "Research progress on the age-related changes in proteins of the synaptic active zone," *Physiology & Behavior*, vol. 101, no. 1, pp. 1–12, 2010.

Functional Connectivity Changes in Behavioral, Semantic, and Nonfluent Variants of Frontotemporal Dementia

P. Reyes,[1,2] M. P. Ortega-Merchan,[1] A. Rueda,[3] F. Uriza,[1] Hernando Santamaria-García,[2,4,5] N. Rojas-Serrano,[2] J. Rodriguez-Santos,[2] M. C. Velasco-Leon,[2] J. D. Rodriguez-Parra,[2] D. E. Mora-Diaz,[2] and D. Matallana[2]

[1]*Departamento de Radiología e Imágenes Diagnósticas, Hospital Universitario San Ignacio, Bogotá, Colombia*
[2]*Facultad de Medicina, Pontificia Universidad Javeriana, Bogotá, Colombia*
[3]*Facultad de Ingeniería, Pontificia Universidad Javeriana, Bogotá, Colombia*
[4]*Centro de Memoria y Cognición Intellectus, Hospital Universitario San Ignacio, Bogotá, Colombia*
[5]*Departamento de Psiquiatría, Universidad Nacional de Colombia, Bogotá, Colombia*

Correspondence should be addressed to P. Reyes; reyes.p@javeriana.edu.co

Academic Editor: Luigi Trojano

Frontotemporal dementia (FTD) affects behavior, language, and personality. This study aims to explore functional connectivity changes in three FTD variants: behavioral (bvFTD), semantic (svPPA), and nonfluent variant (nfvPPA). Seventy-six patients diagnosed with FTD by international criteria and thirty-two controls were investigated. Functional connectivity from resting functional magnetic resonance imaging (fMRI) was estimated for the whole brain. Two types of analysis were done: network basic statistic and topological measures by graph theory. Several hubs in the limbic system and basal ganglia were compromised in the behavioral variant apart from frontal networks. Nonfluent variants showed a major disconnection with respect to the behavioral variant in operculum and parietal inferior. The global efficiency had lower coefficients in nonfluent variants than behavioral variants and controls. Our results support an extensive disconnection among frontal, limbic, basal ganglia, and parietal hubs.

1. Introduction

A major objective in current clinical neuroscience research is to find new and more accurate neural footprints to improve the diagnosis and follow the progression of neurodegenerative disorders [1]. Frontotemporal dementia (FTD) is a group of clinically and pathologically heterogeneous diseases [2–4]. It has variants with different kinds of manifestations in behavior, language, metacognition, and personality. This clinical heterogeneity makes it difficult to obtain an accurate diagnosis [5].

FTD has been associated with regional atrophy in the frontal and temporal lobes [6]. It usually appears in the age group 45–64 years [7] with prevalence of 0.01–4.6 per 1000 persons [8]. Moreover, the clinical and genetic features are heterogeneous and there is still no treatment available for these conditions [4]. FTD encompasses three main phenotypes characterized by specific clinical symptoms. The behavioral variant FTD (bvFTD) is characterized by changes in personality [2], alteration in social cognition [9], disinhibition, and apathy. Nonfluent/agrammatic variant primary progressive aphasia (nfvPPA) is characterized by agrammatism and fluency impairment mainly [10]. Patients with the semantic variant (svPPA) have a loss of semantic knowledge and relative preservation of grammatical aspects of language and episodic memory [5]. A clinically similar linguistic variant, differentiated by the etiology, is the logopenic variant of PPA (lvPPA); it is an atypical variant of Alzheimer's disease with anomia, hesitant speech, and alterations in episodic memory [11].

Several biomarkers have been suggested to aid the clinical diagnosis and treatment. Neuroimaging biomarkers have

Table 1: Sociodemographic characteristics.

Group	bvFTD	svPPA	nfvPPA	Controls	p value	Post hoc
Number (n)	50	14	12	32	—	—
Gender (F/M)	17/23	7/7	5/7	12/20	—	—
Age	65.85 (8.1)	60.3 (7.65)	63.63 (6.87)	61.25 (7.28)	0.02	ns
Disease duration (years)	7.27 (5.89)	5.85 (3.15)	4.28 (2.5)	—	—	—
Education (years)	12.92 (4.66)	12.3 (5.85)	11.62 (6.32)	14.4 (5.13)	0.33	ns

ns: no significant difference with Holm-Sidak.

been derived from structural magnetic resonance imaging (MRI), FDG-PET, SPECT, and functional MRI such as the resting state and functional activation imaging [12]. Structural MRI studies have consistently reported frontotemporal atrophy with a relative sparing of posterior cortical areas in bvFTD [13]. Semantic dementia involves a large area of the temporal lobe; nevertheless, there is a marked degeneration in the rostral fusiform gyrus and ventral temporal lobe bilaterally [14, 15]. In nfvPPA, imaging studies showed atrophy mainly involving the left inferior frontal lobe, insula, and premotor cortex [13, 16–18].

Another biomarker of FTD based on neuroimaging is resting-state fMRI [13, 19]. Resting-state fMRI can be used to show functionally connected brain networks by measuring synchronized time-dependent changes in blood oxygenation levels [20]. Prior research reported a reduction in limbic connectivity and the insula, putamen, anterior thalamus, and middle cingulate cortex in svPPA and bvFTD with respect to controls [21]. Another result showed an increased and diffused prefrontal hyperconnectivity, and it was significantly associated with apathy [21]. Longitudinal studies report a functional connectivity decrease over time in bvFTD between the supramarginal gyrus and the right frontoparietal network [22].

Recent studies showed that svPPA has a disrupted functional connectivity between the anterior temporal lobe [23, 24] and a broad range of regions including primary cortices (sulcus, Heschl's gyrus, precentral and postcentral gyri, and dorsal posterior insula (primary interoceptive cortex)) and auditory and visual association regions [25]. Both svPPA and bvFTD patients show a reduced functional connectivity in limbic areas of the executive network. However, svPPA patients also exhibit a reduced functional connectivity in the bilateral lateral prefrontal cortex and anterior cingulate [21]. In nfvPPA, previous studies have demonstrated compelling evidence that motor speech and grammatical deficits are associated with deficits in the left frontoinsular-striatal structures involved in speech production, a finding related to a reduced activation of a ventral portion of the left inferior cortex during attempts to understand grammatically challenging aspects of a sentence [26–29]. One study with resting-state fMRI analysis in nfvPPA showed connectivity changes in three subnetworks, namely, (a) the left inferior frontal gyrus and the left supplementary motor area, (b) inferior and superior parietal gyri between both hemispheres, and (c) striatum with the supplementary motor area in both hemispheres [30].

The functional connectivity among frontotemporal subvariants has been explored in a few studies. In the literature, usually, there are comparisons between controls and patients with bvFTD or with Alzheimer's disease [21, 31]. This study attempts to describe the alterations in functional connectivity networks among frontotemporal dementia variants to find specific connectivity alteration in each variant. First, we compared the functional connectivity of the whole brain among the variants. Second, topologic measures such as global efficiency, degree, path length, and clustering from each patient and between variants were compared.

2. Methods

2.1. Participants. Seventy-six patients with FTD were selected from Hospital Universitario San Ignacio including thirty-two healthy controls. The FTD diagnosis was initially made by a group of experts, and each case was individually reviewed at a multidisciplinary clinical meeting (neurologist, neuropsychologist, psychiatrist, and geriatrician). The sample included 50 patients with bvFTD, 14 with svPPA, and 22 with nfvPPA diagnosis. Patients were diagnosed with bvFTD based on recent guidelines [3]. These patients showed prominent changes in personality and social behavior as verified by a caregiver during their initial assessment. svPPA diagnosis were done based on international guidelines [18], and these patients included here had important semantic failures. Patients with nfvPPA have an evaluation by an expert in linguistic, and diagnosis was done based on international guidelines [11].

Control subjects were matched with bvFTD, svPPA, and nfvPPA patients (see Table 1). Matching criteria were gender, age, and years of education. An analysis of variance with Holm-Sidak's multiple comparison test did not show differences among groups to age and years of education. Subjects were recruited from a larger pool of volunteers who did not have a neurodegenerative disease diagnosis or psychiatric disorders. All the participants provided written informed consent in accordance with the institutional review board of the Hospital Universitario San Ignacio and Pontificia Universidad Javeriana.

2.2. Cognitive and Behavioral Assessment. Neuropsychological evaluation was performed in patients and controls. The test battery included screening tests, Montreal Cognitive Assessment (MoCA) [32, 33], mini-mental state examination

(MMSE), and INECO Frontal Screening (IFS) test [34]. Verbal inhibitory control was measured by Hayling test [35]. We used Wisconsin Card Sorting Test (WCST) modified to evaluate executive functions [36]. Rey-Osterrieth complex figure (ROCF) test was employed to assess visuomotor skills [37]. Frontal system behavior scale (FrSBe) [38] was used to measure behavioral changes. This test had two sections investigating premorbid or current behavior. Apathy, inhibition, and dysexecutive function subscales were estimated by FrSBe.

Verbal and design fluency tests were used to assess recall, self-monitoring and cognitive flexibility strategies, phonological (words with P and M), and semantic fluency (animals and fruits) [39]. Finally, proverbs test [40] was used to assess verbal comprehension.

2.3. Image Acquisition. Images from patients with FTD and controls were obtained using a Philips Achieva 3T scanner with a 16-channel SENSE coil. The anatomical and 3D T1-weighted images had the following parameters: TR = 7.9 ms, TE = 3.8 ms, acquisition matrix = 220 × 220, voxel size = 0.5 × 0.5 × 0.5 mm, and 310 slices, and these images were resliced to 1 × 1 × 1 mm. The blood oxygenation-dependent sequences of the entire brain were acquired in 25 axial slices by using an echoplanar imaging sequence TR = 2000, TE = 30 ms, and voxel size = 2.3. The fMRI lasted 6 minutes and the instruction to the patient was to keep their open eyes.

2.4. Data Analysis

2.4.1. Behavioral Analysis. Demographic information and scores from clinical tests were compared among groups with ANOVA tests and post hoc test for multiple comparisons and correction of p values by Sidak.

2.4.2. Processing and Analysis. Preprocessing was performed with a combination of the Statistical Parametric Mapping [39] software (http://www.fil.ion.ucl.ac.uk/spm/software/spm12/) (Wellcome Department of Cognitive Neurology, University College London, UK), the Resting-State fMRI Data Analysis Toolkit (REST) version 1.8 (http://www.restfmri.net) [40], and Data Processing Assistant for Resting-State fMRI (DPABI) version 2.1 (http://rfmri.org/DPABI).

2.4.3. Resting-State Preprocessing. The main preprocessing procedure was done with DPABI [41], and the pipeline was (1) removal of the first 10 time points, (2) slice timing, (3) head motion correction, (4) nonlinear registration of the high-resolution T1 structural images to the Montreal Neurological Institute (MNI) template, in which T1 structural images were segmented as white matter, gray matter, and cerebrospinal fluid using a new segment algorithm with DARTEL (diffeomorphic anatomical registration through exponentiated lie algebra), (5) smoothing with a 6 mm full-width-half-maximum Gaussian kernel, (6) removal of the linear trend of the time series, (7) temporal band-pass filtering (0.01–0.08 Hz) to decrease the effects of low-frequency drifts and high-frequency noise, and (8) linear detrending and nuisance signal removal, white matter, cerebrospinal fluid, global signal, 6-head motion parameters, 6-head motion parameters at one time point earlier, and the 12 corresponding squared items (Friston 24-parameter model as covariates) via multiple regression. The general pipeline was reported in another research [19].

2.4.4. Seed-Based Analysis. The functional connectivity was estimated with a seed-based analysis. Regions of interest (ROIs) or seeds were selected according to automated anatomical labeling (AAL) atlas [42]. The diameter of the sphere ROI was 10 mm (approximately 27 cubic voxels). The seed analysis only included the brain. Pearson correlation coefficients were calculated between the mean time course of the ROI and the time courses for all other brain voxels. Fisher's z transform analysis was applied to the Pearson correlation coefficients to obtain an approximate normal distribution to enable the subsequent statistical analysis.

2.4.5. Network-Based Analysis. Global differences in interconnected network components between patients and controls were examined with an F-test by network-based statistics (NBS) [43] based on 10,000 permutations. The p value threshold was set at 0.01 and it was corrected by family-wise error (FWE). Contrasts between groups were bvFTD versus controls, nfvPPA + svPPA versus controls, and bvFTD versus nfvPPA + svPPA.

2.4.6. Graph Theory Analysis. In a secondary analysis, the connectivity metrics such as path length, degree, cluster, and global efficiency were estimated by the Brain Connectivity Toolbox [44]. The correlation between ROIs was graphically represented by a collection of nodes and edges (nodes represent anatomical elements like brain regions and the edges represent the connectivity between those regions). In these graphs, the degree represents the number of edges connected to a node. A cluster is an extension of local interconnectivity. The path length is the number of edges that connect a node with another node, and global efficiency measures the ability of a network to transmit information at a global level. Network centrality (NC) measures the numbers of the shortest paths that go through a node and link the other node pairs across the network [45]. It indicates the importance of a node for efficient communication and integration across a network [45]. Several studies have already used NC (also called "betweenness centrality") to identify changed connections in disconnection syndromes [31, 46, 47]. Finally, an analysis of variance between groups with connectivity metrics was used to evaluate differences among groups.

3. Results

An analysis of variance (ANOVA) on MOCA, MMSE, ROFC, semantic and phonological and fluency, and proverb scores yielded significant variation among groups ($p < 0.05$ in all cases) (see Table 2). There were no differences among variants (bvFTD, svPPA, and nfvPPA) on FrSBe before or currently ($p > 0.05$ in all cases). A post hoc test with Sidak

Table 2: Clinical findings in patients and healthy controls.

	Controls	nfvPPA	svPPA	bvFTD	p value	Post hoc
MOCA	26.32 (2.57)	8.73 (7.26)	8.8 (6.58)	15.61 (7.53)	<0.001	1, 2, 3
MMSE	28.86 (1.27)	16.9 (6.92)	16.67 (7.66)	22.47 (6.5)	<0.001	1, 2, 3
IFS	22.3 (3.37)	6.20 (6.06)	10.8 (6.94)	10.7 (6.76)	<0.001	1, 2
Hayling	—	22.1 (11.09)	18 (13.52)	24.19 (12.66)	0.607	—
Errors WSCT	10.64 (8.14)	28 (7.77)	29.63 (8.88)	21.5 (10.18)	<0.001	1
ROFC	32.66 (5.05)	17.2 (11.86)	27.89 (9.35)	20.79 (12.26)	<0.001	1
FrSBe before	—	77.13 (18.63)	74.91 (29.39)	71.67 (18.79)	0.136	—
FrSBe currently	—	121.47 (32.22)	130.73 (42.66)	129.15 (31.65)	0.449	—
FrSBe apathy before	—	21.69 (4.92)	21 (10.28)	21.14 (7.57)	0.969	—
FrSBe apathy currently	—	46.46 (11.44)	46.55 (16.9)	44 (12.46)	0.76	—
FrSBe inhibition before	—	23.15 (5.68)	22.55 (9.17)	20.65 (5.36)	0.391	—
FrSBe inhibition currently	—	28.54 (7.66)	31.18 (10.05)	32.46 (11.46)	0.516	—
FrSBe DE before	—	32.08 (11.95)	31.27 (13.14)	29.38 (9.62)	0.702	—
FrSBe DE currently	—	50.92 (16.09)	52.55 (17.31)	53.95 (15.28)	0.833	—
Semantic fluency	16.68 (3.58)	5.91 (2.86)	4.20 (3.47)	10.45 (5.26)	<0.001	1, 2, 3
Phonological fluency	14.93 (5.05)	4.69 (3.31)	3.83 (2.79)	9.75 (5.47)	<0.001	1, 2, 3
Proverbs	8.54 (2.05)	2.53 (3.06)	1.4 (2.37)	4.09 (3.49)	<0.001	1

Mean and standard deviation were reported. p value from ANOVA. FrSBe DE: FrSBe dysfunction executive; nfvPPA: primary nonfluent aphasia; svPPA: semantic dementia; BV: behavioral variant; post hoc with Holm-Sidak (<0.05); 1: controls ≠ (bvFTD or svPPA or nfvPPA); 2: bvFTD ≠ nfvPPA; 3: bvFTD ≠ svPPA; 4: svPPA ≠ nfvPPA.

correction showed higher scores in bvFTD than nfvPPA and svPPA on MOCA, semantic, and phonological fluency ($p < 0.05$ in all cases). Besides, the scores on MMSE and IFS were significantly higher in bvFTD with respect to nfvPPA ($p < 0.05$ in all cases). There were no differences among variants on Hayling, FrSBe, errors in WSCT, ROFC, and proverbs.

The results with network-based statistics showed significant differences between the control group and bvFTD, svPPA, nfvPPA, and svPPA + nfvPPA groups. The first comparison between control and bvFTD (Figure 1(a)) showed significant differences in networks with nodes mainly in the left hemisphere in the frontal and temporal lobes (Table S1). Almost 15 nodes located in the left hemisphere in different regions (anterior and posterior) had a higher disconnection than controls. Moreover, in the right hemisphere, the nodes disconnected were anterior cingulate cortex, inferior temporal gyrus, superior occipital gyrus, middle temporal gyrus, putamen, amygdala, inferior frontal triangular gyrus, and fusiform gyrus.

With respect to results with linguistic variants, there were more differences in nfvPPA than svPPA. The comparison between control and svPPA groups showed only connectivity differences between the right operculum and the left putamen (Figure 1(b) and Table S2). The analysis between control and nfvPPA showed differences mainly in the left hemisphere (Figure 1(c) and Table S3). The nodes with disconnection were the inferior temporal gyrus, fusiform gyrus, amygdala, operculum, temporo-parieto-occipital junction, caudate nuclei, inferior parietal gyrus, putamen, and insula. Also, in the right hemisphere, there were nodes disconnected such as the anterior cingulate and the putamen.

The analysis between FTD variants showed differences between bvFTD and nfvPPA into the left hemisphere to the connection between operculum with parietal and cuneus left with occipital superior gyrus (Figure 2(a)). There were no differences between controls and svPPA patients. The comparison between bvFTD and all patients with linguistic alterations showed a disconnection of the left superior occipital, left middle occipital, and right middle temporal gyri (Figure 2(b)). Finally, the comparison between controls and all linguistic variants (Figure 2(c)) showed a major disconnection in Heschl's left gyrus, left amygdala, left fusiform, left inferior temporal gyrus, right middle temporal gyrus, and left temporal pole (Table S4).

An analysis of variance based on topological metrics showed differences in global efficiency ($F(3, 65) = 11.48$, $p < 0.001$) and path length ($F(3, 65) = 3.27$, $p = 0.026$) (Figure 3). In the post hoc test, the global efficiency in bvFTD was significantly higher than nfvPPA; in addition, this measure was higher in controls than nfvPPA patients ($p < 0.05$ in both cases). Finally, we computed Pearson correlations, with correction for multiple correlational analysis [48], between topological metrics and clinical scores in all patients (Figure 4). We found significant associations of topological measures with FrSBe scores related to current behavior. The path length had significant and negative correlations with total FrSBe ($r = -0.27$), apathy ($r = -0.3$), and inhibition ($r = -0.34$). The clustering had significant and positive correlations with total FrSBe ($r = 0.33$), apathy ($r = 0.3$), and inhibition ($r = 0.41$). Also, the degree had similar correlations with total FrSBe ($r = 0.32$), apathy ($r = 0.31$), and inhibition ($r = 0.4$). Finally, the global efficiency had positive correlations with total FrSBe ($r = 0.33$), apathy ($r = 0.31$), and inhibition ($r = 0.42$).

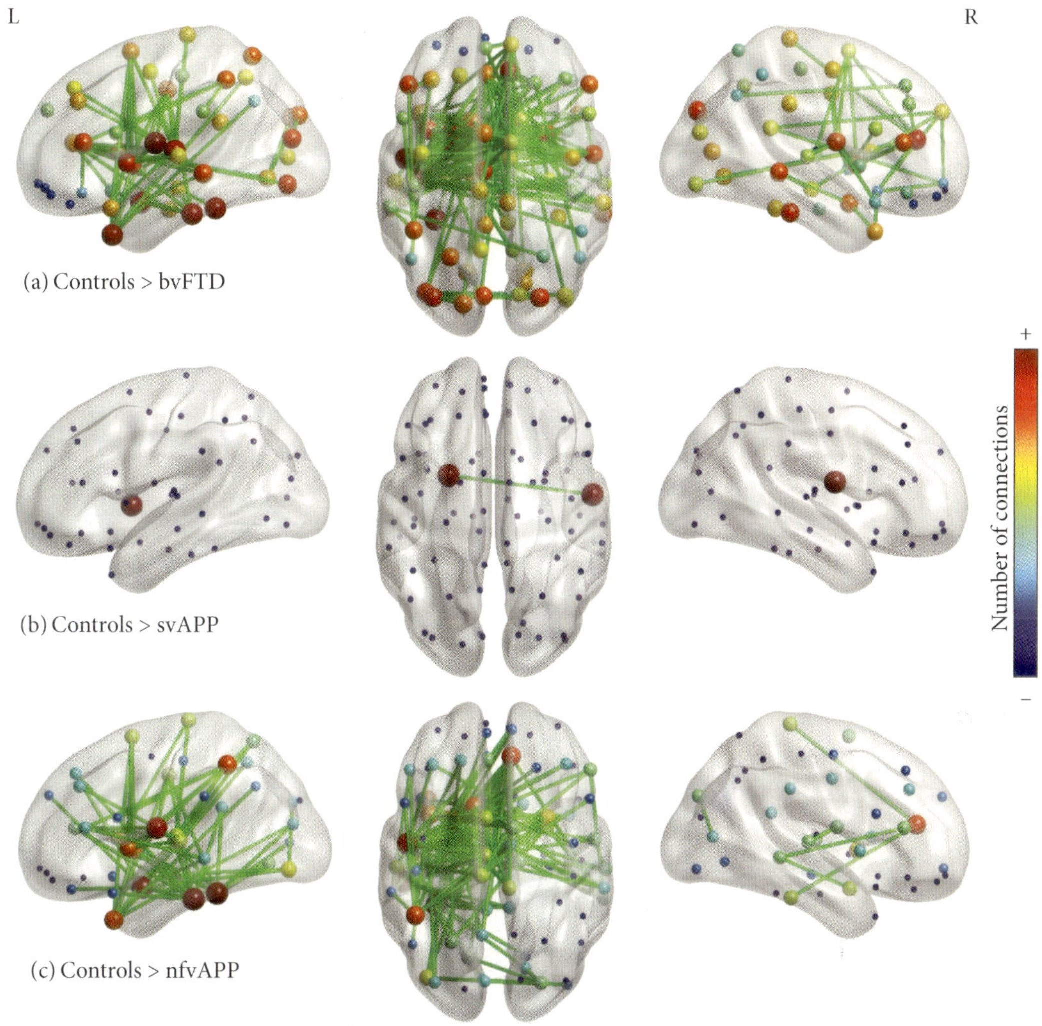

FIGURE 1: NBS results between controls and FTD variants. The edges are the result of F-test between groups. To nodes, the color corresponds to disconnection number.

3.1. Discussion. The study on connectivity based on resting-state functional MRI has the potential to identify differences among variants of FTD. The present study offers some contributions to understand the alterations in connectivity based on changes in networks and topological metrics. The approach based on network analysis showed more accuracy to detect differences than topological metrics of the whole brain with weighted matrices.

In this study, the bvFTD has a bilateral disconnection with a major tendency to nodes into the left hemisphere. Asymmetric results were reported in other studies, for example, a decrease in connectivity in the left frontoparietal network in bvFTD has been reported in comparison with controls [22]. Also, a decrease in connectivity between the right superior temporal gyrus and cuneal cortex was showed in bvFTD with respect to Alzheimer's disease [49]. Our results showed an extended bilateral disconnection between the frontal and limbic areas and the basal ganglia. A decrease between the frontal and limbic hubs was reported in another study [21]; this alteration could be associated with the disruption between affective and self-referential brain systems [21]. Also, the present results show alterations in the cingulum and insula network bilaterally. The cingulum has been associated with motivation and behavior control [50]. The anterior insula is a network hub to human emotional awareness and behavioral guidance networks [51]. Finally, in this report, the analysis supports alteration in posterior nodes in bvFTD, namely, there were disconnections in the middle occipital, inferior, and middle temporal gyri. Alterations in posterior regions in FTD are not frequent but have been reported previously [52].

The results support a connectivity decrease in linguistic variants in comparison with controls. The number of disconnected nodes was higher in nfvPPA than svPPA. In svPPA, the disconnection in the network between putamen and operculum has not been reported previously. However, one study reported atrophy in the putamen in svPPA [53], and the operculum has been associated with phonological processes that support reading [54]. In nfvPPA, a disconnection was found in networks involving hubs such as prerolandic

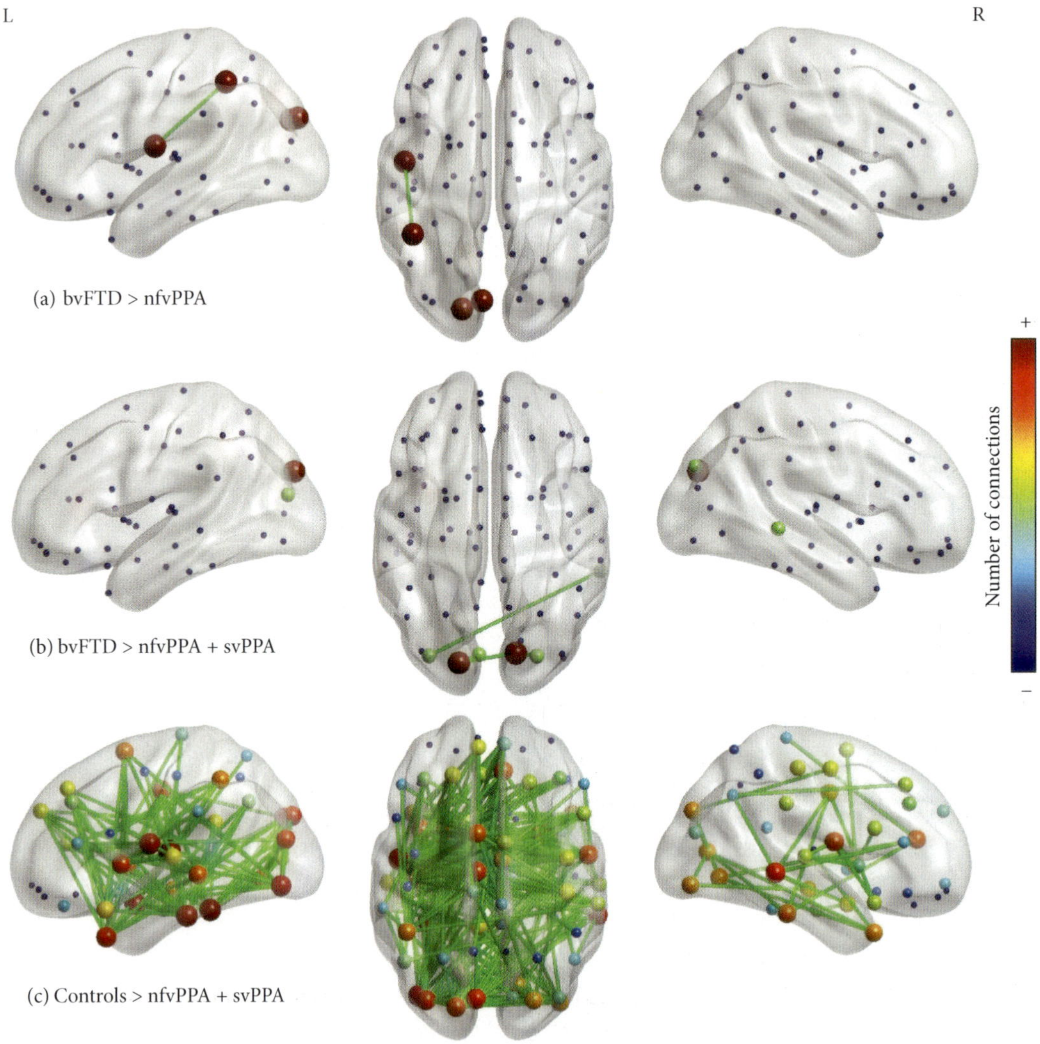

FIGURE 2: NBS results between FTD variants and controls.

areas and basal ganglia, regions related with speech production and syntactic process [55–57]. The topological metrics, global efficiency, and path length were useful to discriminate linguistic variants since global efficiency allows a differentiation between nfvPPA and bvFTD while path length differentiates svPPA and controls. Similar results were reported in a recent study; the path length in svPPA was higher in comparison with controls and similar to Alzheimer's disease patients, and it was correlated with the disease progression [58].

There was similarity among FTD variants in both clinical and neuroimaging analyses. Also, in this study, there were no differences between the linguistic variants (svPPA and nfvPPA). Nevertheless, nfvPPA was the variant with more differences than svPPA, both as the network analysis as topological metrics with respect to bvFTD. nfvPPA showed a worse measure in global efficiency and tends to have more degree and clustering than svPPA and bvFTD.

The behavioral changes measured by FrSBe did not show differences among variants. This result could indicate the presence of behavioral disturbances between linguistic variants and can support the presence of frontal alterations in nfvPPA and bvFTD. All patients had important behavioral changes in FrSBe scores related to premorbid and current behavior. However, only the current scores in apathy and inhibition (FrSBE subscales) were associated with topological measures. Therefore, global changes in functional connectivity could be associated with the presence of disturbances in behavior at least in these variants. The behavioral disturbances have been more reported in svPPA than nfvPPA [59–61]. Only one study reported behavioral changes in nfvPPA, and these behavioral changes were similar to Alzheimer's disease [62].

The limitations of this study are related to sample size, use of topological metrics from weighted matrices, and AAL atlas to create the seeds. The reduced sample size of nfvPPA was due to requirement of a second evaluation by an expert in order to exclude lvPPA. According to several reports, lvPPA is associated with the Alzheimer's variant [63–65]. With respect to topological metrics, these correspond to general

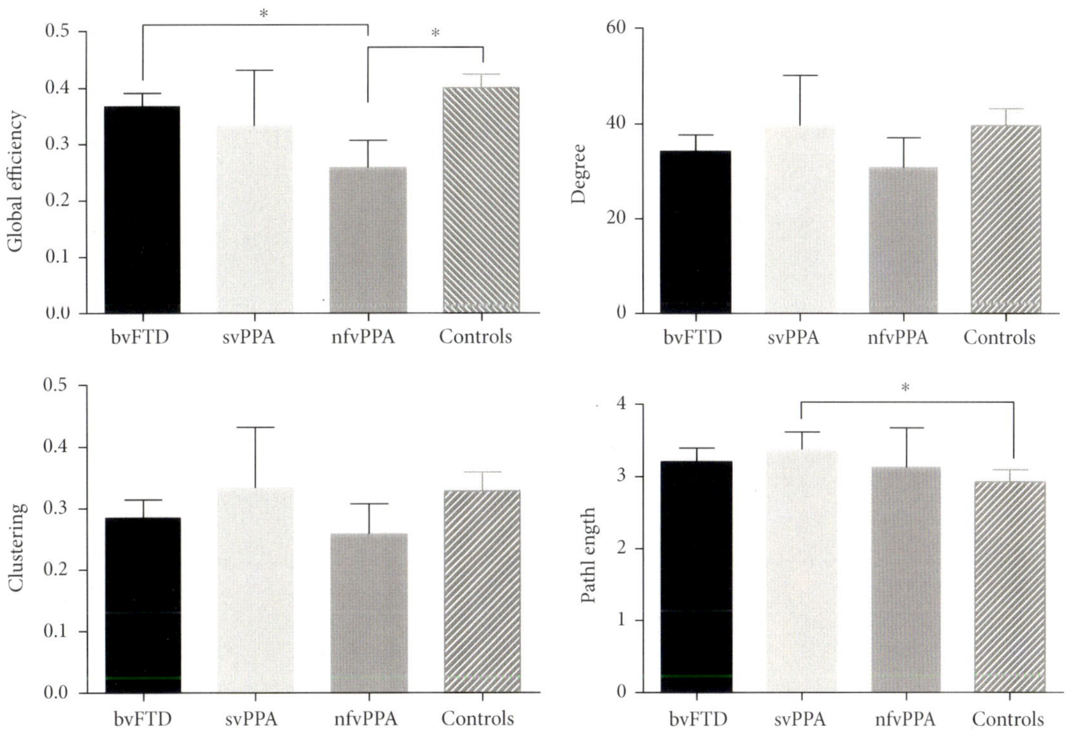

Figure 3: Mean bar of metrics from graph theory analysis by each group (global efficiency, degree, clustering, and path length). The bar represents the mean and error bars are a 95% confidence interval. *Significantly different with $p < 0.05$.

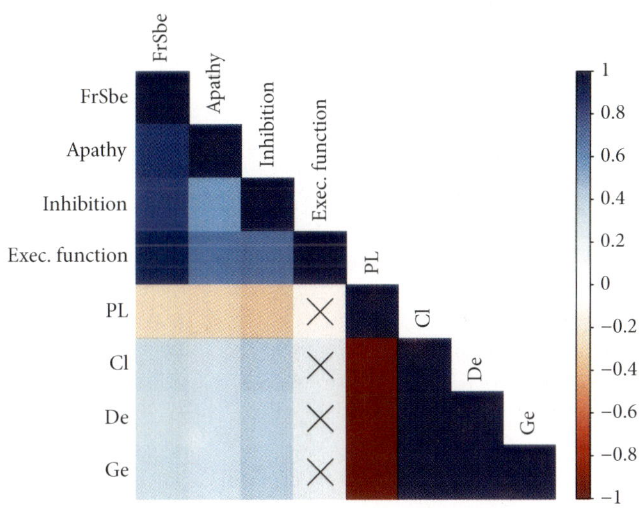

Figure 4: Matrix correlation among topological measures and clinical scores. The bar color indicates the Pearson value coefficient. Symbol X indicates p values > 0.05 with BH correction; FrSBE: total FrSBE currently; apathy: FrSBE apathy currently; inhibition: FrSBE inhibition currently; Exec. function: FrSBE dysexecutive functions currently; PL: path length; Cl: clustering; De: degree; Ge: global efficiency.

measures from graph theory [44]. Both acquisition and image preprocessing could affect the analysis and measures. However, there is no gold standard method and applied protocols similar to those used in previous studies [66]. Finally, some studies show a scale effect in graph analysis related to the number of nodes [67–69], but we used AAL standard atlas to make our results comparable with those from other studies.

In conclusion, our result supports the use of global metrics from graph theory and network analysis to explore differences among some FTD variants. The nfvPPA showed more alterations in networks and global metrics than other variants, and also, alterations in bvFTD involve hubs in frontal lobes, limbic lobes, and basal ganglia. However, there are no differences between svPPA and nfvPPA in either NBS or topological measures. This preliminary study among variants in FTD allows us to identify several hubs and networks, and these can be used in the future to build biomarkers based on fMRI. Finally, the functional connectivity was associated with disturbances in behavior. New studies should explore the association among different biomarkers from multimodal neuroimaging, such as structural and functional connectivity, in order to obtain increased accuracy about networks with changes or alterations due to early onset dementia.

Acknowledgments

The authors want to thank the patients, their families, and healthy controls, as well as the research center of memory and cognition in Hospital Universitario San Ignacio and Pontificia Universidad Javeriana. This research was partially supported by a COLCIENCIAS grant (697-2014). P. Reyes also received a scholarship grant from Hospital Universitario San Ignacio.

References

[1] A. Horn, D. Ostwald, M. Reisert, and F. Blankenburg, "The structural-functional connectome and the default mode network of the human brain," *NeuroImage*, vol. 102, Part 1, pp. 142–151, 2014.

[2] D. Neary, J. S. Snowden, L. Gustafson et al., "Frontotemporal lobar degeneration: a consensus on clinical diagnostic criteria," *Neurology*, vol. 51, no. 6, pp. 1546–1554, 1998.

[3] K. Rascovsky, J. R. Hodges, C. M. Kipps et al., "Diagnostic criteria for the behavioral variant of frontotemporal dementia (bvFTD): current limitations and future directions," *Alzheimer Disease & Associated Disorders*, vol. 21, no. 4, pp. S14–S18, 2007.

[4] S. Gazzina, M. A. Manes, A. Padovani, and B. Borroni, "Clinical and biological phenotypes of frontotemporal dementia: perspectives for disease modifying therapies," *European Journal of Pharmacology*, vol. 817, pp. 76–85, 2017.

[5] J. S. Snowden, D. Bathgate, A. Varma, A. Blackshaw, Z. C. Gibbons, and D. Neary, "Distinct behavioural profiles in frontotemporal dementia and semantic dementia," *Journal of Neurology, Neurosurgery & Psychiatry*, vol. 70, no. 3, pp. 323–332, 2001.

[6] M. Boccardi, M. P. Laakso, L. Bresciani et al., "The MRI pattern of frontal and temporal brain atrophy in fronto-temporal dementia," *Neurobiology of Aging*, vol. 24, no. 1, pp. 95–103, 2003.

[7] C. U. Onyike and J. Diehl-Schmid, "The epidemiology of frontotemporal dementia," *International Review of Psychiatry*, vol. 25, no. 2, pp. 130–137, 2013.

[8] D. B. Hogan, N. Jetté, K. M. Fiest et al., "The prevalence and incidence of frontotemporal dementia: a systematic review," *The Canadian Journal of Neurological Sciences*, vol. 43, Supplement 1, pp. S96–S109, 2016.

[9] H. Santamaría García, P. Reyes, J. Santacruz, S. Baez, A. Ibañez, and D. Matallana, "Clinical, neuropsychological and neural correlates underlying the first symptoms in behavioral variant of fronto temporal dementia (bvFTD)," *Journal of the Neurological Sciences*, vol. 357, Supplement 1, pp. e12–e13, 2015.

[10] M. L. Gorno-Tempini and S. M. Brambati, "The logopenic/phonologic variant of primary progressive aphasia," *AAN Enterprise*, vol. 2008, pp. 1227–1234, 2016.

[11] F. M. Elahi and B. L. Miller, "A clinicopathological approach to the diagnosis of dementia," *Nature Reviews Neurology*, vol. 13, no. 8, pp. 457–476, 2017.

[12] N. Sheikh-Bahaei, S. A. Sajjadi, and A. L. Pierce, "Current role for biomarkers in clinical diagnosis of Alzheimer disease and frontotemporal dementia," *Current Treatment Options in Neurology*, vol. 19, no. 12, p. 46, 2017.

[13] J. D. Rohrer and H. J. Rosen, "Neuroimaging in frontotemporal dementia," *International Review of Psychiatry*, vol. 25, no. 2, pp. 221–229, 2013.

[14] H. Botha, J. R. Duffy, J. L. Whitwell et al., "Classification and clinicoradiologic features of primary progressive aphasia (PPA) and apraxia of speech," *Cortex*, vol. 69, pp. 220–236, 2015.

[15] C. J. Mummery, K. Patterson, C. J. Price, J. Ashburner, R. S. J. Frackowiak, and J. R. Hodges, "A voxel-based morphometry study of semantic dementia: relationship between temporal lobe atrophy and semantic memory," *Annals of Neurology*, vol. 47, no. 1, pp. 36–45, 2000.

[16] K. A. Josephs, J. R. Hodges, J. S. Snowden et al., "Neuropathological background of phenotypical variability in frontotemporal dementia," *Acta Neuropathologica*, vol. 122, no. 2, pp. 137–153, 2011.

[17] M. Catani, M. M. Mesulam, E. Jakobsen et al., "A novel frontal pathway underlies verbal fluency in primary progressive aphasia," *Brain*, vol. 136, no. 8, pp. 2619–2628, 2013.

[18] M. L. Gorno-Tempini, A. E. Hillis, S. Weintraub et al., "Classification of primary progressive aphasia and its variants," *Neurology*, vol. 76, no. 11, pp. 1006–1014, 2011.

[19] L. Sedeño, O. Piguet, S. Abrevaya et al., "Tackling variability: a multicenter study to provide a gold-standard network approach for frontotemporal dementia," *Human Brain Mapping*, vol. 38, no. 8, pp. 3804–3822, 2017.

[20] E. Gordon, J. D. Rohrer, and N. C. Fox, "Advances in neuroimaging in frontotemporal dementia," *Journal of Neurochemistry*, vol. 138, pp. 193–210, 2016.

[21] N. A. S. Farb, C. L. Grady, S. Strother et al., "Abnormal network connectivity in frontotemporal dementia: evidence for prefrontal isolation," *Cortex*, vol. 49, no. 7, pp. 1856–1873, 2013.

[22] A. Hafkemeijer, C. Möller, E. G. P. Dopper et al., "A longitudinal study on resting state functional connectivity in behavioral variant frontotemporal dementia and Alzheimer's disease," *Journal of Alzheimer's Disease*, vol. 55, no. 2, pp. 521–537, 2017.

[23] R. Landin-Romero, R. Tan, J. R. Hodges, and F. Kumfor, "An update on semantic dementia: genetics, imaging, and pathology," *Alzheimer's Research & Therapy*, vol. 8, no. 1, p. 52, 2016.

[24] Q. Yang, Q. H. Guo, and Y. C. Bi, "The brain connectivity basis of semantic dementia: a selective review," *CNS Neuroscience & Therapeutics*, vol. 21, no. 10, pp. 784–792, 2015.

[25] C. C. Guo, M. L. Gorno-Tempini, B. Gesierich et al., "Anterior temporal lobe degeneration produces widespread network-driven dysfunction," *Brain*, vol. 136, no. 10, pp. 2979–2991, 2013.

[26] J. E. Peelle, A. Cooke, P. Moore, L. Vesely, and M. Grossman, "Syntactic and thematic components of sentence processing in progressive nonfluent aphasia and nonaphasic frontotemporal dementia," *Journal of Neurolinguistics*, vol. 20, no. 6, pp. 482–494, 2007.

[27] A. Cooke, C. DeVita, J. Gee et al., "Neural basis for sentence comprehension deficits in frontotemporal dementia," *Brain and Language*, vol. 85, no. 2, pp. 211–221, 2003.

[28] K. G. Ranasinghe, L. B. Hinkley, A. J. Beagle et al., "Distinct spatiotemporal patterns of neuronal functional connectivity in primary progressive aphasia variants," *Brain*, vol. 140, no. 10, pp. 2737–2751, 2017.

[29] M. L. Mandelli, E. Caverzasi, R. J. Binney et al., "Frontal white matter tracts sustaining speech production in primary progressive aphasia," *The Journal of Neuroscience*, vol. 34, no. 29, pp. 9754–9767, 2014.

[30] M. L. Mandelli, E. Vilaplana, J. A. Brown et al., "Healthy brain connectivity predicts atrophy progression in non-fluent variant of primary progressive aphasia," *Brain*, vol. 139, no. 10, pp. 2778–2791, 2016.

[31] M. Filippi, F. Agosta, E. Scola et al., "Functional network connectivity in the behavioral variant of frontotemporal dementia," *Cortex*, vol. 49, no. 9, pp. 2389–2401, 2013.

[32] L. Gil, C. Ruiz De Sánchez, F. Gil, S. J. Romero, and F. Pretelt Burgos, "Validation of the Montreal Cognitive Assessment (MoCA) in Spanish as a screening tool for mild cognitive impairment and mild dementia in patients over 65 years old in Bogotá, Colombia," *International Journal of Geriatric Psychiatry*, vol. 30, no. 6, pp. 655–662, 2015.

[33] Z. S. Nasreddine, N. A. Phillips, V. Bédirian et al., "The Montreal Cognitive Assessment, MoCA: a brief screening tool for mild cognitive impairment," *Journal of the American Geriatrics Society*, vol. 53, no. 4, pp. 695–699, 2005.

[34] T. Torralva, M. Roca, E. Gleichgerrcht, P. López, and F. Manes, "INECO frontal screening (IFS): a brief, sensitive, and specific tool to assess executive functions in dementia," *Journal of the International Neuropsychological Society*, vol. 15, no. 5, p. 777, 2009.

[35] P. W. Burgess and T. Shallice, "Response suppression, initiation and strategy use following frontal lobe lesions," *Neuropsychologia*, vol. 34, no. 4, pp. 263–272, 1996.

[36] H. E. Nelson, "A modified card sorting test sensitive to frontal lobe defects," *Cortex*, vol. 12, no. 4, pp. 313–324, 1976.

[37] P.-A. Osterrieth, "Le test de copie d'une figure complexe; contribution à l'étude de la perception et de la mémoire [Test of copying a complex figure; contribution to the study of perception and memory]," *Archives de Psychologie*, vol. 30, pp. 206–356, 1944.

[38] J. P. Niemeier, P. B. Perrin, M. G. Holcomb, K. S. Nersessova, and C. D. Rolston, "Factor structure, reliability, and validity of the frontal systems behavior scale (FrSBe) in an acute traumatic brain injury population," *Rehabilitation Psychology*, vol. 58, no. 1, pp. 51–63, 2013.

[39] M. M. Benito-Cuadrado, S. Esteba-Castillo, P. Böhm, J. Cejudo-Bolívar, and J. Peña-Casanova, "Semantic verbal fluency of animals: a normative and predictive study in a Spanish population," *Journal of Clinical and Experimental Neuropsychology*, vol. 24, no. 8, pp. 1117–1122, 2002.

[40] S. J. Báez, L. Mendoza, P. Reyes, D. Matallana, and P. Montañés, "Interpretación de refranes y enfermedad de Alzheimer," *Revista de Neurologia*, vol. 49, no. 11, pp. 566–572, 2009.

[41] C. G. Yan, X.-D. Wang, X. N. Zuo, and Y. F. Zang, "DPABI: data processing & analysis for (resting-state) brain imaging," *Neuroinformatics*, vol. 14, no. 3, pp. 339–351, 2016.

[42] N. Tzourio-Mazoyer, B. Landeau, D. Papathanassiou et al., "Automated anatomical labeling of activations in SPM using a macroscopic anatomical parcellation of the MNI MRI single-subject brain," *NeuroImage*, vol. 15, no. 1, pp. 273–289, 2002.

[43] A. Zalesky, A. Fornito, and E. T. Bullmore, "Network based statistic: identifying differences in brain networks," *NeuroImage*, vol. 53, no. 4, pp. 1197–1207, 2010.

[44] M. Rubinov and O. Sporns, "Complex network measures of brain connectivity: uses and interpretations," *NeuroImage*, vol. 52, no. 3, pp. 1059–1069, 2010.

[45] L. C. Freeman, "A set of measures of centrality based on betweenness," *Sociometry*, vol. 40, no. 1, p. 35, 1977.

[46] R. L. Buckner, J. Sepulcre, T. Talukdar et al., "Cortical hubs revealed by intrinsic functional connectivity: mapping, assessment of stability, and relation to Alzheimer's disease," *The Journal of Neuroscience*, vol. 29, no. 6, pp. 1860–1873, 2009.

[47] C. J. Goch, B. Stieltjes, R. Henze et al., "Quantification of changes in language-related brain areas in autism spectrum disorders using large-scale network analysis," *International Journal of Computer Assisted Radiology and Surgery*, vol. 9, no. 3, pp. 357–365, 2014.

[48] Y. Benjamini and Y. Hochberg, "Controlling the false discovery rate: a practical and powerful approach to multiple testing," *Journal of the Royal Statistical Society Series B (Methodological)*, vol. 57, pp. 289–300, 1995.

[49] A. Hafkemeijer, C. Möller, E. G. P. Dopper et al., "Resting state functional connectivity differences between behavioral variant frontotemporal dementia and Alzheimer's disease," *Frontiers in Human Neuroscience*, vol. 9, p. 474, 2015.

[50] M. Hoffmann, "The human frontal lobes and frontal network systems: an evolutionary, clinical, and treatment perspective," *ISRN Neurology*, vol. 2013, Article ID 892459, 34 pages, 2013.

[51] W. W. Seeley, "Anterior insula degeneration in frontotemporal dementia," *Brain Structure and Function*, vol. 214, no. 5-6, pp. 465–475, 2010.

[52] J. D. Rohrer, J. D. Warren, M. Modat et al., "Patterns of cortical thinning in the language variants of frontotemporal lobar degeneration," *Neurology*, vol. 72, no. 18, pp. 1562–1569, 2009.

[53] R. R. Davies, G. M. Halliday, J. H. Xuereb, J. J. Kril, and J. R. Hodges, "The neural basis of semantic memory: evidence from semantic dementia," *Neurobiology of Aging*, vol. 30, no. 12, pp. 2043–2052, 2009.

[54] J. A. Fiez, D. Tranel, D. Seager-Frerichs, and H. Damasio, "Specific reading and phonological processing deficits are associated with damage to the left frontal operculum," *Cortex*, vol. 42, no. 4, pp. 624–643, 2006.

[55] K. A. Josephs, J. R. Duffy, T. R. Fossett et al., "Fluorodeoxyglucose F18 positron emission tomography in progressive apraxia of speech and primary progressive aphasia variants," *Archives of Neurology*, vol. 67, no. 5, pp. 596–605, 2010.

[56] J. R. Booth, L. Wood, D. Lu, J. C. Houk, and T. Bitan, "The role of the basal ganglia and cerebellum in language processing," *Brain Research*, vol. 1133, no. 1, pp. 136–144, 2007.

[57] S. A. Kotz, S. Frisch, D. Y. von Cramon, and A. D. Friederici, "Syntactic language processing: ERP lesion data on the role of the basal ganglia," *Journal of the International Neuropsychological Society*, vol. 9, no. 7, pp. 1053–1060, 2003.

[58] J. Andreotti, T. Dierks, L. O. Wahlund, and M. Grieder, "Diverging progression of network disruption and atrophy in Alzheimer's disease and semantic dementia," *Journal of Alzheimer's Disease*, vol. 55, no. 3, pp. 981–993, 2017.

[59] Y.-H. Jeon, J. Sansoni, L.-F. Low et al., "Recommended measures for the assessment of behavioral disturbances associated with dementia," *The American Journal of Geriatric Psychiatry*, vol. 19, no. 5, pp. 403–415, 2011.

[60] J. Diehl-Schmid, C. Pohl, R. Perneczky, H. Förstl, and A. Kurz, "Behavioral disturbances in the course of frontotemporal dementia," *Dementia and Geriatric Cognitive Disorders*, vol. 22, no. 4, pp. 352–357, 2006.

[61] J. J. Hsiao, N. Kaiser, S. S. Fong, and M. F. Mendez, "Suicidal behavior and loss of the future self in semantic dementia," *Cognitive and Behavioral Neurology*, vol. 26, no. 2, pp. 85–92, 2013.

[62] H. J. Rosen, S. C. Allison, J. M. Ogar et al., "Behavioral features in semantic dementia vs other forms of progressive aphasias," *Neurology*, vol. 67, no. 10, pp. 1752–1756, 2006.

[63] S. Ahmed, C. A. de Jager, A.-M. F. Haigh, and P. Garrard, "Logopenic aphasia in Alzheimer's disease: clinical variant or clinical feature?," *Journal of Neurology, Neurosurgery & Psychiatry*, vol. 83, no. 11, pp. 1056–1062, 2012.

[64] C. E. Leyton, O. Piguet, S. Savage, J. Burrell, and J. R. Hodges, "The neural basis of logopenic progressive aphasia," *Journal of Alzheimer's Disease*, vol. 32, no. 4, pp. 1051–1059, 2012.

[65] M. F. Bonner, S. Ash, and M. Grossman, "The new classification of primary progressive aphasia into semantic, logopenic, or nonfluent/agrammatic variants," *Current Neurology and Neuroscience Reports*, vol. 10, no. 6, pp. 484–490, 2010.

[66] M. Dottori, L. Sedenõ, M. Martorell Caro et al., "Towards affordable biomarkers of frontotemporal dementia: a classification study via network's information sharing," *Scientific Reports*, vol. 7, no. 1, p. 3822, 2017.

[67] A. Zalesky, A. Fornito, I. H. Harding et al., "Whole-brain anatomical networks: does the choice of nodes matter?," *NeuroImage*, vol. 50, no. 3, pp. 970–983, 2010.

[68] A. Fornito, A. Zalesky, and E. T. Bullmore, "Network scaling effects in graph analytic studies of human resting-state fMRI data," *Frontiers in Systems Neuroscience*, vol. 4, p. 22, 2010.

[69] B. C. M. van Wijk, C. J. Stam, and A. Daffertshofer, "Comparing brain networks of different size and connectivity density using graph theory," *PLoS One*, vol. 5, no. 10, article e13701, 2010.

Dynamic Evaluation of Notch Signaling-Mediated Angiogenesis in Ischemic Rats using Magnetic Resonance Imaging

Jia-qi Tian,[1] Jia-jun Zheng,[2] Xiao-zhu Hao,[1] Le-kang Yin,[3] Xiao-xue Zhang,[4] Chan-chan Li,[1] Xiao-yuan Feng,[1] Min Jiang,[5] Hua-ping Sun,[1] Kang Zheng,[2] and Yan-mei Yang[1]

[1]*Department of Radiology, Huashan Hospital, Fudan University, Shanghai 200040, China*
[2]*Department of Neurosurgery, Huashan Hospital, Fudan University, Shanghai 200040, China*
[3]*Department of Radiology, Shanghai Chest hospital, Shanghai Jiao Tong University, Shanghai 200030, China*
[4]*Department of Radiotherapy, Shanghai Eastern Hepatobiliary Surgery Hospital, Shanghai 310114, China*
[5]*Institutes of Science and State Key Laboratory of Medical Neurobiology, Fudan University, Shanghai 200030, China*

Correspondence should be addressed to Hua-ping Sun; sunhuaping@sohu.com, Kang Zheng; huashan_zhengkang@126.com, and Yan-mei Yang; yym9876@sohu.com

Academic Editor: Anatol Manaenko

Objective. The Notch signaling pathway is involved in angiogenesis induced by brain ischemia and can be efficiently inhibited by the γ-secretase inhibitor N-[N-(3,5-difluorophenacetyl)-1-alanyl]-S-phenylglycine t-butyl ester (DAPT). The aim of the present study was to noninvasively investigate the effect of DAPT treatment on angiogenesis in brain repair after stroke using magnetic resonance imaging (MRI). *Methods.* Sprague-Dawley rats ($n = 40$) were subjected to 90 minutes of transient middle cerebral artery (MCA) occlusion and treated with PBS ($n = 20$) or DAPT ($n = 20$) at 72 hours after the onset of ischemia. MRI measurements including T2-weighted imaging (T2WI), susceptibility-weighted imaging (SWI), and cerebral blood flow (CBF) were performed at 24 hours after reperfusion and weekly up to 4 weeks using a 3-Tesla system. Histological measurements were obtained at each time point after MRI scans. *Results.* SWI showed that DAPT treatment significantly enhanced angiogenesis in the ischemic boundary zone (IBZ) with respect to the control group, with local CBF in the angiogenic area elevated, along with increases in vascular density confirmed by histology. *Conclusion.* Treatment of ischemic stroke with DAPT significantly augments angiogenesis, which promotes poststroke brain remodeling by elevating CBF level, and these processes can be dynamically monitored and evaluated by MRI.

1. Introduction

Stroke is a major cause of mortality and disability globally while thrombolytic therapy as a fundamental treatment is not ideal for various restrictions and complications [1]. Obviously, there is a pressing need to develop effective strategies for the treatment of brain ischemia.

Neuroprotection as an alternative approach, which targets the cerebral parenchyma, is aimed at preserving cerebral tissue viability from reduced CBF. It seems to be a promising option for acute ischemic stroke (AIS) treatment. Unfortunately, most potentially neuroprotective drugs have failed to show benefit in clinical trials. At present, there is an increasing amount of studies that focus on the endogenous brain repair processes after stroke, which constitute the basis of neurorestorative therapy. As an essential part of biological substrates for poststroke brain remodeling, angiogenesis induced by brain ischemia enhances blood flow and nutrient supply to the affected tissue, which may benefit functional recovery [2, 3]. In rodents, neurorestorative treatments of either cell-based or pharmacological therapies promote angiogenesis, which is associated with

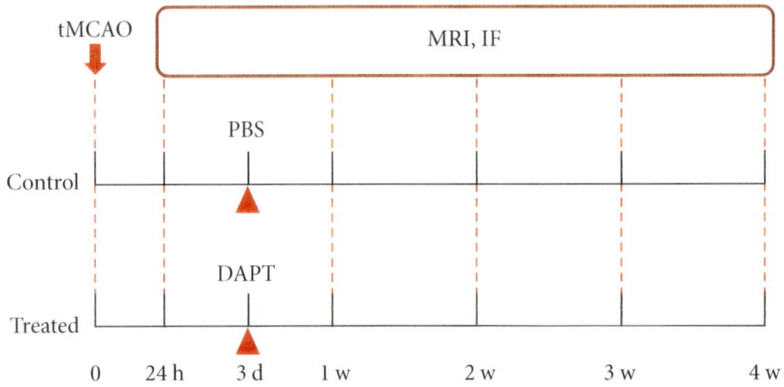

Figure 1: Experimental design. Forty rats were subjected to 90 minutes of transient middle cerebral artery occlusion (tMCAO) and then treated with PBS or DAPT at 3 days after ischemia. MRI was performed at 24 hours and weekly up to 4 weeks, after which four rats of each group were decapitated, respectively, for IF.

improvements in functional outcome [4, 5]. Patients with higher density of blood vessels seem to survive longer than patients with lower vascular density [6]. Moreover, angiogenesis and neurogenesis might be closely and causally linked together [7]. Therefore, the modulation of the endogenous angiogenesis could be a potential therapeutic intervention that promotes functional recovery after stroke.

The Notch signaling pathway plays multiple roles during vascular development, physiology, and disease [8]. Increasing evidence has pointed out that this pathway appears to regulate several steps of the reparative process occurring in ischemic tissues [9, 10]. However, the association between Notch signaling-mediated angiogenesis and poststroke brain remodeling via the improved CBF has not been investigated.

Magnetic resonance imaging (MRI) acts as a useful tool to noninvasively assess the evolution of various indices that can characterize postischemic angiogenic processes, which have been demonstrated from a variety of studies in experimental stroke models [11–13]. The aim of this study was to dynamically evaluate the temporal and spatial changes of angiogenesis modulated by Notch signaling in cerebral ischemia with noninvasive MRI methods.

2. Materials and Methods

All experimental procedures were performed in accordance with the National Institutes of Health Guide for the Care and Use of Laboratory Animals and approved by the Institutional Animal Care and Use Committee of Fudan University. Every effort was made to minimize the number of animals used and their suffering.

2.1. Animal Model and Experimental Design. Adult male Sprague-Dawley rats ($n = 40$) weighing 260–270 g were subjected to 90 minutes of transient middle cerebral artery occlusion (tMCAO) [14]. Briefly, rats were anesthetized with 10% chloral hydrate (350–400 mg/kg) intraperitoneally. The body temperature of $37 \pm 0.5^\circ$C was kept. The left MCA was occluded with a 4.0 silicon-coated nylon filament (Beijing Cinontech Biotech Co. Ltd., Beijing, China). It was inserted into the internal carotid artery (ICA) through the left common carotid artery (CCA) to occlude the origin of the MCA. After 90 minutes, the animals were reperfused by removing the filament.

We randomly divided the rats into control ($n = 20$) and treated groups ($n = 20$). DAPT (Sigma-Aldrich, St. Louis, MO, USA) powder was dissolved in DMSO at the concentrations of 8.3 mg/ml and stereotactically injected into the lateral cerebral ventricle (LV) for the treated group rats (0.03 mg/kg) at 3 days after stroke [15]. The detailed experimental procedure had been previously described [16]. The same volume of PBS was given to the control group rats at 3 days.

Four rats of each group were decapitated at 1 day and weekly up to 4 weeks after MRI scan, respectively, for immunofluorescence staining (IF). Figure 1 shows the time schedule for the experimental design.

2.2. Magnetic Resonance Imaging Measurements. All rats received MR scanning using a 3-Tesla MR system (Discovery MR750; GE Medical Systems, Milwaukee, WI, USA) with a 60 mm diameter gradient coil (Magtron Inc., Jiangyin, China). The total acquisition time was 18 minutes. Anesthesia was maintained during the imaging procedure as mentioned above. Body temperature was kept at $37 \pm 0.5^\circ$C. Blood oxygen saturation and heart rate were monitored.

MR images including T2-weighted imaging (T2WI), susceptibility-weighted imaging (SWI), and three-dimensional arterial spin labeling (3D-ASL) were acquired for all animals in both groups at 1 day and weekly up to 4 weeks after the onset of stroke.

T2WI images were scanned using a fast spin-echo sequence by multiple slices (15 slices; 1.8 mm slice thickness and 1 mm interslice distance). Repetition time (TR) and echo time (TE) were 4000 ms and 96 ms, respectively. Images were produced using a 6×6 cm FOV and a 256×256 matrix. The scan time was 3 min.

SWI employed a 3D gradient echo imaging sequence by multiple slices (30 slices; 1 mm slice thickness and 1 mm interslice distance). RT and ET were 56 ms and 32 ms, respectively. The matrix was set as 300×300 for the 7×7 cm FOV. The flip angle is 10°. The sequence time was approximately 10 minutes.

3D-ASL was acquired by a 3D spiral fast spin-echo sequence with the following parameters: repetition time

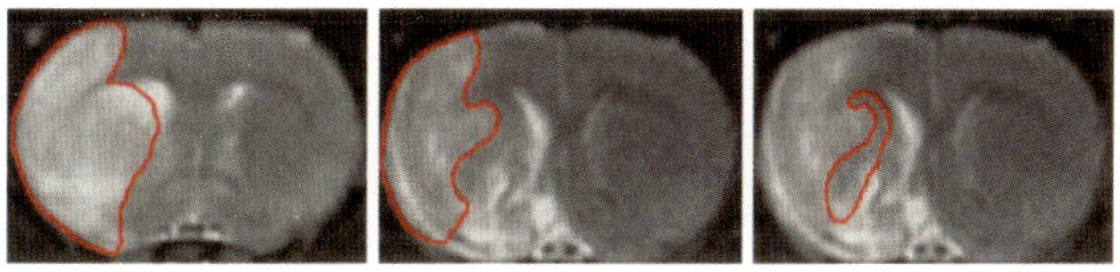

FIGURE 2: Representative T2 maps indicating the ROI. (a) Ischemic lesion size was identified by the T2 map acquired at 24 h after stroke. (b) The final infarction area was determined by the T2 map acquired at 4 weeks. (c) The difference was referred to as the recovery region, the ROI.

(RT) = 4214 ms (PLD = 1.5 s) and 5285 ms (PLD = 2.5 s), labeling duration = 1500 ms, echo time (ET) = 11.948 ms, scan time = 4 min, field of view (FOV) = 4 × 4 cm, slice thickness (ST) = 3 mm, and interslice distance = 3 mm.

2.3. MRI Data Analysis. The MR images were postprocessed using the Functool software based on GE Advanced Workstation 4.6 (GE Medical Systems, Milwaukee, WI). Ischemic lesion size was determined by T2 maps acquired after stroke with values above mean plus two standard deviations (SD) of contralateral measurements [11]. The region of interest (ROI), identified by the difference of the ischemic lesion sizes in T2 maps acquired at 24 h (Figure 2(a)) and 4 weeks (Figure 2(b)) after stroke, was referred to as the recovery region (Figure 2(c)). This region and the mirrored area in the contralateral hemisphere were chosen to measure MRI values, and ratios were obtained. All the ROI were animal dependent.

2.4. Histology. After MRI measurements at each time point, rats were euthanized and transcardially perfused with 200 ml of 0.9% saline followed by 200 ml of 4% paraformaldehyde. The brains were removed and postfixed in 4% paraformaldehyde at 4°C overnight. Coronal brain sections (20 μm) were obtained using a cryostat (RM2135; Leica, Mannheim, Germany) and stained for histological evaluation. The detailed procedure had been previously described [16]. Primary antibodies of rabbit polyclonal anti-NICD (1 : 500; Abcam, Cambridge, MA, USA) and mouse monoclonal anti-CD31 (1 : 100; Abcam, Cambridge, MA, USA) were used to evaluate the cerebral vascular density and Notch signal inhibition. Alexa Fluor 488- and 568-conjugated donkey anti-rabbit and anti-mouse (1 : 200; Life Technologies, Carlsbad, CA, USA) were used as secondary antibodies. Sections were then counterstained with DAPI (1 : 1000; Sigma-Aldrich, St. Louis, MO, USA).

Histological images were scanned using a fluorescence microscope (Olympus PX51; Olympus Corporation, Shinjuku-ku, Japan). The acquired images were quantified using ImageJ (National Institutes of Health, Bethesda, MD, USA) by measuring optical density of positively stained cells of the ROI selected at the recovery region. Five sections of each brain from each group were used for cell counting at 40x objective in three randomly selected views per section. The ipsilateral-versus-contralateral differences in gray levels were converted to a percentage of the contralateral value.

2.5. Statistical Analysis. All values were presented as mean ± SD. The temporal patterns of MRI data between two groups, including CBF and SWI, were analyzed using two-way analysis of variance (ANOVA) with Sidak's multiple comparison test. The differences of histological measurements between the 2 groups were analyzed by *t*-test. A value of $P < 0.05$ was considered statistically significant. Statistical analysis was performed using Prism, version 6.0 (GraphPad Software Incorporated, La Jolla, CA, USA).

3. Results

3.1. MRI Measurements. Figure 3 shows the evolution of an axial section of MRI maps from the representative control rat (a–c) and treated rat (d–f). Ischemic lesion and temporal evolution of the two groups after ischemia were identified by T2 images (Figures 3(a) and 3(d)). Elevated CBF was observed in cortical regions since 24 h in both groups (Figures 3(c) and 3(f)). Elevation of CBF values had appeared at 1 week in striatum regions in the control rats and treated rats, as indicated by white arrows. These areas were detected as having low intensity on the SWI map (Figures 3(b) and 3(e)), which had appeared at 2 weeks in the two groups, as indicated by red arrows. For the treated rats, the size of the hyperintensity areas on the CBF map and hypointensity regions on the SWI map was larger than that in the control rats.

Quantitative longitudinal MRI measurements demonstrated temporal features of CBF and SWI for restorative cerebral tissue after stroke with or without DAPT treatment (Figure 4). As shown in Figure 4(b), elevated CBF ratios had a good consistency between the two groups at 24 h following ischemia. For the control rats, CBF increased starting from 1 to 2 weeks and then regressed toward normal from 3 weeks. For the treated rats, CBF increased starting from 1 to 3 weeks and then decreased at 4 weeks. Compared to the control rats, CBF of cerebral tissue in IBZ in the treated group had consistently higher values during 1 to 4 weeks after stroke. The differences were significant at 2 and 3 weeks ($P < 0.05$ and 0.01, resp.).

Temporal changes of SWI ratios for both treated and control groups were shown in Figure 4(a). It demonstrated a good consistency between the two groups at 24 h. SWI ratios monotonically decreased during 4 weeks after stroke for the control group. For the treated rats, SWI ratios decreased starting from 1 week and reached to minimum at

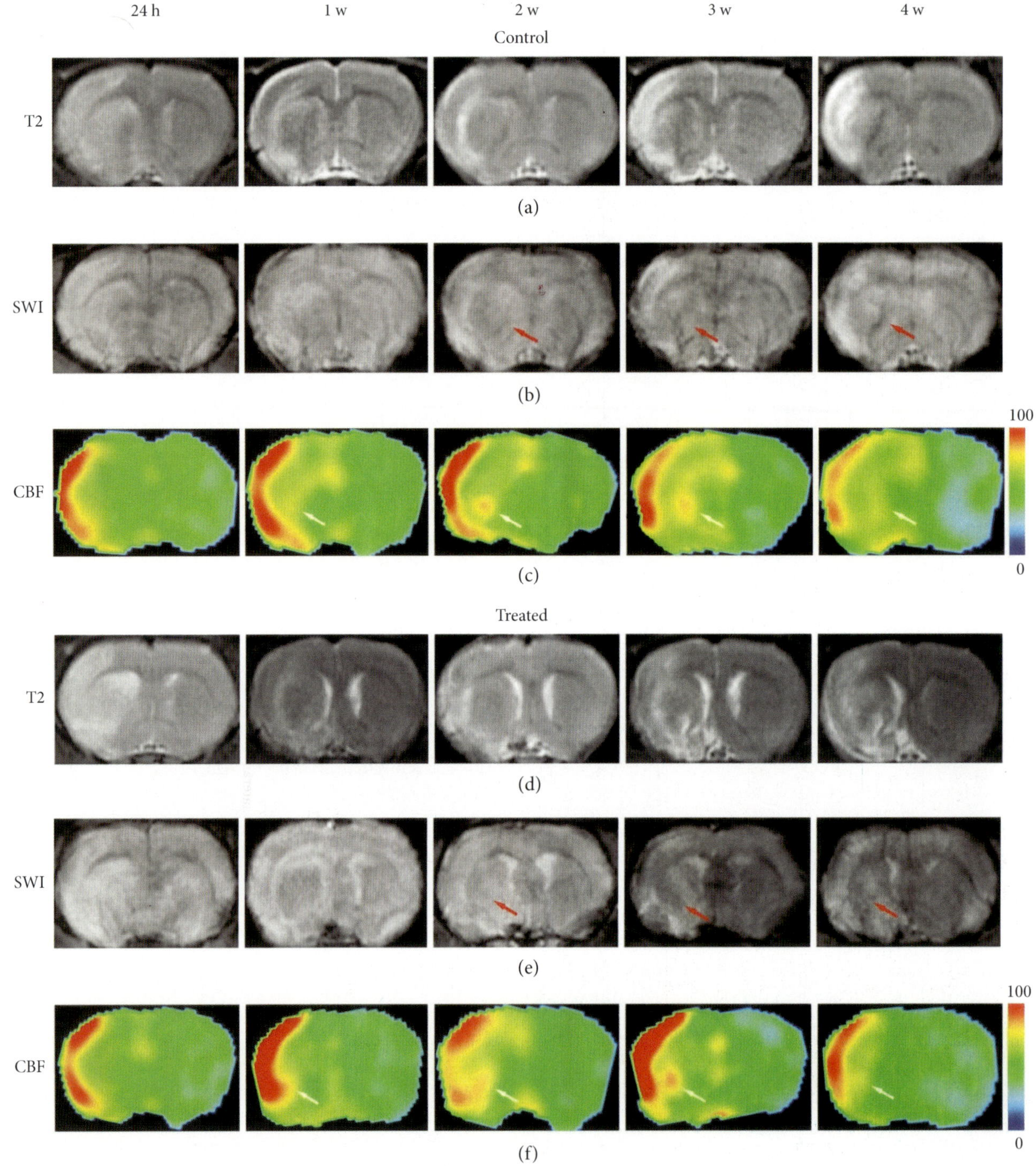

FIGURE 3: MRI maps of representative control (a–c) and treated (d–f) rats. (c, f) Elevated CBF (white arrows) was found in the recovery region. (b, e) SWI showed hypointensity in the same area (red arrows) indicating angiogenesis. The area where angiogenesis might happen in the control rat was smaller than that in the treated one.

3 weeks and then elevated at 4 weeks. Compared to the control rats, SWI ratios in the treated group had consistently lower values during 1 to 4 weeks. The differences were significant at 2 and 3 weeks ($P < 0.05$).

3.2. Histological Measurements. Double immunofluorescent staining (Figures 5(a)–5(c)) showed the NICD-positive microvessels in IBZ in both groups at 1 week (40x microscope). Quantitative analysis of NICD-positive microvessels showed that the number was higher in the control group than in the treated group (Figure 5(d), $P < 0.01$), which indicated that the Notch signal was blocked by DAPT.

MRI data for detecting angiogenesis in this study were confirmed by histological measurements using CD31 staining, as shown in Figure 6. A CD31-stained slice (Figure 6(a))

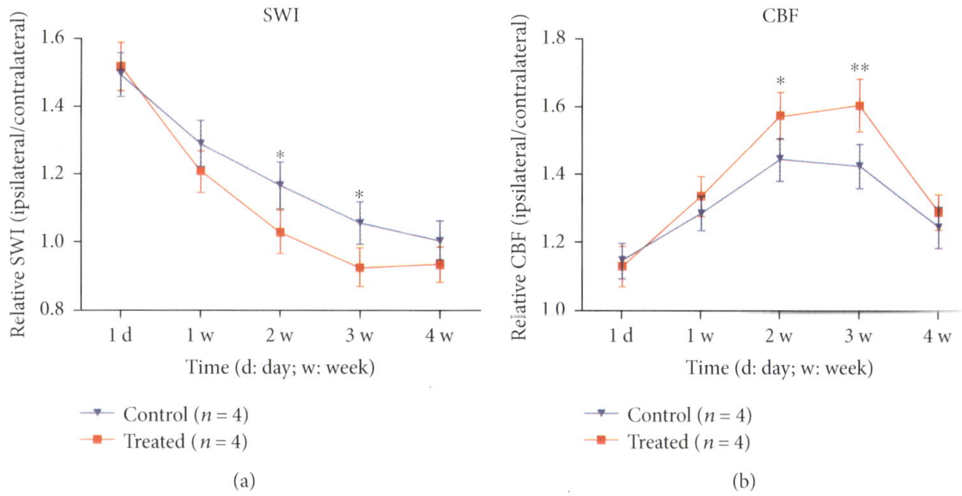

FIGURE 4: Quantitative MRI data demonstrating temporal features of SWI and CBF for both groups. (a) SWI ratios of cerebral tissue in the DAPT-treated group had lower values during 4 weeks after stroke compared to those in the control group; the differences were significant at 2 weeks and 3 weeks. (b) Higher CBF ratios were observed in the DAPT-treated group compared to control rats during 4 weeks; the differences were significant at 2 weeks and 3 weeks. $^{*}P < 0.05$; $^{**}P < 0.01$.

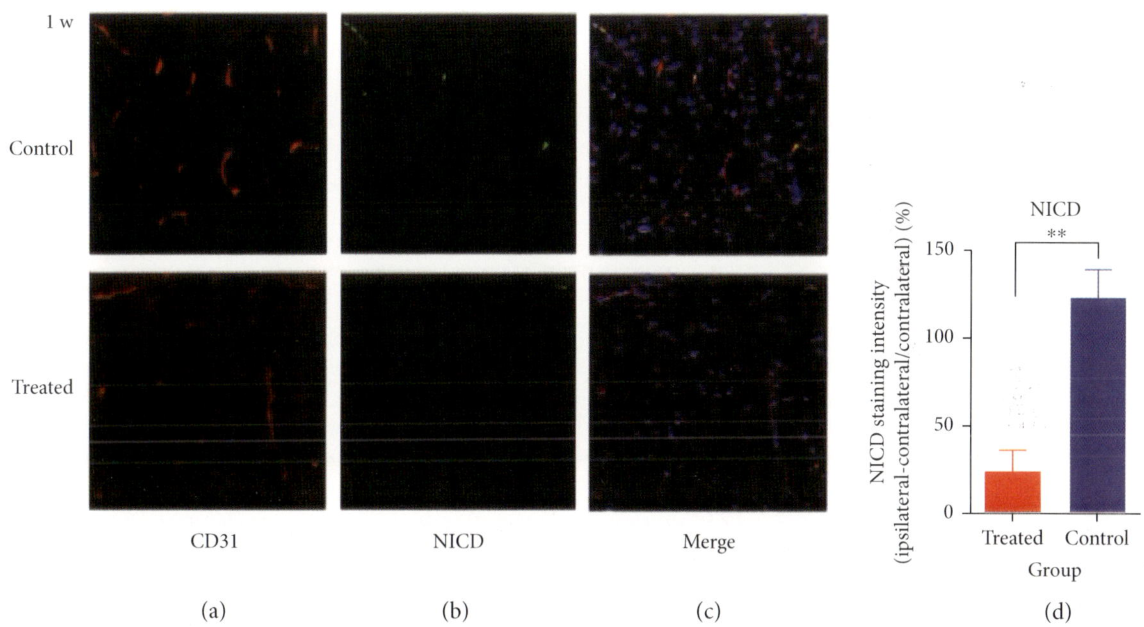

FIGURE 5: Expression of CD31 and NICD indicating the Notch signal blocked by DAPT. (a–c) Immunostaining of NICD-positive microvessels in IBZ for both groups obtained 1 week after stroke (40x). (d) Quantification of NICD fluorescence intensity. $^{**}P < 0.01$.

of a treated rat was obtained at 4 weeks after stroke. The T2 image (Figure 6(b)), SWI map (Figure 6(c)), and CBF map (Figure 6(d)) obtained 4 weeks after stroke detected the angiogenic area in the IBZ (red arrows). This area closely matched the histological result (white arrow).

Figures 6(e) and 6(f) show the representative pictures (20x microscope) of CD31-immunoreactive cerebral vessels for ipsilateral slices of control and DAPT-treated rats in the IBZ area obtained 4 weeks after stroke, respectively. Compared to the control rats, treatment with DAPT significantly increased cerebral vessel density (Figure 6(g), $P < 0.01$).

4. Discussion

Our study showed that the number of NICD-positive microvessels in the control group was higher than that in the treated group at 1 week, which indicated that the Notch signal was blocked by DAPT at 3 days. Cerebral vessel density was significantly enhanced in treated rats at 4 weeks after stroke compared to the control rats, suggesting that inhibition of the Notch signal significantly promoted angiogenesis. It is now becoming clear that the Notch signaling pathway plays a significant role in both developmental and pathological angiogenesis [9, 17]. Ischemia triggers endogenous

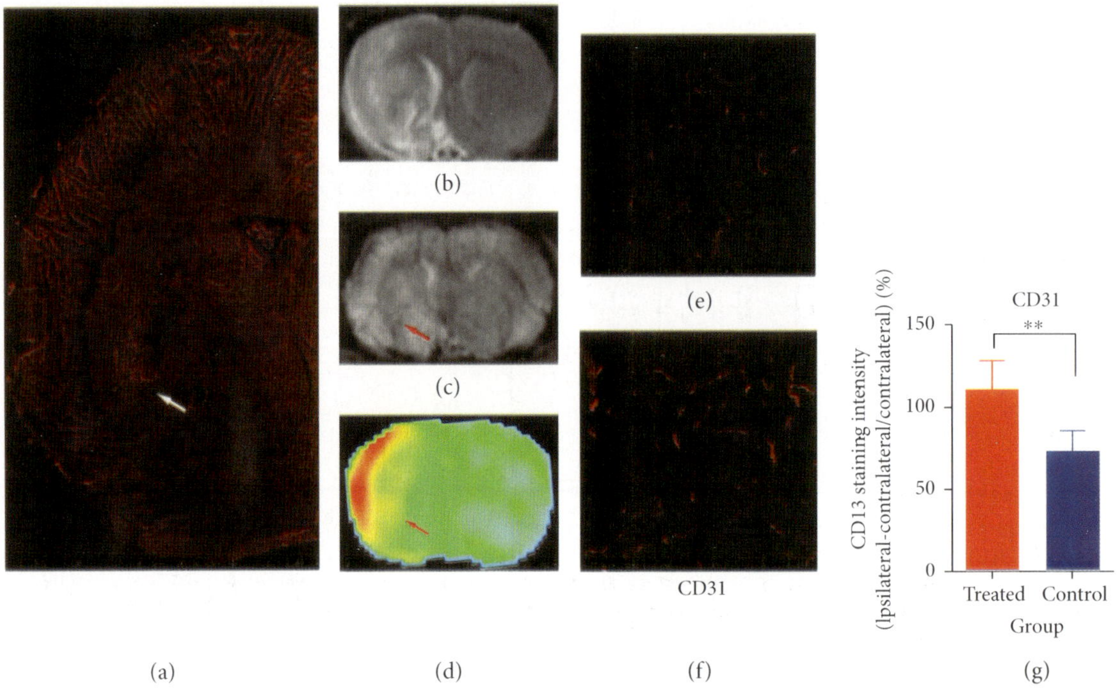

FIGURE 6: Histology and MRI matched the area indicating angiogenesis. (a) A CD31-stained slice and (b–d) MR images of a treated rat obtained at 4 weeks after stroke. These areas are close matched (arrows). (e, f) Immunostaining of CD31-positive cerebral vessels in IBZ for both groups obtained 4 weeks after stroke (20x). (g) Quantification of CD31 fluorescence intensity. $^{**}P < 0.01$.

angiogenesis, involving the new capillaries sprouting from previously existing blood vessels. The current model of endothelial angiogenesis centers on the interplay between "tip" and "stalk" cell characters, and Notch signaling acts as a key regulator of endothelial tip cell formation and function during this process [10, 18]. Suppression of Notch signaling leads to increased endothelial cell proliferation with augmented sprouting and excessive vascular branching [19, 20]. Our study is consistent with previous studies that angiogenesis after ischemia was enhanced by blocking Notch signaling. Together, Notch signaling seems to be essential in building up a proper neovascularization, and the detailed process of how exactly Notch signaling regulates angiogenesis requires further investigations.

Experimental studies suggest that cell-based and pharmacological neurorestorative treatments can promote brain plasticity and benefit functional recovery [2, 3]. However, the current understanding of these processes after stroke derives mainly from regional histological measurements, which do not allow dynamic assessment of tissue remodeling [21]. The high spatial and temporal resolution, safety, and versatility make MRI particularly suitable to monitor the dynamic profiles of events involved in poststroke brain reorganization. After proliferation of endothelial cells, newly formed vessels in the ischemic border zone lead to alterations in vascular density and hemodynamic parameters such as cerebral blood flow (CBF), which can be measured with perfusion MR imaging techniques such as arterial spin labeling (ASL) [22]. MRI-based measurements of elevated CBF were evident in ischemic boundary regions with neural progenitor cell-induced angiogenesis in an embolic stroke model [12]. Similarly, Ding et al. [11] and Li et al. [23] have reported that treatment with sildenafil enhanced angiogenesis and selectively increased the CBF level in the ischemic boundary in rats after embolic stroke. Newly generated venous structures can be identified with susceptibility-weighted images. The local magnetic field disturbances caused by the relatively high magnetic susceptibility of deoxygenated hemoglobin result in a lower signal intensity on the SWI map, which has been used to detect perilesional angiogenesis in sildenafil- or erythropoietin-treated rats after ischemia [13, 24]. Our dynamic measurements revealed that elevation of CBF values appeared at 1 week in striatum regions in the two groups and the closely matched area with low intensity on the SWI map appeared at 2 weeks in the two groups. The size of the hyperintensity areas on the CBF map and hypointensity regions on the SWI map was larger in treated rats compared to the control group. CBF of cerebral tissue in IBZ in the treated group had consistently higher values during 1 to 4 weeks after stroke while SWI ratios had lower values during 1 to 4 weeks. These results suggest that poststroke angiogenesis is augmented by blocking Notch signaling, and this process can be evaluated by noninvasive MRI methods.

Compensatory angiogenesis after ischemic brain injury is considered an intrinsic process of the brain for neuroplasticity. It is essential for poststroke brain repair, as this event stimulates blood flow and nutrient supply to the affected tissue [25]. In stroke patients, the extent of angiogenesis is associated with survival and improved neurological recovery [6]. In animal stroke models, neurorestorative treatments of either cell-based or pharmacological therapies promoted angiogenesis, which is associated with improvements in functional outcome [4, 5]. Our previous study showed that suppression of Notch signaling resulted in ameliorated brain edema at the subacute stage and recovered brain tissue at the chronic stage in the ipsilateral striatum, as indicated by MRI data [16]. Evidently, this is partially due to the ischemia-induced angiogenesis. In addition, the benefits probably come through the interplay between neurorestorative events (angiogenesis, neurogenesis, and synaptic plasticity), which will be investigated in our future experiment.

5. Conclusion

The current study demonstrates that treatment of ischemic stroke with DAPT by suppression of the Notch signal significantly augments angiogenesis, which promotes poststroke brain remodeling by elevating CBF level. Noninvasive MRI methods can be used to investigate and evaluate cerebral tissue undergoing angiogenesis and can be helpful in estimating the potential in functional recovery, all of which may provide new insight into clinical trials of angiogenic therapy for cerebral ischemia.

Disclosure

Portion of this work has been presented in the form of oral presentation at the European Congress of Radiology 2018, European Society of Radiology, Vienna, Austria, March 1, 2018.

Authors' Contributions

Jia-qi Tian and Jia-jun Zheng contributed equally to this work.

Acknowledgments

This work was supported by the grant from National Natural Science Foundation of China (nos. 81771788 and 81371521).

References

[1] A. Moretti, F. Ferrari, and R. F. Villa, "Neuroprotection for ischaemic stroke: current status and challenges," *Pharmacology & Therapeutics*, vol. 146, pp. 23–34, 2015.

[2] D. M. Hermann and M. Chopp, "Promoting brain remodelling and plasticity for stroke recovery: therapeutic promise and potential pitfalls of clinical translation," *The Lancet Neurology*, vol. 11, no. 4, pp. 369–380, 2012.

[3] Z. G. Zhang and M. Chopp, "Neurorestorative therapies for stroke: underlying mechanisms and translation to the clinic," *The Lancet Neurology*, vol. 8, no. 5, pp. 491–500, 2009.

[4] L. Wang, M. Chopp, S. R. Gregg et al., "Neural progenitor cells treated with EPO induce angiogenesis through the production of VEGF," *Journal of Cerebral Blood Flow & Metabolism*, vol. 28, no. 7, pp. 1361–1368, 2008.

[5] L. Wang, Z. Zhang, Y. Wang, R. Zhang, and M. Chopp, "Treatment of stroke with erythropoietin enhances neurogenesis and angiogenesis and improves neurological function in rats," *Stroke*, vol. 35, no. 7, pp. 1732–1737, 2004.

[6] J. Krupinski, J. Kaluza, P. Kumar, S. Kumar, and J. M. Wang, "Role of angiogenesis in patients with cerebral ischemic stroke," *Stroke*, vol. 25, no. 9, pp. 1794–1798, 1994.

[7] L. Ruan, B. Wang, Q. ZhuGe, and K. Jin, "Coupling of neurogenesis and angiogenesis after ischemic stroke," *Brain Research*, vol. 1623, pp. 166–173, 2015.

[8] A. Louvi and S. Artavanis-Tsakonas, "Notch and disease: a growing field," *Seminars in Cell & Developmental Biology*, vol. 23, no. 4, pp. 473–480, 2012.

[9] T. Gridley, "Chapter nine - Notch signaling in the vasculature," *Current Topics in Developmental Biology*, vol. 92, pp. 277–309, 2010.

[10] L. K. Phng and H. Gerhardt, "Angiogenesis: a team effort coordinated by Notch," *Developmental Cell*, vol. 16, no. 2, pp. 196–208, 2009.

[11] G. Ding, Q. Jiang, L. Li et al., "Magnetic resonance imaging investigation of axonal remodeling and angiogenesis after embolic stroke in sildenafil-treated rats," *Journal of Cerebral Blood Flow & Metabolism*, vol. 28, no. 8, pp. 1440–1448, 2008.

[12] Q. Jiang, Z. G. Zhang, G. L. Ding et al., "Investigation of neural progenitor cell induced angiogenesis after embolic stroke in rat using MRI," *NeuroImage*, vol. 28, no. 3, pp. 698–707, 2005.

[13] G. Ding, Q. Jiang, L. Li et al., "Angiogenesis detected after embolic stroke in rat brain using magnetic resonance T2 * WI," *Stroke*, vol. 39, no. 5, pp. 1563–1568, 2008.

[14] X. Hao, L. K. Yin, X. X. Zhang et al., "Combining systemic and stereotactic MEMRI to detect the correlation between gliosis and neuronal connective pathway at the chronic stage after stroke," *Journal of Neuroinflammation*, vol. 13, no. 1, p. 156, 2016.

[15] S. Li, X. Zhang, Y. Wang, H. Ji, Y. Du, and H. Liu, "DAPT protects brain against cerebral ischemia by down-regulating the expression of Notch 1 and nuclear factor kappa B in rats," *Neurological Sciences*, vol. 33, no. 6, pp. 1257–1264, 2012.

[16] X. Z. Hao, J. Q. Tian, L. K. Yin et al., "MRI detects protective effects of DAPT treatment with modulation of microglia/macrophages at subacute and chronic stages following cerebral ischemia," *Molecular Medicine Reports*, vol. 16, no. 4, pp. 4493–4500, 2017.

[17] T. Kume, "Novel insights into the differential functions of Notch ligands in vascular formation," *Journal of Angiogenesis Research*, vol. 1, no. 1, p. 8, 2009.

[18] A. A. H. Zen and P. Madeddu, "Notch signalling in ischaemia-induced angiogenesis," *Biochemical Society Transactions*, vol. 37, no. 6, pp. 1221–1227, 2009.

[19] S. Suchting, C. Freitas, F. le Noble et al., "The Notch ligand delta-like 4 negatively regulates endothelial tip cell formation and vessel branching," *Proceedings of the National Academy of Sciences of the United States of America*, vol. 104, no. 9, pp. 3225–3230, 2007.

[20] M. Hellström, L. K. Phng, J. J. Hofmann et al., "Dll4 signalling through Notch1 regulates formation of tip cells during angiogenesis," *Nature*, vol. 445, no. 7129, pp. 776–780, 2007.

[21] Q. Jiang, Z. G. Zhang, and M. Chopp, "MRI of stroke recovery," *Stroke*, vol. 41, no. 2, pp. 410–414, 2010.

[22] D. S. Williams, J. A. Detre, J. S. Leigh, and A. P. Koretsky, "Magnetic resonance imaging of perfusion using spin inversion of arterial water," *Proceedings of the National Academy of Sciences of the United States of America*, vol. 89, no. 1, pp. 212–216, 1992.

[23] L. Li, Q. Jiang, L. Zhang et al., "Angiogenesis and improved cerebral blood flow in the ischemic boundary area detected by MRI after administration of sildenafil to rats with embolic stroke," *Brain Research*, vol. 1132, no. 1, pp. 185–192, 2007.

[24] G. Ding, Q. Jiang, L. Li et al., "Cerebral tissue repair and atrophy after embolic stroke in rat: a magnetic resonance imaging study of erythropoietin therapy," *Journal of Neuroscience Research*, vol. 88, no. 14, pp. 3206–3214, 2010.

[25] H. Beck and K. H. Plate, "Angiogenesis after cerebral ischemia," *Acta Neuropathologica*, vol. 117, no. 5, pp. 481–496, 2009.

Sleep Quality and Emotion Regulation Interact to Predict Anxiety in Veterans with PTSD

Janna Mantua,[1,2] Steven M. Helms,[3,4] Kris B. Weymann,[3,4] Vincent F. Capaldi II,[2] and Miranda M. Lim[3,4]

[1]*Neuroscience & Behavior Program, University of Massachusetts, Amherst, Amherst, MA 01003, USA*
[2]*Behavioral Biology Branch, Walter Reed Army Institute of Research, Silver Spring, MD 20910, USA*
[3]*VA Portland Health Care System, Portland, OR 97239, USA*
[4]*Oregon Health & Science University, Portland, OR 97239, USA*

Correspondence should be addressed to Miranda M. Lim; lmir@ohsu.edu

Academic Editor: Laura Piccardi

Posttraumatic stress disorder (PTSD) is a debilitating and common consequence of military service. PTSD is associated with increased incidence of mood disturbances (e.g., anxiety). Additionally, veterans with PTSD often have poor-quality sleep and poor emotion regulation ability. We sought to assess whether such sleep and emotion regulation deficits contribute to mood disturbances. In 144 veterans, using a double moderation model, we tested the relationship between PTSD and anxiety and examined whether sleep quality and emotion regulation interact to moderate this relationship. We found that PTSD predicts higher anxiety in veterans with poor and average sleep quality who utilize maladaptive emotion regulation strategies. However, there was no relationship between PTSD and anxiety in individuals with good sleep quality, regardless of emotion regulation. Similarly, there was no relationship between PTSD and anxiety in individuals with better emotion regulation, regardless of sleep quality. Results were unchanged when controlling for history of traumatic brain injury (TBI), despite the fact that those with both PTSD and TBI had the poorest emotion regulation overall. Taken together, these results suggest that good-quality sleep may be protective against poor emotion regulation in veterans with PTSD. Sleep may therefore be a target for therapeutic intervention in veterans with PTSD and heightened anxiety.

1. Introduction

Posttraumatic stress disorder (PTSD), which can occur after a traumatic event, is characterized by negative alterations in cognition, mood, and arousal/reactivity [1]. PTSD is prevalent in post-9/11 veteran populations; roughly 1 in 7 deployed veterans and 1 in 10 nondeployed veterans carry a diagnosis of PTSD [2]. Additionally, PTSD can have lasting negative consequences and significant disability. Compared to age- and gender-matched veterans without PTSD, veterans with PTSD have a significantly poorer functioning in a number of tested domains. For example, veterans with PTSD are less likely to be working, more likely to have physical limitations, and more likely to have committed violence in the past several years [3]. Therefore, identifying contributing factors to impairment in PTSD is critical to designing effective therapies.

Given the prevailing physiological hyperarousal present in PTSD, it is perhaps not surprising that sleep issues are common in this population. In fact, insomnia is the most commonly reported symptom of PTSD [4]. Yet, sleep issues are not simply the product of hyperarousal, as they also seem to be causal in exacerbating PTSD symptomatology. For instance, in PTSD populations, treating insomnia (via cognitive behavioral therapy) reduces PTSD symptomatology [5] and treating of obstructive sleep apnea (OSA), which is also common in PTSD, reduces symptoms as well [6]. Taken together, these results suggest that sleep quality is an important and modifiable factor that can influence PTSD severity.

Individuals with PTSD also suffer from impaired emotion regulation, which involves the voluntary or involuntary process of modulating one's own emotional experience [7]. The process of emotion regulation is implemented using a number of well-characterized cognitive techniques or strategies. These strategies are not all equally valuable. That is, some emotion regulation strategies tend to be helpful or adaptive, while others are not. For instance, "expressive suppression" (trying to hold back or hide emotions) is predictive of poor emotional outcomes (e.g., anxiety), while "cognitive reappraisal" (reframing emotional situations to make them less emotional) is predictive of healthy emotional functioning [8]. Individuals with PTSD tend to utilize more expressive suppression than cognitive reappraisal [9], and the overuse of expressive suppression may exacerbate poor psychological functioning in this population.

Importantly, the type of strategy used for emotion regulation seems to be moderated by sleep quality. Vantieghem and colleagues recently showed that individuals with sleep issues (i.e., insomnia) suppress emotions more frequently and are less likely to use cognitive reappraisal than those without insomnia [10]. A separate study showed that poorer sleep quality (e.g., higher scores on the Pittsburgh Sleep Quality Index) predicted less cognitive reappraisal use and more expressive suppression use [10]. These studies suggest that there is a potential interaction between sleep quality and emotion regulation strategy use, such that sleep quality influences emotion regulation or vice versa.

The current study therefore is aimed at examining the potential relationship between sleep quality and emotion regulation in veterans with and without PTSD. We specifically focus on a core feature of PTSD, that is, anxiety symptomatology, and examine how sleep quality and emotion regulation interact to moderate this relationship. Using a cohort of veterans with and without PTSD, we hypothesized the following: (1) Individuals with PTSD would have higher anxiety than veterans without PTSD. (2) Individuals with PTSD would have poorer sleep quality than veterans without PTSD. (3) Individuals with PTSD would utilize higher levels of expressive suppression and lower levels of cognitive reappraisal than veterans without PTSD. (4) Sleep quality and emotion regulation strategy use would interact to moderate the link between PTSD and anxiety. Furthermore, given that PTSD is often comorbid with TBI in the veteran population, we also examined the effects of TBI on these hypotheses as a contributing factor.

2. Materials and Methods

2.1. Sample. In total, 144 veterans from the Veterans Affairs (VA) Portland Healthcare System participated under a VA IRB approved protocol (MIRB number 3641, PI: Lim). Twenty-four individuals met criteria for PTSD on the basis of self-reported symptoms (cluster criteria in the PTSD Checklist 5 or PCL-5, total score > 33 [11]) ("PTSD only" group). Twenty-three individuals carried a diagnosis of TBI confirmed in the medical record ("TBI only" group). Eleven veterans met criteria for PTSD and carried a diagnosis of TBI ("PTSD + TBI" group). Eighty-six veterans without a history of trauma exposure (neither PTSD nor TBI) served as matched controls ("control" group).

2.2. Questionnaires. The main analyses were conducted using several self-reported questionnaires: (1) Emotion Regulation Questionnaire (ERQ) [12], (2) National Institutes of Health Patient-Reported Outcomes Measurement Information System (NIH PROMIS) anxiety items [13], and (3) Insomnia Severity Index (ISI) [14]. We also included two questionnaires for descriptive purposes: (1) Patient Health Questionnaire-9 (PHQ-9) [15] and (2) the Functional Outcomes of Sleep Questionnaire-10 (FOSQ-10) [16].

2.2.1. ERQ. The ERQ is a 10-item scale that measures an individual's tendency to use specific emotion regulation strategies [12]. Two emotion regulation strategies in particular (expressive suppression and cognitive reappraisal) are assessed by this questionnaire. Individual items are 7-point Likert scales: 1 = "strongly disagree", 4 = "neutral", and 7 = "strongly agree". A higher number indicates that the participant utilizes the given emotion regulation strategy more frequently.

2.2.2. NIH PROMIS. The NIH PROMIS battery is a multidomain test with a range of outcomes pertaining to physical, mental, and social wellbeing. Participants were asked to rate to what extent four items about anxiety symptoms described them (e.g., "In the past 7 days, my worries overwhelmed me."). Items are 5-point Likert scales: 5 = "never", 4 = "rarely", 3 = "sometimes", 2 = "often", and 1 = "always". A lower number indicates higher dysfunction.

2.2.3. ISI. The ISI is a 7-item measure assessing insomnia severity (i.e., difficulty initiating and staying asleep). Individual items are 5-point Likert scales: 0 = "none", 1 = "mild", 2 = "moderate", 3 = "severe", and 4 = "very severe". A higher score indicates higher dysfunction.

2.2.4. FOSQ-10. The FOSQ-10 is a 10-item measure assessing whether an individual has poor quality of life due to poor sleep quality. Individual items are 4-point Likert scales: 1 = "yes, extreme difficulty", 2 = "yes, moderate difficulty", 3 = "yes, a little difficulty", and 4 = "no difficulty"; however, half of the items are a 5-point Likert scale that includes a rating of 0 = "I do not do this activity for other reasons". The survey has 5 subscales: (1) activity level, (2) vigilance, (3) intimacy and sexual relationships, (4) general productivity, and (5) social outcomes. A lower score indicates higher dysfunction.

2.2.5. PHQ-9. The PHQ-9 is a 10-item measure assessing the presence of depressive symptoms. Individual items, which enquire about how frequently participants experience the presented symptoms, are a 4-point Likert scale: 0 = "not at all", 1 = "several days", 2 = "more than half the days", and 3 = "nearly every day." A higher score indicates higher dysfunction.

2.3. PTSD Diagnosis. Individuals met criteria for PTSD on the basis of symptoms reported in the Posttraumatic Stress Disorder Checklist (PCL-5) [11], using a combination of cluster criteria, and total score > 33 [11]. The PTSD Checklist for DSM-5 (PCL-5) is a 20-item measure used for the screening and provisional diagnosis of PTSD, as well as assessing symptom severity. Individual items are 5-point Likert scales: 0 = "not at all", 1 = "a little bit", 2 = "moderately", 3 = "quite a bit", and 4 = "extremely". In the current study, PTSD status was used as a categorical variable (1 = presence of PTSD, 0 = no PTSD).

2.4. TBI Diagnosis. Two trained researchers reviewed medical records from the Portland VA electronic medical record system to determine whether veterans had a history of TBI. Individuals with self-reported TBI that was not confirmed in the medical record were excluded from the sample.

2.5. Protocol. Consecutive veterans who entered the Portland VA Sleep Clinic for a clinical diagnostic sleep study were recruited to participate as part of a larger study (MIRB number 3641, factors that affect adherence to treatment for sleep apnea, PI: Lim). All participants were in the lab for overnight sleep assessments and were asked by a trained research coordinator whether they would like to participate. Veterans who wished to participate completed all questionnaires either in person, via mail, or by phone, between the time of consent and 12 months later.

2.6. Statistical Analyses. IBM SPSS Statistics 23 (Armonk, NY) was used to conduct statistical analyses. Analyses were conducted in several phases. First, descriptive statistical tests were conducted to determine whether groups differed at cross section in meaningful ways. One-way ANOVA tests were used to determine whether groups differed for demographic factors (e.g., age), objective sleep characteristics (e.g., TST and sleep staging), and self-reported functioning (e.g., via the FOSQ-10 and PHQ-9). If a significant difference between groups was detected, post hoc Tukey tests were used to determine which groups differed.

Next, 2×2 ANOVA tests (TBI versus non-TBI, PTSD versus non-PTSD) were used to assess whether groups differed for the outcome measures of interest. For this set of analyses, a 2×2 ANOVA was utilized rather than a one-way ANOVA so that we could examine whether PTSD and TBI interacted to synergistically affect outcomes of interest. Outcome measures were cognitive reappraisal (higher = more use of that strategy), expressive suppression (higher = more use of that strategy), ISI scores (sleep quality; higher = more sleep problems), and NIH PROMIS anxiety scores (anxiety; lower = more anxiety). In addition, an emotion regulation ratio was calculated, which consists of cognitive reappraisal divided by expressive suppression (higher = more cognitive reappraisal use, lower = more expressive suppression use), so both strategies could be assessed in one continuous outcome measure.

Lastly, given our a priori hypotheses about sleep quality interacting with emotion regulation to affect anxiety symptomatology in individuals with PTSD, moderation analyses were conducted to determine whether sleep (ISI scores) and emotion regulation (emotion regulation ratio) both moderate the relationship between PTSD (yes/no diagnosis) and

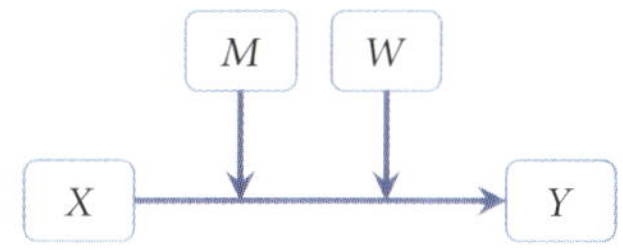

FIGURE 1: Conceptual model of the relationship between PTSD status, sleep quality, emotion regulation strategy use, and anxiety symptoms. X = PTSD status; M = sleep quality (ISI scores); W = emotion regulation strategy use (emotion regulation ratio); Y = anxiety symptoms (PROMIS anxiety items).

anxiety (NIH PROMIS scores) (see Figure 1 for schematic). Analyses were conducted with and without TBI as a covariate to determine whether the presence of TBI impacts the relationship between PTSD, sleep, emotion regulation, and anxiety. A moderation model was chosen over a mediation model due to our a priori focus on the interaction between factors [17].

Moderation analyses, discussed directly above, were conducted using the SPSS PROCESS macro (Model 3). PROCESS calculates statistical significance using 95% confidence intervals to determine the effect of the predictor on the outcome measure. PROCESS also calculates the interaction effects of the moderators by testing the predictive effect of each factor at different levels (e.g., a low emotion regulation ratio and good sleep quality or a high emotion regulation ratio with poor sleep quality). Each predictor level was determined by values plus or minus 1 standard deviation from the centered mean. In order to eliminate both statistical power limitations and concerns about statistical assumption violations, 5000 bootstrap iterations were used within the macro (at least 2000 bootstrap iterations are recommended [18]).

Given the potential bias in our sample, which was referred for evaluation of sleep disorders, polysomnography- (PSG-) derived measures of sleep were assessed for group differences using ANOVA tests and results are reported below.

3. Results and Discussion

3.1. Preliminary Analyses. Demographic information is listed in Table 1. Notably, consistent with the demographics of veterans, the sample was predominantly male. There were no significant group differences for age, sex, or BMI between groups, although the mean age of the PTSD + TBI group was notably lower than that of the other groups. There were no group differences between objective PSG-derived sleep metrics (total sleep time (TST), sleep efficiency, sleep staging, and apnea-hypopnea index (AHI)).

There were several mental health/quality-of-life questionnaires for which groups differed. For example, there was a significant difference between groups for the NIH PROMIS anxiety items (Figure 2(a)). Consistent with our hypotheses, post hoc tests showed that the control group had significantly lower anxiety symptomatology than the PTSD-only group (mean difference = 2.95, $p = 0.002$) and the PTSD + TBI group (mean difference = 5.05, $p < 0.001$). The TBI-only group had significantly lower anxiety than the PTSD + TBI group (mean difference = 3.46, $p = 0.03$).

Table 1: Demographics (mean ± standard deviation). BMI = body mass image; PHQ-9 = Patient Health Questionnaire version 9; FOSQ-10 = Functional Outcomes of Sleep Questionnaire version 10; NIH PROMIS = National Institutes of Health Patient-Reported Outcomes Measurement Information System anxiety items; TST = total sleep time; SE = sleep efficiency; NREM1 (%) = percent of the night in non-REM sleep stage 1; NREM2 (%) = percent of the night in non-REM sleep stage 2; SWS (%) = percent of the night in slow wave sleep; REM (%) = percent of the night in rapid eye movement sleep; AHI = apnea/hypopnea index.

	Controls	TBI only	PTSD only	PTSD + TBI	*F* value	*p* value
Demographics						
Age	59.1 ± 13.3	56.2 ± 15.3	55.7 ± 13.5	48.8 ± 21.3	1.6	0.13
BMI	33.0 ± 6.8	33.0 ± 7.5	32.2 ± 5.4	29.3 ± 5.0	1.0	0.42
Gender (% male)	89.4	90	80.1	100	2.7	0.45
Mental health and quality of life						
NIH PROMIS	16.0 ± 3.1	14.4 ± 4.3	13.0 ± 3.6	10.9 ± 4.0	10.6	<0.001
PHQ-9	6.6 ± 4.8	8.7 ± 4.7	13.3 ± 5.6	14.0 ± 7.1	15.0	<0.001
FOSQ-10	15.9 ± 3.1	14.9 ± 3.7	10.9 ± 3.0	12.3 ± 4.3	15.6	<0.001
ISI	12.0 ± 6.1	13.7 ± 5.04	17.2 ± 5.9	18.5 ± 5.4	6.8	<0.001
Objective PSG-derived sleep metrics						
TST (min)	294.3 ± 101.1	313.4 ± 67.9	311.2 ± 89.0	286.4 ± 113.5	0.4	0.76
SE (%)	69.0 ± 18.7	72.9 ± 13.9	71.5 ± 18.6	65.4 ± 22.7	0.5	0.69
NREM1 (%)	12.1 ± 5.7	12.7 ± 4.9	11.6 ± 5.4	10.1 ± 3.8	0.6	0.65
NREM2 (%)	42.5 ± 15.7	46.1 ± 15.3	46.2 ± 13.7	38.7 ± 20.3	0.8	0.49
SWS (%)	1.7 ± 4.2	1.2 ± 3.1	1.3 ± 3.8	1.5 ± 2.5	0.1	0.94
REM (%)	11.7 ± 7.4	11.8 ± 6.9	11.0 ± 5.7	13.7 ± 9.5	0.3	0.81
AHI	19.5 ± 20.0	13.7 ± 11.1	16.5 ± 11.7	18.5 ± 15.5	0.7	0.57

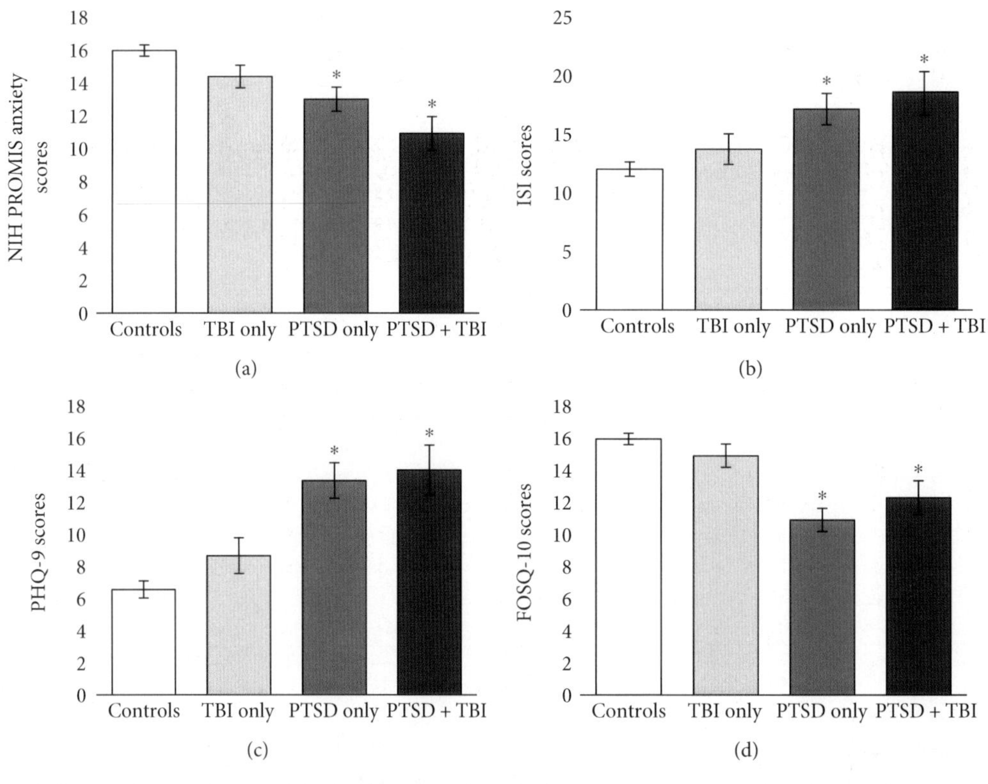

Figure 2: Groups differ on sleep and mental health based on TBI and PTSD status. Asterisk indicates that a given group differed significantly from veteran controls. (a) National Institutes of Health Patient-Reported Outcomes Measurement Information System (NIH PROMIS) anxiety items; (b) Insomnia Severity Index (ISI) scores; (c) Patient Health Questionnaire version 9 (PHQ-9) scores; (d) Functional Outcomes of Sleep Questionnaire version 10 (FOSQ-10) scores.

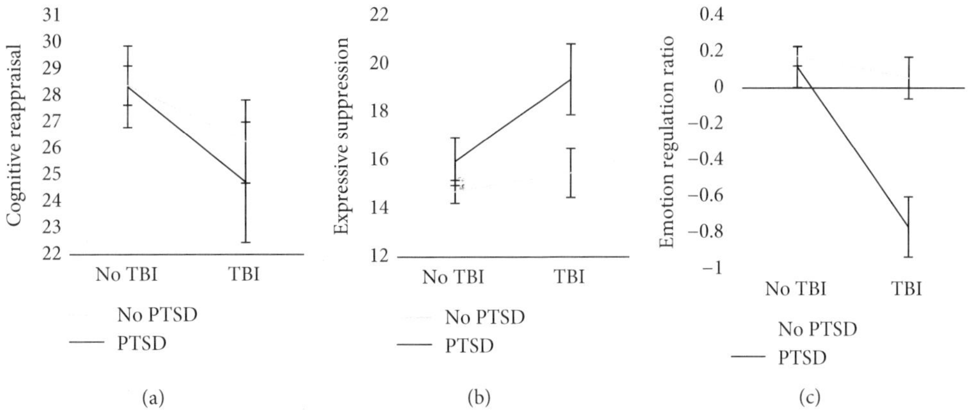

Figure 3: PTSD and TBI interact to predict certain outcomes. Black lines = PTSD; gray lines = no PTSD. (a) Usage of cognitive reappraisal (higher = more use of that strategy); (b) usage of expressive suppression (higher = more use of that strategy); (c) the ER ratio comprising both emotion regulation strategies (higher indicates more use of cognitive reappraisal, less use of expressive suppression).

Next, as hypothesized, groups differed significantly on the ISI (Figure 2(b)). Post hoc tests showed that the veteran control group had significantly lower ISI scores than the PTSD-only group (mean difference = −5.15, $p = 0.003$) and the PTSD + TBI group (mean difference = −6.49, $p = 0.006$), suggesting that subjective sleep quality was particularly poor in the PTSD and PTSD + TBI populations.

Groups also differed significantly on the PHQ-9 questionnaire (Figure 2(c)). Post hoc tests showed that the control group had significantly fewer depressive symptoms than the PTSD-only group (mean difference = 6.78, $p < 0.001$) and the PTSD + TBI group (mean difference = 7.45, $p < 0.001$). The TBI-only group also had significantly fewer depressive symptoms than the PTSD-only group (mean difference = 4.68, $p = 0.02$) and the PTSD + TBI group (mean difference = 5.35, $p = 0.03$).

Lastly, groups differed significantly on the FOSQ-10 (Figure 2(d)). Follow-up tests showed that the control group had significantly higher functioning than the PTSD-only group (mean difference = 5.03, $p < 0.001$) and the PTSD + TBI group (mean difference = 3. 64, $p = 0.006$). Additionally, the TBI-only group had significantly higher functioning than the PTSD-only group (mean difference = 3.89, $p = 0.001$).

3.2. Primary Analyses. We next conducted 2 × 2 ANOVA tests to determine whether emotion regulation strategies differed between groups. Contrary to hypotheses, when using cognitive reappraisal as an outcome measure, there was no main effect of PTSD, a trending main effect of TBI ($F(1,158) = 3.11, p = 0.08$; Figure 3(a)), and no interaction between the two factors. However, as predicted, for expressive suppression, there was a main effect of PTSD ($F(1,158) = 6.04$, $p = 0.01$; Figure 3(b)) and TBI ($F(1,158) = 3.98$, $p = 0.048$), such that those with PTSD and TBI used expressive suppression, a maladaptive strategy, more than controls. However, there was no interaction between these factors. Finally, the emotion regulation ratio was used as an outcome measure. There was a main effect of both PTSD ($F(1,158) = 13.90, p < 0.001$; Figure 3(b)) and TBI ($F(1,158) = 17.95, p < 0.001$), such that both the PTSD-only and TBI-only groups had a lower emotion regulation ratio than controls (indicating greater expressive suppression usage). There was also a significant interaction between the two factors, such that individuals in the PTSD + TBI group ($F(1,158) = 10.35$, $p = 0.002$) had the lowest emotion regulation ratio among the groups. Taken together, these results indicate that veterans with PTSD and TBI have an overall poorer emotion regulation profile. Additionally, PTSD and TBI cumulatively interact to create the poorest profile (i.e., the lowest emotion regulation ratio in the PTSD + TBI group).

We next conducted moderation analyses to determine the conditional effect of PTSD on anxiety symptomatology at different levels of the moderators (sleep and emotion regulation). In the omnibus model, as expected, having PTSD was a significant predictor of higher anxiety symptomatology ($B = -1.83$, 95% CI: −3.53, −0.13, $p = 0.04$). Poor sleep quality also significantly predicted higher anxiety ($B = -1.77$, 95% CI: −0.27, −0.07, $p = 0.0005$). Emotion regulation ratio significantly predicted anxiety, but in the opposite manner as predicted ($B = -1.27$, 95% CI: −2.43, −0.10, $p = 0.03$). That is, greater utilization of cognitive reappraisal (rather than expressive suppression) predicted higher anxiety. However, as described below, this main effect of emotion regulation is qualified by a significant interaction with sleep quality.

Table 2 demonstrates interactive effects between sleep quality and emotion regulation in individuals with PTSD. Notably, because these factors are moderators, a significant interaction indicates that those specific conditions must be met in order for PTSD to predict anxiety symptomatology. PTSD diagnosis significantly predicted higher anxiety in individuals who (1) utilize expressive suppression to a greater extent than cognitive reappraisal and also (2) have poor and average sleep quality. Similarly, PTSD significantly predicts higher anxiety symptomatology in individuals who (1) utilize both emotion regulation strategies equally and (2) have poor or average sleep quality. On the other hand, consistent with the above, for individuals with good sleep quality (and for individuals that predominantly utilize cognitive reappraisal, regardless of sleep quality), PTSD is not predictive of anxiety symptoms.

Table 2: PTSD presence predicts higher anxiety symptoms at each level of the moderators. Bold indicates statistical significance.

Emotion regulation strategy	Sleep quality	Beta	SE of beta	t	p	Lower CI	Upper CI
Suppression	Good	−2.26	1.56	−1.44	0.15	−5.36	0.83
Suppression	**Average**	**−2.31**	**1.09**	**−2.11**	**0.03**	**−4.48**	**−0.15**
Suppression	**Poor**	**−2.37**	**1.06**	**−2.23**	**0.02**	**−4.47**	**−0.27**
Equal utilization	Good	−1.77	1.40	−1.26	0.20	−4.55	1.00
Equal utilization	**Average**	**−1.82**	**0.85**	**−2.12**	**0.03**	**−3.52**	**−0.12**
Equal utilization	**Poor**	**−1.88**	**0.82**	**−2.27**	**0.02**	**−3.51**	**−0.24**
Reappraisal	Good	−1.28	1.47	−0.87	0.38	−4.19	1.62
Reappraisal	Average	−1.33	0.97	−1.37	0.17	−3.26	0.58
Reappraisal	Poor	−1.39	0.95	−1.45	0.14	−3.27	0.49

We conducted the same set of analyses while including TBI status as a covariate. Contrary to predictions, results were nearly identical to those noted above, indicating that the conditional effect of PTSD on anxiety symptomatology is not impacted by history of TBI.

3.3. Discussion

3.3.1. Links between Sleep, Emotion Regulation, PTSD, and Anxiety. Our results demonstrate the strong and complex links between PTSD, anxiety, sleep quality, and emotion regulation. As expected, we found that individuals with PTSD reported more anxiety and poorer subjective sleep compared to control subjects. With regard to emotion regulation, individuals with PTSD used emotion suppression (maladaptive) more so than cognitive reappraisal (adaptive) compared to control subjects. Individuals with PTSD + TBI showed the lowest emotion regulation scores (most maladaptive) across groups.

In particular, we found that the diagnosis of PTSD predicted higher anxiety in individuals who both (1) utilize expressive suppression to a greater extent than cognitive reappraisal or utilize expressive suppression and cognitive reappraisal equally and (2) report less than good sleep quality. Thus, although anxiety was significantly correlated with poor sleep quality, there was also an interaction between sleep quality and emotion regulation strategy use. The interaction suggests that PTSD predicts anxiety symptoms *only when certain conditions are met.* That is, PTSD predicts higher anxiety in the context of different combinations of sleep quality and emotion regulation strategy use. Specifically, poor emotion regulation (i.e., greater expressive suppression use and equal utilization of expressive suppression and cognitive reappraisal) is linked with maladaptive anxiety symptoms only in the context of less than good sleep quality. When an individual is a good sleeper, the link between PTSD and anxiety is not present, regardless of emotion regulation. Therefore, having better sleep quality may be protective against poor emotion regulation.

Our findings are consistent with the results of a recent longitudinal study that examined the relationship between sleep, emotion regulation, and depression. Poor emotion regulation was found to mediate the relationship between poor sleep at baseline and depression at 6-month follow-up. The authors suggested that sleep was a causal factor in influencing emotion regulation and depression. Although our model examines anxiety and not depression, we believe that these models are not mutually exclusive, as depression and anxiety are highly comorbid [19, 20]. Thus, our findings confirm and add to a growing body of literature which suggests that emotion regulation difficulties link sleep with poor emotional health.

It is important to note that opposite causality (or bidirectional causality) is possible, as better emotion regulation could be protective against poor sleep quality. Individuals utilizing poor emotion regulation skills may have maladaptive thought processes that could disturb sleep. For instance, higher use of expressive suppression has been linked with higher levels of rumination [21], which can exacerbate sleep issues [22, 23]. Therefore, it is possible that the modification of either sleep or emotion regulation could causally reduce downstream anxiety symptomatology in veterans with PTSD.

3.3.2. The Role of Comorbid TBI in Individuals with PTSD. In this study, we also aimed to assess the potentially moderating effect of traumatic brain injury (TBI) on sleep and emotion regulation. Although it is difficult to estimate cooccurrence of PTSD and TBI, a large cohort study found that one-third of veterans who had a TBI also have comorbid PTSD symptoms [24] and a separate study found that as many as 73% of individuals with TBI also had PTSD [25]. TBI and PTSD have separate but overlapping effects on psychopathology [26] and independent of PTSD; TBI has been linked with poor sleep quality [27, 28] and anxiety [29]. Therefore, when examining PTSD in a veteran population, TBI should also be considered to determine the potential influence of this factor on prolonged PTSD symptoms.

Many of the symptoms experienced during the chronic phase of recovery following TBI are similar in clinical presentation to PTSD symptoms. Specifically, anxiety, depression, irritability, and anger have been associated with both diagnoses [26]. Sleep issues are also common in both TBI and PTSD [28]. Consequently, individuals with both diagnoses tend to have a poorer functional status than individuals with only one diagnosis. For instance, veterans with both PTSD and TBI were shown to be more psychologically distressed and had poorer neurocognitive functioning than those with only

PTSD or TBI [30]. Several other studies have detected neurocognitive differences between PTSD + TBI groups and TBI-only or PTSD-only groups [31, 32]. In line with these findings, for the first time, we have shown that individuals with both PTSD + TBI exhibit the most maladaptive profile of emotion regulation strategies. Individuals in the PTSD + TBI group utilize expressive suppression to the greatest extent across groups. These results indicate that the PTSD + TBI population has particularly poor emotion regulation.

However, unexpectedly, inclusion of TBI in our moderation model did not impact the outcomes of interest. In other words, the relationship between PTSD and anxiety symptomatology (and conditional the effects at each level of the moderators) was not affected by TBI history. It is possible that the effect of PTSD is "overriding" that of TBI, which is consistent with previous literature on these topics. Vanderploeg and colleagues tested a model several years ago to determine whether PTSD and TBI independently or concurrently predicted tested outcomes (e.g., cognitive and emotional symptoms) [33]. The authors of this work noted that PTSD had a much larger effect on outcomes than TBI. In accordance, our results suggest that TBI status was of little influence relative to PTSD. Another similar explanation is that PTSD alone already confers a ceiling effect on anxiety and emotion regulation, such that addition of TBI (or any other factors) will not show discernable effects.

3.3.3. The Central Role of Sleep Disturbances and Anxiety in PTSD. Sleep disturbances are often thought of as a hallmark feature in individuals with PTSD. However, the impact of these sleep issues on quality of life—and the possible interrelationships between sleep and other factors—remains relatively unexplored. Our findings that sleep and emotion regulation interact to moderate the relationship between PTSD and anxiety symptoms could have meaningful implications for understanding barriers to treatment in veterans with PTSD.

For example, previous work has shown that improving poor-quality sleep improves PTSD severity. Treating sleep disorders (e.g., insomnia and OSA) lowers PTSD symptoms, such as nightmare frequency, unwanted thoughts, and distress [5, 6, 34, 35], suggesting that poor sleep actively contributes to PTSD symptomatology. Poor sleepers tend to utilize maladaptive emotion regulation strategies, potentially because poor sleep limits communication between emotion-regulating brain regions (e.g., the amygdala and the prefrontal cortex [36, 37]). Therefore, poor sleep may lead to poor emotion regulation, which could ultimately impact PTSD severity. Future work should be aimed at improving sleep and assessing whether emotion regulation also improves in individuals with PTSD.

Individuals with PTSD are 10 times more likely to have generalized anxiety disorder than those without PTSD [38]. Furthermore, veterans with both PTSD and high levels of anxiety have poorer quality of life than those with only PTSD [39, 40]. Focusing on anxiety symptomatology in PTSD could therefore provide valuable information to improve quality of life in individuals with PTSD.

3.3.4. Limitations. The results of this study must be interpreted in the context of the study limitations. Our cohort was recruited from a single site from a single clinic, the Portland VA Sleep Clinic. By definition, these subjects are referred for evaluation of sleep complaints, which presents potential sample bias in our results. Thus, the sleep characteristics of our sample (and related factors) may not be generalizable to the population at large.

Similarly, our sample was predominantly male, as is generally representative of the veteran population. Because most veterans are male, we believe that our results have external validity and some generalizability to other veteran populations. However, due to this bias, we were unable to assess sex as a biological variable. Given that females tend to have more military-related mental health issues than males [41, 42], identifying poor mental health contributors in the female population is critical. Future studies should attempt to include a more diverse population.

Lastly, this study utilized a cross sectional design, limiting causal and directional interpretability. Although we surmise, based on previous literature, that sleep is causally impacting emotion regulation, it is possible that emotion regulation is impacting sleep. Poor emotion regulation itself may lead to mental health issues [12], which, in turn, could worsen sleep quality. In the absence of sampling these factors at multiple time points, any hypotheses of directionality are speculative.

3.3.5. Implications and Future Directions. Given our results, there are two clear foreseeable steps that could be taken to follow up on this work. First, a longitudinal study should be conducted to determine whether sleep issues precede emotion regulation issues or vice versa. There is ample evidence to support the idea that poor sleep worsens emotional functioning, and in particular, there is evidence that poor sleep precedes the development of PTSD (but notably, PTSD does not precede the development of sleep disturbances) [43]. However, as mentioned, it is certainly possible that poor emotion regulation, which can contribute to mood disturbances, precedes poor sleep. Therefore, future work should be aimed at clarifying directionality.

After directionality is established, interventions could be implemented and assessed for efficacy. As discussed, there are many treatments for sleep disruption in individuals with PTSD, such as cognitive behavioral therapy for insomnia, image rehearsal therapy for nightmares, and medications [5, 35]. Implementing such sleep interventions may help support emotion regulation and improve anxiety symptomatology in veterans with PTSD. It is notable that subjective sleep, rather than objective sleep, was particularly poor in this population. Therefore, subjective sleep quality should be a point of intervention even in the absence of poor objective sleep. Alternatively, or perhaps concurrently, cognitive behavioral therapy focusing on emotion regulation strategies could perhaps be implemented to change emotional experience. Emotion regulation strategy modification (e.g., merely instructing individuals to use a different strategy) has been shown to be effective both experimentally [44] and therapeutically [45]. Taken together, modifying both sleep and emotion regulation could potentially lead to improved emotional outcomes, which could ultimately enhance quality of life in individuals with PTSD.

4. Conclusions

We found a relationship between PTSD and anxiety in veterans with poor/average sleep quality who utilize maladaptive emotion regulation strategies (i.e., utilizing expressive suppression more than cognitive reappraisal or using both strategies equally). However, in veterans who sleep well, there was no relationship between PTSD and anxiety, even when emotion regulation was poor. We posit that good-quality sleep is protective against poor emotion regulation in veterans with PTSD. Improving sleep could, in effect, improve anxiety symptomatology in this population. Future experimental work should implement sleep intervention techniques (e.g., cognitive behavioral therapy) in veterans in order to enhance wellbeing and quality of life in this group.

Disclosure

The contents do not represent the views of the U.S. Department of Veterans Affairs or the United States Government. Material has been reviewed by the Walter Reed Army Institute of Research. There is no objection to its presentation and/or publication. The opinions or assertions contained herein are the private views of the author and are not to be construed as official or as reflecting true views of the Department of the Army or the Department of Defense. The investigators have adhered to the policies for protection of human subjects as prescribed in AR 70–25.

Acknowledgments

The authors would like to express their sincere appreciation and gratitude for the participation of all subjects, to the staff at the VA Portland Health Care System Sleep Disorders Clinic. Specific acknowledgements go to Ryan A. Opel for assistance with data curation and Alexander Q. Chau and Matthew R. Gieger for assistance with chart review. This work was supported by the Sleep Research Society Mentor-Mentee Program award, awarded to Janna Mantua. This work was also supported with resources and the use of facilities at the VA Portland Health Care System, VA Career Development Award no. IK2 BX002712, NIH EXITO Institutional Core, no. UL1GM118964, the Portland VA Research Foundation to Miranda M. Lim, and VA OAA Post-doctoral Nursing Research Fellowship to Kris B. Weymann.

References

[1] American Psychiatric Association, *Diagnostic and Statistical Manual of Mental Disorders*, American Psychiatric Association, Washington, DC, USA, 5th edition, 2013.

[2] E. K. Dursa, M. J. Reinhard, S. K. Barth, and A. I. Schneiderman, "Prevalence of a positive screen for PTSD among OEF/OIF and OEF/OIF-era veterans in a large population-based cohort," *Journal of Traumatic Stress*, vol. 27, no. 5, pp. 542–549, 2014.

[3] D. F. Zatzick, C. R. Marmar, D. S. Weiss et al., "Posttraumatic stress disorder and functioning and quality of life outcomes in a nationally representative sample of male Vietnam veterans," *The American Journal of Psychiatry*, vol. 154, no. 12, pp. 1690–1695, 1997.

[4] R. N. McLay, W. P. Klam, and S. L. Volkert, "Insomnia is the most commonly reported symptom and predicts other symptoms of post-traumatic stress disorder in U.S. service members returning from military deployments," *Military Medicine*, vol. 175, no. 10, pp. 759–762, 2010.

[5] C. S. Ulmer, J. D. Edinger, and P. S. Calhoun, "A multi-component cognitive-behavioral intervention for sleep disturbance in veterans with PTSD: a pilot study," *Journal of Clinincal Sleep Medicine*, vol. 7, no. 1, pp. 57–68, 2011.

[6] S. Tamanna, J. D. Parker, J. Lyons, and M. I. Ullah, "The effect of continuous positive air pressure (CPAP) on nightmares in patients with posttraumatic stress disorder (PTSD) and obstructive sleep apnea (OSA)," *Journal of Clinical Sleep Medicine*, vol. 14, no. 5, p. 631, 2014.

[7] J. J. Gross, "The emerging field of emotion regulation: an integrative review," *Review of General Psychology*, vol. 2, no. 3, pp. 271–299, 1998.

[8] J. J. Gross, "Emotion regulation: affective, cognitive, and social consequences," *Psychophysiology*, vol. 39, no. 3, pp. 281–291, 2002.

[9] M. T. Boden, S. Westermann, K. McRae et al., "Emotion regulation and posttraumatic stress disorder: a prospective investigation," *Journal of Social and Clinical Psychology*, vol. 32, no. 3, pp. 296–314, 2013.

[10] I. Vantieghem, N. Marcoen, O. Mairesse, and M. Vandekerckhove, "Emotion regulation mediates the relationship between personality and sleep quality," *Psychology & Health*, vol. 31, no. 9, pp. 1064–1079, 2016.

[11] F. W. Weathers, B. T. Litz, D. S. Herman, J. A. Huska, and T. M. Keane, "The PTSD Checklist (PCL): reliability, validity, and diagnostic utility," in *Annual Convention of the International Society for Traumatic Stress Studies*, San Antonio, TX, USA, 1993.

[12] J. J. Gross and O. P. John, "Individual differences in two emotion regulation processes: implications for affect, relationships, and well-being," *Journal of Personality and Social Psychology*, vol. 85, no. 2, pp. 348–362, 2003.

[13] J. Broderick, E. M. DeWit, N. Rothrock, P. Crane, and C. B. Forrest, "Advances in patient-reported outcomes: the NIH PROMIS® measures," *eGEMs*, vol. 1, no. 1, 2013.

[14] C. H. Bastien, A. Vallières, and C. M. Morin, "Validation of the Insomnia Severity Index as an outcome measure for insomnia research," *Sleep Medicine*, vol. 2, no. 4, pp. 297–307, 2001.

[15] B. Löwe, K. Kroenke, W. Herzog, and K. Gräfe, "Measuring depression outcome with a brief self-report instrument: sensitivity to change of the Patient Health Questionnaire (PHQ-9)," *Journal of Affective Disorders*, vol. 81, no. 1, pp. 61–66, 2004.

[16] E. R. Chasens, S. J. Ratcliffe, and T. E. Weaver, "Development of the FOSQ-10: a short version of the Functional Outcomes of Sleep Questionnaire," *Sleep*, vol. 32, no. 7, pp. 915–919, 2009.

[17] A. F. Hayes, *PROCESS: A Versatile Computational Tool for Observed Variable Mediation, Moderation, and Conditional Process Modeling*, University of Kansas, Lawrence, KS, USA, 2012.

[18] T. J. DiCiccio and B. Efron, "Bootstrap confidence intervals," *Statistical Science*, vol. 11, no. 3, pp. 189–212, 1996.

[19] L. A. Clark and D. Watson, "Tripartite model of anxiety and depression: psychometric evidence and taxonomic implications," *Journal of Abnormal Psychology*, vol. 100, no. 3, pp. 316–336, 1991.

[20] M. E. den Hollander-Gijsman, E. de Beurs, N. J. A. van der Wee, Y. R. van Rood, and F. G. Zitman, "Distinguishing between depression and anxiety: a proposal for an extension of the tripartite model," *European Psychiatry*, vol. 25, no. 4, pp. 197–205, 2010.

[21] S. Nolen-Hoeksema, B. E. Wisco, and S. Lyubomirsky, "Rethinking rumination," *Perspectives on Psychological Science*, vol. 3, no. 5, pp. 400–424, 2008.

[22] M. A. Kompier, T. W. Taris, and M. Van Veldhoven, "Tossing and turning-insomnia in relation to occupational stress, rumination, fatigue, and well-being," *Scandinavian Journal of Work, Environment & Health*, vol. 38, no. 3, pp. 238–246, 2012.

[23] J. Fernández-Mendoza, A. Vela-Bueno, A. N. Vgontzas et al., "Cognitive-emotional hyperarousal as a premorbid characteristic of individuals vulnerable to insomnia," *Psychosomatic Medicine*, vol. 72, no. 4, pp. 397–403, 2010.

[24] G. Sheppes and N. Meiran, "Divergent cognitive costs for online forms of reappraisal and distraction," *Emotion*, vol. 8, no. 6, pp. 870–874, 2008.

[25] B. C. Taylor, E. M. Hagel, K. F. Carlson et al., "Prevalence and costs of co-occurring traumatic brain injury with and without psychiatric disturbance and pain among Afghanistan and Iraq War Veteran VA users," *Medical Care*, vol. 50, no. 4, pp. 342–346, 2012.

[26] M. B. Stein and T. W. McAllister, "Exploring the convergence of posttraumatic stress disorder and mild traumatic brain injury," *The American Journal of Psychiatry*, vol. 166, no. 7, pp. 768–776, 2009.

[27] J. Mantua, A. Grillakis, S. Mahfouz et al., "A systematic review and meta-analysis of sleep architecture and chronic traumatic brain injury," *Sleep Medicine Reviews*, 2018.

[28] D. K. Sandsmark, J. E. Elliott, and M. M. Lim, "Sleep-wake disturbances after traumatic brain injury: synthesis of human and animal studies," *Sleep*, vol. 40, no. 5, article zsx044, 2017.

[29] A. C. Scholten, J. A. Haagsma, M. C. Cnossen, M. Olff, E. F. Van Beeck, and S. Polinder, "Prevalence of and risk factors for anxiety and depressive disorders after traumatic brain injury: a systematic review," *Journal of Neurotrauma*, vol. 33, no. 22, pp. 1969–1994, 2016.

[30] H. L. Combs, D. T. R. Berry, T. Pape et al., "The effects of mild traumatic brain injury, post-traumatic stress disorder, and combined mild traumatic brain injury/post-traumatic stress disorder on returning veterans," *Journal of Neurotrauma*, vol. 32, no. 13, pp. 956–966, 2015.

[31] L. A. Brenner, S. E. Ladley-O'Brien, J. E. F. Harwood et al., "An exploratory study of neuroimaging, neurologic, and neuropsychological findings in veterans with traumatic brain injury and/or posttraumatic stress disorder," *Military Medicine*, vol. 174, no. 4, pp. 347–352, 2009.

[32] L. A. Nelson, R. E. Yoash-Gantz, T. C. Pickett, and T. A. Campbell, "Relationship between processing speed and executive functioning performance among OEF/OIF veterans: implications for postdeployment rehabilitation," *Journal of Head Trauma Rehabilitation*, vol. 24, no. 1, pp. 32–40, 2009.

[33] R. D. Vanderploeg, H. G. Belanger, and G. Curtiss, "Mild traumatic brain injury and posttraumatic stress disorder and their associations with health symptoms," *Archives of Physical Medicine and Rehabilitation*, vol. 90, no. 7, pp. 1084–1093, 2009.

[34] S. O. Margolies, B. Rybarczyk, S. R. Vrana, D. J. Leszczyszyn, and J. Lynch, "Efficacy of a cognitive-behavioral treatment for insomnia and nightmares in Afghanistan and Iraq veterans with PTSD," *Journal of Clinical Psychology*, vol. 69, no. 10, pp. 1026–1042, 2013.

[35] L. M. Swanson, T. K. Favorite, E. Horin, and J. T. Arnedt, "A combined group treatment for nightmares and insomnia in combat veterans: a pilot study," *Journal of Traumatic Stress*, vol. 22, no. 6, pp. 639–642, 2009.

[36] Y. Motomura, S. Kitamura, K. Oba et al., "Sleep debt elicits negative emotional reaction through diminished amygdala-anterior cingulate functional connectivity," *PLoS One*, vol. 8, no. 2, article e56578, 2013.

[37] Y. Motomura, R. Katsunuma, M. Yoshimura, and K. Mishima, "Two days' sleep debt causes mood decline during resting state via diminished amygdala-prefrontal connectivity," *Sleep*, vol. 40, no. 10, 2017.

[38] J. R. Davidson, D. Hughes, D. G. Blazer, and L. K. George, "Post-traumatic stress disorder in the community: an epidemiological study," *Psychological Medicine*, vol. 21, no. 3, pp. 713–721, 1991.

[39] K. Ginzburg, T. Ein-Dor, and Z. Solomon, "Comorbidity of posttraumatic stress disorder, anxiety and depression: a 20-year longitudinal study of war veterans," *Journal of Affective Disorders*, vol. 123, no. 1–3, pp. 249–257, 2010.

[40] M. G. Warshaw, E. Fierman, L. Pratt et al., "Quality of life and dissociation in anxiety disorder patients with histories of trauma or PTSD," *The American Journal of Psychiatry*, vol. 150, no. 10, pp. 1512–1516, 1993.

[41] A. E. Street, S. E. Gilman, A. J. Rosellini et al., "Understanding the elevated suicide risk of female soldiers during deployments," *Psychological Medicine*, vol. 45, no. 4, pp. 717–726, 2015.

[42] S. Maguen, B. Cohen, L. Ren, J. Bosch, R. Kimerling, and K. Seal, "Gender differences in military sexual trauma and mental health diagnoses among Iraq and Afghanistan veterans with posttraumatic stress disorder," *Womens Health Issues*, vol. 22, no. 1, article e61–e66, pp. e61–e66, 2012.

[43] K. M. Wright, T. W. Britt, P. D. Bliese, A. B. Adler, D. Picchioni, and D. Moore, "Insomnia as predictor versus outcome of PTSD and depression among Iraq combat veterans," *Journal of Clinical Psychology*, vol. 67, no. 12, pp. 1240–1258, 2011.

[44] J. J. Gross, "Antecedent-and response-focused emotion regulation: divergent consequences for experience, expression, and physiology," *Journal of Personality and Social Psychology*, vol. 74, no. 1, pp. 224–237, 1998.

[45] M. Berking, P. Wupperman, A. Reichardt, T. Pejic, A. Dippel, and H. Znoj, "Emotion-regulation skills as a treatment target in psychotherapy," *Behaviour Research and Therapy*, vol. 46, no. 11, pp. 1230–1237, 2008.

Permissions

All chapters in this book were first published in BN, by Hindawi Publishing Corporation; hereby published with permission under the Creative Commons Attribution License or equivalent. Every chapter published in this book has been scrutinized by our experts. Their significance has been extensively debated. The topics covered herein carry significant findings which will fuel the growth of the discipline. They may even be implemented as practical applications or may be referred to as a beginning point for another development.

The contributors of this book come from diverse backgrounds, making this book a truly international effort. This book will bring forth new frontiers with its revolutionizing research information and detailed analysis of the nascent developments around the world.

We would like to thank all the contributing authors for lending their expertise to make the book truly unique. They have played a crucial role in the development of this book. Without their invaluable contributions this book wouldn't have been possible. They have made vital efforts to compile up to date information on the varied aspects of this subject to make this book a valuable addition to the collection of many professionals and students.

This book was conceptualized with the vision of imparting up-to-date information and advanced data in this field. To ensure the same, a matchless editorial board was set up. Every individual on the board went through rigorous rounds of assessment to prove their worth. After which they invested a large part of their time researching and compiling the most relevant data for our readers.

The editorial board has been involved in producing this book since its inception. They have spent rigorous hours researching and exploring the diverse topics which have resulted in the successful publishing of this book. They have passed on their knowledge of decades through this book. To expedite this challenging task, the publisher supported the team at every step. A small team of assistant editors was also appointed to further simplify the editing procedure and attain best results for the readers.

Apart from the editorial board, the designing team has also invested a significant amount of their time in understanding the subject and creating the most relevant covers. They scrutinized every image to scout for the most suitable representation of the subject and create an appropriate cover for the book.

The publishing team has been an ardent support to the editorial, designing and production team. Their endless efforts to recruit the best for this project, has resulted in the accomplishment of this book. They are a veteran in the field of academics and their pool of knowledge is as vast as their experience in printing. Their expertise and guidance has proved useful at every step. Their uncompromising quality standards have made this book an exceptional effort. Their encouragement from time to time has been an inspiration for everyone.

The publisher and the editorial board hope that this book will prove to be a valuable piece of knowledge for researchers, students, practitioners and scholars across the globe.

List of Contributors

Vasiliy V. Reshetnikov
Laboratory of Gene Expression Regulation, Institute of Cytology and Genetics, Siberian Branch of the Russian Academy of Sciences,10 Prospect Lavrentyeva, Novosibirsk 630090, Russia
Novosibirsk National Research State University, 2 Pirogova Street, Novosibirsk 630090, Russia

Natalya P. Bondar and Arina A. Lepeshko
Laboratory of Gene Expression Regulation, Institute of Cytology and Genetics, Siberian Branch of the Russian Academy of Sciences, 10 Prospect Lavrentyeva, Novosibirsk 630090, Russia
Novosibirsk National Research State University, 2 Pirogova Street, Novosibirsk 630090, Russia

Ray-Chang Tzeng, Ching-Fang Tsai and Ching-Tsu Wang
Department of Neurology, Tainan Municipal Hospital (Managed by Show Chwan Medical Care Corporation), Tainan, Taiwan

Tzu-Yuan Wang
Division of Endocrinology and Metabolism, Department of Internal Medicine, China Medical University Hospital,

Pai-Yi Chiu
Department of Neurology, Show Chwan Memorial Hospital, Changhua, Taiwan

Xiaojing Long, Chunxiang Jiang and Lijuan Zhang
Paul C. Lauterbur Research Center for Biomedical Imaging, Shenzhen Institutes of Advanced Technology, Chinese Academy of Sciences, 1068 Xueyuan Avenue, Shenzhen 518055, China

Laura Scott, Maryanne McPhee, Susan Mathers, Marie-Claire Davis, Roxanne Maule and Fiona Fisher
Calvary Health Care Bethlehem, South Caulfield, VIC, Australia

Nicholas P. Ryan
Calvary Health Care Bethlehem, South Caulfield, VIC, Australia
Melbourne School of Psychological Sciences, The University of Melbourne, Parkville, VIC, Australia

Pablo Cruz Gonzalez and Kenneth N. K. Fong
Department of Rehabilitation Sciences, The Hong Kong Polytechnic University, Hong Kong, Hong Kong

Ted Brown
Department of Occupational Therapy, Monash University, Melbourne, VIC, Australia

Ling-yun Wu, Zong Zhuang, Yongyue Gao, Chao Tang, Chen-hui Zhou, Chun-xi Wang, Xiang-sheng Zhang, Guang-bin Xie, Meng-liang Zhou and Ji-xin Shi
Department of Neurosurgery, Jinling Hospital, School of Medicine, Nanjing University, 305 East ZhongShan Road, Nanjing, Jiangsu Province 210002, China

Chun-hua Hang
Department of Neurosurgery, Jinling Hospital, School of Medicine, Nanjing University, 305 East ZhongShan Road, Nanjing, Jiangsu Province 210002, China
Department of Neurosurgery, Jinling Hospital, School of Medicine, Southern Medical University (Guangzhou), Nanjing

Zhen-nan Ye
Department of Neurosurgery, the Second Affiliated Hospital of Guangzhou Medical University, Guangzhou, Guangdong Province 510260, China
Department of Neurosurgery, Jinling Hospital, School of Medicine, Southern Medical University (Guangzhou), Nanjing,Jiangsu Province 210002, China

Jing-peng Liu
Department of Neurosurgery, Jinling Hospital, School of Medicine, Southern Medical University (Guangzhou), Nanjing, Jiangsu Province 210002, China

Nathan J. Wilson
School of Nursing and Midwifery, Western Sydney University, Hawkesbury Campus, Locked Bag 3, Richmond, NSW 2753, Australia

Hoe C. Lee, Sharmila Vaz, Priscilla Vindin and Reinie Cordier
School of Occupational Therapy Social Work and Speech Pathology, Faculty of Health Sciences, Curtin University, Perth, WA 6845, Australia

I-Chen Li, Li-Ya Lee, Wan-Ping Chen and Yen-Po Chen
Grape King Bio Ltd, Zhong-Li Dist., Taoyuan City, Taiwan

Chin-Chu Chen
Grape King Bio Ltd, Zhong-Li Dist., Taoyuan City, Taiwan
Institute of Food Science and Technology, National Taiwan University, Taipei City, Taiwan
Department of Food Science, Nutrition and Nutraceutical Biotechnology, Shih Chien University, Taipei City, Taiwan
Institute of Biotechnology, National Changhua University of Education, Changhua, Taiwan

Tsai-Teng Tzeng and Young-Ju Shiao
Institute of Biopharmaceutical Sciences, National Yang-Ming University, Taipei City, Taiwan

Hui-Chi Lin
Department of Neurology, MacKay Memorial Hospital, Taipei, Taiwan

Pei-Hao Chen
Department of Neurology, MacKay Memorial Hospital, Taipei, Taiwan
Department of Medicine, Mackay Medical College, New Taipei City, Taiwan
Graduate Institute of Mechanical and Electrical Engineering, National Taipei University of Technology, Taipei, Taiwan

Shih-Jung Cheng
Department of Neurology, MacKay Memorial Hospital, Taipei, Taiwan
Department of Medicine, Mackay Medical College, New Taipei City, Taiwan
Department of Physical Therapy and Assistive Technology, National Yang-Ming University, Taipei, Taiwan

Chuo-Yu Lee
Department of Neurology, MacKay Memorial Hospital, Taipei, Taiwan
Department of Medicine, Mackay Medical College, New Taipei City, Taiwan
Graduate Institute of Chemistry, Tamkang University, New Taipei City, Taiwan

Chih-Ho Chou
Department of Neurology, Chi-Mei Medical Center, Tainan, Taiwan
Chia Nan University of Pharmacy and Science, Tainan, Taiwan

Paul Bosch and Mauricio Herrera
Facultad de Ingeníera, Universidad del Desarrollo, Av. Plaza 700, Las Condes, Santiago, Chile

Julio López
Facultad de Ingeniería y Ciencias, Universidad Diego Portales, Ejército 441, Santiago, Chile

Sebastián Maldonado
Facultad de Ingeniería y Ciencias Aplicadas, Universidad de los Andes, Monseñor Álvaro del Portillo 12455, Las Condes, Santiago, Chile

Foteini Christidi
First Department of Neurology, Aeginition Hospital, Medical School, National and Kapodistrian University of Athens, Athens, Greece

Raffaella Migliaccio
INSERM U 1127, CNRS UMR 7225, Sorbonne Universités, and Université Pierre et Marie Curie-Paris 6, UMRS 1127, Institut du Cerveau et de la Moelle Épinière (ICM), 75013 Paris, France

Hernando Santamaría-García
Pontificia Universidad Javeriana Bogotá, Colombia, Centro de Memoria y Cognición Intellectus Hospital Universitario San Ignacio, Bogotá, Colombia

Gabriella Santangelo
Department of Psychology, University of Campania "Luigi Vanvitelli", Caserta, Italy

Francesca Trojsi
Department of Medical, Surgical, Neurological, Metabolic, and Aging Sciences, University of Campania "Luigi Vanvitelli",Naples, Italy

Serpil Özmen
Narman Technical College, Atatürk University, Erzurum, Turkey

Afife Yurttaş
Faculty of Nursing, Atatürk University, Erzurum, Turkey

Mi Li and Hongpei Xu
Laboratory of Intelligent Scienceand Technology, Department of Automation, Faculty of Information Technology,Beijing University of Technology, Beijing 100024, China
Beijing International Collaboration Base on Brain Informatics and Wisdom Services, Beijing 100024, China

Shengfu Lu
Laboratory of Intelligent Scienceand Technology, Department of Automation, Faculty of Information Technology, Beijing University of Technology, Beijing 100024, China
Beijing International Collaboration Base on Brain Informatics and Wisdom Services, Beijing 100024, China
Beijing Advanced Innovation Centre for Future Internet Technology, Beijing University of Technology, Beijing 100024, China

Marcia Belas dos Santos, Arly dos Santos and Ricardo Mario Arida
Physiology Department, Universidade Federal de São Paulo (UNIFESP), São Paulo, SP, Brazil

Clarissa Barros de Oliveira and Viviana Dylewski
Physiotherapy Department, Associação de Assistência a Criança Deficiente (AACD), São Paulo, SP, Brazil

Cristhiane Garabello Pires
Faculty of Medicine, University of Sao Paulo (USP), São Paulo, SP, Brazil

Linlin Zhang and Wenliang Ji
Capital University of Physical Education and Sports, Beijing 100191, China

Yi Feng
Beijing Xicheng District Desheng Community Health Service Center, Beijing 100120, China

Jianzhang Liu
Peking University School and Hospital of Stomatology, Beijing 100081, China

Kun Liu
Capital University of Physical Education and Sports, Beijing 100191, China
Department of Psychiatry, Yale University School of Medicine, New Haven, CT 06511, USA

Caroline Neely and Jane Flinn
Department of Psychology, George Mason University, 4400 University Drive, Fairfax, VA 22030, USA

Christina Lane and Julio Torres
Interdisciplinary Program in Neuroscience, George Mason University, 4400 University Drive, Fairfax, VA 22030, USA

Masahito Takahashi, Hideaki Ohne, Atsushi Hasegawa, Shunsuke Sato and Shoichi Ichimura
Department of Orthopaedic Surgery, Kyorin University, 6-20-2 Shinkawa, Mitaka-shi, Tokyo 181-0004, Japan

Takumi Takeuchi
Department of Orthopaedic Surgery, Kyorin University, 6-20-2 Shinkawa, Mitaka-shi, Tokyo 181-0004, Japan
Department of Orthopaedic Surgery, Kugayama Hospital, 2-14-20 Kitakarasuyama, Setagaya-ku, Tokyo 157-0061, Japan

Kazuhiko Satomi
Department of Orthopaedic Surgery, Kugayama Hospital, 2-14-20 Kitakarasuyama, Setagaya-ku, Tokyo 157-0061, Japan

Shasha Yang, Daien Liu, Bin Zeng, Zhiqing Liu and Haoran Kang
Chengdu University of Traditional Chinese Medicine, Chengdu, Sichuan province, China

Jing Wu
Guiyang College of Traditional Chinese Medicine, Guiyang, Guizhou province, China

Qinxiu Zhang and Xinrong Li
Department of Otorhinolaryngology, Head and Neck Surgery, Teaching Hospital of Chengdu University of Traditional Chinese Medicine, Chengdu, Sichuan province, China

Zhendong Zhong
Sichuan Academy of Medical Sciences and Sichuan Provincial People's Hospital, Chengdu, China

Chih-Kuang Cheng
Stroke Center and Department of Neurology, Linkou Medical Center, Chang Gung Memorial Hospital and College of Medicine, Chang Gung University, Taoyuan, Taiwan

Yu-Chien Tsao
Department of Internal Medicine, Yonghe Cardinal Tien Hospital, Taipei, Taiwan
Department of Neurology, Neurological Institute, Taipei Veterans General Hospital, Taipei, Taiwan
School of Medicine, National Yang-Ming University, Taipei, Taiwan

Yuan-Chih Su
Management Office for Health Data, China Medical University Hospital, Taichung, Taiwan
College of Medicine, China Medical University, Taichung, Taiwan

Fung-Chang Sung
Department of Public Health, China Medical University, Taichung, Taiwan

Hsu-Chih Tai
Department of Exercise and Health Promotion, College of Education, Chinese Culture University, Taipei, Taiwan

Woon-Man Kung
Department of Exercise and Health Promotion, College of Education, Chinese Culture University, Taipei, Taiwan
Division of Neurosurgery, Department of Surgery, Taipei Tzu Chi Hospital, Buddhist Tzu Chi Medical Foundation, New Taipei City, Taiwan
Department of Surgery, School of Medicine, Buddhist Tzu Chi University, Hualien, Taiwan

Danyan Chen and Hucheng Zhou
Shanghai Institute for Advanced Communication and Data Science, Shanghai University, Shanghai, China

Jiehui Jiang
Shanghai Institute for Advanced Communication and Data Science, Shanghai University, Shanghai, China
Institute of Biomedical Engineering, Shanghai University, Shanghai, China

Jiaying Lu, Ping Wu, Jingjie Ge and Huiwei Zhang
PET Center, Huashan Hospital, Fudan University, Shanghai, China

Chuantao Zuo
PET Center, Huashan Hospital, Fudan University, Shanghai, China
Institute of Functional and Molecular Medical Imaging, Fudan University, Shanghai, China

Qihao Guo
Department of Neurology, Huashan Hospital, Fudan University, Shanghai, China

Kuangyu Shi
Department of Nuclear Medicine, Technische Universität München, Munich, Germany

Shaoyang Cui
Department of Rehabilitation, Shenzhen Hospital of Guangzhou University of Chinese Medicine, Shenzhen, China
Stroke Biological Recovery Laboratory, Spaulding Rehabilitation Hospital, Harvard Medical School, Charlestown, MA 02129, USA

Mingzhu Xu and Qing Mei Wang
Stroke Biological Recovery Laboratory, Spaulding Rehabilitation Hospital, Harvard Medical School, Charlestown, MA 02129, USA

Jianting Huang
Stroke Biological Recovery Laboratory, Spaulding Rehabilitation Hospital, Harvard Medical School, Charlestown, MA 02129, USA
Clinical Medical College of Acupuncture and Rehabilitation, Guangzhou University of Chinese Medicine, Guangzhou, China

Chunzhi Tang
Clinical Medical College of Acupuncture and Rehabilitation, Guangzhou University of Chinese Medicine, Guangzhou, China

Binbin Nie and Baoci Shan
Key Laboratory of Nuclear Analysis Techniques, Beijing Engineering Research Center of Radiographic Techniques and Equipment, Institute of High Energy Physics, Chinese Academy of Sciences, Beijing, China

Xun Luo
Kerry Rehabilitation Medicine Research Institute, Shenzhen, China

John Wong
School of Nursing, MGH Institute of Health Professions, Boston, MA 02129, USA
Department of Occupational Therapy, MGH Institute of Health Professions, Boston, MA 02129, USA

Andrew R. Carr
VA Greater Los Angeles Healthcare System, Los Angeles, CA, USA
Department of Neurology, David Geffen School of Medicine, University of California at Los Angeles, Los Angeles, CA, USA

Elvira E. Jimenez
VA Greater Los Angeles Healthcare System, Los Angeles, CA, USA
Department of Neurology, David Geffen School of Medicine, University of California at Los Angeles, Los Angeles, CA, USA

Mario F. Mendez
VA Greater Los Angeles Healthcare System, Los Angeles, CA, USA
Department of Neurology, David Geffen School of Medicine, University of California at Los Angeles, Los Angeles, CA, USA
Department of Psychiatryand Biobehavioral Sciences, David Geffen School of Medicine, University of California at Los Angeles, Los Angeles, CA, USA

Mark M. Ashla
Department of Neurology, David Geffen School of Medicine, University of California at Los Angeles, Los Angeles, CA, USA

Paul B. Perrin
Department of Psychology, Virginia Commonwealth University, Richmond, VA, USA
Department of Physical Medicineand Rehabilitation, Virginia Commonwealth University School of Medicine, Richmond, VA, USA

Melody N. Mickens
Department of Psychology, Virginia Commonwealth University, Richmond, VA, USA
Department of Physical Medicineand Rehabilitation, Virginia Commonwealth University School of Medicine, Richmond, VA, USA

Brenda Rabago and Miguel A. Macías-Islas
Department of Neuroscience, CUCS, University of Guadalajara, Guadalajara, JAL, Mexico

Adriana Aguayo
Department of Neuroscience, CUCS, University of Guadalajara, Guadalajara, JAL, Mexico
Department of Psychology, Enrique Diaz de Leon University, Guadalajara, JAL, Mexico

Juan Carlos Arango-Lasprilla
BioCruces Health Research Institute, Cruces University Hospital Barakaldo, Bizkaia, Spain
IKERBASQUE, Basque Foundation for Science, Bilbao, Spain

Xiang-Dong Xiong
Department of Neurology, The First Affiliated Hospital of Anhui Medical University, Hefei, 230022 Anhui, China
Lu'an Affiliated Hospital of Anhui Medical University, People's Hospital of Lu'an City, Lu'an, 237005 Anhui, China

Wei-Dong Xiong and Shang-Shen Xiong
Department of Neurology, The First Affiliated Hospital of Anhui Medical University, Hefei, 230022 Anhui, China
Hefei National Level High and New Technology Development Zone, Hefei, 230088 Anhui, China

Gui-Hai Chen
Department of Neurology, The First Affiliated Hospital of Anhui Medical University, Hefei, 230022 Anhui, China
Department of Neurology, The Affiliated Chaohu Hospital of Anhui Medical University, Chaohu, 238000 Anhui, China

M. P. Ortega-Merchan, F. Uriza and P. Reyes
Departamento de Radiología e Imágenes Diagnósticas, Hospital Universitario San Ignacio, Bogotá, Colombia
Facultad de Medicina, Pontificia Universidad Javeriana, Bogotá, Colombia

N. Rojas-Serrano, J. Rodriguez-Santos, M. C. Velasco-Leon, J. D. Rodriguez-Parra, D. E. Mora-Diaz and D. Matallana
Facultad de Medicina, Pontificia Universidad Javeriana, Bogotá, Colombia

Hernando Santamaria-García
Facultad de Medicina, Pontificia Universidad Javeriana, Bogotá, Colombia
Centro de Memoria y Cognición Intellectus, Hospital Universitario San Ignacio, Bogotá, Colombia
Departamento de Psiquiatría, Universidad Nacional de Colombia, Bogotá, Colombia

A. Rueda
Facultad de Ingeniería, Pontificia Universidad Javeriana, Bogotá, Colombia

Jia-qi Tian, Xiao-zhu Hao, Chan-chan Li, Xiao-yuan Feng, Hua-ping Sun and Yan-mei Yang
Department of Radiology, Huashan Hospital, Fudan University, Shanghai 200040, China

Jia-jun Zheng and Kang Zheng
Department of Neurosurgery, Huashan Hospital, Fudan University, Shanghai 200040, China

Le-kang Yin
Department of Radiology, Shanghai Chest hospital, Shanghai Jiao Tong University, Shanghai 200030, China

Xiao-xue Zhang
Department of Radiotherapy, Shanghai Eastern Hepatobiliary Surgery Hospital, Shanghai 310114, China

Min Jiang
Institutes of Science and State Key Laboratory of Medical Neurobiology, Fudan University, Shanghai 200030, China

Janna Mantua
Neuroscienceand Behavior Program, University of Massachusetts, Amherst, Amherst, MA 01003, USA
Behavioral Biology Branch, Walter Reed Army Institute of Research, Silver Spring, MD 20910, USA

Vincent F. Capaldi II
Behavioral Biology Branch, Walter Reed Army Institute of Research, Silver Spring, MD 20910, USA

Steven M. Helms, Kris B. Weymann and Miranda M. Lim
VA Portland Health Care System, Portland, OR 97239, USA
Oregon Healthand Science University, Portland, OR 97239, USA

Index

A

Acupoint Group, 203-204, 209

Acupuncture, 203-207, 209-212

Allergic Rhinitis, 176-177, 181-182

Alzheimer's Disease, 14, 20-23, 29-30, 40-41, 52-53, 81, 85-92, 94-95, 97, 115-117, 121, 125-126, 129, 137, 153-155, 157, 183, 185-187, 189-192, 201-203, 209-211, 213-214, 224, 228, 241

Amyotrophic Lateral Sclerosis, 115-116, 118, 126-127

Angiogenesis, 247-248, 250-254

Angular Gyri, 138, 143-144

Anxiety Symptomatology, 257, 259-262

Ataxia, 147-152

Atrophy, 22-23, 25, 28-30, 115, 117-121, 123, 126, 206-207, 211, 215, 218, 237-238, 241, 244-246

Autism Spectrum, 64-67, 70, 78-80, 114, 122-123, 130, 245

Autopsy, 14-15, 19-20, 201

B

Basal Ganglia, 15, 120, 192, 237, 241-243, 245-246

Behavioral Variant Frontotemporal Dementia, 113, 116, 124-125, 213, 216-218

Benzodiazepine, 92, 97

Bilateral Anterior Cingulate, 138, 141

C

Central Nervous System, 81-82, 89, 131, 165, 172, 174, 188, 191

Cerebral Blood Flow, 190, 199, 201, 247, 253-254

Cervical Cord Hemisection, 165-166, 171

Cognitive Rehabilitation, 40, 42, 52

Cognitive Stimulation, 40-44

Compound Muscle Action Potentials, 165-166, 168, 171-172

Corticospinal Tract, 165, 170-175

Cytokine, 59, 179, 182

D

Dementia, 14-22, 29-32, 34-36, 38-42, 44, 52-53, 81-82, 85-97, 113-116, 118, 121-127, 129, 137, 148, 155, 157-158, 183-192, 198-199, 201-204, 209-211, 213-218, 222, 227-228, 240

Dementia with Lewy Bodies, 14, 17-18, 20-21, 92, 97, 183, 185-187, 189-191, 201-202

Depression, 1-2, 6, 10-12, 15, 18-19, 32-33, 39, 42, 44, 53, 77, 81, 86-87, 90, 93-97, 120, 126, 134-135, 138-146, 156, 158, 160, 163-164, 176, 179, 181, 188, 211, 219-220, 222-228, 260, 262-263

Dopamine, 15, 19, 81, 86-87, 153-158, 207

F

Forelimb Motor Function, 165, 172-174

Frontotemporal Dementia, 41, 85, 91, 113, 116, 123-127, 129, 157, 213, 216-218, 237, 244-246

Fusiform Gyrus, 114, 118, 138, 143-144, 191, 197, 199, 238, 240

H

Hericium Erinaceus, 81-82, 88-90

Hippocampus, 6, 19, 21-24, 27, 29, 82, 86-87, 144, 156-157, 164, 176-183, 191, 199, 206-207, 210-212

Hyperlipidemia, 15, 18, 91, 94-95, 184-188

Hypermetabolism, 203, 206-207, 209

Hypertension, 15, 18, 20, 91-93, 95, 184-188

I

Inferior Frontal Gyrus, 116, 120, 123, 138, 141-144, 191, 197, 238

Insomnia Severity Index (ISI), 256, 258

Ischemia, 55, 62, 82, 85, 89, 157, 189-190, 247-249, 251-254

Ischemic Stroke, 61, 81, 85, 87-88, 183, 186-188, 247, 253

M

Magnetic Resonance Imaging, 22, 30, 138, 146, 181, 188, 192, 202, 237-238, 247-248, 253-254

Medulla Oblongata, 165-166, 172

Microdialysis, 153-154, 157

Midbrain Tegmentum, 203, 206, 209

Mild Cognitive Impairment, 20, 22, 29-30, 40, 52-53, 82, 89, 91, 96-97, 116, 129, 211, 245

Motor Neurone Disease, 31, 127

Multiple Sclerosis, 31, 35, 38, 131, 135-137, 219-220, 222, 227-229

N

Nerve, 81-82, 86-90, 140, 145, 157, 171, 173, 177, 207

Neural Synchronization, 98-100

Neurodegenerative Diseases, 87, 94, 96, 113, 116, 123, 189

Neuroimaging, 22-23, 29-30, 92, 111, 119-120, 125, 129, 139-140, 146, 157, 190, 203, 218, 237-238, 242, 244, 263

Neuroimmune Mechanisms, 176

Neurology, 14, 19-20, 30, 38-39, 52-53, 88-91, 96-97, 110-111, 113, 122-129, 132-133, 136-137, 151, 157-158, 173-174, 183, 189-191, 201-202, 210-211, 213, 217-218, 222, 230, 239, 253

Neuron, 42-43, 60, 85-86, 90, 110, 114, 118-119, 123, 126, 172-173, 182

Neuronal Apoptosis, 54-56, 61-62, 85

Neuropsychiatric Inventory, 15, 17-18, 20, 33, 39, 116, 121
Neuroscience, 11-13, 22, 30, 52-53, 63, 98, 100-101, 104, 110-112, 122-129, 137, 145-146, 156-159, 163-164, 173-174, 182, 189, 201-202, 211-212, 217-219, 227, 236-237, 244-246, 254
Neurotransmitter, 153, 156, 207
Nonacupoint Group, 203-204, 209

O
Occipital Gyrus, 24, 28, 138, 141, 143-144, 197, 240
Olfactory Cortex, 191, 199, 202
Open-field Test, 2, 7-8
Orbital Cortex, 203, 206-207

P
Parietal Lobule, 24, 26-28, 114, 197
Posttraumatic Stress Disorder, 255, 262-263
Progressive Neurological Diseases, 31-32, 35
Psychosis, 10, 15, 17-18, 21, 81, 110

R
Radial Six-armed Water Maze, 230-231
Regional Homogeneity, 138-139, 141-146
Robot-assisted Gait Training, 147-148, 151

S
Sleep Apnea, 183, 255, 257, 262
Striatal Dopamine Level, 153-156
Striatum, 87, 116-117, 120, 153-156, 171, 188, 203, 206-207, 211, 238, 249, 252-253
Stroke, 15, 19-20, 52, 61-63, 81-82, 85-90, 92, 94, 96-97, 125-126, 137, 147-152, 157-158, 183-189, 227, 247-249, 251-254
Structural Equation Model, 219, 222
Subarachnoid Hemorrhage, 54, 62-63
Synaptic Plasticity, 153, 156-157, 203, 207, 209, 253

T
Theory of Mind, 113-114, 117-118, 120, 122-130
Therapist-assisted Gait Training,
147-149
Transcranial Direct Current
Stimulation, 40-42, 44, 52-53
Traumatic Brain Injury, 62-63, 183, 255, 260, 263

V
Vascular Dementia, 14-15, 19-20, 41, 53, 91, 94-95, 158, 211
Vertex-based Thickness Analysis, 24, 28
Voxel-based Morphometry, 22-24, 27, 30, 244